Handbook of Exotic Pet Medicine

Handbook of Exotic Pet Medicine

Edited by

Marie Kubiak
West Midland Safari Park
Bewdley, UK

WILEY Blackwell

Registered Offices
John Wiley & Sons, Inc., 111 River Street, Hoboken, NJ 07030, USA
John Wiley & Sons Ltd, The Atrium, Southern Gate, Chichester, West Sussex, PO19 8SQ, UK

Editorial Office
9600 Garsington Road, Oxford, OX4 2DQ, UK

For details of our global editorial offices, customer services, and more information about Wiley products visit us at www.wiley.com.

Wiley also publishes its books in a variety of electronic formats and by print-on-demand. Some content that appears in standard print versions of this book may not be available in other formats.

Library of Congress Cataloging-in-Publication Data

Names: Kubiak, Marie, author.
Title: Handbook of exotic pet medicine / Marie Kubiak.
Description: Hoboken, NJ : Wiley-Blackwell, 2021. | Includes
    bibliographical references and index.
Identifiers: LCCN 2020013120 (print) | LCCN 2020013121 (ebook) | ISBN
    9781119389941 (paperback) | ISBN 9781119389996 (adobe pdf) | ISBN
    9781119389958 (epub)
Subjects: MESH: Animals, Exotic | Animal Diseases | Evidence-Based Practice
Classification: LCC SF997.5.E95 (print) | LCC SF997.5.E95 (ebook) | NLM
    SF 997.5.E95 | DDC 591.6/2–dc23
LC record available at https://lccn.loc.gov/2020013120
LC ebook record available at https://lccn.loc.gov/2020013121

Cover Design: Wiley
Cover Image: Courtesy of Marie Kubiak

Set in 9.5/12.5pt STIXTwoText by SPi Global, Pondicherry, India
Printed and bound in Singapore by Markono Print Media Pte Ltd

10 9 8 7 6 5 4 3 2 1

For Ben
Stand tall, be kind, work hard and you will find your way.

Contents

List of Contributors *ix*

Acknowledgments *xi*

About the Companion Website *xiii*

1   Ground Squirrels *1*
Marie Kubiak

2   African Pygmy Hedgehogs *13*
Nathalie Wissink-Argilaga

3   Common Marmosets *27*
Jane Hopper

4   Striped Skunk *43*
Clive Munns

5   Degus *57*
Marie Kubiak

6   Mongolian Gerbils *71*
Marie Kubiak

7   Hamsters *83*
Marie Kubiak

8   Rats *99*
Richard Saunders

9   Sugar Gliders *125*
Marie Kubiak

10   Budgerigars and Cockatiels *141*
Marie Kubiak

11   Grey Parrots *165*
Marie Kubiak

12   Birds of Prey *189*
Alberto Rodriguez Barbon and Marie Kubiak

13 Bearded Dragons *219*
Marie Kubiak

14 Geckos *241*
Marie Kubiak

15 Chameleons *263*
Marie Kubiak

16 Corn Snakes *283*
Marie Kubiak

17 Boas and Pythons *305*
Joanna Hedley

18 Mediterranean Tortoises *327*
Sarah Brown

19 African Tortoises *361*
Marie Kubiak and Sarah Pellett

20 Terrapins *387*
Ian Sayers and Marie Kubiak

21 Amphibians *415*
Stephanie Jayson

22 Koi Carp *437*
Lindsay Thomas

23 Tarantulas *459*
Sarah Pellett and Steven A. Trim

24 Giant African Land Snails *477*
Sarah Pellett and Michelle O'Brien

Index *487*

List of Contributors

Marie Kubiak BVSc CertAVP(ZM) DZooMed MRCVS
RCVS Recognised Specialist in Zoo and Wildlife Medicine
West Midland Safari Park
Bewdley, UK

Alberto Rodriguez Barbon LdoVet CertZooMed DipECZM
(Avian Non practising) MRCVS
Staff veterinarian, Durrell Wildlife Conservation Trust
Trinity, UK

Sarah Brown MA VetMB Cert ZooMed GPCert(ExAP)
MRCVS, Advanced Practitioner in Zoological Medicine
Holly House Veterinary Hospital
Leeds, UK

Joanna Hedley BVM&S DZooMed (Reptilian) DipECZM
(Herpetology) MRCVS
RVC Exotics Service
Beaumont Sainsbury Animal Hospital
Royal Veterinary College
London, UK

Jane Hopper MA VetMB CertZooMed MRCVS
RCVS Advanced practitioner in Zoological Medicine
Head of Veterinary Services, The Aspinall Foundation
Lympne, UK

Stephanie Jayson MA Vet MB CertAVP(ZM) MVetMed
MRCVS
Senior Scientific Officer, Exotics and Wildlife Trade,
Wildlife Department, Science and Policy Group, RSPCA
Southwater, UK

Clive Munns BVSc CertZooMed MRCVS
RCVS Advanced Practitioner in Zoological Medicine
Montgomery Veterinary Clinic
Smeeth, UK

Michelle O'Brien, BVetMed CertZooMed
DipECZM(ZHM) MRCVS
RCVS and European specialist in Zoo and Wildlife Medicine
Wildfowl & Wetlands Trust
Slimbridge, UK

Sarah Pellett BSc(Hons) MA VetMB CertAVP(ZM)
DZooMed (Reptilian) MRCVS
RCVS Recognised Specialist in Zoo and Wildlife Medicine
Veterinary Advisor, BIAZA Terrestrial Invertebrate
Working Group
Exotics Manager, Animates Veterinary Clinic
Thurlby, UK

Richard Saunders BSc (Hons) BVSc FRSB CBiol DZooMed
(Mammalian) DipECZM(ZHM) MRCVS
RCVS Specialist in Zoo and Wildlife Medicine (Mammalian)
European Specialist in Zoological Medicine
Bristol Zoo Gardens
Bristol, UK

Ian Sayers BVSc CertZooMed MRCVS
RCVS Advanced Practitioner in Zoological Medicine
South Devon Exotics
Torquay UK

Lindsay Thomas BVSc MSc CertAVP(ZM) MRCVS
Montgomery Veterinary Clinic
Smeeth, UK

Steven A. Trim BSc CBiol MRSB
Founder, Chief Scientific Officer, Managing Director
Venomtech
Chair – Veterinary Invertebrate Society
Sessional Lecturer in Drug Discovery
Canterbury Christ Church University
Sandwich, UK

Nathalie Wissink-Argilaga Lic.Vet CertAVP(ZM) DZooMed
(Reptilian) MRCVS
RCVS Recognised Specialist in Zoo and Wildlife Medicine
Head of Exotics and Zoo Medicine, Scott Veterinary Clinic
Bedford, UK

Acknowledgments

This book has been several decades in the making and it makes all the trials and tribulations along the way worthwhile to finally see it in print. My interest in exotic animals started long before my veterinary career was even a consideration, back in the early days of childhood. Many days then were spent hunting and studying invertebrates and reptiles in the garden much to the despair of my family. The fascination only intensified through university and post-graduate training as a small zoo gradually accumulated at home alongside the developing clinical work. It delights me that in the current day I see that same spark of enthusiasm about both animals and learning in my son and can only hope he gains as much fulfillment and joy from them as I have done.

To all those people who have supported me and fostered my interest in exotic animals, from my exceptionally resilient and tolerant friends and family to my incredible colleagues through the years, I am more grateful than I could ever express. Ghislaine Sayers, who gave me the push I needed as a student to follow my dreams, Rai Janz for providing me with my first job and supporting me quietly and calmly until I found my feet in the veterinary world, then the fellow residents and interns who provided the solidarity we needed to get through, particularly Pru, Eli and Richard – we got there in the end! And to all the vets and nurses at Manor over the years who made those years so much fun and so rewarding, especially Toby, Steph, Lindsay, Jack, Sam, Annabel, Teresa and Laura – you became like family and I'm so proud of what you have all achieved.

This book itself could never have been completed without the help and support of so many people. I am indebted to everyone who willingly wrote, read, let me turn up to take photos, made cups of tea and listened, or cajoled me until we got to this stage! Thank you all and I hope you are as proud as I am of the book we have created.

About the Companion Website

Don't forget to visit the companion website for this book:

www.wiley.com/go/kubiak/exotic_pet_medicine

There you will find valuable material designed to enhance your learning, including case reports and care sheets.

Scan this QR code to visit the companion website

1

Ground Squirrels
Marie Kubiak

1.1 Introduction

Ground squirrels make up the subfamily of Xerinae, within the Sciuridae (squirrel) family and include a variety of well-known species such as the groundhog and marmot. The species within this subfamily that are more commonly kept as pets, and are covered in this chapter, are prairie dogs, Richardson's ground squirrels and Siberian chipmunks. Biological parameters for these species are included in Table 1.1.

1.2 Husbandry

1.2.1 Siberian Chipmunks

Siberian chipmunks (*Tamias sibiricus*) are squirrel-like rodents originating primarily from Northern Asia. Although common in the pet trade in Europe in the late twentieth and early twenty-first century, in 2015 this species was added to EU Invasive Alien Species (IAS) Regulation (1143/2014), resulting in a ban within the European Union on importation, keeping, breeding, transport, trade, and accidental or intentional release of this species, though an exemption is made for animals to be transported for veterinary care. As such this species can only be kept by existing owners for their natural lifespan, or under licence for medical, research, or conservation purposes. At present these restrictions remain in place for the United Kingdom. Pet Siberian chipmunk numbers are declining as animals reach the end of their life and no new animals are able to be acquired or bred. Other species of chipmunks may be legally kept but are extremely rare as pets. The Pallas squirrel (*Callosciurus erythraeus*) and Fox squirrel (*Sciurus niger*), both rarely kept as pets, have also been listed as invasive species and are subject to the same restrictions.

Chipmunks are terrestrial though have good climbing capabilities and will use the full height of enclosures. They are inquisitive and highly active so enclosures should be secure – such as large aviaries with narrow spaced mesh. Nest boxes should be provided (at least one per animal) with hay substrate and branches, tunnels, hides and wheels provided for enrichment and to encourage activity. Chipmunks will chew plastics, wood, wires and other materials and this should be taken into account when planning enclosure construction, and when toys or décor are added. They are omnivores and can be fed a rodent pellet diet but this should be supplemented with seeds, vegetables, insects, and hay. Food may be stored in substrate or nest boxes so it is important to check and clean enclosures thoroughly on at least a weekly basis to prevent spoilage. Fresh water should always be available and water bottles are generally accepted well. Free range access within a house is not advisable due to potential for escape, injury, or damage inflicted to household possessions. In winter wild chipmunks do not exhibit true hibernation but have fluctuating torpor, with several days of dormancy followed by a period of normothermia, activity, and feeding. In torpor their body temperature drops to around 5 °C and heart rate slows to 4 beats/min. In captivity there is no drive for torpor as temperatures tend to remain stable through seasons and food is abundant. There is no evidence that absence of torpor has any negative impact.

1.2.2 Prairie Dogs

Prairie dogs (*Cynomys* spp.) are large, North American members of the squirrel family and have five recognised species. Of these only the black-tailed prairie dog (*Cynomys ludovicianus*) is encountered with any frequency as a pet in the UK. Well-socialised individuals can make good pets but even the tamest prairie dog can become aggressive during their breeding season.

Captive animals require deep substrate to form their burrows as well as a large overground area for activity, sufficient to enable a group of animals to be kept together.

Table 1.1 Biological parameters (for animals not undergoing torpor).

	Body weight	Lifespan	Body temperature (°C)	Respiratory rate (/min)	Heart rate (/min)	Sexual maturity	Gestation
Siberian Chipmunk (*Tamias sibiricus*)	50–150 g	5–10 years	37–38	70–80	250–350	8–14 months	30–31 days
Black tailed-prairie dog (*Cynomys ludovicianus*)	0.7–2 kg	7–10 years	35.3–39	40–60	200–318	2 yrs	30–35 days
Richardson's Ground Squirrel (*Urocitellus richardsonii*)	0.4–0.6 kg	4 years	37.5–39.5	40–100	245–275	11 months	23 days

Enclosure size requirements have been detailed as 2×2×2.5 ft (L×W×H) per animal (Pilny and Hess 2004) but this should be regarded as an absolute minimum and 4×4×2.5 ft would be considered more suitable as a minimum to allow animals to display normal behaviour. An area of deep substrate should be provided to allow creation of burrows and can be hay, shredded paper, or soil. Artificial burrows and shelters such as drain pipes or wooden boxes can be provided for hide and sleeping areas. Cage bars should be no further than 1 inch apart to prevent escape. An elevated observation shelf should be provided as prairie dogs are inquisitive and will often climb to investigate activity in the surrounding area (Pilny and Hess 2004). Plastic should be avoided as it is likely to be chewed. Chosen toilet areas will be well defined allowing easy daily cleaning of urine and faeces and a litter tray can be placed in the chosen site. A warm room or supplemental heating is necessary to provide temperatures of 20–22 °C as prairie dogs may enter torpor at cooler temperatures (Johnson-Delaney 2006). Torpor is not obligatory in prairie dogs but is a facultative response to temperature drop and lack of available food and water. Although body temperatures reduce, they remain significantly higher than ambient environmental temperature at approximately 19 °C even in deep torpor bouts. These deep torpor bouts are interspersed with periods of activity and normothermia when environmental conditions improve (Lehmer et al. 2001). As torpor is facultative there is no need to replicate the conditions in captivity and to date no adverse effects have been reported with absence of torpor in prairie dogs.

Prairie dogs are hindgut fermenters and require a high fibre intake to maintain intestinal health. Where a normal appetite is present, provision of a variety of grasses, hay, flowers, herbs, fresh vegetables and leaves and occasional invertebrates is appropriate (Orcutt 2005). Pelleted diets designed for rabbits or rodents can be convenient food source for owners but should make up no more than 10% of the diet, with high fibre material making up the majority of food provided. Seeds and grains can be offered in small quantities as treats or to increase body condition but can lead to obesity or disruption to normal intestinal function if fed in excess.

1.2.3 Ground Squirrels

Ground squirrel species are uncommon as companion animals though Richardson's Ground squirrels (*Urocitellus richardsonii*) (RGS) are occasionally kept. This species is native to the grasslands of the Northern United States of America and Southern Canada and do cross over territory with prairie dogs. In the wild, female familial groups exist with solitary males only being tolerated during breeding. In captivity they can be maintained in social single-sex colonies or mixed sex colonies with males being neutered. Though destructive and with a tendency to bite defensively, RGS tend to make good companion animals with regular handling and interaction.

Captive animals have similar requirements to prairie dogs, though as a smaller species enclosures can be less extensive, with 3×2×1.5 ft advised per animal. Cage bars should be no more than 0.75 inch apart. The observation shelf should not be placed more than 18 inches above the ground as RGS are not good climbers. Ambient temperatures of 18–25 °C are advisable but they are adapted to cooler temperatures and will not enter torpor unless temperatures drop to below 7 °C (Michener 1983). In the wild RGS are obligate hibernators and will spend up to nine months of the year in true torpor, with body temperature dropping to close to environmental temperature as heart and respiratory rates slow dramatically (Michener and Koeppl 1985). Brief periods of around 12 hours of warming to normal body temperature occur during this torpor (Michener and Koeppl 1985). In captivity temperatures are stable and food is readily available and torpor rarely occurs. These less harsh conditions aid overall longevity but the lack of torpor and high metabolic rate all year round may be associated with higher rates of neoplasia seen in RGS in captivity.

RGS are omnivorous with their dietary requirements intermediate between prairie dogs and chipmunks. Seeds should be limited to occasional treats to avoid obesity.

1.3 Clinical Evaluation

1.3.1 History-Taking

A full review of husbandry is essential as inappropriate conditions are common causes of health concerns. Contact with other animals, diet, previous medical history, enclosure size and set-up, and reproductive status are all key information. It is prudent to ascertain familiarity of individual animals with handling before attempting restraint.

For individual health complaints, the duration of symptoms, number of animals affected, and any changes made to environment in the period preceding clinical disease should be ascertained.

1.3.2 Handling

Chipmunks are fast moving, adept at climbing and jumping, and rarely habituated to handling. It is often easiest to catch them in their enclosure or carry box with a small towel and gently grasp them around the neck and thorax with one hand for examination. Avoid restraining the tail as degloving injuries can result.

Many prairie dogs and RGS are familiar with handling and are comfortable being restrained by owners. For more reluctant animals, firm restraint with one hand around the neck and one underneath the abdomen, or wrapping the patient in a towel may be necessary. Prairie dogs in particular can inflict painful bites with their long incisor teeth and secure restraint is advised before any procedures are carried out.

1.3.3 Sex Determination

The shorter anogenital distance in female sciuromorphs is key for determining sex. Female prairie dogs have close association of the vulva and anus, male prairie dogs have a clear separation of at least 1 cm (Figures 1.1 and 1.2). Males will only have visible descended testes in breeding season and morphology and pelage does not vary between sexes.

Adult male RGS tend to be larger than females, but otherwise sexing is carried out as for prairie dogs.

Mature male chipmunks have testes descended for most of the year and the prepuce is well defined so sexing is more straightforward. In juveniles and in winter anogenital distance is used to differentiate between sexes.

1.3.4 Clinical Examination

Clinical examination should be carried out in a systematic approach as for any species. Particular areas of focus include dental evaluation – with attention to incisor

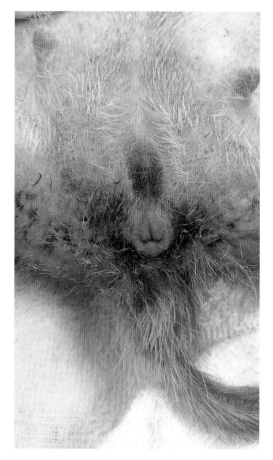

Figure 1.1 Female prairie dog.

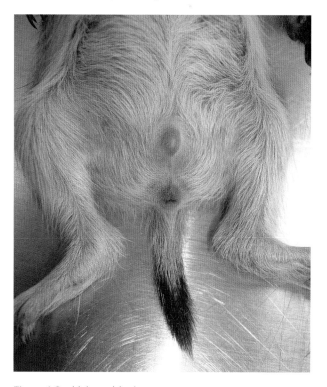

Figure 1.2 Male prairie dog.

structure and uniformity due to potential presence of elodontoma in prairie dogs and RGS, presence of wounds, assessment of respiratory effort or noise, evaluation of joints (especially stifles) for swelling and reduced range of movement, and abdominal palpation for masses. Nail overgrowth and obesity are common findings. It is prudent to weigh animals at each visit and to be aware of seasonal variation in weight – males tend to lose weight during the Spring breeding season and all animals gain weight prior to expected hibernation in Autumn and subsequently lose this during winter torpor. It is useful for owners to keep records that document the typical weight changes of individuals through the seasons and previous maximum and minimum values.

1.4 Basic Techniques

1.4.1 Sample Collection

In prairie dogs the saphenous and cephalic veins can be used to collect small volume blood samples of less than 0.2 ml and this may be possible under manual restraint in tame animals. For larger samples the cranial vena cava is accessed under general anaesthesia (Head et al. 2017). A needle is inserted just cranial to the manubrium and directed caudolaterally at an angle of 30° from the midline (Figure 1.3). The vein is typically superficial and volumes of up to 6 ml/kg can be collected in healthy animals (Head et al. 2017), but this should be reduced to 1.5 ml/kg in debilitated patients. The jugular vein is an alternative in this species but may not be visible or palpable.

In RGS and chipmunks the smaller veins are harder to access and the cranial vena cava is the usual site with venepuncture carried out under general anaesthesia. In small individuals where sample size required exceeds the recommended maximum volume, crystalloid replacement can be used to restore volume.

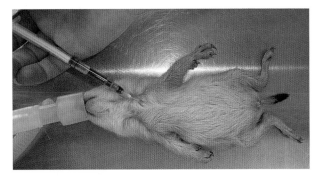

Figure 1.3 Blood sample collection from the vena cava in a juvenile prairie dog.

1.4.2 Nutritional Support

For anorexic patients, a high fibre liquid feed designed for herbivorous species such as rabbits is appropriate for nutritional support, following manufacturers' recommendations. A maximum of 10 ml/kg bodyweight can be administered at a single feed. Syringe feeding is generally tolerated well though nasogastric intubation should be considered for cases where extensive recovery periods are likely or orofacial disease affects feeding ability.

1.4.3 Fluid Therapy

Maintenance fluid requirements for sciuromorphs are estimated to be 50–100 ml/kg/day, based on requirements for similar sized rodent species (Lichtenberger 2007).

Fresh water should be available in sipper bottles or bowls at all times where animals are voluntarily drinking. Subcutaneous fluids are suitable for mild–moderately dehydrated animals and 10–15 ml/kg can be injected as a bolus between scapulae (Johnson-Delaney 2006).

Intravenous access can be difficult in a hypotensive animal and patient interference with cannulas is common. Where used, the cephalic or saphenous veins are most readily accessible in prairie dogs and RGS. Intraosseous catheters are alternative options in severely dehydrated animals, or for chipmunks where vessel size limits access, and placement is via the greater trochanter of the femur, preferably under sedation and with ongoing analgesia.

1.4.4 Anaesthesia

Fasting before anaesthesia is unnecessary and should be avoided.

Many different anaesthetic protocols have been detailed (see formulary), and an injectable combination is preferred over gaseous anaesthesia alone in prairie dogs and RGS as in all but the most debilitated animals mask or chamber induction is resented. In chipmunks, their small size and difficulty gaining an accurate weight complicates accurate, safe dosing of injectable agents and volatile agents may be used as the sole anaesthetic agent but it must be remembered that this provides no analgesia. Once immobilised under volatile anaesthesia, weight measurement can be carried out and appropriate analgesics administered based on weight.

Endotracheal intubation of sciuromorphs is possible using blind or endoscope assisted techniques but is challenging so oxygen and volatile agent anaesthesia are typically provided by mask.

1.4.5 Euthanasia

Humane euthanasia is best achieved with intracardiac injection of pentobarbitone after induction of general anaesthesia. Intracardiac or intraperitoneal injection in a conscious patient is not appropriate. The apex beat of the heart is both visible and palpable in the caudoventral thorax and rapid intracardiac injection of 80–160 mg/kg is sufficient to euthanase animals effectively.

1.4.6 Hospitalisation requirements

Prey species like sciuromorphs should be kept separate from predators, including cats and dogs, to minimise stress. Where possible hospitalised individuals should be maintained with their normal social group to maintain social bonds and avoid the negative effects of social isolation.

Husbandry within the hospital should approximate conditions recommended for companion animals although cage size can be reduced if necessary given the short-term nature of housing. For chipmunks in particular it is important to check cages are entirely secure due to their ability to escape through small apertures and the ensuing legal ramifications. Often owners will be able to provide a cage and food and this should be encouraged as familiarity will result in more relaxed patients and a closer approximation of normal behaviour.

1.5 Common Medical and Surgical Conditions

1.5.1 Neoplasia

Neoplasia appears uncommon in chipmunks. Two osteosarcomas have been described as have a mammary adenocarcinoma and a single report of hepatic carcinoma (Wadsworth et al. 1982; Morera 2004; Tamaizumi et al. 2007; Oohashi et al. 2009).

Spontaneous neoplasia has been reported as uncommon in Richardson's ground squirrels with limited case reports comprising a mast cell tumour and several adenocarcinomas (Yamate et al. 2007; He et al. 2009; Carminato et al. 2012). However, this author has seen a high incidence of soft tissue and hepatic neoplasms in RGS, with females predominantly affected (Figures 1.4 and 1.5). Excision of masses is advisable where possible for diagnosis and attempted curative treatment (Figure 1.6). A hepadnavirus induced syndrome of hepatitis progressing to hepatic carcinoma has been recognised in RGS (Tennant et al. 1991) as well as wood chucks (*Marmota monax*), Californian ground squirrels (*Spermophilus beecheyi*) and Arctic

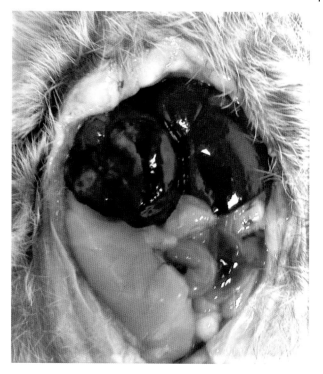

Figure 1.4   Hepatic carcinoma in an RGS.

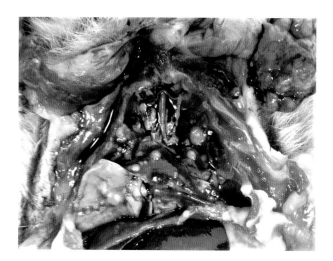

Figure 1.5   Pulmonary metastases of a hepatic carcinoma in an RGS.

squirrels (*Spermophilus parryi*) (Testut et al. 1996). The hepadnaviruses appear to be highly host-specific with no cross-infection between squirrel species.

A high prevalence of hepatic carcinomas has been reported in Prairie dogs, presumed to be associated with hepadnavirus but testing has not confirmed viral presence (Garner et al. 2004). Otherwise neoplasia in prairie dogs appears uncommon with sparse case reports comprising lymphoma, lipoma, and osteosarcoma (Rogers and Chrisp 1998; Miwa et al. 2006; Mouser et al. 2006).

(a)

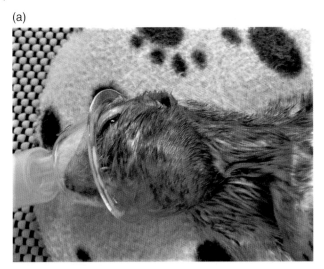

(b)

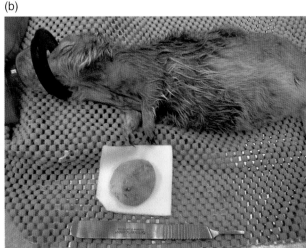

Figure 1.6   (a) Facial mass in a Richardson's ground squirrel. (b) RGS following removal of facial mass, determined on histopathology to be a lipoma.

1.5.2   Dental Disease

Sciuromorphs have a typical dental formula of I 1/1, C 0/0, P 1-2/1 M 3/3. Incisors are long and chisel-shaped with a pattern of continuous growth whereas the premolars and molars have closed anelodont roots and do not have a pattern of ongoing growth and attrition (Legendre 2003). There are well formed cheek pouches for food collection and storage that extend down the neck (Mancinelli and Capello 2016).

Acquired dental disease leading to incisor malocclusion has been described as common in chipmunks and is also regularly seen in other sciuromorphs (Girling 2002). Incisor extraction is preferred over repeat incisor trims due to the stress to the patient and progression of dental changes over time. It is prudent to radiograph those animals presenting with incisor malocclusion as elodontoma presence may be the cause of the coronal alteration.

High sugar diets are associated with dental caries, periodontal disease, and tooth decay (Mancinelli and Capello 2016) and often extraction is the only option remaining due to advanced disease at the time of presentation. Trimming or reduction in crown height of premolar or molar teeth should not be carried out as these are closed-rooted teeth.

1.5.2.1   Elodontomas

Elodontomas are a benign but progressive accumulation of mixed alveolar bone and odontogenic material at the apices of elodont teeth and are considered to be hamartomas. As squirrels have elodont incisors but closed rooted premolars and molars, this dysplasia can only affect incisor apices. The resulting space-occupying mass is painful and, when upper incisors are involved, the accu-

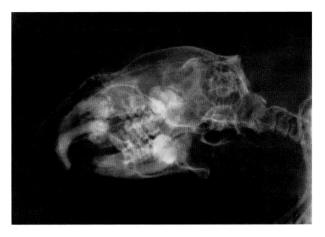

Figure 1.7   Elodontoma formation affecting apices of all four incisors in an RGS.

mulated material can obstruct nasal air flow. Elodontomas have been widely reported in sciuromorphs in the literature, including in chipmunks and the author has also confirmed presence of elodontomas in several RGS using both radiography and CT imaging (Figure 1.7). Possible inciting factors include trauma, chronic inflammation, advanced acquired dental disease, and toxin exposure. In prairie dogs a similar phenomenon is observed as a degenerative process in older animals, predominantly affecting the apices of the maxillary incisors and these are more accurately termed pseudo-odontomas. Dystrophy of the germinal tissue results in development of a plicated mass of dentine with damage to surrounding tissues (Mancinelli and Capello 2016). Nasal air flow is obstructed and eruption of affected incisors may cease.

Treatment options attempt to alleviate the secondary respiratory consequences of elodontomas or pseudo-odontomas and include extraction of incisors and associated dysplasia, or surgical creation of a dorsally or laterally placed stoma to allow air flow into the sinuses, bypassing the compressed nasal passages (Bulliot and Mentre 2013; Smith et al. 2013). Surgery is more challenging in squirrels and chipmunks compared to prairie dogs given the smaller patient size and disproportionally narrower nasal passages.

1.5.3 Respiratory Tract Disease

Although respiratory distress is commonly associated with elodontoma presence, upper and lower respiratory tract infections are also seen as a cause of dyspnoea. Primary pathogens have been implicated, e.g. *Pasteurella multocida* in prairie dogs (Figure 1.8), and *Pasteurella haemolytica* in Siberian chipmunks (Astorga et al. 1996). However, in many cases, especially in chipmunks, husbandry failings leading to stress and immunosuppression are thought to be the primary inciting factor for development of opportunistic bacterial pneumonia. Ideally therapy is based on a firm diagnosis made from radiography, and culture and cytology of a tracheal or bronchoalveolar lavage sample. In many cases this is not possible, due to patient status or size, and broad spectrum antibiotic therapy alongside nebulisation is a compromise made.

Metastatic hepatic carcinoma can cause severe pulmonary changes with dyspnoea that is non-responsive to supportive or attempted treatment options.

Dilated cardiomyopathy is reported as common in prairie dogs of over three years of age (Funk 2004) and may present with respiratory signs. Treatment follows that of the domestic mammals but response to therapy appears to be poor.

1.5.4 Arthritides

Stifle swelling, new bone formation, and altered range of movement have been seen by the author in several geriatric RGS and less commonly in prairie dogs (Figures 1.9 and 1.10). Management using meloxicam and glucosamine/chondroitin appeared to assist with mobility alongside husbandry modification to house affected animals in a single tier cage. In one case acupuncture in a prairie dog with osteoarthritis resulted in a perceived marked improvement by the owner but given the variable presentation of osteoarthritis further data would be needed before making a recommendation for this treatment modality.

A single case of mycobacterial synovitis has also been seen by the author but no infectious joint conditions have been reported in the literature to date.

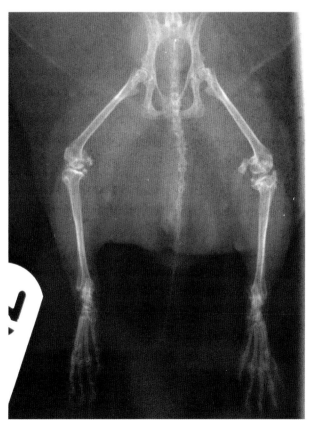

Figure 1.9 RGS with stifle osteoarthritis. On clinical examination there was a marked reduction in the range of movement of both stifles.

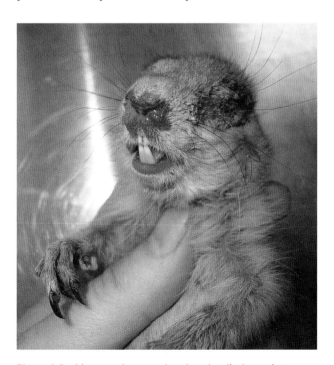

Figure 1.8 Mucopurulent nasal and ocular discharge in a juvenile prairie dog with acute pasteurellosis.

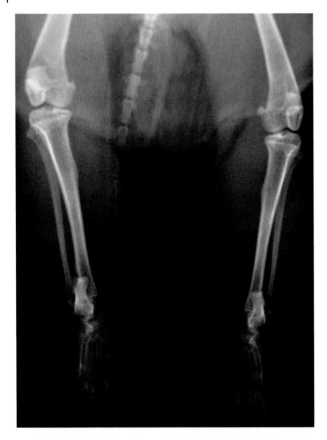

Figure 1.10 Normal appearance to stifles of an adult prairie dog.

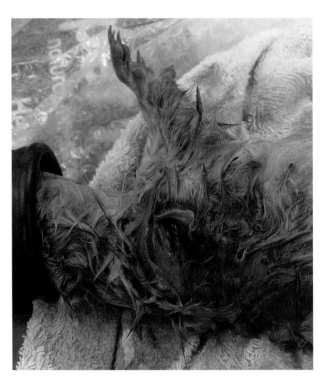

Figure 1.11 Conspecific bite injuries in a prairie dog following a territorial dispute. This animal was euthanased after confirmation of an open scapular fracture.

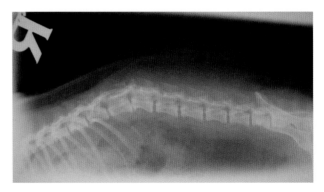

Figure 1.12 Intervertebral disc rupture in a geriatric prairie dog following a fall. Hind limb paresis was present initially but function returned over a three month period.

1.5.5 Traumatic Injury

In rut, male prairie dogs may compete for territory, inflicting bite wounds on other animals – typically affecting the tail base, scrotum, and dorsum. Most wounds are relatively superficial but may require suturing. Intradermal sutures are advisable to prevent premature suture removal by the patient. Occasionally territorial disputes can result in more serious injuries (Figure 1.11)

Significant trauma has been seen following a fall from cage tier, or drop from owners' hands. Limb and spinal fractures have both been seen by the author, as well as intervertebral disc rupture in a geriatric prairie dog following a fall (Figure 1.12).

1.5.6 Miscellaneous Infectious Conditions

Siberian chipmunks were found to be a significant host for Borreliosis (Lyme Disease) in one study of an introduced population in France (Vourc'h et al. 2007) and may serve as a reservoir of infection.

Historically many prairie dogs are wild caught as free-living populations are extensive, not currently under threat, and captive breeding is hard to achieve at commercially viable levels. Sporadic infectious disease outbreaks have been identified in wild populations and subsequently in wild caught individuals introduced into the pet trade.

Yersinia pestis is the bacterial cause of bubonic plague and prairie dogs and ground squirrels are both highly susceptible. An outbreak has been reported in captive prairie dogs collected from the wild for the pet trade and wild populations may also suffer high mortality in outbreaks (Phalen 2004). The peracute form of disease results in rapid death, whereas in slower progressing cases only lethargy and anorexia may be evident. Post-mortem examination can be unrewarding but in some cases lymph node enlargement or abscessation may be evident. Where outbreaks of high mortality occur in imported animals, or those in contact with recently imported animals, Yersiniosis should be considered as a potential cause and a post-mortem carried out in a laboratory with suitable biosecurity measures to manage the potential zoonotic risks.

Tularaemia is caused by the bacterium *Francisella tularensis,* and both prairie dogs and ground squirrels are susceptible. Humans can be infected by direct contact with animals, aerosol inhalation, bacterial contamination of an open wound, or indirectly through arthropod vectors. Granulomatous infection of liver, spleen, lymph nodes, lungs, and bone marrow results (Phalen 2004). Disease has not been reported in the UK but is established in North America and parts of Europe. An outbreak in North America was reported to have resulted in extensive mortality in wild-caught prairie dogs and prairie dog to human transmission was confirmed. Clinical presentation was high mortality with a predominance of oropharangeal lesions noted at post-mortem examination (Avashia et al. 2004).

Prairie dogs have been infected with Monkeypox following contact with rodents imported from Ghana. Symptoms included pyrexia, coughing, conjunctivitis, lymphadenopathy, and dermal pox-like lesions. Disease was transmitted from prairie dogs to humans, including veterinary staff resulting in flu-like symptoms and a papular rash (Guarner et al. 2004). Prairie dogs are also susceptible to cowpox, resulting in similar lesions.

As a result of the zoonotic disease outbreaks associated with prairie dogs, it is now illegal in the USA to capture, transport, sell, or release into the wild any of this species (Phalen 2004). No trade restrictions currently apply in the UK.

Mycobacterium avium avium has been reported in an RGS (Juan-Sallés et al. 2009). The individual presented hypothermic and dehydrated, and died. Granulomatous inflammation within the lungs and lymph nodes was noted at gross post-mortem and extensive inflammatory changes associated with acid-fast bacteria were noted on histological examination of spleen, liver, mediastinal fat, pleura, and peritoneum in addition. Polymerase chain reaction (PCR) analysis supported *M. a. avium* as the causative bacterium (Juan-Sallés et al. 2009).

1.6 Preventative Health Measures

A variety of endoparasites have been reported at low levels in wild prairie dog populations (Pfaffenberger et al. 1984) and wild chipmunks have reported infestations with *Brevistriata skrjabini* and *Syphabulea maseri* in their natural range (Schulz and Lubimov 1932; Pisanu et al. 2007). A wider variety of nematodes (Ascarids, Trichostrongyles, Oxyurids, and Trichurids) have been reported, as well as *Eimeria* coccidia, in regions where this species is considered a non-native species (Chapuis et al. 2012). Asymotomatic carriage of

Cryptosporidium muris has been reported in pet Siberian chipmunks (Hůrková et al. 2003). The rodent tapeworm *Hymenolepis nana* has been reported as a cause of protein losing enteropathy and death in prairie dogs and it should be noted that this is zoonotic (Thas 2010). Endoparasitism still remains rare in captive animals and so prophylactic use of antiparastic agents is not advisable. Faecal microscopy to detect endoparasites is advisable for new animals, or those exhibiting signs consistent with endoparasitism.

Prairie dogs have fast growing nails due to the need for extensive digging in the wild. In captivity trimming of nails may be necessary to prevent overgrowth which often results in fractures at the nail base and mild–moderate haemorrhage. Guillotine type nail clippers tend to work well and cautery materials should be available in case of inadvertent damage to the vascular core of the nail.

1.6.1 Neutering Technique

It is important to note that legislation mandates that precautions must be taken to prevent Siberian chipmunks from breeding. This can involve maintaining this species as single individuals which is often well tolerated, as single sex groups or utilising surgical neutering. Little information is available on chemical contraception in this species.

All three species can often be maintained as single sex groups though during their breeding season ('the rut') prairie dogs in particular can become aggressive to conspecifics and human handlers, necessitating separation.

Where animals are being kept as a mixed sex group then neutering of males is the simplest way to control breeding. Open inguinal canals in these species necessitate a closed castration technique and the author prefers a midline abdominal approach with retraction of testes into the abdomen prior to ligation and removal. This results in a single incision compared with two scrotal incisions and has reduced potential for post-operative infection as scrotal wounds tend to be heavily contaminated due to their ventral and peri-anal position. Wound closure is in three layers with intradermal skin sutures used to minimise wound interference.

Females can be spayed following a similar approach to other small mammals but elective neutering of females is less commonly carried out.

Elective neutering is best carried out in prairie dogs at an age of less than one year, and in summer time when animals are at their lowest body weight. In older animals, or at winter weight, large adipose deposits make surgery more challenging.

1.6.2 Radiographic Imaging

Radiography is invaluable for investigation of dental lesions and is best carried out under sedation or general anaesthesia for optimal positioning. Whole body laterolateral views are commonly used for survey radiographs (Figure 1.13). A series of views (typically dorsoventral, laterolateral and left and right oblique views) are used to assess dental anatomy fully. Elodontomas or pseudo-odontomas are best evaluated on slightly oblique lateral views where incisors are not superimposed (Figure 1.7). Computed Tomography can provide greater detail on size and location of lesions prior to planning any surgical intervention.

Radiographs are also valuable in detection of articular changes, intraabdominal soft tissue masses, detection of lung lesions, and evaluation of extent of injuries.

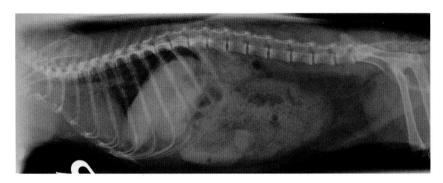

Figure 1.13 Laterolateral survey view of an adult prairie dog.

Formulary

Medication	Dose	Dosing interval	Additional comments
Anaesthesia			
Buprenorphine	0.03 mg/kg SC		30 mins prior to induction
Ketamine	10 mg/kg IM		
Midazolam	1–2 mg/kg IM		(Pilny and Hess 2004)
Medetomidine	0.1–0.3 mg/kg IM		(Johnson-Delaney 2006)
Diazepam	1–5 mg/kg IM		(Johnson-Delaney 2006)
Ketamine	40 mg/kg IM		
ACP	0.4 mg/kg IM		(Sinclair 2007)
Medetomidine	0.1 mg/kg IM		Reversal with 0.5 mg/kg atipamezole
Ketamine	2–5 mg/kg IM		
Butorphanol	1 mg/kg IM		
Ketamine	85 mg/kg		High ketamine doses may lead to protracted recovery
Xylazine	10 mg/kg IM		(Olson and McCabe 1986)
Analgesia			
Butorphanol	2 mg/kg SC	q2–4h	(Sinclair 2007)
Buprenorphine	0.05–0.1 mg/kg SC	q6–12h	(Smith and Burgmann 1997)
Meloxicam	0.4 mg/kg SC or PO	q12h	(Wright et al. 2017)
Tramadol	10 mg/kg PO	q12h	(Mayer 2012)
Antibiotics			
Enrofloxacin	5–10 mg/kg PO	once daily	(Morrissey and Carpenter 2004)
Chloramphenicol	50 mg/kg PO	q12h	(Morrissey and Carpenter 2004)
Metronidazole	20 mg/kg PO	q12h	(Adamcak and Otten 2000)
Trimethoprim sulfa	30 mg/kg PO SC	q12h	(Collins 1988)
Doxycycline	2.5 mg/kg PO	q12h	(Morrissey and Carpenter 2004)

Avoid oral penicillins, cephalosporins and clindamycin

(Continued)

Medication	Dose	Dosing interval	Additional comments
Antiparasitics			
Ivermectin	0.2–0.4 mg/kg SC	q10-14d	(Ness 2005)
Fenbendazole	25 mg/kg PO	q24h for 5d	(Allen et al. 1993)
Metronidazole	40 mg/kg PO	q24h for 5d	(Ness 2005)
Miscellaneous			
Enalapril	0.25–0.5 mg/kg PO	q12h	(Funk 2004)
Furosemide	0.3–0.4 mg/kg PO, SC, IM, IV	q12–24h	(Mayer 2012)

References

Adamcak, A. and Otten, B. (2000). Rodent therapeutics. *The Veterinary Clinics of North America. Exotic Animal Practice* 3 (1): 221–237.

Allen, D.G., Pringle, X., Smith, D. et al. (1993). *Handbook of Veterinary Drugs*. Philadelphia: Lippincott.

Astorga, R.J., Carrasco, L., Luque, I. et al. (1996). Pneumonic pasteurellosis associated with *Pasteurella haemolytica* in chipmunks (*Tamias sibiricus*). *Journal of Veterinary Medicine Series B* 43 (1–10): 59–62.

Avashia, S.B., Petersen, J.M., Lindley, C.M. et al. (2004). First reported prairie dog-to-human tularemia transmission, Texas, 2002. *Emerging Infectious Diseases* 10 (3): 483–486.

Bulliot, C. and Mentre, V. (2013). Original rhinostomy technique for the treatment of pseudo-odontoma in a prairie dog (*Cynomys ludovicianus*). *Journal of Exotic Pet Medicine* 22: 76–81.

Carminato, A., Nassuato, C., Vascellari, M. et al. (2012). Adenocarcinoma of the dorsal glands in 2 European ground squirrels (*Spermophilus citellus*). *Comparative Medicine* 62 (4): 279–281.

Chapuis, J.-L., Obolenskaya, E., Pisanu, B. et al. (2012). *Tamias sibiricus* (Siberian chipmunk). CABI Invasive Species Compendium. http://www.cabi.org/isc/datasheet/62788 (accessed 5 May 2017).

Collins, B.R. (1988). Common diseases and medical management of rodents and lagomorphs. In: *Contemporary Issues in Small Animal Practice: Exotic Animals* (eds. E.R. Jacobson and G.V. Kollias), 261–316. New York: Churchill Living-stone.

Funk, R. (2004). Medical management of prairie dogs. In: *Ferrets, Rabbits and Rodents Clinical Medicine and Surgery* (eds. K.E. Quesenberry and J.W. Carpenter), 266–273. St. Louis, MO: Saunders.

Garner, M.M., Raymond, J.T., Toshkov, I. et al. (2004). Hepatocellular carcinoma in black-tailed prairie dogs (*Cynomys ludivicianus*): tumor morphology and immunohistochemistry for hepadnavirus core and surface antigens. *Veterinary Pathology* Online 41 (4): 353–361.

Girling, S. (2002). Mammalian anatomy and Imaging. In: *BSAVA Manual of Exotic Pets* (eds. A. Meredith and S. Redrobe), 1–12. Gloucester, UK: BSAVA.

Guarner, J., Johnson, B.J., Paddock, C.D. et al. (2004). Monkeypox transmission and pathogenesis in prairie dogs. *Emerging Infectious Diseases* 10 (3): 426–431.

He, X.J., Uchida, K., Tochitani, T. et al. (2009). Spontaneous cutaneous mast cell tumor with lymph node metastasis in a Richardson's ground squirrel (*Spermophilus richardsonii*). *Journal of Veterinary Diagnostic Investigation* 21 (1): 156–159.

Head, V., Eshar, D., and Nau, M.R. (2017). Techniques for nonterminal blood sampling in black-tailed prairie dogs (*Cynomys ludovicianus*). *Journal of the American Association for Laboratory Animal Science* 56 (2): 210–213.

Hůrková, L., Hajdušek, O., and Modrý, D. (2003). Natural infection of Cryptosporidium muris (Apicomplexa: Cryptosporiidae) in Siberian chipmunks. *Journal of Wildlife Diseases* 39 (2): 441–444.

Johnson-Delaney, C.A. (2006). Common procedures in hedgehogs, prairie dogs, exotic rodents, and companion marsupials. *The Veterinary Clinics of North America. Exotic Animal Practice* 9 (2): 415–435.

Juan-Sallés, C., Patrício, R., Garrido, J. et al. (2009). Disseminated *Mycobacterium avium* subsp. *avium* infection in a Captive Richardson's ground squirrel (*Spermophilus richardsonii*). *Journal of Exotic Pet Medicine* 18 (4): 306–310.

Legendre, L.F. (2003). Oral disorders of exotic rodents. *The Veterinary Clinics of North America. Exotic Animal Practice* 6: 601–628.

Lehmer, E.M., Van Horne, B., Kulbartz, B. et al. (2001). Facultative torpor in free-ranging black-tailed prairie dogs (*Cynomys ludovicianus*). *Journal of Mammalogy* 82 (2): 551–557.

Lichtenberger, M. (2007). Shock and cardiopulmonary-cerebral resuscitation in small mammals and birds. *The Veterinary Clinics of North America. Exotic Animal Practice* 10 (2): 275–291.

Mancinelli, E. and Capello, V. (2016). Anatomy and disorders of the oral cavity of rat-like and squirrel-like rodents. *The Veterinary Clinics of North America. Exotic Animal Practice.* 19 (3): 871–900.

Mayer, J. (2012). Rodents. In: *Exotic Animal Formulary*, 4e (ed. J.W. Carpenter), 494. St. Louis: Elsevier.

Michener, G.R. (1983). Spring emergence schedules and vernal behavior of Richardson's ground squirrels: why do males emerge from hibernation before females? *Behavioral Ecology and Sociobiology* 14 (1): 29–38.

Michener, G.R. and Koeppl, J.W. (1985). Spermophilus richardsonii. *Mammalian Species* (243): 1–8.

Miwa, Y., Matsunaga, S., Nakayama, H. et al. (2006). Spontaneous lymphoma in a prairie dog (*Cynomys ludovicianus*). *Journal of the American Animal Hospital Association* 42 (2): 151–153.

Morera, N. (2004). Osteosarcoma in a Siberian chipmunk. *Exotic DVM* 6 (1): 11–12.

Morrissey, J.K. and Carpenter, J.W. (2004). Formulary. In: *Ferrets, Rabbits and Rodents: Clinical Medicine and Surgery*, 2e (eds. K.E. Quesenberry and J.W. Carpenter), 436–444. St Louis: WB Saunders.

Mouser, P., Cole, A., and Lin, T.L. (2006). Maxillary osteosarcoma in a prairie dog (*Cynomys ludovicianus*). *Journal of Veterinary Diagnostic Investigation* 18 (3): 310–312.

Ness, R.D. (2005). Rodents. In: *Exotic Animal Formulary*, 3e (ed. J.W. Carpenter), 375–408. St. Louis, MO: Elsevier/Saunders.

Olson, M.E. and McCabe, K. (1986). Anesthesia in the Richardson's ground squirrel: comparison of ketamine, ketamine and xylazine, droperidol and fentanyl, and sodium pentobarbital. *Journal of the American Veterinary Medical Association* 189 (9): 1035–1037.

Oohashi, E., Kangawa, A., and Kobayashi, Y. (2009). Mammary adenocarcinoma in a chipmunk (*Tamias sibiricus*). *Journal of Veterinary Medical Science* 71 (5): 677–679.

Orcutt, C. (2005). Prairie dogs, hedgehogs and sugar gliders. Proceeding of the NAVC North American Veterinary Conference 8–12 January 2005, Orlando, Florida, 1361–1363.

Pfaffenberger, G.S., Nygren, B., de Bruin, D. et al. (1984). Parasites of the black-tailed prairie dog (*Cynomys ludovicianus*) from eastern New Mexico. *Proceedings of the Helminthological Society of Washington* 51 (2): 241–244.

Phalen, D.N. (2004). Prairie dogs: vectors and victims. *Seminars in Avian and Exotic Pet Medicine* 13 (2): 105–107.

Pilny, A.A. and Hess, L. (2004). Prairie dog care and husbandry. *The Veterinary Clinics of North America. Exotic Animal Practice* 7 (2): 269–282.

Pisanu, B., Jerusalem, C., Huchery, C. et al. (2007). Helminth fauna of the Siberian chipmunk, *Tamias sibiricus* Laxmann (Rodentia, Sciuridae) introduced in suburban French forests. *Parasitology Research* 100 (6): 1375–1379.

Rogers, K.L. and Chrisp, C.E. (1998). Lipoma in the mediastinum of a prairie dog (*Cynomys ludovicianus*). *Journal of the American Association for Laboratory Animal Science* 37 (1): 74–76.

Schulz, R.E. and Lubimov, M.P. (1932). *Longistriata skrjabini* n. sp. (Nematoda, Trichostrongylidae) from the Ussuri squirrel. *Parasitology* 24: 50–53.

Sinclair, K. (2007). Richardson's ground squirrel (*Spermophilus richardsonii*). *Exotic DVM* 9 (4): 6–7.

Smith, D.A. and Burgmann, P.M. (1997). Formulary. In: *Ferrets, Rabbits and Rodents: Clinical Medicine and Surgery* (eds. E.V. Hilyer and K.E. Quesenberry), 392–404. Phildelphia: WB Saunders.

Smith, M., Dodd, J.R., Hobson, H. et al. (2013). Clinical techniques- surgical removal of elodontomas in the black tailed prairie dog (*Cynomys ludovicianus*) and the eastern fox squirrel (*Sciurus niger*). *Journal of Exotic Pet Medicine* 22: 258–264.

Tamaizumi, H., Kondo, H., Shibuya, H. et al. (2007). Tail root osteosarcoma in a chipmunk (*Tamias sibiricus*). *Veterinary Pathology* Online 44 (3): 392–394.

Tennant, B.C., Mrosovsky, N., McLean, K. et al. (1991). Hepatocellular carcinoma in Richardson's ground squirrels (*Spermophilus richardsonii*): evidence for association with hepatitis B–like virus infection. *Hepatology* 13 (6): 1215–1221.

Testut, P., Renard, C.A., Terradillos, O. et al. (1996). A new hepadnavirus endemic in arctic ground squirrels in Alaska. *Journal of Virology* 70 (7): 4210–4219.

Thas, I. (2010). Hymenolepis nana in Black-tailed Prairie Dogs (*Cynomys ludivicianus*). In: Proceedings of Association of Avian Veterinarians, San Diego, August, 69. Teaneck, NJ: Association of Avian Veterinarians.

Vourc'h, G., Marmet, J., Chassagne, M. et al. (2007). *Borrelia burgdorferi* sensu lato in Siberian chipmunks (*Tamias sibiricus*) introduced in suburban forests in France. *Vector Borne and Zoonotic Diseases* 7 (4): 637–642.

Wadsworth, P.F., Jones, D.M., and Pugsley, S.L. (1982). Primary hepatic neoplasia in some captive wild mammals. *The Journal of Zoo Animal Medicine* 13 (1): 29–32.

Wright, T.L., Eshar, D., McCullough, C. et al. (2017). Pharmacokinetics of single-dose subcutaneous meloxicam injections in black-tailed prairie dogs (*Cynomys ludovicianus*). *Journal of the American Association for Laboratory Animal Science* 56 (5): 539–543.

Yamate, J., Yamamoto, E., Nabe, M. et al. (2007). Spontaneous adenocarcinoma immunoreactive to cyclooxygenase-2 and transforming growth factor-. BETA. 1 in the buccal salivary gland of a Richardson's ground squirrel (*Spermophilus richardsonii*). *Experimental Animals* 56 (5): 379–384.

2

African Pygmy Hedgehogs

Nathalie Wissink-Argilaga

Hedgehogs belong to the order Insectivora and the family Erinaceidae. The most commonly presented pet hedgehog species is the African pygmy hedgehog (APH) (*Atelerix albiventris*) (Figure 2.1), also known as the white-bellied, central African or four-toed hedgehog. APH are native to equatorial Africa, where they inhabit steppes, savannas, grassland, and agricultural fields from Senegal to Ethiopia and south to the Zambezi River. They are widely used in biomedical research but are also becoming more popular in the exotic pet trade (Santana et al. 2010) and this chapter will focus on this species. The North African hedgehog (*Atelerix algirus*) may also be seen in practice infrequently (Figure 2.2). Native European hedgehogs may present as wildlife casualties but are readily differentiated by their larger size and darker colouration.

2.1 Anatomy and Physiology

Biological parameters for this species are shown in Table 2.1. Hedgehog anatomy is remarkably similar to other small mammals. The most striking difference is the presence of several thousand smooth cutaneous spines (quills). These range in size from 0.5 to 2 cm in length (Smith 1999). In most hedgehogs these are brown and white although colour variants do exist. They are not present on small areas over the head, ventrum, feet, and muzzle where they have sparse hair instead (Ivey and Carpenter 2012). These spines are not barbed and do not detach. They are very strong but are filled with small air-filled chambers to minimise weight (Mori and O'Brien 1997). The spines are attached to the skin and, at the base, they possess a muscle to allow erection of the spine. When a hedgehog is scared or frightened, they raise the spines and assume a defensive posture. The panniculus muscle over the back enables the hedgehog to roll into a ball and the circular orbicularis muscle contracts to appose the skin of the skirt over the withdrawn limbs and head (Mori and O'Brien 1997; Ivey and Carpenter 2012). The spines become erect at different angles creating a very effective protective barrier (Santana et al. 2010) (Figure 2.3). The spines can last up to 18 months and are replaced individually, a process known as quilling (Ivey and Carpenter 2012).

The adult dental formula is I3/2:C1/1:P3/2:M3/3, and the teeth are brachydont (closed-rooted) (Ivey and Carpenter 2012). They possess a typical insectivore gastrointestinal tract with a simple stomach, absent caecum, and non complex colon (Santana et al. 2010).

Eyesight in hedgehogs is poor and monochromatic (Reeve 1994) and they rely heavily on their sense of smell and hearing (Mori and O'Brien 1997). The sense of smell is very important for the location of food items, avoidance of predators and communication with other hedgehogs (Johnson 2006). Hedgehogs can emit a variety of different sounds including snorting and huffing (aggressive or warning sounds), screaming (severe distress), twittering (sound emitted by neonates), whistling (emitted by hoglets to attract the female's attention), clucking (made by males during courtship) and other sounds inaudible to human ears (Smith 1999; Johnson 2006; Ivey and Carpenter 2012).

A unique behaviour exhibited by both genders of captive and free-ranging hedgehogs is self-anointing (Figure 2.4). This behaviour can be elicited by a variety of strong-smelling substances. The hedgehog takes it into their mouth, produces mouthfuls of frothy saliva and then applies this to their spines using the tongue (Simone-Freilicher and Hoefer 2004; Ivey and Carpenter 2012). The exact purpose of this behaviour is unknown but it seems to be to give an individual smell to the hedgehog and it's environment that can last for minutes or hours (Reeve 1994). Other theories for this behaviour include: production of strong odours with a sexual function, cleaning of the

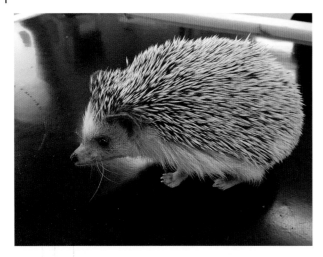

Figure 2.1 African pygmy hedgehog (*A. albiventris*).

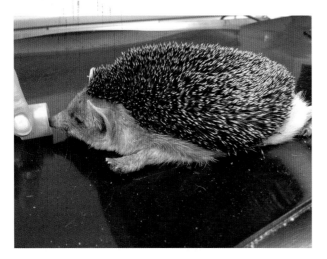

Figure 2.2 North African hedgehog (*A. algirus*).

spines, reduction of parasites on the skin and predator deterrent by depositing distasteful substances on the skin (Mori and O'Brien 1997).

2.2 Husbandry

It is important to understand the aspects of natural history and behaviour of the species to ensure the correct husbandry is provided.

APH are nocturnal and hide in burrows during the day. At night they spend most of their time predating on invertebrates such as insects, earthworms, slugs, and snails. They can also consume small vertebrates such as snakes, lizards, frogs, young and eggs of ground-nesting birds and very occasionally will consume plant material (Santana et al. 2010).

A. albiventris have a low metabolic rate and can go into torpor if kept too warm (above 30 °C) or too cold (below 7 °C) (Mori and O'Brien 1997). Hedgehogs are unlikely to experience this in the wild, and therefore it is considered undesirable in captive individuals (Ivey and Carpenter 2012).

Hedgehogs tend to be solitary in the wild and, although they aren't typically territorial, they mutually avoid each other to prevent direct competition for resources (Smith 1999). They will only come together during courtship and when a female has young (Santana et al. 2010).

2.2.1 Captive Housing

Hedgehogs are best housed singly. They are very active and a large cage should be provided with minimum dimensions of 0.6×0.9 m recommended (Ivey and Carpenter 2012). They can climb and escape easily so this should be considered in the design of the enclosure. Generally, cages with a plastic base and wire mesh walls are used as they are easily cleaned and achieve good ventilation. A litter tray with wood based cat litter can be provided and some animals can be trained to use it. Stress can be a common problem in this species so a hiding place should always be available. This can be in the form of a hollowed log, cardboard, plastic, or wooden box (Smith 1999). The bedding should be soft and absorbent such as newspaper, shavings, alfalfa pellets, or hay. Deep bedding should be provided to allow digging and foraging. A lot of owners still use cloths/towel substrates but limb entanglement from loose threads can be a problem. Bedding should be cleaned frequently as hedgehogs are very messy.

In the wild, hedgehogs travel long distances so exercise is important to avoid problems in captivity such as obesity. An exercise wheel is highly recommended and one with solid walls will avoid limb injury. Hedgehogs can also be allowed to roam outside of the cage in a safe area under constant supervision.

The preferred temperature for hedgehogs is 24–30 °C to avoid torpor or heat stroke. This temperature can be achieved by using thermostatically controlled heat mats or radiant heat bulbs. Direct contact with any heat source should be prevented. Humidity should be low, at around 40%. Being nocturnal animals, they prefer quiet and dim environments, however a day cycle of 10–14 hours of low level light should be provided (Ivey and Carpenter 2012).

Some owners like to bath their hedgehogs to remove faecal soiling; this can be done using a mild pet shampoo.

APH are monogastric insectivores/omnivores. In the wild they feed on a variety of invertebrates, small vertebrate prey, and plants (Reeve 1994) however, their exact dietary requirements are not documented. A study by

Table 2.1 Biological parameters.

Body weight	Male: 400–600 g Female: 300–600 g
Average life expectancy	4–7 years, up to 10 years (Hoefer 1994)
Rectal temperature	35.4 °C–37.2 °C
Heart rate (beats/minute)	180–280
Respiratory rate (breaths/minute)	25–50
Adult dental formula	2(I3/2:C1/1:P3/2:M3/3) = 36
Gastrointestinal transit time	12–16 hours
Age at sexual maturity	2–8 months
Oestrus cycle	Seasonally polyoestrus (wild), breed all year round (captive)
Duration of oestrus	3–17 days (Johnson 2010)
Gestational period	34–37 days
Litter size	1–7 (average 3)
Birth weight	8–13 g
Eyes open	13–16 days
Ears open	10 days
Weaning	4–6 weeks (start eating solids at 3 weeks)

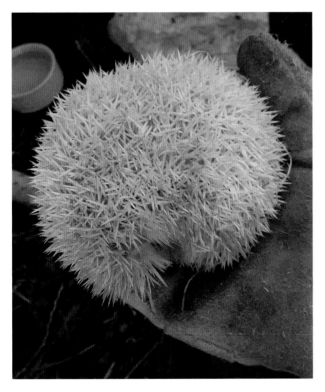

Figure 2.3 Rolled up albino APH. Note the criss-crossing of the spines, creating a very effective protective barrier.

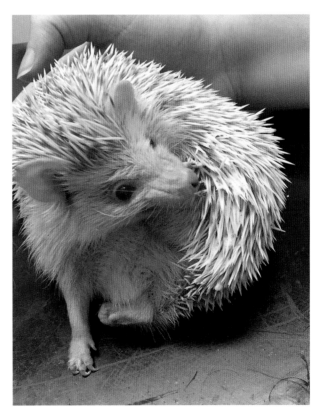

Figure 2.4 Self-anointing behaviour.

Graffam et al. (1998) concluded that APH were able to digest 64–68% of chitin compared to only 38% of cellulose suggesting a tendency towards an insectivorous diet. Captive hedgehogs tend to become obese (Smith 1999) and

to combat this, cellulose (plant matter) can be added to the diet to dilute nutrient density (Graffam et al. 1998). Due to their nocturnal activity patterns, hedgehogs should be fed at night and any uneaten food should be removed in the morning (Hedley 2014).

In captivity, hedgehogs have been successfully maintained on a variety of moderately high-protein (30–50%, dry matter basis) moderate fat (10–20%) diets (Ivey and Carpenter 2012). These include canned and dry dog and cat foods, kitten foods, ferret foods, commercial hedgehog foods and dry and semi-moist insectivore diets supplemented with earthworms, insects, and small quantities of vegetables and fruit (Graffam et al. 1998; Smith 1999). Treats can include hard-boiled or scrambled eggs and pinky mice. Dairy products should be avoided because of reports of lactose intolerance in hedgehogs (Hoefer 1994; Stocker 2003). Metabolic bone disease has been reported in hedgehogs fed only on larval insects and the calcium to phosphorus ratio in the diet should be 1.2–1.5 : 1.0 (Mori and O'Brien 1997; Johnson 2010). Nuts and grains should be avoided as they can become lodged against the hard palate (Hoefer 1994). Dry foods and uncooked produce are preferred over soft dietary items due to the tendency to develop tartar and gingivitis (Dierenfeld 2009).

Fresh water should always be available either in a sipper bottle or a shallow bowl, and replaced daily.

2.2.2 Breeding

APH breed well in captivity (Santana et al. 2010). The females reach sexual maturity at two to eight months with males maturing at six to eight months (Mori and O'Brien 1997). Females should not be bred from before six months as early breeding is associated with a higher risk of dystocia (Mori and O'Brien 1997). They are polyoestrus and can breed throughout the year with an average of one litter per year (Santana et al. 2010; Ivey and Carpenter 2012). Ovulation is thought to be induced and occurs 16–23 hours post-mating (Bedford et al. 2000) although many texts still report ovulation to be spontaneous (Mori and O'Brien 1997; Smith 1999). The gestation period is 34–37 days although delayed implantation might occur extending this period to 40 days (Reeve 1994). Litters sizes vary from one to seven hoglets, with an average of three (Mori and O'Brien 1997). Pregnancy diagnosis can be difficult but a breeding female can be assumed to be pregnant if she experiences a weight gain of 50 g or more in the two weeks after copulation (Santana et al. 2010). Abdominal and mammary enlargement can be noted from day 30 (Ivey and Carpenter 2012). Birth weight of the hoglets is between 8 and 13 g and they are born with closed ears and eyes and without hair or spines; these erupt within 24 hours. The ears open at 10 days and the eyes at 13–16 days. Hair appears by three weeks of age. The deciduous teeth appear at four weeks and the adult teeth erupt at seven to nine weeks. Weaning should occur at four to six weeks of age. If the hoglets are orphaned, puppy or kitten milk can be used as a replacer and feeding should occur every three to four hours. Massaging of the ventrum and anus will stimulate passing or urine and faeces (Mori and O'Brien 1997).

Infanticide and cannibalism are not uncommon, and the male should be kept separate from the neonates (Ivey and Carpenter 2012). Giving the female strict privacy and a hiding place may also reduce stress and the risk of abandonment or cannibalism (Smith 1999; Ivey and Carpenter 2012).

2.3 Clinical Evaluation

2.3.1 History-Taking

Due to their nocturnal habits it is preferable to arrange appointments for the evening. Owners should be asked to transport the animal in a sturdy box with a hiding place to reduce stress. It is also useful to instruct the owners to bring any pictures of the enclosure, samples of the diet offered and a recent faecal sample. In the author's practice, the reception team are trained to request this when making an appointment.

A thorough history should be taken from the owner including all aspects of husbandry (housing, temperature provision, diet and supplements provided) and behaviour. This is extremely important as many health problems seen in exotic pets are due to suboptimal husbandry and diet provision. Annual examinations are recommended.

2.3.2 Handling

APH can be challenging patients to handle, as even the tamest animals will tend to curl up in a ball when frightened or stressed in unfamiliar surroundings. It can help to dim the lights in the consulting room and avoid any loud noises. Hedgehogs don't tend to bite but the spines can be uncomfortable to the handler and latex or thin leather gloves can be used to facilitate handling. Very well handled APH can be examined briefly without too much trouble and some are even amenable to oral examination using a wooden tongue depressor. If the hedgehog is walking around on the examination table a brief visual inspection of the face, feet and dorsum can be performed. Placing the hedgehog on a clear plastic tray and observing it from underneath can aid evaluation of the ventrum and feet. There are also several ways described to uncurl a hedgehog; these include placing it in shallow water (<2 cm deep), gently extending the hind limbs in a wheelbarrow fashion

(Johnson 2010), gently rocking it in your hands until the head comes out and then pressing on the back of the neck and dorsum to prevent it curling up again or stroking the spines on the back in a caudal fashion (Ivey and Carpenter 2012). The main advice is to have patience.

2.3.3 Sex Determination

APH are sexually dimorphic. Males can be identified by the presence of the preputial opening cranially on the ventral abdomen. The testicles are intra-abdominal, located in a para-anal recess (Bedford et al. 2000) and they have no scrotal sac. In females the anogenital distance is very short and the vulva is slit-shaped (Hedley 2014) (Figure 2.5).

(a)

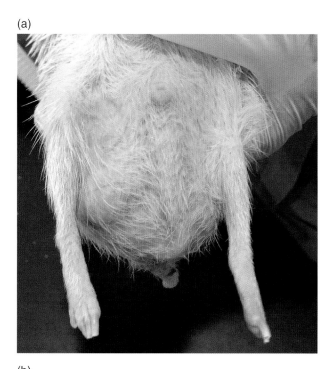

(b)

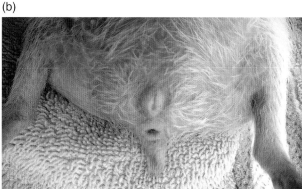

Figure 2.5 (a) male genitalia. (b) Female genitalia (*Source:* Courtesy of Sarah Pellett).

2.3.4 Clinical Examination

The physical examination of a hedgehog should follow the usual head-to-tail process employed for domestic species.

Healthy hedgehogs should be active and inquisitive (Ivey and Carpenter 2012). They may make a variety of snorting and grunting noises during the examination and these must not be confused with signs of respiratory disease. The eyes should be bright and free of any discharge or ocular pathology, the skin and spines should be assessed for any signs of dermatological disease and auscultation of the heart and chest performed listening for the presence of murmurs or abnormal respiratory sounds. Where possible, the mouth should be checked for the presence of any masses or dental disease, the colour of the mucous membranes assessed, the lymph nodes palpated for any enlargement, palpation of the abdomen carried out to detect any masses or organomegaly, the genitalia examined, femoral pulses palpated, the anus examined for discharge or abnormal stool remnants, rectal temperature obtained and the toes and feet should be examined. Often sedation or anaesthesia is required to carry out a full clinical examination.

2.4 Basic Techniques

2.4.1 Sample Collection

Blood: A safe volume of blood to withdraw in small exotic mammals is often estimated at 1% body weight (1 ml/100 g) (Joslin 2009). However, in sick or debilitated animals it is better to reduce this amount to 0.5% (Pilny 2008). Sedation or anaesthesia is generally necessary to obtain a blood sample. The author's preferred veins to obtain larger volumes of blood in this species are the cranial vena cava or the jugular vein. For smaller amounts the cephalic, femoral, and medial saphenous veins can also be used. The approach to the cranial vena cava is very similar to the one used in other small mammals. A short and narrow gauge needle (1/2–5/8 inch, 25 or 27 gauge) attached to a 1 or 2.5 ml syringe is inserted cranially to the clavicle and directed towards the opposite hip (Figure 2.6). Care must be taken to not puncture the heart as this is more cranially located than in the ferret. The jugular is not easily visible and can be difficult to locate due to the accumulation of fat around the neck.

Reference intervals for haematology and biochemistry are presented in Tables 2.2 and 2.3.

Urine: can be obtained by free catch during a physical examination. The bladder can also be expressed by gentle digital pressure. More invasive techniques include

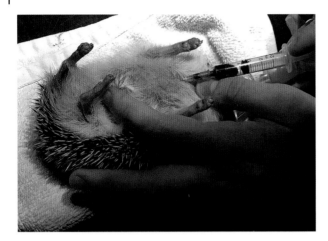

Figure 2.6   Cranial vena cava venepuncture.

Table 2.2   Haematologic reference intervals for African Pygmy Hedgehogs (Species360- 2017).

Measurement	Units	Reference interval	Range
Red blood cell count	×10¹² cells/l	2.44–7.12	0.14–8.98
Haemoglobin	g/l	57–156	15–205
Haematocrit	%	20.5–47	6–56
MCV	fL	52.4–102.6	52–110
MCH	pg	17.9–32.2	12.1–35.6
MCHC	g/l	221–399	200–430
Platelets	×10¹² cells/l	0.030–0.597	0.09–0.85
White blood cell count	×10⁹ cells/l	2.87–21.93	0.7–26.5
Lymphocytes	×10⁹ cells/l	0.79–9.06	0.03–12.46
Monocytes	×10⁹ cells/l	0.032–1.31	0–1.5
Segmented neutrophils	×10⁹ cells/l	0.71–11.8	0.27–15.3
Band neutrophils	×10⁹ cells/l	0–0.76	0–0.79
Eosinophils	×10⁹ cells/l	0.052–3.36	0–4.04
Basophils	×10⁹ cells/l	0–0.88	0–1.2

Table 2.3   Biochemical reference intervals for African Pygmy Hedgehogs (Species360- 2017).

Measurement	Units	Reference interval	Range
Sodium	mmol/l	134–156	131–164
Potassium	mmol/l	3.6–6.4	2.8–6.8
Chloride	mmol/l	94–124	92–126
Calcium	mmol/l	1.6–2.9	1.4–3.3
Phosphorus	mmol/l	0.94–2.95	0.1–3.88
Glucose	mmol/l	0.6–7.7	0–10.5
BUN	mmol/l	4.9–20.2	3.2–23.9
Creatinine	μmol/l	9–73	0–115
Alanine aminotransferase	U/l	21–152	11–185
Aspartase aminotransferase	U/l	6–120	4–140
Lactate dehydrogenase	U/l	33–1318	27–1335
Alkaline phosohatase	U/l	3–96	0–137
Gamma-glutamyltransferase	U/l	0–14	0–18
Amylase	U/l	147–982	27–1067
Lipase	U/l	6–263	0–385
Creatinine kinase	U/l	180–1937	0–2294
Total bilirubin	μmol/l	0–13.7	0–15.4
Total protein	g/l	42–75	30–90
Albumin	g/l	18–43	13–47
Globulin	g/l	17–44	6–51
Cholesterol	mmol/l	1.9–6.6	0.4–7.4
Triglyceride	mmol/l	0–1.4	0–1.5

catheterization or cystocentesis and for these anaesthesia will be necessary. Reference values have not been established for hedgehogs but neoplastic cells, crystals, white blood cells and red blood cells may be considered abnormal depending on the method of urine collection (Evans and Souza 2010).

Faeces: cytology and culture can be performed on fresh faecal samples. This can be obtained by voluntary voidance or using a small swab directly introduced into the rectum (Klaphake 2006). Parasitology can be carried out using direct smear analysis and faecal flotation.

Cytology: samples can be obtained from masses or fluid accumulations in the thorax or abdomen. Both cytology and culture and sensitivity should be carried out if appropriate.

2.4.2   Nutritional Support

APH are insectivores/omnivores and commercial insectivore mixes or omnivore mixes can be used. These are fed according to manufacturer's guidelines, though in critically ill animals the first feed should be reduced at 1% bodyweight (BW) progressing up to recommended feeding volumes in successive feeds. These feeds can be given via gavage or

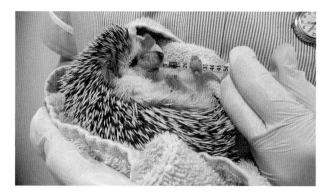

Figure 2.7 Tame hedgehog accepting syringe feeding. (*Source:* Courtesy of Sarah Pellett).

assisted feeding through a syringe. Tame hedgehogs may be amenable to syringe feeding but most patients will pose a challenge (Figure 2.7). For longer term nutritional support the placement of an oesophagostomy tube can be considered (Adamovicz et al. 2016). Live crickets and mealworms can also be used to stimulate feeding. It is very important that the patient is hydrated and normothermic before commencing nutritional support (Johnson-Delaney 2006).

2.4.3   Fluid Therapy

Fluid requirements have not been established for APH but maintenance requirements are assumed to be 50–100 ml/kg/day following guidelines for other small mammals. Fluid therapy can be administered via the subcutaneous (SC), intravenous (IV), intraosseous (IO) or intraperitoneal (IP) routes. The SC route is useful only for mildly dehydrated animals. Absorption of SC fluids can be erratic due to the differences in vascularization between the spiny and the furred skin (Ivey and Carpenter 2012). The area where spiny and furred skin join mid-body provides a reliable and accessible site (Johnson-Delaney 2006). IV catheters can be very difficult to maintain in place if the hedgehog tightens into a ball but in severely debilitated animals the cephalic, lateral saphenous, or jugular vein can be used (Johnson 2010). The IO route might be a better option for severely dehydrated or shocked patients. Sedation and aseptic placement will be necessary. An IO catheter can be placed in the tibial crest or the femur following the same procedure as for rabbits and rodents (Mader 2004). The IP route can be used unless the patient has an acute abdomen, a gastrointestinal disorder, or an abdominal surgery is planned (Johnson-Delaney 2006). The procedure is similar to that described in rats, in the lower right quadrant of the abdomen (Bihun and Bauck 2004). Five to ten ml can be given via this route but sedation is generally necessary (Johnson-Delaney 2006) and there is potential for visceral perforation with blind placement.

2.4.4   Anaesthesia

Most APH, with the exception of extremely docile individuals, will not allow a full examination without the use of sedation or anaesthesia. Anaesthesia or sedation will also be required to perform most diagnostic testing and surgical procedures. The patient must undergo a clinical assessment and be stabilised before any anaesthetic event and thermal and fluid support should be continued during anaesthesia. Fasting for 4–6 hours is recommended for anaesthetic procedures that will last longer than 20 minutes (Heatley 2009a).

The most common method of anaesthesia induction is by the administration of volatile anaesthetics (typically isofluorane or sevoflurane) via facemask or chamber induction after pre-oxygenation (Figure 2.8). Maintenance of anaesthesia can be achieved either with the use of a facemask or by tracheal intubation, using 1.0–1.5 mm endotracheal tube or an adapted IV catheter or feeding tube (Johnson 2010). Monitoring of anaesthesia follows the same principles as for any other small mammals and additional equipment such as pulseoximetry and capnography should be used. The use of injectable anaesthetics has been reported in hedgehogs but induction is variable and recovery is usually prolonged (Pye 2001). Analgesia should be considered for any painful procedures.

Sedation has been gaining popularity in exotic pet medicine and can be beneficial in some cases. Drugs used for sedation in APH include midazolam with or without the addition of an opioid (such as buprenorphine or butorphanol), ketamine, or alfaxalone. Combinations of Midazolam/opioid/ketamine can be combined in the same syringe and given IM in the epaxial muscles. If using alfaxalone, this can be given after the administration of midazolam/opioid (Lennox and Miwa 2016).

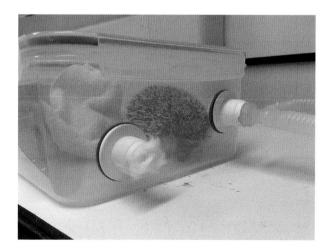

Figure 2.8   Hedgehog anaesthesia induction in chamber.

2.4.5 Euthanasia

Euthanasia can be achieved by IV, IP, or intracardiac injection of a barbiturate. The patient should be anaesthetised prior to euthanasia unless vascular access is available.

2.4.6 Hospitalisation Requirements

A quiet area with subdued lighting will help reduce the stress in these patients. APH fall into the category of prey species and so they should be separated from sight, sound, and smell of predators (Longley 2008). As they like to burrow, a substrate of shredded paper can be used. A hiding place should also be provided. Ambient temperature should be maintained at 27–29 °C (80–85 °F) for weak or debilitated patients (Ivey and Carpenter 2012). This can be achieved using a thermostatically controlled heat-pad under the cage or by hospitalising them in a secure incubator. Low humidity at less than 40% is advisable (Ivey and Carpenter 2012). Getting hospitalised patients to eat may be difficult and familiar food items brought in by the owner can help with this. A variety of suitable diets and invertebrates should also be available and supportive nutrition should be instigated if voluntary feeding does not occur. Fluid therapy is often necessary and syringe drivers and fluid warmers should be available.

2.5 Common Medical and Surgical Conditions

As prey species, APH are good at hiding signs of illness. The presenting signs can often be vague rather than system-specific and might include lethargy, weakness, and/or anorexia. These can be caused by a variety of underlying medical and/or environmental conditions. This fact highlights the importance of good history taking as well appropriate diagnostic testing.

2.5.1 Ocular Conditions

The specific anatomy of the hedgehog's eye, with shallow orbits and large palpebral fissures, predisposes them to proptosis and ocular injuries (Wheler et al. 2001). Proptosis of the globe is considered an emergency and enucleation is often necessary. Ocular injuries leading to ulceration and keratitis can be caused by trauma or occur secondary to tooth root abscesses, retro-bulbar abscessation or neoplasia, and ectoparasites (Johnson 2010). Diagnosis and treatment is as for other small animals. The author has diagnosed cataracts on various occasions, the underlying cause is unknown but could be age and/or nutrition related

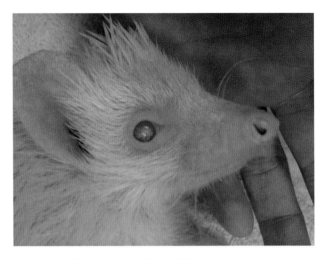

Figure 2.9 Cataract in an albino APH.

as happens in European hedgehogs (Williams et al. 2017) and albino APH seem to be over-represented (Figure 2.9).

2.5.2 Dermatologic and Otic Conditions

Dermatological conditions were the most commonly reported problem in a retrospective study on disease occurrence in APH, accounting for 66.04% of presenting cases (Gardhouse and Eshar 2015). Acariasis, dermatophytosis, and external parasites are commonly encountered. Mite infestations with *Caparinia, Chorioptes,* and *Notoedres* cause white/brown crusting at the base of the quills, quill loss, and hyperkeratosis. Diagnosis is via mite identification on skin scrapes. Dermatitis of the pinna is often seen in APH and can present with erythema, secretions, crusting, and ragged pinnal edges. Differential diagnosis include ectoparasitism (*Caparinia tripilis* [Moreira et al. 2013], *Notoederes cati* [Pantchev and Hofmann 2006]), dermatophytosis, nutritional deficiencies, and otitis externa (bacterial or yeast). Diagnostic approach and treatment follows the same principles as other small mammals including cytology, skin scrapings, bacteriology, and topical and/or systemic antimicrobial and anti-inflammatory therapy (Figure 2.10). Antiparasitics such as ivermectin, selamectin, imidacloprid/moxidectin (Pantchev and Hofmann 2006; Kim et al. 2012) and fluralaner (Romero et al. 2017) have all been suggested treatments for acariasis.

Middle aged to older APH can be affected by skin neoplasia (Ellis and Mori 2001).

2.5.3 Dental and Oral Conditions

Dental disease is observed commonly including calculus, periodontitis, gingivitis, gingival recession, and tooth fractures. Clinical signs of dental disease include anorexia,

(a)

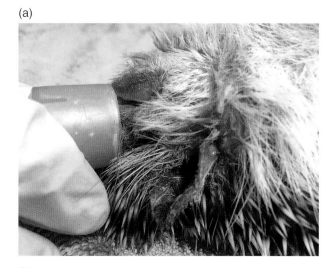

(b)

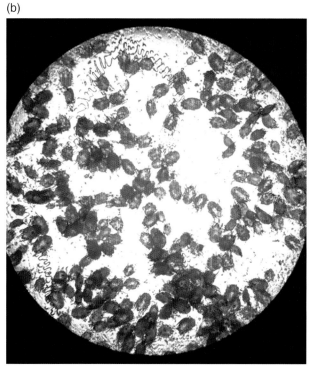

Figure 2.10   (a) Severe otitis externa with discharge secondary to acariasis. (b) Cytology from the above otic discharge revealing mite proliferation.

salivation, halitosis, and pawing at the mouth. Inappropriate diet is thought to be a causative factor (Hoefer 1994). Routine oral examinations (likely under sedation/anaesthesia), home dental care, appropriate diet and dental radiography, descaling and extractions under anaesthesia are paramount to deal with this problem. Secondary abscessation and osteomyelitis has also been described and culture of any abscesses is recommended to allow targeted therapy (Martínez et al. 2005).

Oral squamous cell carcinoma is seen frequently and is listed as one of the most common neoplasms in the species (Pei-Chi et al. 2015; Raymond and Garner 2001). One description of an odontogenic fibroma has also been published (Wozniak-Biel et al. 2015). Any masses in the oral cavity should be biopsied and histopathology should be performed.

Trauma of the oral cavity due to a fall, blunt facial trauma or chewing inappropriate objects, has also been observed by the author. Foreign objects can become lodged between the dental arcades (Ivey and Carpenter 2012).

2.5.4   Respiratory Conditions

Respiratory infections due to *Corynebacterium* (Raymond et al. 1998) have been reported in this species. They are also believed to be susceptible to *Bordetella bronchiseptica* and *Pasteurella multocida* (Ivey and Carpenter 2012). Work up and treatment would follow the same guidelines as for other small mammals. Other differentials for dyspnoea include cardiac disease and neoplasia. APH make a variety of snorting and wheezing noises as part of their communication and these should not be confused with respiratory pathology.

2.5.5   Cardiovascular and Haematologic Conditions

The incidence of cardiomyopathy in APH is significant, approaching 40% in one study (Raymond and Garner 2000). It is more commonly seen in geriatric males (>3 years old) but has been described in animals as young as 1 year of age. Clinical signs of heart disease are generally similar to those in other species although they can be very vague with symptoms such as weight loss and lethargy. Causes of heart disease are thought to include diet, toxins, stress, obesity, and genetics (Heatley 2009b). Diagnostic testing should include radiography, echocardiography, and ECG. A detailed protocol for cardiac assessment has been published (Black et al. 2011). Treatment of these cases is generally extrapolated from other species and can include furosemide, enalapril, pimobendan, and L-carnitine (Delk et al. 2014).

Haematologic disorders such as congenital erythropoietic porphyria (Wolff et al. 2005) and anaemia secondary to uterine tumours can also be encountered (Johnson 2010).

2.5.6   Gastrointestinal and Hepatic Conditions

Diarrhoea is commonly seen in APH. *Salmonella* spp. and other bacteria (Chomel et al. 2007), intestinal parasitism, intestinal neoplasia (lymphoma/lymphosarcoma) (Raymond and Garner 2001), and dietary inadequacies are all possible causes. APH are inquisitive and intestinal foreign bodies such as hair, carpet, or rubber are occasionally seen (Ivey and Carpenter 2012). Diagnostics and treatment follow the same guidelines as for other mammals.

Hepatic lipidosis is commonly seen as a sequel to chronic diseases (Ivey and Carpenter 2012). Hepatic neoplasia (either primary or metastatic) is an important cause of liver failure in this species (Lightfoot 2000). A case of liver failure due to human herpes simplex virus 1 has also been reported (Allison et al. 2002).

2.5.7 Urinary Conditions

Signs of cystitis include haematuria, stranguria, pollakuria, anorexia, and/or lethargy. Urolithiasis with possible urethral obstruction has also been reported (Johnson 2010). Kidney diseases including nephritis, tubular necrosis, polycystic kidneys, and neoplasia have all been identified on histology (Fisher 2006). Diagnosis follows the same guidelines as for other mammals and treatment includes correction of the underlying cause, fluid therapy, and supportive care.

2.5.8 Reproductive Conditions

Uterine neoplasia is very commonly seen in this species and often presents with bloody vulval discharge. Ultrasonography is useful in the diagnosis of this condition. Treatment primarily consists of ovariohysterectomy (OVH). Histopathology is recommended to decide on prognosis as different neoplasms have been described including adenosarcomas, endometrial stroma sarcomas and endometrial polyps (Mikaelian and Reavill 2004).

Pyometra, metritis, and dystocia have all been reported (Ivey and Carpenter 2012). Entrapment of substrate around the prepuce can cause posthitis in males (Ivey and Carpenter 2012).

2.5.9 Musculoskeletal Conditions

Lameness is commonly seen and can be caused by fractures, osteoarthritis, nail overgrowth, pododermatitis, annular constriction or necrosis of a digit or foot due to foreign material, neurological disease, and neoplasia. Full physical examination is paramount to achieve a diagnosis (Johnson 2010).

2.5.10 Neurologic Conditions

Ataxia is commonly seen in APH. Differential diagnosis for these cases should include:

- *Torpor*: this is a state of dormancy that hedgehogs can enter when they experience extremes of temperatures or are ill. In this state, respiratory rate and heart rate are reduced but they still remain sensitive to touch. This can last several weeks but the affected animals can have periods of activity with ataxia (Johnson 2006). Treatment consists in providing adequate temperature support, fluid therapy, and nutritional support.
- *Trauma*: spinal or head trauma can present with neurological signs.
- *Toxins*: no species-specific susceptibility to intoxication is reported but it would be expected that agents that cause neurotoxicity in other mammal species would affect hedgehogs similarly.
- *Metabolic*: hepatic failure and hepatic encephalopathy can be the cause of neurological signs. Hypocalcaemia due to postpartum eclampsia has also been described (Ivey and Carpenter 2012)
- *Weakness* due to cardiac disease or malnutrition could present as ataxia.
- *Neoplasia*: Several neoplasms involving the nervous system have been reported including Schwannomas (Heatley et al. 2005), anaplastic astrocytomas (Gibson et al. 2008) and gliomas (Benneter et al. 2014)
- *Intervertebral disc disease (IVDD)*: a case series was reported in 2009 with four APH with IVDD. The clinical signs included hindlimb ataxia, urinary stasis, proprioceptive deficits, and lameness. Narrowing of the cervical intravertebral canal and spondylosis were noted on radiographs in two cases. The animals were four years or older and both males and females were affected (Raymond et al. 2009). The clinical signs are very similar to the signs of wobbly hedgehog syndrome (WHS) and disc disease should therefore, be included in the list of differential diagnosis in ataxic hedgehogs.
- *WHS*: This is a neurodegenerative disease that has been described since the mid-1990s and occurs in approximately 10% of pet APH in North America (Graesser et al. 2006). The initial clinical sign is the inability to ball up and progresses to mild ataxia that can wax and wane initially. Over a period of several months, the signs progress to falling over, tremors, and seizures. The paralysis is generally ascending from hindlimbs to forelimbs (Graesser et al. 2006). As the signs progress they are normally accompanied by weight loss despite good appetite. The end stage is tetraplegia and aphagia. It most frequently occurs in animals younger than two years of age but both younger and older animals have been affected. The progression of the disease varies from weeks to months; 60% of affected hedgehogs were immobile within nine months of presenting ataxic and 90% were immobile after 15 months (Graesser et al. 2006). Diagnosis can only be made post-mortem and histological examination with vacuolization of the white matter tract of the cerebrum, cerebellum, brain stem, and throughout the spinal cord. The demyelination

responsible for the initial clinical signs is followed by axonal degeneration and loss and finally neuronal degeneration (Garner and Graesser 2006). The aetiology is unknown but an inherited component is suspected. Treatment is supportive including hand feeding and supportive care. The disease has a poor prognosis and is invariably fatal.

Head tilt and circling due to otitis media or central lesions and infectious causes of neurological signs such as rabies and *Baylisascaris* have also been reported (Lightfoot 2000; Gardhouse and Eshar 2015).

2.5.11 Neoplastic Conditions

Neoplasia is commonly encountered in this species and several reviews on neoplastic conditions have been published with prevalence ranging from 29–52% of necropsied cases (Raymond and Garner 2001; Heatley et al. 2005). A wide range have been reported with mammary gland adenocarcinomas, lymphoma, and oral squamous cell carcinomas most commonly identified (Figure 2.11) (Heatley et al. 2005).

2.5.12 Nutritional Conditions

Obesity is commonly seen in captive APH and is exacerbated by overfeeding and inactivity. Gradual food reduction with withdrawal of high fat foods (mealworms, waxworms), regular weighing and increased exercise are all part of the treatment regime.

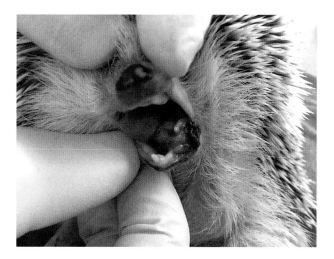

Figure 2.11 Oral swelling subsequently confirmed on histopathology as a squamous cell carcinoma in the oral cavity of an APH.

2.5.13 Preventative Health Measures

Yearly general health checks are recommended at the author's practice. These include a review of husbandry and diet as well as a physical exam, paying especial attention to the oral cavity and body condition. In older animal these checks are recommended bi-annually and further diagnostic testing might be recommended.

Nail trimming can be performed at these checks but may require sedation in nervous individuals.

There are currently no advised vaccinations or routine worming protocols for this species.

As APH are generally kept as solitary animals, routine neutering is not necessary to prevent reproduction. Routine OVH might become more commonplace due to the high incidence of uterine pathology in this species.

2.5.14 Neutering Technique

Although routine neutering is rarely performed the surgical approach is similar to that used in other small mammals.

For females, the midline abdominal approach is used and OVH is performed as for other mammalian species. Skin closure using an intradermal pattern in the skin is the author's favoured technique.

For castration of males, bilateral inguinal incisions are used, similar to those used in guinea pigs (Johnson 2010). A closed technique is advisable as APH have open inguinal canals.

2.5.15 Radiographic Imaging

Radiography generally requires anaesthesia or sedation to obtain good quality images. The routine views are the same as for other small mammals, including a full body dorso-ventral (DV) and a latero-lateral (LL) view. A more centred approach to the oral cavity can be achieved with the use of dental radiography; and further projections such as oblique and ventro-dorsal will also be useful for specific areas. The overlay of spines can hinder correct interpretation, especially of the DV view. On the LL view, this can be improved by pulling the mantle dorsally (Figure 2.12).

Radiography is useful for the assessment of fractures/dislocations, pulmonary, and cardiac disease, digestive and urinary/reproductive problems and visualisation of organomegaly. It often needs to be combined with other imaging techniques such as ultrasonography and more recently computed tomography (CT) and magnetic resonance imaging (MRI).

(a)

(b)

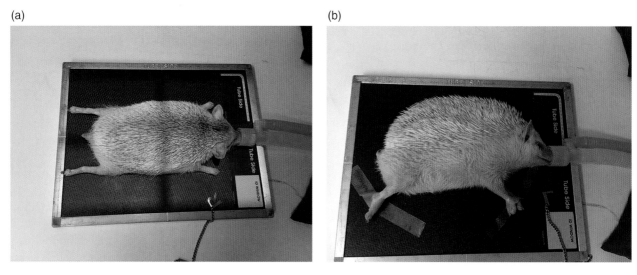

Figure 2.12 (a) Positioning for the dorsoventral radiographic view. (b) Positioning for the laterolateral radiographic view.

Formulary

Medication	Dose	Dosing interval	Additional comments
Anaesthesia and Analgesia			
Midazolam/Butorphanol/ Ketamine	0.5–1 mg/kg (M) + 0.4 mg/kg (B) + 5–7 mg/kg (K) IM		(Lennox and Miwa 2016)
Alfaxalone	1–2 mg/kg IM		(Lennox and Miwa 2016)
Buprenorphine	0.01–0.5 mg/kg SC, IM	q8–12h	(Lennox 2007)
Meloxicam	0.2 mg/kg PO, SC	q24h	(Johnson-Delaney 2006)
Antibiotics			
Amoxicillin/clavulanic acid	12.5 mg/kg PO	q 12 h	(Morrisey and Carpenter 2012)
Clindamycin	5.5–10 mg/kg PO	q12h	(Lightfoot 2000)
Metronidazole	20 mg/kg PO	q12h	(Morrisey and Carpenter 2012)
Trimethoprim /sulfa	30 mg/kg PO, SC, IM	q12h	(Smith 1992)
Antiparasitics			
Fenbendazole	10–30 mg/kg PO	q24h × 5 days	(Smith 2000)
Ivermectin	0.2 mg/kg PO, SC	q14d × 3 treatments	(Morrisey and Carpenter 2012)
Selamectin	6 mg/kg topically		(Fehr and Koestlinger 2013)
Fluralaner (Bravecto)	15 mg/kg PO	once	(Romero et al. 2017)
10% imidacloprid +1% moxidectin (Advocate for cats)	0.1 ml/kg topically	once	(Kim et al. 2012)
Miscellaneous			
Enalapril	0.5 mg/kg PO	q24h	(Lightfoot 2000)
Furosemide	2.5–5 mg/kg PO, SC, IM	q8h	(Morrisey and Carpenter 2012)

References

Adamovicz, L., Bullen, L., Saker, K. et al. (2016). Use of an esophagostomy tube for management of traumatic subtotal glossectomy in an African pygmy hedgehog (*Atelerix albiventris*). *Journal of Exotic Pet Medicine* 25: 231–236.

Allison, N., Chang, T.C., Steele, K.E. et al. (2002). Fatal herpes simplex infection in a pygmy African hedgehog (*Atelerix albiventris*). *Journal of Comparative Pathology* 126: 76–78.

Bedford, J.M., Mock, O.B., Nagdas, S.K. et al. (2000). Reproductive characteristics of the African pygmy hedgehog, *Atelerix albiventris*. *Journal of Reproduction and Fertility* 120: 143–150.

Benneter, S.S., Summers, B.A., Schulz-Schaeffer, W.J. et al. (2014). Mixed glioma (Oligoastrocytoma) in the brain of an African hedgehog (*Atelerix albiventris*). *Journal of Comparative Pathology* 151: 420–424.

Bihun, C. and Bauck, L. (2004). Basic anatomy, physiology, husbandry, and clinical techniques. In: *Ferrets, Rabbits and Rodents. Clinical Medicine and Surgery* (eds. K.E. Quesenberry and J.W. Carpenter), 286–198. St. Louis, MO: Saunders Elsevier.

Black, P.A., Marshall, C., Seyfried, A.W. et al. (2011). Cardiac assessment of African hedgehogs (*Atelerix albiventris*). *Journal of Zoo and Wildlife Medicine* 42: 49–53.

Chomel, B.B., Belotto, A., and Meslin, F.-X. (2007). Wildlife, exotic pets, and emerging zoonoses. *Emerging Infectious Diseases* 13: 6–11. https://doi.org/10.3201/eid1301.060480.

Delk, K.W., Eshar, D., Garcia, E. et al. (2014). Diagnosis and treatment of congestive heart failure secondary to dilated cardiomyopathy in a hedgehog. *The Journal of Small Animal Practice* 55: 174–177.

Dierenfeld, E.S. (2009). Feeding behavior and nutrition of the african pygmy hedgehog (*Atelerix albiventris*). *The Veterinary Clinics of North America. Exotic Animal Practice* 12: 335–337.

Ellis, C. and Mori, M. (2001). Skin diseases of rodents and small exotic mammals. *The Veterinary Clinics of North America. Exotic Animal Practice* 4: 493–542.

Evans, E.E. and Souza, M.J. (2010). Advanced diagnostic approaches and current management of internal disorders of select species (rodents, sugar gliders, hedgehogs). *The Veterinary Clinics of North America. Exotic Animal Practice* 13: 453–469.

Fehr, M. and Koestlinger, S. (2013). Ectoparasites in small exotic mammals. *The Veterinary Clinics of North America. Exotic Animal Practice* 16: 611–657. https://doi.org/10.1016/j.cvex.2013.05.011.

Fisher, P.G. (2006). Exotic mammal renal disease: causes and clinical presentation. *The Veterinary Clinics of North America. Exotic Animal Practice* 9: 33–67.

Gardhouse, S. and Eshar, D. (2015). Retrospective study of disease occurrence in captive African pygmy hedgehogs (*Atelerix albiventris*). *Israel Journal of Veterinary Medicine* 143: 532–534.

Garner, M. and Graesser, D. (2006). Wobbly Hedgehog Syndrome: a neurodegenerative disease of African and European hedgehogs. In: *Procedings of the Association of Avian Veterinarians*. Session 133, 67–68. Teaneck, NJ: Association of Avian Veterinarians.

Gibson, C.J., Parry, N.M.A., Jakowski, R.M. et al. (2008). Anaplastic astrocytoma in the spinal cord of an African pygmy hedgehog (*Atelerix albiventris*). *Veterinary Pathology* 45: 934–938. https://doi.org/10.1354/vp.45-6-934.

Graesser, D., Spraker, T.R., Dressen, P. et al. (2006). Wobbly hedgehog syndrome in African pygmy hedgehogs (*Atelerix* spp.). *Journal of Exotic Pet Medicine* 15: 59–65.

Graffam, W.S., Fitzpatrick, M.P., and Dierenfeld, E.S. (1998). Fiber digestion in the African white-bellied hedgehog (*Atelerix albiventris*): a preliminary evaluation. *The Journal of Nutrition* 128: 2671S–2673S.

Heatley, J.J. (2009a). Hedgehogs. In: *Manual of Exotic Pet Practice* (eds. M.A. Mitchell and T.N. Tully), 433–455. St. Louis, MO: Saunders Elsevier.

Heatley, J.J. (2009b). Cardiovascular anatomy, physiology, and disease of rodents and small exotic mammals. *The Veterinary Clinics of North America. Exotic Animal Practice* 12: 99–113.

Heatley, J.J., Mauldin, G.E., and Cho, D.Y. (2005). A review of neoplasia in the captive African hedgehog (*Atelerix albiventris*). *Seminars in Avian and Exotic Pet Medicine* 14: 182–192. https://doi.org/10.1053/j.saep.2005.07.002.

Hedley, J. (2014). African pygmy hedgehogs: general care and health concerns. *Companion Animal* 19: 40–44. https://doi.org/10.12968/coan.2014.19.1.40.

Hoefer, H.L. (1994). Hedgehogs. *The Veterinary Clinics of North America. Small Animal Practice* 24: 113–120.

Ivey, E. and Carpenter, J.W. (2012). African hedgehogs. In: *Ferrets, Rabbits and Rodents. Clinical Medicine and Surgery* (eds. K. Quesenberry and J.W. Carpenter), 411–427. St. Louis, MO: Saunders Elsevier.

Johnson, D.H. (2006). Miscellaneous small mammal behaviour. In: *Exotic Pet Behavior: Birds, Reptiles, and Small Mammals* (eds. T.B. Bays, T. Lightfoot and J. Mayer), 263–344. St. Louis, MO: Saunders Elsevier.

Johnson, D.H. (2010). African pygmy hedgehogs. In: *BSAVA Manual of Exotic Pets, A Foundation Manual* (eds. C. Johnson-Delaney and A. Meredith), 139–147. Quedgeley, Gloucester: British Small Animal Veterinary Association.

Johnson-Delaney, C.A. (2006). Common procedures in hedgehogs, prairie dogs, exotic rodents, and companion marsupials. *The Veterinary Clinics of North America. Exotic Animal Practice* 9: 415–435.

Joslin, J.O. (2009). Blood collection techniques in exotic small mammals. *Journal of Exotic Pet Medicine* 18: 117–139.

Kim, K.R., Ahn, K.S., Oh, D.S. et al. (2012). Efficacy of a combination of 10% imidacloprid and 1% moxidectin against *Caparinia tripilis* in African pygmy hedgehog (*Atelerix albiventris*). *Parasites & Vectors* 5 (1): 158.

Klaphake, E. (2006). Common rodent procedures. *The Veterinary Clinics of North America. Exotic Animal Practice* 9: 389–413.

Lennox, A.M. (2007). Emergency and critical care procedures in sugar gliders (*Petaurus breviceps*), African hedgehogs (*Atelerix albiventris*), and prairie dogs (*Cynomys* spp). *The Veterinary Clinics of North America. Exotic Animal Practice* 10: 533–555.

Lennox, A.M. and Miwa, Y. (2016). Anatomy and disorders of the Oral cavity of miscellaneous exotic companion mammals. *The Veterinary Clinics of North America. Exotic Animal Practice* 19: 929–945.

Lightfoot, T.L. (2000). Therapeutics of African pygmy hedgehogs and prairie dogs. *The Veterinary Clinics of North America. Exotic Animal Practice* 3: 155–172.

Longley, L. (2008). Mammal anaesthesia. In: *Anaesthesia of Exotic Pets* (ed. L. Logley), 27–35. St. Louis, MO: Saunders Elsevier.

Mader, D. (2004). Basic approach to veterinary care. In: *Ferrets, Rabbits and Rodents. Clinical Medicine and Surgery* (eds. K.E. Quesenberry and J.W. Carpenter), 147–155. St. Louis, MO: Saunders Elsevier.

Martínez, L.S., Juan-Sallés, C., Cucchi-Stefanoni, K. et al. (2005). *Actinomyces naeslundii* infection in an African hedgehog (*Atelerix albiventris*) with mandibular osteomyelitis and cellulitis. *The Veterinary Record* 157: 450–451.

Mikaelian, I. and Reavill, D.R. (2004). Spontaneous proliferative lesions and tumors of the uterus of captive African hedgehogs (*Atelerix albiventris*). *Journal of Zoo and Wildlife Medicine* 35: 216–220.

Moreira, A., Troyo, A., and Calderón-Arguedas, O. (2013). First report of acariasis by *Caparinia tripilis* in African hedgehogs, (*Atelerix albiventris*), in Costa Rica. *Revista Brasileira de Parasitologia Veterinária* 22: 155–158.

Mori, M. and O'Brien, S.E. (1997). Husbandry and medical management of African hedgehogs. *Iowa State University Veterinarian* 59: 5.

Morrisey, J. and Carpenter, J.W. (2012). Formulary. In: *Ferrets, Rabbits and Rodents. Clinical Medicine and Surgery* (eds. K. Quesenberry and J.W. Carpenter), 566–575. St. Louis, MO: Saunders Elsevier.

Pantchev, N. and Hofmann, T. (2006). Notoedric mange caused by *Notoedres cati* in a pet African pygmy hedgehog (*Atelerix albiventris*). *The Veterinary Record* 158 (2): 59.

Pei-Chi, H., Jane-Fang, Y., and Lih-Chiann, W. (2015). A retrospective study of the medical status on 63 African hedgehogs (*Atelerix Albiventris*) at the Taipei zoo from 2003 to 2011. *Journal of Exotic Pet Medicine* 24: 105–111.

Pilny, A.A. (2008). Clinical hematology of rodent species. *The Veterinary Clinics of North America. Exotic Animal Practice* 11: 523–533.

Pye, G.W. (2001). Marsupial, insectivore, and chiropteran anesthesia. *The Veterinary Clinics of North America. Exotic Animal Practice* 4: 211–237.

Raymond, J.T. and Garner, M.M. (2000). Cardiomyopathy in captive African hedgehogs (*Atelerix albiventris*). *Journal of Veterinary Diagnostic Investigation* 12: 468–472.

Raymond, J.T. and Garner, M.M. (2001). Spontaneous tumours in captive African hedgehogs (*Atelerix albiventris*):

a retrospective study. *Journal of Comparative Pathology* 124: 128–133. https://doi.org/10.1053/jcpa.2000.0441.

Raymond, J.T., Williams, C., and Wu, C.C. (1998). Corynebacterial pneumonia in an African hedgehog. *Journal of Wildlife Diseases* 34: 397–399.

Raymond, J.T., Aguilar, R., Dunker, F. et al. (2009). Intervertebral disc disease in African hedgehogs (*Atelerix albiventris*): four cases. *Journal of Exotic Pet Medicine* 18: 220–223. https://doi.org/10.1053/j.jepm.2009.06.007.

Reeve, N. (1994). *Hedgehogs*. London: T & AD Poyser (Natural History).

Romero, C., Sheinberg, W.G., Pineda, J. et al. (2017). Fluralaner as a single dose oral treatment for *Caparinia tripilis* in a pygmy African hedgehog. *Veterinary Dermatology* 28 (6): 622.

Santana, E.M., Jantz, H.E., and Best, T.L. (2010). *Atelerix albiventris* (Erinaceomorpha: Erinaceidae). *Mammalian Species* 42: 99–110.

Simone-Freilicher, E.A. and Hoefer, H.L. (2004). Hedgehog care and husbandry. *The Veterinary Clinics of North America. Exotic Animal Practice* 7: 257–267.

Smith, A.J. (1992). Husbandry and medicine of African hedgehogs (*Atelerix albiventris*). *Journal of Small Exotic Animal Medicine* 2: 21–28.

Smith, A.J. (1999). Husbandry and nutrition of hedgehogs. *The Veterinary Clinics of North America. Exotic Animal Practice* 2: 127–141.

Smith, A.J. (2000). General husbandry and medical care of hedgehogs. *KIRKS Current Veterinary Therapy* 13: 1128–1132.

Stocker, L. (2003). The St.Tiggywinkles hedgehog fact sheet. Haddenham, UK: The Wildlife Hospital Trust.

Wheler, C.L., Grahn, B.H., and Pocknell, A.M. (2001). Unilateral proptosis and orbital cellulitis in eight African hedgehogs (*Atelerix albiventris*). *Journal of Zoo and Wildlife Medicine* 32: 236–241. https://doi.org/10.1638/1042-7260(2001)032[0236:UPAOCI]2.0.CO;2.

Williams, D., Adeyeye, N., and Visser, E. (2017). Ophthalmological abnormalities in wild European hedgehogs (*Erinaceus europaeus*): a survey of 300 animals. *Open Veterinary Journal* 7: 261–267. https://doi.org/10.4314/ovj.v7i3.10.

Wolff, F.C., Corradini, R.P., and Cortés, G. (2005). Congenital erythropoietic porphyria in an African hedgehog (*Atelerix albiventris*). *Journal of Zoo and Wildlife Medicine* 36: 323–325.

Wozniak-Biel, A., Janeczek, M., Janus, I. et al. (2015). Surgical resection of peripheral odontogenic fibromas in African pygmy hedgehog (*Atelerix albiventris*): a case study. *BMC Veterinary Research* 11: 145.

3

Common Marmosets

Jane Hopper

The common marmoset (*Callithrix jacchus*) is a small cal-litrichid primate originating from Brazil. Their natural habitat is varied and includes scrub, swamps, and tree plantations (Schiel and Souto 2017). In the wild common marmosets are active in the early morning and late evening, and they spend the rest of the day grooming and sleeping (De la Fuente et al. 2014). Their social structure is complex with a typical natural group size of 8, but ranging up to 20 individuals (Schiel and Souto 2017). The common marmoset conservation status is listed as 'least concern' by the International Union for the Conservation of Nature's red list of threatened species (IUCN 2018). Biological parameters for this species are shown in Table 3.1.

3.1 Husbandry

Free-living common marmosets form social groups and demonstrate monogamy, and so in captivity they should not be housed alone but with at least one conspecific. A compatible pair (and their offspring if breeding) is an appropriate family group. Most marmoset groups will have a dominance hierarchy, and housing should be designed so that hierarchical stress can be minimised. Areas for the marmosets to avoid visual contact with others are essential and hide boxes at various heights should be provided (Figure 3.1). Primates require a complex and stimulating arboreal environment and regular enrichment (such as puzzle feeders, complex cage furniture such as swings, suspended feeders, and branches to gnaw) should be part of normal husbandry (French and Fite 2005).

Marmosets should be provided with both indoor and outdoor accommodation with their arboreal activity accommodated. Suitable outdoor enclosures should have a minimum height of 2.5 m (Ruivo 2010), and the total three dimensional space available should be no less than 22.5 m³

(Masters 2010) (Figure 3.2). More space should be provided if the group size is larger than five. Both indoor and outdoor housing should be kept at a minimum temperature of 18 °C, and a heated area of 24–29 °C should be provided to allow thermoregulation (Ruivo 2010). All heat sources and wiring must be adequately protected to prevent animal injury. Humidity in the indoor quarters should be maintained at 60% (Ruivo 2010), and low humidity can cause poor skin and coat condition. Wire mesh used for the enclosure should be welded stainless steel with no sharp edges, and should not be big enough for the primate to put its arm through.

All new world monkeys have a high vitamin D3 requirement (Yamaguchi et al. 1986) and will obtain this from the ultraviolet-B (UVB) component of sunlight in the wild. In captivity in temperate climes, outdoor enclosure access in the summer may be sufficient but in winter UVB exposure is likely to be inadequate. Provision of artificial UVB lighting (and oral supplementation) is necessary to maintain Vitamin D3 and enable calcium homeostasis year round.

Primate accommodation should be regularly cleaned with non-toxic viricidal and bactericidal disinfectants, using dedicated tools, to avoid the transfer of disease between the primates and their owners. Disposable gloves should always be worn when cleaning primate enclosures and their equipment such as food dishes.

When keeping primates effective rodent control is essential, as rodents are potential vectors of diseases such as *Yersinia pseudotuberculosis* (Bielli et al. 1999). Both the accommodation and food store areas should be rodent-proof with active monitoring.

The primary food item in the wild is gum (Cunha et al. 2006) but they feed opportunistically on a wide variety of items. Marmosets are primarily frugivore-insectivores in captivity (French and Fite 2005; Ruivo 2010). The base diet is typically a balanced marmoset pellet and marmoset gum, alongside a variety of fruit, soft or cooked vegetables, and

Handbook of Exotic Pet Medicine, First Edition. Edited by Marie Kubiak.
© 2021 John Wiley & Sons Ltd. Published 2021 by John Wiley & Sons Ltd.
Companion website: www.wiley.com/go/kubiak/exotic_pet_medicine

Table 3.1 Biological parameters of common marmosets, (Thornton 2002; Ludlage and Mansfield 2003; Masters 2010).

Parameter	Unrestrained
Heart rate (bpm)	230 ± 26 (restrained 348 ± 51)
Respiratory rate (breaths/min)	36–44
Rectal body temperature (°C)	38.4–39.1
Mean arterial pressure (mmHg)	95 ± 9 (restrained 107 ± 16)
Average weight	Males 350 g Females 300 g
Average length	188 mm (280 mm with tail)
Lifespan in captivity	Up to 15 years
Gestation	148 days

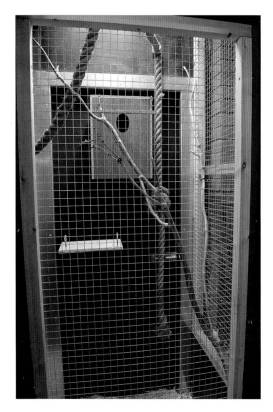

Figure 3.1 Indoor enclosure compartment with nest box.

invertebrates (Crissey et al. 2003). Dividing this into two feeds, and offering the less palatable pellets in the morning feed, when animals are most hungry, tends to result in reliable intake. Marmoset gum should be placed in holes drilled into wood as this allows natural gnawing behaviour.

Captive marmosets over-express binding proteins that reduce Vitamin D receptor density, rendering them at high risk of developing vitamin D deficiency (Abbott et al. 2003). As such, dietary supplementation with vitamin D3

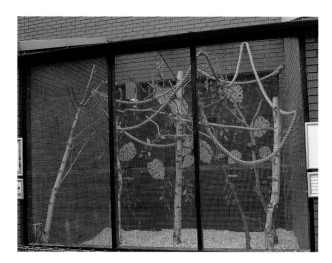

Figure 3.2 Outdoor quarters with climbing apparatus and protected basking lamp.

is advisable. The recommended dose for an adult male common marmoset is 250 IU/day (Masters 2010).

All primates require pre-formed dietary vitamin C as they are unable to make their own. Adequate levels of vitamin C should be provided by marmoset pellets, fresh fruit and vegetables.

Fresh water should be available ad lib, typically in several small bowls in elevated positions within the enclosure.

3.1.1 Breeding

The oestrous cycle in common marmosets lasts 28 days and gestation is 148 days (Tardif et al. 2003). Females reach sexual maturity at 12 months and males at 15 months (Abbott et al. 2003). Females give birth to their first offspring at 20–24 months and breeding can occur with a 5–6 month interval (Tardif et al. 2003). Pregnancy diagnosis is possible by means of visual examination, abdominal palpation, radiography, or ultrasound (Ruivo 2010). Usually they have twins, but one, three or even four offspring may result from pregnancy (Tardif et al. 2003). The birth weight of a common marmoset infant should be 35–40 g (Tardif et al. 2003). Postpartum oestrus occurs within 9–10 days after a birth (Ruivo 2010).

3.2 Clinical Evaluation

3.2.1 History

The majority of the presenting conditions of pet primates to vets in the UK are associated with husbandry problems. One UK study found that 50% of pet primates presented had clinical conditions as a consequence of husbandry deficiencies (Kubiak 2015). It is therefore very important to take a thorough history of the marmoset's husbandry that should include as a minimum: origin of the animal, social group, housing, diet (including any supplements), UV light provision, rodent control, and hygiene protocols. When considering diet, ascertain what is consumed of the diet provided. A nutritionally balanced diet provided may be rendered inadequate by selective feeding.

A thorough history of presenting medical problems should also be taken as for other species.

3.2.2 Handling

As even the smallest callitrichid can inflict deep bites, if handling is required it should always be done with gloves – preferably leather, as if the animal does bite on the glove the material will be soft enough to minimise the risk of tooth damage whilst still preventing the keeper's skin from being broken (French and Fite 2005; Fowler 2008). Bites from primates carry the risk of disease transmission both from the animal to the handler and from handler to animal. However, new world primates, such as marmosets, carry fewer zoonotic diseases of concern compared to old world primates (Abbott et al. 2003).

When the marmoset is being handled one hand should stabilise the upper body with the thumb and the forefinger around the neck; the other hand holds the hind legs (Figure 3.3) (Fowler 2008).

It is very important for animal as well as human health that steps are taken to prevent disease transfer between primates and humans (Joslin 1993) – e.g. herpes simplex virus is present in 90% of humans, and is fatal to callitrichids (Huemer et al. 2002; Wald and Corey 2007). No-one with an active cold sore should therefore be in contact with primates. Veterinary staff should always wear latex exam gloves when handling primates and their samples, and the environment should always be cleaned with a suitable disinfectant.

Veterinary surgeons who treat primates should ensure their staff are appropriately vaccinated against a range of zoonotic diseases carried by primates (e.g. *Mycobacterium tuberculosis*, measles, Hepatitis A, and Hepatitis B) (National Research Council 2003).

3.2.3 Sex Determination

Common marmosets can be difficult to sex as neonates. Male infants have a longer anogenital distance than female infants. In males the testes can be palpated in either in the scrotal or inguinal region (Stein 1978). It should also be possible to differentiate the male prepuce (with the glans penis visible within it) and the female vestibular opening. Figures 3.4 and 3.5 show the differences in external genitalia inadult animals.

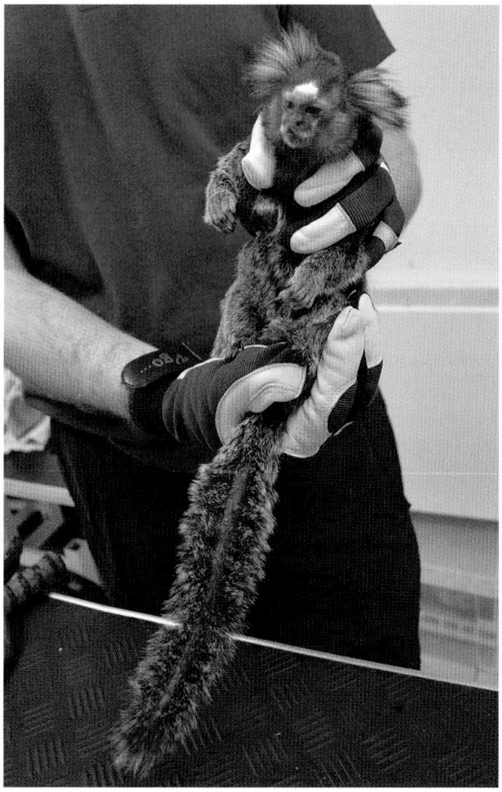

Figure 3.3   Restraint of a common marmoset.

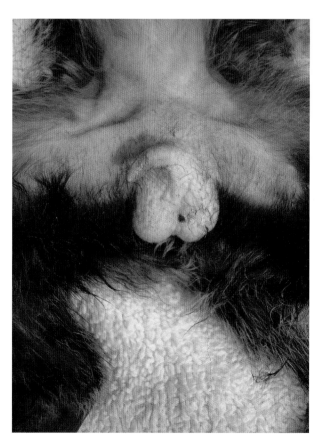

Figure 3.4   Male common marmoset with penis exteriorised.

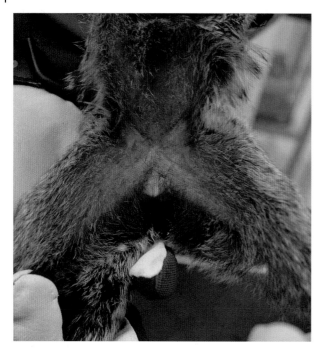

Figure 3.5 Female common marmoset.

3.2.4 Clinical Exam

The primate will need to be restrained for close examination and this is typically resented. Examination should be performed as quickly as possible in order to avoid extended stress. In many cases anaesthesia may be required for a detailed clinical examination. An examination should include careful examination of the oral cavity, mucosal membranes and lymph nodes, as well as thoracic auscultation, palpation of the abdominal cavity, and palpation and manipulation of the bones and joints. Marmosets should always be weighed and body condition assessed as part of a clinical exam.

3.3 Basic Techniques

3.3.1 Sample Collection

The most convenient site for blood sampling is the femoral vein. To locate the femoral vein, the femoral artery should first be palpated. The vein is superficial to the artery in the femoral triangle (Figure 3.6). A 25 gauge needle should be used with a 1 ml or 2 ml syringe (Ludlage and Mansfield 2003). Single samples of 0.57% body weight can be safely collected from healthy animals, with regeneration of volume taking one week (Diehl et al. 2001). Most marmosets will need to be sedated to collect a blood sample.

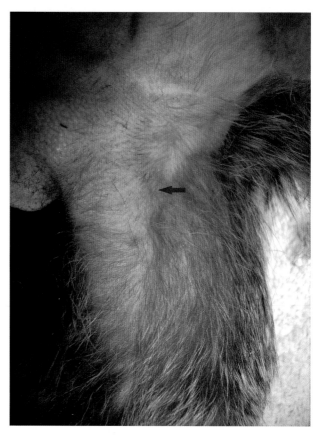

Figure 3.6 The femoral vein is located in a shallow groove in the proximal medial thigh.

3.3.2 Nutritional Support

As previously mentioned, marmosets are frugivore-gummivore-insectivores, and nutritional support should reflect this. It is always advisable to ask the owner to bring in food for a hospitalised marmoset with details of what it normally eats as unfamiliar food items are particularly likely to be rejected by the marmoset when it is unwell. When an ill marmoset will not accept a normal diet, marmoset jellies can be provided as a palatable option. These are high-protein, high-energy and designed to provide the majority of the primate's daily requirements. The jelly can be mixed with pieces of fruit to further enhance its palatability.

3.3.3 Fluid Therapy

Assessing dehydration in marmosets is similar to other species. Marmosets over 10% dehydrated will have a skin tent and dry mucus membranes. At 5–6% dehydrated marmosets will show a subtle loss in skin elasticity.

Maintenance fluid requirements for non-human primates are estimated to be 50 ml/kg/day (Wolfensohn and Honess 2005). For mild to moderately dehydrated animals warmed fluids can very easily be given subcutaneously at two to three sites, to a maximum of 5 ml per site (Diehl et al. 2001). Intravenous infusions are possible but difficult to perform due to the size of marmoset veins and patient interference with cannulae and infusion equipment. The most commonly cannulated vein is the saphenous vein (Ludlage and Mansfield 2003). In severely dehydrated animals intra-osseous catheters can be placed via the greater trochanter of the femur but only if the marmoset is sedated and is receiving the appropriate pain medication.

3.3.4 Anaesthesia

Common marmosets should only be fasted for six to eight hours before anaesthesia (Olberg and Sinclair 2014). Small primates are easiest to induce using isoflurane in a chamber (Longley 2008), or a mask can be held over the head of a restrained marmoset (Figure 3.7). Isoflurane has been used for induction of common marmosets at 4% (Prestes et al. 2014). For maintenance, the minimum alveolar concentration for isoflurane is 1.28–1.46% (Soma et al. 1998) and for sevoflurane is 2% (Horne 2001) and both have a wide margin of safety.

After induction the marmoset should be intubated. The marmoset is placed in dorsal recumbency with the mouth held open and the tongue gently extended forward. A local anaesthetic is sprayed onto the larynx to reduce the chance of laryngospasm and a laryngoscope is used to enhance visibility (Morris et al. 1997). For common marmosets a 2–2.5 mm diameter and 5–7 cm long ET tube is used routinely by the author and this length of tube avoids passing the tracheal bifurcation and intubating only a single bronchus (Horne 2001).

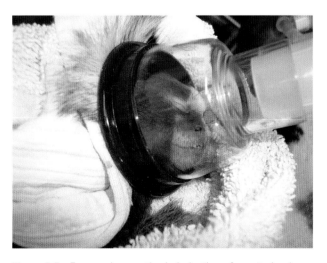

Figure 3.7 Facemask anaesthesia induction of a restrained marmoset.

If it is not possible to sedate the marmoset in a chamber or with a mask then injectable agents can be used (Bakker et al. 2013).

Due to the small size of marmosets, heat loss under anaesthesia is a concern. Body temperature should be closely monitored, and all animals should be given supplemental heat, e.g. from a heat pad or exam gloves filled with warm water, although careful attention should be paid to avoiding burns (Longley 2008). Alcohol and sterile preparation solutions should be used cautiously to maximise antibacterial properties but minimise heat loss.

Monitoring of cardiac and respiratory parameters is the same as for other small mammals. Pulse oximeter probes can be attached to the tongue or ear, and ECG leads can be attached to feet using pads (Longley 2008).

The marmoset should be placed in a small, warm, padded area for anaesthetic recovery. If part of a social group, it should be returned as soon as possible after resumption of normal behaviour to minimise potential problems of re-acceptance.

3.3.5 Euthanasia

Due to the stress usually caused by manually restraining primates and the fragility and small size of veins, it is best to anaesthetise a marmoset before euthanasia. Once the animal is anaesthetised, pentobarbitone at 60 mg/kg can be injected into the femoral vein or directly into the heart (UFAW 1978).

Euthanasia using high concentrations of carbon dioxide has been described in marmosets but causes significant distress in these animals and is not advisable (UFAW 1978). No physical methods of euthanasia are considered acceptable for this species (Reilly 2001).

3.3.6 Hospitalisation Requirements

Marmosets should be hospitalised in a quiet area away from other species that may cause them stress (e.g. barking dogs). They require a warm cage (minimum 18 °C, preferably with a basking lamp) and a UV-B light. The cage should be above ground level and offer hide areas for the marmoset and shelves or branches that the marmosets can climb on, mimicking an arboreal habitat. They should be offered the diet listed previously, but it is advisable to ask the owner to bring in food for the marmoset, or details of what it normally eats. Very commonly marmosets presenting to veterinary practices in the UK are fed unsuitable diets however when the marmoset is sick is not the best time to try to alter the diet. Slow dietary modification is required once health status has normalised. Hospitalised marmosets should still be offered various forms of enrichment. They should always be handled with gloves and strict hygiene practices should be used.

3.4 Common Medical and Surgical Conditions

3.4.1 Husbandry Related Diseases

3.4.1.1 Nutritional Secondary Hyperparathyroidism (NSHP)

One of the most frequently identified diseases in pet marmosets is NSHP, and it is recognised as the most common bone deformity seen in callitrichids (Yamaguchi et al. 1986). This syndrome of demineralisation of bone and disruption of calcium homeostasis develops if the diet consumed is not properly balanced, specifically if the dietary calcium to phosphorus ratio is less than 1, or the diet is deficient in vitamin D3 or protein (Masters 2010). Absence of UV-B lighting compounds the dietary inadequacies by preventing endogenous Vitamin D3 formation.

Clinical signs of NSHP include lethargy, inappetence, weight loss, inability to jump, skeletal deformities, fractures and paralysis of the hind legs (Hatt and Sainsbury 1998; Potkay 1992). Marmosets with suspected cases of NSHP should always be handled very carefully as they are prone to pathological fractures. Diagnosis should involve radiographs, biochemistry, and haematology. Reported radiographic lesions included kyphosis, decreased bone density, bone fractures, subperiosteal bone resorption in the bones of the hand, and a lack of lamina dura (alveolus) of the tooth socket (Olson et al. 2015) (Figure 3.8). Serum calcium levels are usually decreased, and phosphorus levels may be increased, however, in some cases, levels are normal (Hatt and Sainsbury 1998). Serum alkaline phosphatase levels are elevated in any condition involving osteoblastic or osteoclastic activity, including NSHP (Hatt and Sainsbury 1998). If it is possible to take a large enough blood sample vitamin D3 levels can also be run – normal circulating levels of 1 alpha, 25-dihydroxyvitamin D3 are 4–10 times higher than in other primates (Shinki et al. 1983). The 1 alpha, 25-dihydroxyvitamin D3 level of marmosets in the wild has been found to be 20.1–103.3 ng/ml (Teixeira et al. 2012). However, results vary between different assays and this can complicate interpretation (Ziegler et al. 2015).

Treatment options depend on the severity of the NSHP and whether fractures are present. Marmosets with fractured vertebrae causing spinal cord compression have a very poor prognosis and euthanasia is advisable. Marmosets with other fractures where welfare is not significantly compromised and healing will result in reasonable mobility

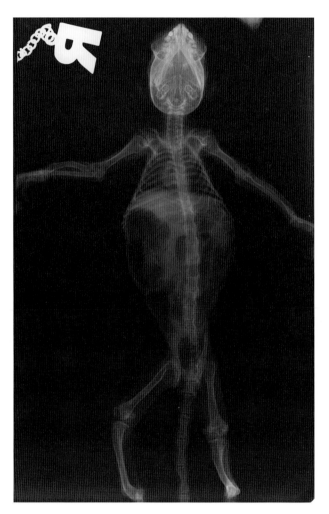

Figure 3.8 NSHP in a common marmoset – note the long bone asymmetry, reduced mineralisation of bone and gastrointestinal stasis. *Source:* Courtesy of Manor vets.

may be treated conservatively. This includes correcting the diet, supplementing with vitamin D, calcium, additional protein, and cage rest with appropriate pain relief. They should be re-evaluated after six weeks of rest. Plenty of enrichment should be given during the period of cage rest, and ideally the marmoset should at least be able to see a nearby conspecific. It is not advisable to attempt surgical repair of fractures caused by NSHP due to the poor quality of the bone (Thornton 2002).

Changes made to diet and husbandry should be applied to any other primates kept in the same household to avoid further cases of NSHP.

3.4.1.2 Hepatic Haemochromatosis

Hepatic iron accumulation with secondary inflammatory disease is an important cause of debility and premature death in captive marmosets. Clinical signs are usually non-specific and include decreased appetite, weakness, and weight loss (Sanchez et al. 2004). Serum iron, transferrin saturation, and serum ferritin values appear to be good indicators of systemic iron stores (Crawford et al. 2005). These values can be used together with serum biochemistry and liver biopsy to diagnose haemochromatosis. Treatment in primates includes regular peripheral blood removal by phlebotomy or the use of iron chelators to reduce total body iron content (Sanchez et al. 2004). Studies indicate that dietary iron intake can directly influence hepatic iron concentration in these primates. The National Research Council's recommended value is 100 mg/kg of diet (dry matter). One must also consider that vitamin C enhances intestinal absorption of iron and dietary fruit content should be reduced in clinically affected animals.

3.4.1.3 Vitamin C Deficiency

Primates are dependent on dietary vitamin C as they are incapable of endogenous synthesis (Nishikimi and Yagi 1996). Deficiency of vitamin C is rare in marmosets but can occur with chronic malnutrition. It causes a range of clinical signs including widespread haemorrhage on serosal surfaces, in subcutaneous tissues, and from the gums, as well as joint swelling. A predisposition to infections, particularly enteritis and pneumonia, has been associated with deficiency of vitamin C in macaques (Sabin 1939). For clinical cases vitamin C should be supplemented by giving 250 mg per day – chewable formulations for children are usually most readily accepted (Masters 2010). Long-term dietary improvement is needed to prevent recurrence.

3.4.1.4 Wasting Marmoset Syndrome

Wasting marmoset syndrome (WMS) is one of the leading causes of morbidity and mortality in captive marmosets (Otovic et al. 2015). There are a wide variety of clinical changes associated with, but not limited to WMS. These include decreased body weight ($\geq$30% loss), alopecia, chronic diarrhoea, chronic lymphocytic enteritis, muscle atrophy, and anaemia (Logan and Khan 1996). A comprehensive investigation is required including bloodwork, faecal culture and parasitology, and imaging as this is a diagnosis of exclusion.

Treatment typically includes supportive therapy, improvement of any husbandry deficiencies and targeted therapies for factors identified during the diagnostic process. A widely acknowledged protocol established at Jersey Zoo stages therapy according to weight loss, with increasing intervention as weight loss progresses (Ruivo 2010). Suspected cases are initially prescribed sulphasalazine (Madara et al. 1985), and in any individual that has lost 25% of its body weight, ciprofloxacin, metronidazole, vitamin B12, rehydration salts and probiotics are also used. A more aggressive treatment is used where weight loss exceeds 33% and includes subcutaneous fluids, enrofloxacin, metronidazole, multivitamins and probiotics (Ruivo 2010). It is accepted that therapy is often broad and clinical benefit is poorly defined but many cases lack a clear diagnosis to allow targeted therapy.

It is probable that many factors contribute to the development of WMS in a given animal. At present, no one specific aetiology is known. Some of the factors that have been proposed as predisposing conditions or causative agents include non-specific nutritional factors (e.g. protein deficiency, excessive fruit in the diet, excessive dietary simple sugars, and conversely, insufficient simple sugars in the diet), stress, overcrowding, lack of social coprophagy, infectious agents including *Trichospirura leptostoma*, food allergies, inappropriate spectrum of natural light, autoimmune disease, and anorexia (Otovic et al. 2015; Cabana et al. 2018). A recent survey of over 200 zoos holding marmosets concluded that stress minimisation and the provision of adequate fibre in the diet were important in preventing the development of WMS (Cabana et al. 2018). Therefore a thorough husbandry review with supportive symptomatic therapy for affected animals is recommended.

3.4.2 Bacterial Diseases

3.4.2.1 *Yersinia pseudotuberculosis*

Y. pseudotuberculosis may cause acute disease with lethargy and diarrhoea or, more commonly, a chronic infection with loss of weight. At post-mortem an ulcerative enterocolitis and the presence of numerous small necrotic foci in the mesenteric lymph nodes, liver, and spleen are noted (Allchurch 2003). The route of *Y. pseudotuberculosis* infection is oral, by consuming food contaminated by rodent or bird faeces (Bielli et al. 1999). This bacterium grows particularly well at cold temperatures, and outbreaks typically occur in the autumn (Bielli et al. 1999). Food hygiene (at both storage and preparation) is the best way to avoid infection. Diagnosis of clinical cases is often made post-mortem but suspected clinical cases should be treated with amoxicillin-clavulanate or fluoroquinolones and prognosis is guarded. Some zoological collections have produced vaccines against endemic strains of *Y. pseudotuberculosis* but their efficacy is not proven.

3.4.2.2 Enteritis

Salmonella, *Shigella*, and *Campylobacter* are classically involved in severe enteritis (Cooper and Needham 1976; Ludlage and Mansfield 2003). They can be diagnosed by faecal culture and therapy necessitates antibiotics (based on a sensitivity profile) as well as fluids and gastrointestinal protectants. As the faecal-oral route is the common mode of infection, hygiene and sanitation are of utmost importance for other primates and for keepers as all three of these bacteria are zoonotic.

It is common to detect enteric protozoans in marmoset faeces analysed by direct examination but not all of them are pathogenic. *Entamoeba, Cryptosporidium*, and *Giardia* have been associated with enteritis in marmosets and can be treated with metronidazole (Ludlage and Mansfield 2003).

Several viral infections can cause enteritis in marmosets, including coronavirus, rotavirus, adenovirus, and paramyxovirus (Courtney 2013; Yu et al. 2013). The main treatment is supportive care.

Fungal causes of enteritis are rare in primates, but cryptococcal enteritis has been reported in a common marmoset, associated with weight loss, abdominal distension, and death (Juan-Salles et al. 1998).

Rectal prolapse can be seen in marmosets with chronic diarrhoea. Many cases involve intussusception (which may be palpated manually and confirmed with imaging) and urgent surgical treatment should be considered. A marmoset with a rectal prolapse should quickly separated from other primates as they may traumatise the prolapse. Simple rectal prolapses can be replaced and treated with an absorbable purse string suture. In severe recurrent cases a coloplexy can be performed, but the key treatment is to find and treat the cause of diarrhoea otherwise recurrence is inevitable.

3.4.2.3 Bacterial Pneumonia

Streptococcus, Klebsiella, Haemophilus, Bordetella, Pasteurella, and *Staphylococcus* are relatively common causes of pneumonia in marmosets (Ludlage and Mansfield 2003; Masters 2010). These infections are often associated with lack of access to an outside enclosure, over heated accommodation, and low humidity. Treatment includes antibiotics and supportive care.

3.4.2.4 Tuberculosis

Mycobacterium bovis and *M. tuberculosis* are infrequently diagnosed in callitrichids (Masters 2010) and two cases of *Mycobacterium avium* infection have been reported (Urbain 1951; Hatt and Guscetti 1994). Clinical signs are varied but include weight loss, weakness, anorexia, and lethargy. Ante-mortem diagnosis involves an intradermal skin test with mammalian old tuberculin (or avian tuberculin for *M. avium*). 0.05 ml of tuberculin is injected intradermally, typically in the palpebrum (Figure 3.9) (Ludlage and Mansfield 2003). To minimise bruising and trauma to the site a 27 gauge needle is recommended. The test result is read 72 hours later and is graded as per Table 3.2.

The zoonotic aspect should be considered for suspect or confirmed cases and euthanasia is advised. Culture

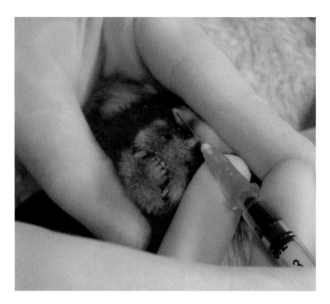

Figure 3.9 Intradermal tuberculin being injected into the palpebrum.

Table 3.2 Interpretation of palpepral intradermal tuberculin test (Butler et al. 1995).

Grade applied	Presentation	Interpretation
Grade 1	Slight bruising of the eyelid	Negative
Grade 2	Erythema of the palpebrum without swelling	Negative
Grade 3	Variable degree of erythema	Intermediate
Grade 4	Obvious swelling with drooping of the eyelid and erythema	Positive
Grade 5	Marked swelling and/or necrosis of the eyelid	Positive

remains the gold standard and is typically used for post-mortem confirmation.

3.4.2.5 Leptospirosis

As in other species leptospirosis causes nephritis, haemolysis, haemoglobinuria, and icterus (Baitchman et al. 2006). Primates can become infected when their food is contaminated by infected rodent urine, or by eating rodents (Baitchman et al. 2006). Treatment is with doxycycline.

3.4.2.6 Septicaemia

Septicaemia can develop after trauma or other bacterial diseases such as enteritis. Treatment should be with appropriate antibiotics (intravenous if possible) and supportive care including intravenous or intraosseous fluids.

3.4.3 Viral Diseases

Several human viruses (e.g. measles [Levy and Mirkovic 1971], influenza, parainfluenza [Flecknell et al. 1983; Sutherland et al. 1986; Potkay 1992]) may cause fatal disease in callitrichids. Humans suffering from respiratory infections should be kept away from marmosets. Sendai virus is carried by mice and can also cause a fatal infection in marmosets. This is another reason that rodents should be excluded from callitrichid enclosures.

3.4.3.1 Lymphocytic Choriomeningitis Virus

This arenavirus causes 'Callitrichid hepatitis' with high mortality (Stephenson et al. 1991). There are few specific clinical signs and animals often present with anorexia, weakness, and lethargy (Ludlage and Mansfield 2003). Necropsy findings include hepatic necrosis, ascites, and occasionally haemorrhages and jaundice. Callitrichids classically become infected by eating infected mice either by being fed rodents (this is therefore not recommended) or by hunting and eating wild mice opportunistically (Montali et al. 1993).

3.4.3.2 Herpes Infection

Various herpes virus infections in callitrichids can be fatal. Contact with humans with open *Herpes simplex* oral lesions, or with squirrel monkeys carrying *Herpes tamarinus* can lead to fatalities in callitrichids (King et al. 1967; Hunt et al. 1973). The first sign is vesicles and ulcers on the skin and mucous membranes (Mätz-Rensing et al. 2003). These lesions may then progress to severe encephalitis, with death within two days.

3.4.4 Parasitic Diseases

3.4.4.1 Helminths

Any marmoset presenting with diarrhoea should have a faecal parasite check. Several nematodes have been associated with morbidity and mortality in callitrichids (Masters 2010). In the case of nematodiasis (e.g. infection by Strongyloides sp.), a drug of the benzimidazole family or ivermectin should be used.

In the case of *Capillaria hepatica* infection, eggs and adults are found in the biliary ducts of the liver. Unembryonated eggs are shed by rodents and must pass through the intestine of a carnivore before becoming infectious to rodents or primates. Treatment is with albendazole.

3.4.4.2 Protozoa

Enteric flagellates such as *Entamoeba histolytica* and *Giardia* can cause diarrhoea in primates (Flynn 1973; Hamlen and Lawrence 1994; Kalishman et al. 1996). Diagnosis can be difficult due to various non-pathogenic protozoa found in primate faeces. Samples can be submitted to specialist labs for a more reliable diagnosis. The treatment for pathogenic protozoa is metronidazole.

Toxoplasma gondii infection is contracted by ingesting food contaminated with cat faeces or eating infected small prey such as rodents and birds. Callitrichids are particularly susceptible (Cunningham et al. 1992; Dietz et al. 1997). Signs of acute pneumonia due to pulmonary oedema are noticed but digestive and nervous system signs may also be recorded. This infection is often fatal. Treatment is with clindamycin, but prevention through cat and rodent control is more successful than treatment.

3.4.4.3 Ectoparasites

Mites (e.g. *Sarcoptes* or sarcoptiform species, *Demodex*) are rare in callitrichids, but have been seen to cause pruritus, alopecia, lichenification of the skin, and even loss of appetite and weight loss (Johnson-Delaney 2009). They are diagnosed using a skin scrape. They are usually acquired from other pets in the household and treatment with ivermectin has been successful (Johnson-Delaney 2009).

Fleas have also been recorded in animals in very poor condition. The fleas have often been acquired through contact with household dogs and cats (Johnson-Delaney 2009).

3.5 Miscellaneous Conditions

3.5.1 Dental Disease

The dental formulary of the common marmoset is I 2/2 C 1/1 P 3/3 M 2/2 (Swindler 2002). Common marmoset incisors form a comb shape (Figure 3.10), as a dental adaptation to enable them to gouge or scrape trees to stimulate the flow of gum (Nash 1986). They have a 'short tusked' cranial dentition and lack enamel on the lingual incisor surfaces (Nash 1986).

Tooth decay is common and is mostly due to inadequate diets, accidents, and age-related degeneration. Marmosets are vulnerable to dental disease if fed a large amount of soft food (Crissey et al. 1999). Signs of dental problems are loss of appetite, salivation, or difficulty when chewing. Root infections of the upper canine often produce a swelling ventral to the eye (Ludlage and Mansfield 2003). These should be treated with antibiotics initially but recurrent or persistent abscesses require extraction of the tooth. Abnormal tooth eruption and teeth abnormally positioned in the jaw can be seen in marmosets suffering from NSHP (Thornton 2002). Primates cope well even if several teeth have to be extracted.

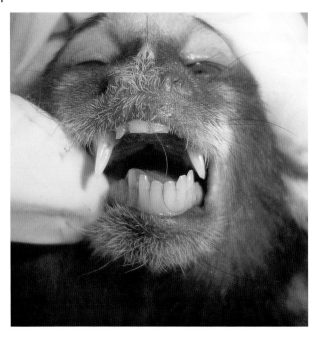

Figure 3.10 Common marmoset incisors forming a comb shape as an adaption to feeding on tree sap.

3.5.2 Cardiovascular Disease

Cardiovascular disease occurs less commonly in the common marmoset than some other species of New World primate (Ludlage and Mansfield 2003). Ventricular dilatation has been recorded in young anaemic animals (Chalmers et al. 1983; Tucker 1984). Myocardial fibrosis and lipofuscinosis have also been recorded (Chalmers et al. 1983; Tucker 1984). Fibrosis and myocardial degeneration have been found fairly commonly in male marmosets and have been seen much less often in females (Okazaki et al. 1996). Pericarditis has been recorded in animals with pneumonia (Chalmers et al. 1983; Tucker 1984). Pericardial effusion has been seen in common marmosets with severe anaemia and hypoproteinaemia (Chalmers et al. 1983).

Femoral artery haematomas can develop if a blood sample is taken from the femoral artery rather than the vein. If a femoral haematoma is seen, a pressure bandage should be immediately applied. In severe cases surgery may be needed to ligate the artery (Ludlage and Mansfield 2003).

3.5.3 Neoplasia

Neoplasia is often seen in older animals and should be considered in any case involving weight loss. There are a wide variety of reported neoplasms in common marmosets including mediastinal sarcoma, thyroid adenoma, kerato-

canthomas, and hepatocellular carcinoma (Kawasako et al. 2014; Morosco et al. 2017; Diaz-Delagdo et al. 2018a, 2018b).

Some cases of neoplasia in the common marmoset seem to be associated with viral infections, notably gamma herpesviruses (Callitrichine herpesvirus-3 and Herpesvirus saimiri) causing lymphoproliferative disease (Ramer et al. 2000; Yamaguchi et al. 2014). Clinical signs are usually non-specific and involve depression, weight loss, and anorexia. On clinical exam a thickened intestinal wall can often be palpated. A biopsy of the intestinal wall is diagnostic. Prognosis for the affected animal is poor, and control should focus on identifying and eliminating the viral cause.

3.5.4 Renal Disease

Renal disease in the common marmoset is not common. A spontaneous progressive nephropathy with glomerular lesions has been identified on histopathology, developing initially in young animals and progressing with age in the absence of clinical signs (Isobe et al. 2012).

Renal amyloid deposition has also been recorded in the common marmoset (Ludlage and Mansfield 2003). Systemic amyloidosis has also been frequently seen though the most common clinical finding is hepatomegaly with a non-regenerative anaemia and hypoalbuminaemia (Ludlage and Mansfield 2003). It appears that marmosets with systemic amyloidosis often do not have an underlying inflammatory condition, and the disorder may be inherited.

3.5.5 Trauma

Bites and resulting abscesses are commonly seen in pet primates. Any bite from a primate is likely to be contaminated by many bacteria, and it is usually best to clean the wound and administer antibiotics before considering wound closure. Wounds are often best left to heal by second intention. External skin sutures are invariably removed by the marmoset and so where primary closure is attempted, absorbable sub-cuticular sutures should be used. Pain relief, such as meloxicam or morphine (Murphy et al. 2012) should always be prescribed for marmosets with painful wounds, and the use of proper analgesia decreases the likelihood that the primate will interfere with a healing wound or sutures.

3.5.6 Reproductive Disease

Pregnant females should be closely monitored. Marmosets usually give birth overnight and without obvious signs of being in labour. If a marmoset is seen to be in labour during the day and is regularly straining then it is likely that there is a problem and that intervention will be necessary. Dystocia is relatively common in pet primates, and it is thought that poor nutrition contributes to the problem (Masters 2010). The only appropriate treatment for dystocia is a caesarean section- other treatments can lead to a high rate of complications.

A caesarean should be carried out under general anaesthesia. Intravenous fluids are recommended but if this not possible then subcutaneous or intraosseous fluids can be used. The marmoset should be intubated and placed in dorsal recumbency. A midline incision is made caudal to the umbilicus. The uterus should be elevated to the skin incision and a longitudinal incision made through the uterine wall over the foetus. The foetus, or foetuses, can then be removed and passed to another member of staff for neonatal care. As soon as the foetus has been delivered the mother should be given analgesia. The uterus should be closed in a continuous two layer inverting pattern. The abdominal musculature should be closed with simple interrupted sutures using material such as polydioxanone. The skin should be closed with a continuous subcuticular layer and then an intradermal layer of simple interrupted sutures.

3.5.7 Hypothermia

Due to their high surface area to volume ratio, marmosets can easily become hypothermic when sick or anaesthetised. Body temperature should always be part of a routine clinical exam and warmth provided if necessary using heat lamps, pads, or a warm air blower.

3.5.8 Hypoglycaemia

Due to marmosets' high metabolic rate and their requirement to feed frequently, sick marmosets can easily become hypoglycaemic. A blood glucose reading should be taken from all depressed looking marmosets and glucose given intravenously or onto the mucous membranes where necessary.

3.6 Preventive Health Measures

Microchips should be placed between the scapulae.

Vaccinations are not routinely given to pet marmosets. A commercial *Y. pseudotuberculosis* vaccine is available from the Utrecht University but its efficacy is still uncertain (Lewis 2000).

Intradermal tests for tuberculosis should be recommended before any animals enter or leave a collection.

A faecal parasitology exam should be carried out every six months (flotation method and direct examination). Only positive animals should be treated and anthelmintics should be used in a targeted, rotational manner to minimise resistance.

3.7 Neutering Technique and Contraception

Primates are usually surgically contracepted by either vasectomy or by ligation of the fallopian tubes so that sexual hormone levels and cycles remain intact. This means that sexual and social behaviours are not affected and social hierarchy is not altered. However, castration of young males can be used to allow them continue to live in a group as low ranking individuals. Castration can result in significant loss of bone mineral density in marmosets as calcium homeostasis is altered by the removal of the gonads (Seidlova-Wuttke et al. 2008).

Vasectomy: The anaesthetised animal should be placed in dorsal recumbency and a surgical site prepared cranial to the scrotum in the midline. A 1 cm skin incision should be made in the ventral midline over the pubic symphysis, 1 cm cranial to the cranial border of the scrotum. The testis can be pushed cranially and an incision made over it before letting the testis fall back. Blunt dissection to the left and right will reveal the vaginal tunic and spermatic cord. This should be dissected free and exteriorised. Further dissection will free the ductus deferens and this should be ligated twice with non-absorbable suture material before a 1 cm section is removed between the ligatures. This is repeated for the other testis. The wound should be closed with absorbable subcuticular sutures. (Morris and David 1993). It is prudent to keep the excised pieces of ductus deferens in formalin to submit for histological confirmation.

Tubal ligation: The anaesthetised animal should be placed in dorsal recumbency and a 2 cm midline skin incision is made caudal to the umbilicus. The uterus and associated fallopian tubes can be located caudally in the abdomen, within the cranial pevic region. Each fallopian tube should be gently ligated with a single non absorbable suture material each side. The wound should then be closed in two layers (muscular and subcuticular) with absorbable suture material.

Pain relief such as buprenorphine and meloxicam should be prescribed post-operatively for these procedures.

Contraceptive implants can be used in marmosets. A short anaesthesia is required to place the implants, and the site used is the inner arm just below the axilla. The implants can then be easily located and removed for reversal to breeding or replacement with a new implant.

Implants of the GnRH agonist deslorelin are considered the safest reversible contraceptives in female callitrichids (Strike and Feltrer 2017). The implants should be placed subcutaneously. A 4.7 mg implant will suppress cycling for a minimum of 6 months, and a 9.4 mg implant for a minimum of 12 months. The implant will be effective within three weeks of placement, and the marmoset should either be separated or given a 5 mg megestrol acetate tablet daily for one week before until one week after the implant has been placed. There is not enough information about the use of deslorelin in marmosets to recommend its use in males, although it has been used to ameliorate aggression in males at high doses (Strike and Feltrer 2017).

Progestagen implants such as etonogestrel 68 mg (Implanon) can also be used in female marmosets (Strike and Feltrer 2017). The implant should be divided in a sterile manner and one third or one quarter of the implant placed subcutaneously. This will suppress cycling for 2–3 years and should be effective within 14 days (Strike and Feltrer 2017).

3.8 Radiographic Imaging

Radiography should be carried out under general anaesthesia. Standard radiographic views are used, left to right lateral and ventrodorsal whole body views (Wagner and Kirberger 2005), see Figures 3.11 and 3.12.

Radiographs are commonly taken in marmosets to assess bone density, and in these cases it is helpful to use a normal bone to aid assessment of skeletal density. It is also possible to age common marmosets by the ossification of their epiphyses (Nassar et al. 1990). Radiographs are useful in the detection of dental disease, gastrointestinal disease, to evaluate injuries, and to assess the reproductive tract.

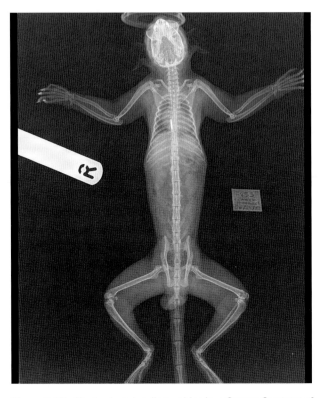

Figure 3.12 Ventrodorsal radiographic view. *Source:* Courtesy of Twycross Zoo.

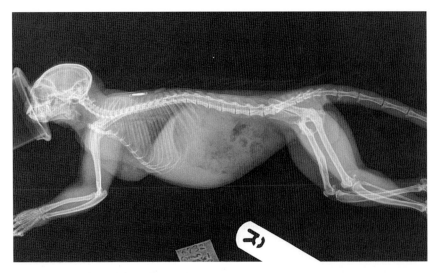

Figure 3.11 Laterolateral radiographic view. *Source:* Courtesy of Twycross Zoo.

Formulary

Drug	Dose
Anaesthetic drugs	
5 mg/kg ketamine +100 µg/kg medetomidine IM. Atipamezole can be used to reverse the medetomidine at 0.5 mg/kg IM.	(Ruivo 2010)
12 mg/kg alphaxalone IM	(Bakker et al. 2013)
25 mg/kg ketamine +0.05 mg/kg medetomidine IM. Atipamezole can be used to reverse the medetomidine at 0.25 mg/kg IM	(Bakker et al. 2013)
18 mg/kg alfaxalone and alphadalone IV	(Phillips and Grist 1975)
8–10 mg/kg zolazepam +8–10 mg/kg tiletamine IM.	(Ruivo 2010)
Analgesic drugs	
Buprenorphine	0.01 mg/kg IV or IM every 8–12 hours (Longley 2008)
Carprofen	2–4 mg/kg PO or SC sid (Longley 2008)
Meloxicam	0.1 mg/kg PO or sid (Murphy et al. 2012)
Morphine	0.1–2 mg/kg SC or IM q3–6h (Murphy et al. 2012)
Antimicrobial and antifungal drugs	
Amoxycillin and clavulanic acid	11 mg/kg PO bid (Baitchman et al. 2006)
Cefovecin	No dose currently recommended. Half-life of this drug in primates is much shorter than in dogs and cats and it is not suitable for use as a long-acting antibiotic
Ceftazidime	50 mg/kg IM or IV tid (Masters 2010)
Clindamycin	12.5 mg/kg PO bid 14 days (Masters 2010)
Ciprofloxacin	10 mg/kg PO sid for 21 days for MWS (Ruivo 2010) 15 mg/kg PO bid
Doxycycline	5 mg/kg PO bid once and then 2.5 mg/kg PO bid (Johnson-Delaney 2009)
Enrofloxacin	5–10 mg/kg PO IM sid for MWS (Ruivo 2010)
Erythromycin	75 mg/kg PO bid for 10 days (Masters 2010)
Fluconazole	18 mg/kg PO bid (Masters 2010)
Itraconazole	10 mg/kg PO sid (Masters 2010)
Marbofloxacin	2–5 mg/kg PO sid (Baitchman et al. 2006)
Metronidazole	20 mg/kg PO sid for 5 days for MWS (Ruivo 2010) 20–50 mg/kg PO bid for 10 days (Baitchman et al. 2006)
Trimethoprim/ sulphamethoxazole	15 mg/kg PO bid (Masters 2010)
Antiparasitic drugs	
Clindamycin	12.5 mg/kg PO bid for 14 days
Fenbendazole	50 mg/kg PO sid for 3 days (Johnson-Delaney 2009)
Ivermectin	0.2–0.4 mg/kg PO IM repeated after 14–21 days (Johnson-Delaney 2009)
Levamisole	10 mg/kg PO as a single dose (Johnson-Delaney 2009) 7.5 mg/kg SC as a single dose
Mebendazole	100 mg/kg PO sid (Johnson-Delaney 2009)
Metronidazole	17–25 mg/kg PO bid for 10 days (Johnson-Delaney 2009)
Praziquantel	15–20 mg/kg PO or IM as a single dose (Johnson-Delaney 2009)
Miscellaneous drugs	
Sulphasalazine	25 mg/kg PO bid (Madara et al. 1985)
Vitamin B12	0.7 mcg/ day PO for 3 months for MWS (Ruivo 2010)

References

Abbott, D.H., Barnett, D.K., Colman, R.J. et al. (2003). Aspects of common marmoset basic biology and life history important for biomedical research. *Comparative Medicine* 53 (4): 339–350.

Allchurch, A. (2003). Yersiniosis in all taxa. In: *Zoo and Wild Animal Medicine*, 5e (eds. M. Fowler and E. Miller), 724–727. Saint Louis, MO: Saunders.

Baitchman, E., Calle, P., James, S. et al. (2006). Leptospirosis in Wied's marmosets (*Callithrix kuhli*). *Journal of Zoo and Wildlife Medicine* 37 (2): 182–185.

Bakker, J., Uilenreef, J., Pelt, E. et al. (2013). Comparison of three different sedative- anaesthetic protocols (ketamine, ketamine- medetomidine and ketamine- medetomidine and alphaxalone) in common marmosets (*Callithrix jacchus*). *BMC Veterinary Research* 9: 113.

Bielli, M., Lauzi, S., Pratelli, A. et al. (1999). Pseudotuberculosis in marmosets, tamarins, and Goeldi's monkeys (Callitrichidae/ callimiconidae) housed at a European zoo. *Journal of Zoo and Wildlife Medicine* 30 (4): 532–536.

Butler, T., Brown, B., Dysko, R. et al. (1995). Medical management. In: *Nonhuman Primates in Biomedical Research, Biology and Management* (eds. B. Bennet, C. Abee and R. Henrickson), 255–333. SanDiego, CA: Academic Press.

Cabana, F., Maguire, R., Hsu, C. et al. (2018). Identification of possible nutritional and stress risk factors in the development of marmoset wasting syndrome. *Zoo Biology* 37: 98–106.

Chalmers, D., Murgatroyd, L., and Wadsworth, P. (1983). A survey of the pathology of marmosets (Callithrix jacchus) derived from a marmoset breeding unit. *Laboratory Animals* 17: 270–279.

Cooper, J. and Needham, J. (1976). An outbreak of shigellosis in laboratory marmosets and tamarins. *The Journal of Hygiene* 76 (3): 415–424.

Courtney, A. (ed.) (2013). Management of gastrointestinal/ abdominal conditions. In: *Pocket Handbook of Nonhuman Primate Clinical Medicine*, 69–102. Florida: CRC Press.

Crawford, G., Andrews, G., Chavey, P. et al. (2005). Survey and clinical application of serum iron, total iron binding capacity, transferrin saturation and serum ferritin in captive black and white lemurs (*Varecia variegate vareiegata*). *Journal of Zoo and Wildlife Medicine* 36 (4): 653–660.

Crissey, S., Lintzenich, B., and Slifka, K. (1999). Diets for callitrichids: management guidelines. In: *SSP Callitrichidae Husbandry Manual* (eds. V. Sodaro and N. Saunders), 53–63. Chicago: Brookfield Zoo.

Crissey, S., Gore, M., Lintzenich, B. et al. (2003). Callitrichids: nutrition and dietary husbandry. In: *AZA: Nutrition Advisory Group Handbook*, Fact sheet 013. Silver Spring, MD: Associaion of Zoos and Aquariums.

Cunha, A.A., Vieira, M.V., and Grelle, C.E. (2006). Preliminary observations on habitat, support use and diet in two non-native primates in an urban Atlantic forest fragment: the capuchin monkey (*Cebus sp.*) and the common marmoset (*Callithrix jacchus*) in the Tijuca forest, Rio de Janeiro. *Urban Ecosystem* 9 (4): 351–359.

Cunningham, A., Buxton, D., and Thomson, K. (1992). An epidemic of toxoplasmosis in a captive colony of squirrel monkeys (*Saimiri sciureus*). *Journal of Comparative Pathology* 107: 207–219.

De la Fuente, M., Souto, A., Sampaio, M. et al. (2014). Behavioural adjustments by a small neotropical primate (*Callithrix jacchus*) in a sermiarid Caatinga environment. *Scientific World Journal* 2014: 326524.

Diaz-Delagdo, J., Sanches, T., Cirqueira, C. et al. (2018a). Multicentric cutaenouos keratoacanthomas in a free-living marmoset (*Callithirx spp.*). *Journal of Medical Primatology* 47 (3): 205–208.

Diaz-Delagdo, J., Sanches, T., Cirqueira, C. et al. (2018b). Hepatocellular carcinoma in a free-living marmoset (*Callithirx spp.*) with concomitant biliary trematodiasis. *Journal of Medical Primatology* 47 (2): 128–131.

Diehl, K., Hull, R., Morton, D. et al. (2001). A good practice guide to the administration of substances and removal of blood, including routes and volumes. *Journal of Applied Toxicology: An International Journal* 21 (1): 15–23.

Dietz, H., Henriksen, P., Bille-Hansen, V. et al. (1997). Toxoplasmosis in a colony of new world monkeys. *Veterinary Parasitology* 68: 299–304.

Flecknell, P., Parry, R., Needham, J. et al. (1983). Respiratory disease associated with parainfluenza type I (Sendai) virus in a colony of marmosets (*Callithrix jacchus*). *Laboratory Animals* 17: 111–113.

Flynn, R. (1973). *Parasites of Laboratory Animals*, 698. Ames, IA: Iowa State Press.

Fowler, M. (ed.) (2008). Non human primates. In: *Restraint and Handling of Wild and Domestic Animals*, 3e, 293–306. Ames. IA: Wiley-Blackwell.

French, J. and Fite, J. (2005). *Marmosets and Tamarins (Callitrichids)*, 7. Maryland, USA: Office of Lab Animal Welfare.

Hamlen, H. and Lawrence, J. (1994). Giardiasis in laboratory house squirrel monkeys: a retrospective study. *Laboratory Animal Science* 44: 235–239.

Hatt, J.M. and Guscetti, F. (1994). A case of mycobacteriosis in a common marmoset (*Callithrix jacchus*). In: *Proceedings of ARAV and AAZV* (ed. R.E. Junge), 241–243. Pittsburgh: American Association of Zoo Veterinarians.

Hatt, J.-M. and Sainsbury, A. (1998). Unusual case of metabolic bone disease in a common marmoset (*Callithrix jacchus*). *Veterinary Record* 143: 78–80.

Horne, W. (2001). Primate anaesthesia. The veterinary clinics of North America. *Exotic Animal Practice* 4: 239–266.

Huemer, H., Larcher, C., Czedick-Eysenberg, T. et al. (2002). Fatal infection of a pet monkey with human herpesvirus. *Emerging Infectious Diseases* 8: 639–642.

Hunt, R., Garcia, F., Barahona, H. et al. (1973). Spontaneous Herpesvirus saimiri lymphoma in an owl monkey. *Journal of Infectious Diseases* 127: 723–725.

Isobe, K., Adachi, K., Hayashi, S. et al. (2012). Sponatneous glomerular and tubulointerstitial lesions in common marmosets (*Callithrix jacchus*). *Veterinary Pathology* 49 (5): 839–845.

IUCN (2018). The IUCN Red List of Threatened Species. Version 2018-1. www.iucnredlist.org. (accessed 5 July 2018).

Johnson-Delaney, C. (2009). Parasites of captive nonhuman primates. *Veterinary Clinics Exotic Animal Practice* 12 (3): 563–581.

Joslin, J. (1993). Zoonotic disease of non human primates. In: *Zoo and Wild Animal Medicine*, 3e (eds. M. Fowler and R.E. Miller), 358–373. Philadelphia: WB Saunders.

Juan-Salles, C., Marco, A., and Domingo, M. (1998). Intestinal Cryptococcosis in a common marmoset (*Callithrix jacchus*). In: *Proceedings of AAZV and AAWV Joint Conference, Omaha, Nebraska, 17–22 October 1998* (ed. C.K. Baer), 516–518. Pittsburgh: American Association of Zoo Veterinarians.

Kalishman, J., Paul-Murphy, J., Scheffler, J. et al. (1996). Survey of cryptosporidium and giardia spp. in a captive population of common marmosets. *Laboratory Animal Science* 46: 116–119.

Kawasako, K., Doi, T., Kanno, T. et al. (2014). Thyroid follicular adenoma with accumulation of collagen type IV in a common marmoset (*Callithrix jacchus*). *Journal of Comparative Pathology* 150 (1): 71–74.

King, N., Hunt, R., Daniel, M. et al. (1967). Overt herpes- T infection in squirrel monkeys. *Laboratory Animal Care* 17: 413–423.

Kubiak, M. (2015). A comparison of presenting complaints and husbandry conditions for privately owned and zoo held primates. In: *Proceedings of BVZS Conference, Bristol, 6–8 November* (ed. F. Molenaar), 17. London: British Veterinary Zoological Society.

Levy, B. and Mirkovic, R. (1971). An epizootic of measles in a marmoset colony. *Laboratory Animal Science* 20: 121–126.

Lewis, J. (2000). Preventative health measures for primates and keeping staff in British and Irish zoological collections. Reports to the British and Irish Primate Taxon Advisory Group. British and Irish Primate TAG meeting May 2000, London UK.

Logan, A. and Khan, N. (1996). Clinical pathologic changes in two marmosets with wasting syndrome. *Toxicologic Pathology* 24: 707–709.

Longley, L. (ed.) (2008). Non human primate anaesthesia. In: *Anaesthesia of Exotic Pets*, 103–111. Philadelphia: Saunders Elsevier.

Ludlage, E. and Mansfield, K. (2003). Clinical care and diseases of the common marmoset (*Callithrix jacchus*). *Comparative Medicine* 53 (4): 369–382.

Madara, J., Podolsky, D., King, N. et al. (1985). Characterisation of spontaneous colitis in cotton top tamarins (*Saguinus Oedipus*) and its response to sulfasalazine. *Gastroenterology* 88 (1): 13–19.

Masters, N. (2010). Primates- callitrichids, cebids and lemurs. In: *BSAVA Manual of Exotic Pets*, 5e (ed. A. Meredith), 148–166. Gloucester: BSAVA.

Mätz-Rensing, K., Jentsch, K.D., Rensing, S. et al. (2003). Fatal herpes simplex infection in a group of common marmosets (*Callithrix jacchus*). *Veterinary Pathology* 40 (4): 405–411.

Montali, R., Scanga, C., Pernikoff, D. et al. (1993). A common source outbreak of callitrichid hepatitis in captive tamarins and marmosets. *Journal of Infectious Diseases* 176: 946–950.

Morosco, D., Cline, C., Owston, M. et al. (2017). Spontaneous mediastinal myeloid sarcoma in a common marmoset (*Callithrix jacchus)* and a review of the veterinary literature. *Journal of Medical Primatology* 46 (2): 42–47.

Morris, T. and David, C. (1993). Illustrated guide to surgical technique for vasectomy of the common marmoset. *Laboratory Animals* 27: 381–384.

Morris, T., Jackson, R., Acker, W. et al. (1997). An illustrated guide to endotracheal intubation in small non-human primates. *Laboratory Animals* 31 (2): 157–162.

Murphy, K., Baxter, M., and Flecknell, P. (2012). Anesthesia and analgesia in nonhuman primates. In: *Nonhuman Primates in Biomedical Research* (eds. C. Abee, K. Mansfield, S. Tardif, et al.). Missouri: Elsevier.

Nash, L. (1986). Dietary, behavioural, and morphological aspects of gumnivory in primates. *Yearbook of Physical Anthropology* 29: 113–137.

Nassar, F., Sainsbury, A.W., Kirkwoord, J.K. et al. (1990). A practical guide for aging common marmoset (*Callithrix* jacchus) by radiographic examination. In: *Proceedings of the American Association of Zoo Veterinarians*, 343–344. Lawrence, KS: AAZV.

National Research Council (US) Committee on Occupational Health and Safety in the Care and Use of Nonhuman Primates (2003). *Occupational Health and Safety in the Care and Use of Non Human Primates*. Washington, DC: Washington Academic Press.

Nishikimi, M. and Yagi, K. (1996). Biochemistry and molecular biology of ascorbic acid biosynthesis. *Sub-Cellular Biochemistry* 25: 17–39.

Okazaki, Y., Kurata, Y., Makinodan, F. et al. (1996). Sponatenous lesions detected in the common cotton-eared marmosets (*Callithrix jacchus*). *Journal of Veterinary Science* 58 (3): 181–190.

Olberg, R. and Sinclair, M. (2014). Monkeys and gibbons. In: *Zoo Animal and Wildlife Immobilisation and Anesthesia* (eds. G. West, D. Heard and N. Caulkett), 561–571. Ames, IA: Wiley.

Olson, E., Shaw, G., Hutchinson, E. et al. (2015). Bone disease in the common marmoset: radiographic and histological findings. *Veterinary Pathology* 52 (5): 883–893.

Otovic, P., Smith, S., and Hutchinson, E. (2015). The use of glucocorticoids in marmoset wasting syndrome. *Journal of Medical Primatology* 44: 53–59.

Phillips, I. and Grist, S. (1975). Clinical use of CT 1341 anaesthetic (Saffan) in marmosets. *Laboratory Animals* 9: 57–60.

Potkay, S. (1992). Diseases of callitrichidae: a review. *Journal of Medical Primatology* 21: 189–236.

Prestes, N.C., Ferreira, J.C.P., Ferraz, M.C. et al. (2014). Caesarean sections in marmosets: white-tufted marmoset (*Callithrix jacchus*). *Veterinaria e Zootecnia*: 92–97.

Ramer, J., Garber, R., Steele, K. et al. (2000). Fatal lymphoproliferative disease associated with a novel gammaherpesvirus in a captive population of common marmosets. *Comparative Medicine* 51 (1): 59–68.

Reilly, J.S. (ed.) (2001). *Euthanasia of Animals Used for Scientific Purposes*, vol. 2. Adelaide: ANZCCART.

Ruivo, E. (2010). *EAZA Husbandry Guidelines for Callitrichidae*. Saint Aignan,France: Beauval Zoo.

Sabin, A.B. (1939). Vitamin C in relation to experimental poliomyelitis with incidental observations on certain manifestations in Macacus rhesus monkeys on a scorbutic diet. *The Journal of Experimental Medicine* 69: 507–515.

Sanchez, C., Murray, S., and Montali, R. (2004). Use of desferoxamine and S-adenosylmethionine to treat haemochromatosis in a red ruffed lemur (*Varecia variegate ruber*). *Comparative Medicine* 54 (1): 100–103.

Schiel, N. and Souto, A. (2017). The common marmoset: an overview of its natural history, ecology and behaviour. *Developmental Neurobiology* 77 (3): 244–262.

Seidlova-Wuttke, D., Schlumbohm, C., Jarry, H. et al. (2008). Orchidectomized marmoset (*Callithrix jacchus*) as a model to study the development of osetopaenia/osteoporosis. *American Journal of Primatology* 70: 294–300.

Shinki, T., Shiina, Y., Takahashi, N. et al. (1983). Extremely high circulating levels of 1 alpha,25-dihydroxyvitamin D3 in the marmoset, a new world monkey. *Biochemical and Biophysical Research Communications* 114 (2): 452–457.

Soma, L., Tierney, W., and Satoh, N. (1998). Sevoflurane anaesthesia in the monkey: the effects of multiples of MAC. *Hiroshima Journal of Anaesthesia* 24: 3–14.

Stein, F. (1978). Sex determination in the common marmoset (*Callithrix jacchus*). *Laboratory Animal Science* 28 (1): 75–80.

Stephenson, C., Jacob, J., Montali, R. et al. (1991). Isolation of an arenavirus from a marmoset with callitrichid hepatitis and its serologic association with the disease. *Journal of Virology* 65: 3995–4000.

Strike, T. and Feltrer, Y. (2017). Guidelines for callitrichidae. http://www.egzac.org/home/viewdocument?filename=Cal litrichid%20EGZAC%20guidelines%202017.pdf (accessed 28 November 2018).

Sutherland, S., Almedia, J., Gardner, P. et al. (1986). Rapid diagnosis and management of parainfluenza I virus infection in common marmosets (*Callithrix jacchus*). *Laboratory Animals* 20: 121–126.

Swindler, D. (2002). Ceboidea. In: *Primate Dentition. An Introduction to the Teeth of Non- human Primates* (ed. D. Swindler), 96–108. Cambridge: Cambridge University Press.

Tardif, S., Smucny, D., Abbott, D. et al. (2003). Reproduction in captive common marmosets (*Callithrix jacchus*). *Comparative Medicine* 53 (4): 364–368.

Teixeira, D., Nobrega, Y., Valencia, C. et al. (2012). Evaluation of 25-hydroxy-vitamin D and parathyroid hormone in *Callithrix penicillata* primates living in their natural habitat in Brazil. *Journal of Medical Primatology* 41: 364–371.

Thornton, S. (2002). Primates. In: *BSAVA Manual of Exotic Pets*, 4e (eds. A. Meredith and S. Redrobe), 127–137. Gloucester: BSAVA.

Tucker, M. (1984). A survey of the pathology of marmosets (*Callithrix jacchus*) under experiment. *Laboratory Animals* 18: 351–358.

UFAW (1978). *Humane Killing of Animals*, 4e. London: UFAW.

Urbain, A. (1951). Deux cas de tuberculose spontanée d'origine aviaire chez un singe africain: Cercopitheque grivet (*Cercopithecus aethiops L.*) et chez un singe américain: Ouistiti à pinceaux blancs (Hapalemur jacchus L.). *Bulletin de l'Académie Vétérinaire de France* 22: 349–351.

Wagner, W. and Kirberger, R. (2005). Radiographic anatomy of the thorax and abdomen of the common marmoset (*Callithrix jacchus*). *Veterinary Radiology & Ultrasound* 46 (3): 217–224.

Wald, A. and Corey, L. (2007). HSV: persistence in the population: epidemiology, transmission. In: *Human Herpesviruses: Biology, Therapy and Immunoprophylaxis* (eds. A. Arvin, G. Campadelli-Fiume, E. Mocarski, et al.), 656–672. Cambridge, UK: Cambridge University Press.

Wolfensohn, S. and Honess, P. (2005). *Handbook of Primate Husbandry and Welfare*. Oxford: Blackwell Publishing Ltd.

Yamaguchi, A., Kohno, Y., Yamazaki, T. et al. (1986). Bone in the marmoset: a resemblance to vitamin D dependent rickets, type II. *Calcified Tissue International* 39 (1): 189–236.

Yamaguchi, S., Marumoto, T., Nil, T. et al. (2014). Characterisation of common marmoset dysgerminoma-like tumour induced by the lentiviral expression of reprogramming factors. *Cancer Science* 105 (4): 402–408.

Yu, G., Yagi, S., Carrion, R. et al. (2013). Experimental cross-species infection of common marmosets by Titi monkey adenovirus. *PLoS One* https://doi.org/10.1371/journal.pone.0068558.

Ziegler, T., Kapoor, A., Hedman, C. et al. (2015). Measurement of 25-hydroxyvitamin D2&3 and 1, 25-dihydroxyvitamin D2&3 by tandem mass spectrometry: a primate multispecies comparison. *American Journal of Primatology* 77 (7): 801–810.

4

Striped Skunk
Clive Munns

4.1 Introduction

There are over 10 species of skunk but only the striped skunk (*Mephitis mephitis*) is commonly kept as a pet and this chapter will focus primarily on this species. Biological parameters for this species are included in Table 4.1. Skunks are part of the order Carnivora and originally were classified within this order as a sub-family of mustelids (along with ferrets, otters, and badgers). Skunks have since been re-classified in their own family, Mephitidae along with the stink badgers (*Mydaus* spp.).

Striped skunks are found throughout North America from Southern Canada to Northern Mexico. They are able to survive in a variety of habitats from grassland to mixed woodland, and even desert (Nowak 1999). Skunks often live in and around cultivated and urban areas, where human-skunk conflict may occur (Dragoo 2009). They are mainly crepuscular or nocturnal (Dragoo 1982), and tend to be solitary animals. Those living in colder climates will gather in groups in winter in underground dens for up to 120 days and undergo an intermittent torpor (Nowak 1999; Dragoo 2009). Skunks are not very territorial but maintain and defend a home range that fluctuates depending on resources and season, from 0.5 km² to over 12 km² (Greenwood et al. 1997; Lariviere and Messier 1998; Bixler and Gittleman 2000). Male-to-male interactions can become aggressive.

Skunks are of a similar size to a domestic cat. They have a dense coat, with a long bushy tail, a small triangular head with a small nose and short ears. They have short stocky legs with five toes on each foot (Dragoo 1982). Their claws are long, especially on the front feet and are used for digging and foraging (Dragoo 1982). The dental formula is I 3/3 C1/1 P3/3 M1/2 = 34 (Dragoo 1982) and they have a simple monogastric intestinal tract, similar to that of mustelids.

Skunks' wild colouration is black with a white 'V' running all the way down their back from the head. A white stripe runs between their eyes from the top of the head to the tip of snout. The young are born with stripes clearly visible on the skin before they are fully furred (Dragoo 2009). Brown, red, grey, cream, apricot, white, and albino variants have been selectively bred and can now also be found in the fur and pet trade (Dragoo 2009).

Skunks are known for their foul-smelling anal gland secretions. A typical fear response in a skunk is shown by vocalisation, raising the tail and turning away from the threat. Only with much provocation will they eject foul-smelling musk from anal-glands (Wood et al. 2002). Skunks can aim and direct their secretion using a nipple at the entrance to the gland and ejections can reach several metres (Dragoo 1982).The secretion is a mixture of sulphur-containing chemicals such as thiols (mercaptans) and other volatile components. The smell has been described as a mixture of rotten eggs, garlic, and burned rubber (Wood et al. 2002). The secretion is very difficult to clear, and it can take days for the smell to disperse.

Skunks are very playful and may be seen giving a fake threat display where they will stamp their front feet and lift their tail but not actually empty their anal glands (Kramer and Lennox 2003).

4.2 Breeding

Skunks have a seasonally mono-oestrus cycle which lasts about 10 days. However, they can come back into oestrus within a few weeks if not pregnant after the first season (Nowak 1999; Dragoo 2009). Males will mate with multiple females if the opportunity arises. In the wild, mating generally occurs from February to April, and young are born between April and June. A brief delayed implantation of

Handbook of Exotic Pet Medicine, First Edition. Edited by Marie Kubiak.
© 2021 John Wiley & Sons Ltd. Published 2021 by John Wiley & Sons Ltd.
Companion website: www.wiley.com/go/kubiak/exotic_pet_medicine

Table 4.1   Biological parameters of striped skunks.

Length	530–810 mm including tail (Tail 170–400 mm)
Weight	2–4 kg
Temperature	37–38.9 °C
Heart Rate	140–190 beats per minute
Respiratory Rate	35–40 breaths per minute
Sexually mature	10–12 months (1st spring)
Oestrus	10 days
Gestation	59–77 days
Litter size	5–7
Eyes open	3–4 weeks
Wean	6–8 weeks
Life span	6–10 years.

up to 20 days can occur, especially if mated early in the season (Wade-Smith et al. 1980). Dams can have up to 12 offspring but on average have 5–7 young. Females usually have 12 mammae but this can vary between individuals (Dragoo 2009).Young are born blind, deaf, and naked. Despite this their anal glands are intact and they can scent within the first week. Eyes and ears are open by day 28 and they are weaned by 6–8 weeks (Dragoo 1982).

Commercial milk replacer can be used for neonates requiring hand-rearing (Johnson-Delaney 1996). Skunks' milk is 32% protein, 45% fat and 10% lactose and canine milk replacers are the closest approximation. Neonates should be fed roughly every two hours and solid food should be offered from four weeks of age. The introduced solid food should equate to an adult skunk diet, but should be finely chopped.

4.3   Husbandry

4.3.1   Environment

If skunks are kept in a home it must be made skunk proof as they can be very resourceful and destructive. An outdoor enclosure may be preferable, or a large dog crate used for temporary confinement when not under supervision, though this greatly limits normal behaviours. Skunks can be trained to use a litter tray and unscented cat litter should be used. Skunks may select their own toileting areas; in those cases place the tray in their chosen spot, and once they are using to the litter tray well, gradually move it to the preferred location (Kubiak 2016).

An outdoor enclosure should be sturdy with a minimum area of 3.7 m² and a height of 0.9 m for a single skunk (Johnson-Delaney 1996), though much larger enclosures

are advisable to allow for activity and expression of normal behaviours. A solid base is necessary for enclosures to prevent escape by digging, and a deep substrate on top of this allows for safe digging and foraging for enrichment. Skunks are poor climbers so there is no need to provide high obstacles to climb due to risk of falling. Providing ramps and shelves will encourage activity and give more usable space in an enclosure. Skunks are inquisitive in nature and like to explore their environment. Therefore environmental and feeding enrichment is important. Enrichment toys need to be robust. Durable dog toys are a suitable example but these should be regularly checked and replaced when damage is noted. More destructive behaviour is more likely to be seen in skunks with inadequate enrichment (Kubiak 2016). Skunks can be harness trained and taken for walks for exercise and enrichment.

Skunks require a sheltered den with solid sides, containing suitable bedding, such as blankets, that can be washed regularly. With such a den, adapted wild skunks can tolerate very low temperatures of up to −40 °C (Aleksiuk and Stewart 1977), but captive skunks are less tolerant of such extremes and additional heated indoor quarters should be available if temperatures are approaching 0 °C.

Skunks are generally solitary animals, and in captivity may fight, particularly if males are housed together (Dragoo 2009). However, they can be kept with other skunks if they are introduced when young and adequate space is provided. If skunks are to be kept as a group it is preferable to use littermates and to not house two entire males together. Once skunks are mature it is very difficult to integrate them.

If handled from an early age skunks can make good, well socialised pets. They can develop strong bonds with humans (Kubiak 2016) and co-habit well with other pets such as dogs.

4.3.2   Diet

Skunks are foragers and eat an omnivorous diet, adapting to available food sources. In the wild their diet would include small rodents, birds and invertebrates, fruits, grains, and vegetables (Dragoo 2009).

Many of the common diseases seen in skunks are related to diet, so a good diet is crucial. Recommended diets consist of dry dog food (reduced calorie formulations are preferred for animals over a year old) plus fruit and vegetables (Johnson-Delaney 1996; Kramer and Lennox 2003). Invertebrates can be used as treats, or to encourage foraging. Schoemaker (2010) suggests that dog food is used for 2/3 of the diet and 1/3 made up of mixed fruits and vegetables. Cat food should be avoided due to the higher fat and protein content which may predispose to obesity, diarrhoea, or even hepatic and renal disease (Dragoo 2009). Day-old chicks and cooked meats can be included in the diet, as can cottage cheese, eggs, and yoghurt. Wild skunk intake equates to approximately 100 g of food per kg bodyweight daily outside of torpor periods (Aleksiuk and Stewart 1977), though it should be appreciated that captive skunks are less active and are exposed to less thermal extremes and intake may need to be lower. Although wild skunks are not normally active in the day, they will become partially diurnal in captivity so can be fed at any time, preferably with multiple small feeds and use of scatter feeding or enrichment devices to encourage foraging behaviours. Water should always be available, offered in a water bottle or spill-proof bowl.

4.4 Clinical Evaluation

4.4.1 History-Taking

As with any species it is important to get a complete history. Particular questions to ask include whether the skunk has been imported (especially with respect to potential infectious diseases or surgical scent gland removal). It is important to get information about diet, housing and general husbandry and any preventative health measures in place such as vaccination.

4.4.2 Handling

This is similar to handling cats or ferrets and many skunks are tolerant of gentle restraint and examination. Most skunks will allow a reasonable conscious clinical exam but it is important to be aware that if they become stressed or agitated they may express their anal glands or give a nasty bite. Gauntlets or a towel can be used to wrap the skunk in if needed or manual restraint can be achieved by grasping the scruff in one hand and extending the hind limbs and tail in the other (see Figure 4.1) (Kramer and Lennox 2003). Firm physical restraint is often resented and should be avoided in compliant animals.

Sedation or anaesthesia may be required for a more thorough examination, diagnostics, and sample collection.

4.4.3 Sex Determination

Skunks have external genitalia similar to those seen in ferrets and sexes are easily differentiated (Figures 4.2 and 4.3). It is important not to confuse the large anal glands with the smaller testes. The anal glands are ventro-lateral to the anus whilst the testes are located on the ventrum (Capello 2006).

4.4.4 Clinical Examination

This is similar to the clinical examination of cats or ferrets, with systematic evaluation and palpation of all body parts, including careful palpation of the scent glands.

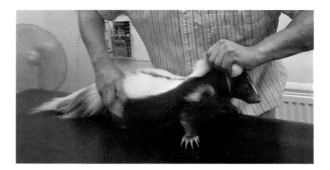

Figure 4.1 Firm manual restraint of a skunk with chocolate brown coat colour variant.

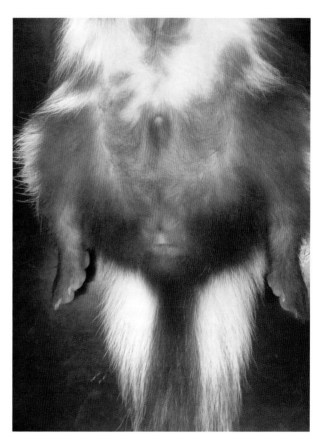

Figure 4.2 Male skunk, note the ventral location of the prepuce and caudal location of the small testes.

4.5 Basic Techniques

4.5.1 Sample Collection

Blood samples are routinely taken from the jugular or cephalic veins. These may be taken conscious in amenable animals but veins may not be visible in overweight animals. Saphenous and femoral veins are also suitable for blood sample collection, as is the cranial vena cava via the sternal notch. The femoral vein may be easiest to access in obese patient, inserting the needle caudal to the palpable pulse of the femoral artery at the level of the proximal third

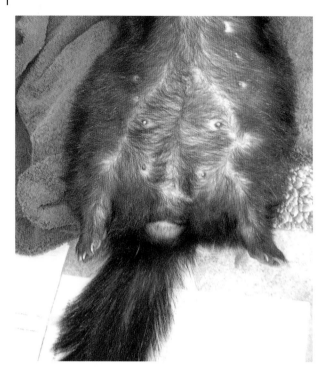

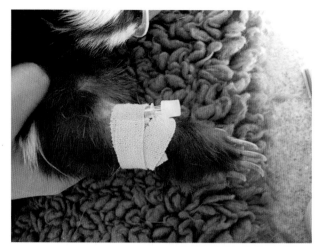

Figure 4.4   Intravenous cannula placed into the cephalic vein.

Figure 4.3   Female skunk, note the short ano-genital distance and prominent nipples. This animal is obese.

of the femur (Kubiak 2016). From healthy adult animals up to 3 ml/kg can be collected but in debilitated patients this should be reduced to 1.5 ml/kg (Diehl et al. 2001).

4.5.2   Nutritional Support

Many skunks can be tempted to feed with strong-smelling, palatable foods. For anorexic patients a commercial convalescent liquid feed can be offered. Most brands recommend a mixture of omnivore and carnivore liquid feeds combined at a specific ratio. Care should be taken when syringe feeding skunks, and in aggressive animals this will not be possible. Pharyngostomy or nasogastric tube placement can be carried out as for domestic species for ongoing nutritional support but is unlikely to be tolerated in active animals.

4.5.3   Fluid Therapy

Maintenance fluid requirements for skunks are estimated to be 50–100 ml/kg/ day, based on requirements for similar species (Kubiak 2016). Oral and subcutaneous routes can be used for animals with up to 5% dehydration. For administration of larger volumes, the cephalic or saphenous veins are the most readily accessible for intravenous fluid therapy (Figure 4.4) but intravenous cannulation may be challenging in obese patients (Kubiak 2016). Intraosseous catheters are alternative

options in severely dehydrated patients. Placement via the greater trochanter of the femur is carried out under sedation and ongoing analgesia should be given if this route is used.

4.5.4   Anaesthesia

Care should be taken during anaesthesia as patients are often overweight or may have undiagnosed heart disease which may increase the anaesthetic risk. Maintaining obese patients in a reverse Trendelenburg position (dorsal recumbency with elevation of the thorax) will help minimise the effects of body mass on respiration (Figure 4.5).

Skunks should be starved for approximately six hours pre-anaesthesia and water should be freely available until the anaesthesia.

Induction of anaesthesia may result in emptying of anal glands so consideration should be given to inducing skunks in an isolated area, or possibly even outside. Anaesthesia has been described using isoflurane via an induction chamber or facemask (Marcilla et al. 2010) although this may induce more stress than injectable methods, and is generally not recommended. Propofol can also be used where intravenous access is possible (Summa et al. 2015). Intravenous or intramuscular injectable induction protocols are also suitable using doses used in ferrets. Protocols are included in the formulary.

Maintenance of anaesthesia is best achieved using inhaled volatile agents following intubation. Intubation is achieved as for cats and ferrets, although a laryngoscope may be required for clear laryngeal visualisation, especially in obese animals. A typical endotracheal tube size used in a skunk is 3–3.5 mm. It is recommended to apply local anaesthesia to the larynx before intubation as laryngospasm has been seen in skunks (Chitty 2015).

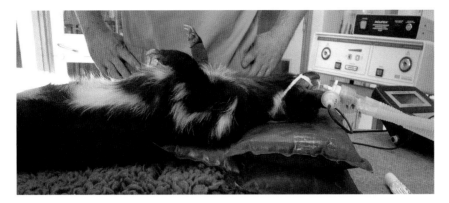

Figure 4.5 Anaesthetised skunk placed in reverse Trendelenburg position to avoid compromising respiratory movements.

Pulse oximeter probes can be attached to the tongue or ear, and ECG leads can be attached to feet using adhesive pads. Body temperature should be closely monitored, and animals given supplemental heat as necessary. Precautions should be taken to prevent burns from heat sources, particularly in obese animals.

4.5.5 Euthanasia

Euthanasia is performed using an intravenous overdose of pentobarbitone, at 150 mg/kg (Reilly 2001). The cephalic vein can often be used in an amenable conscious patient. Sedation or anaesthesia may be necessary if more restraint is needed, or if intracardiac or intraperitoneal injections are necessary due to difficulties with venous access.

4.6 Hospitalisation Requirements

Standard stainless steel cat hospital kennels are usually acceptable for short-term hospitalisation. Skunks are intelligent and inquisitive and additional security such as cage locks may be needed to prevent escape. Fleece pads or towels make suitable bedding but should be monitored for damage from chewing or digging. Keeping skunks in isolation away from other patients will help to reduce their anxiety.

4.7 Common Medical and Surgical Conditions

4.7.1 Obesity

This is one of the most common conditions seen in pet skunks, due to over-feeding, the feeding of inappropriate diets, and minimal exercise (Dragoo 2009). Neutering has been hypothesised as predisposing to obesity but the asso-

ciation is unclear. Obesity can predispose animals to other health problems such as hepatic lipidosis, heart disease, and arthritis. Management is by providing an appropriate diet and encouraging physical activity. There are currently no body condition scoring systems available for skunks but scoring systems for domestic species and regular weight checks can be used to monitor planned weight loss.

4.7.2 Nutritional Secondary Hyperparathyroidism (NSHP)

This is a common problem, especially in young animals. It is linked to excessive growth (such as with over-feeding) and feeding inappropriate diets with a low calcium:phosphorous ratio (Chitty 2015). Clinical signs of NSHP include pain, reluctance to move and long-bone deformities. Skunks with metabolic bone disease often present with pathological fractures (Wissink-Argilaga and Pellett 2014; Chitty 2015). Diagnosis is made on radiography where demineralised bones and fractures may be seen (Figure 4.6). Ionised blood calcium levels may be low and phosphorous high (Schneider 2003). Treatments include changing to an appropriate diet, supplementing with calcium and Vitamin D3, and exposure to daylight or artificial ultra-violet light. Analgesia is required where lesions present in the bone. Calcitonin has also been reported in managing advanced nutritional hypocalcaemia but should only be initiated once serum calcium levels have been stabilised (Schneider 2003).

Malaligned pathological fractures may require surgical correction but this can be problematic since placement of plates or pins can exacerbate damage. Supportive treatment may be all that can be undertaken initially until the bone density improves and surgery becomes an option. This might include analgesia, modification of the home environment (e.g. removing steps) and a supportive dressing if appropriate for the fracture (although a skunk's anatomy and behaviour makes it difficult to keep dressings in place).

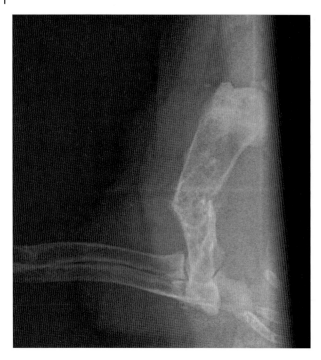

Figure 4.6 Lateral radiographic view of forelimb in a skunk with NSHP, showing marked demineralisation, irregular cortical outlines and a pathological fracture of the humerus.

4.7.3 Musculoskeletal Disease

Cauda equina compression has been described, with no clear cause of compression and treatment by laminectomy (Marcilla et al. 2010). Intervertebral disc disease with herniation has also been reported in skunks (Krauss et al. 2014). The affected skunks showed signs of paraparesis, ataxia, and diminished reflexes and surgical laminectomy was successful.

4.7.4 Dental Disease

Gingivitis, tartar, and periodontal disease are common findings in skunks. It would appear that they have a similar pathogenesis to those found in dogs (Kramer and Lennox 2003). They can be treated similarly with descaling of deposits and extraction of damaged teeth. It is likely that prevention of dental disease would also be similar to that of dogs, such as reduction of soft food, provision of dental treats, or diets and regular brushing.

4.7.5 Cardiac Disease

Myocardial fibrosis, myxomatous valve degeneration, hypertrophic cardiomyopathy, dilated cardiomyopathy, and valvular endocarditis have all been reported in striped skunks (Benato et al. 2014). Chronic granulomatous myocarditis due to *Trypanosoma cruzi* has also been recorded

(Ryan et al. 1985). Dirofilarial infections should be considered in imported animals (Heatley 2009).

Age and obesity are risk factors for cardiac disease in skunks (Rivera 2003; Heatley 2007; Benato et al. 2014). Most skunks with cardiac disease do not present with obvious clinical signs, but auscultation of a cardiac murmur may be noted on examination (Benato et al. 2014). Diagnosis is usually made on radiography or echocardiology. Treatment based on canine and feline regimens may be of benefit but prognosis is poor for skunks in congestive heart failure.

4.7.6 Anal Gland Pathology

Occasionally skunks are presented for clearly distended or painful anal glands, or over-grooming of the peri-anal area. The normal anal gland size is 2.5–4 cm (Aldrich 1896), but abnormal glands may measure up to 10 cm diameter. The content is often normal secretions, consisting of an oily, yellow foul-smelling substance and expressing the glands in an enclosed space without respiratory and ocular protection is not advised. Identifying and treating any contributing factors that may affect gland emptying such as inadequate fibre or parasitic enteritis, may result in resolution but many cases fail to respond. Chronic distension or inflammation results in remodelling and permanent distortion of the anatomy with poor prognosis for return to normal function. Surgical excision of the gland(s) is recommended for these cases and two techniques are recognised.

The ductal approach is only suitable for glands that are not currently distended due to the necessarily small incisions. The skunk is placed in ventral recumbency, with the hindlegs raised and the tail retracted cranially and secured. The gland openings can be located at the junction between anal and rectal mucosa, at 3 o'clock and 9 o'clock (Capello 2006). The gland orifice is grasped with forceps and a circumferential incision of the anal mucosa is made close to the papilla. Traction is used to expose the duct and ligating the duct at this stage can help minimise leakage of the noxious secretions. Blunt dissection is then used to break down the attachments between the gland and the surrounding tissues and enable gland removal through the anal mucosa (Thatcher 1980). The mucosal incision is closed with a single suture of absorbable material (Capello 2006). The primary complication of this technique is anal sphincter incompetence so incisions must be kept as small as possible.

Alternatively, better access can be achieved for removal of distended glands via the extraductal approach. This is carried out with the patient in dorsal recumbency. The skin on each side of the anus is clipped and surgically prepared. The two incisions are made in the skin immediately lateral to the anus, over the distal duct and gland on each side, and soft tissues are bluntly separated (Capello 2006). It is prudent to identify and ligate or clamp the duct prior to

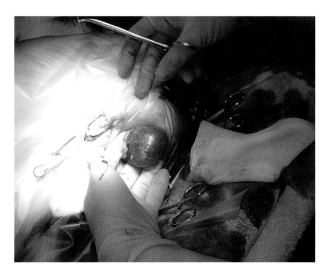

Figure 4.7 Dissection of the gland prior to anal sacculectomy, note the thin wall to the sac.

manipulation to avoid drainage of secretions. The constrictor muscles encircling the gland are very carefully dissected free (Figure 4.7). The gland can then be exteriorised and the duct double ligated. The duct is transected between the ligatures and the gland removed. Surrounding tissues are flushed and the integrity of the rectal wall must be confirmed prior to closure of the soft tissues and skin (Capello 2006). Inadvertent rupture of the gland itself during surgery will release highly noxious secretions into the surgical incision and the environment.

Post-operative complications for both techniques include rectal fistula formation, persistent cellulitis and rectal necrosis (Capello 2006). Care must be taken during surgery to preserve the surrounding tissues. A single case of perineal hernia following the extraductal approach has been reported (Summa et al. 2015).

Analgesia is essential in the post-operative period until healing is complete. Prophylactic antibiotic therapy is often administered as the potential for infection due to faecal contamination of the site or patient interference is high.

Elective sacculectomy may be carried out in juvenile skunks to render them more suitable pets. However in many countries, including the UK, this procedure is not permitted. Removal of glands affected by disease remains acceptable. In these cases it is advisable to record detailed clinical information and consider submitting samples of removed glands for histological analysis to corroborate the clinical grounds for surgical intervention.

4.7.7 Neoplasia

Neoplasia is often seen in older animals, and should be considered as a differential in cases of non-specific signs such as weight loss, or where a mass is evident. There are a wide variety of reported neoplasms in skunks including teratoma, lymphoma, renal adenosarcoma, thyroid adenoma, intestinal adenocarcinoma, interstitial cell tumour, phaeochromocytoma, squamous cell carcinoma, and mesothelioma. (Smith and Barker 1983; Miller et al. 1985; Pang et al. 1998; Munday et al. 2004; Kim et al. 2016; Liptovszky et al. 2017). Treatment mirrors that of domestic species and no species-specific chemotherapy protocols have been reported.

4.7.8 Renal Disease

Renal disease may be underdiagnosed in pet skunks. Reports in the literature are scant but leptospirosis, viral pathogens, idiopathic amyloidosis, and reactive amyloidosis have been identified as causes of renal lesions in wild and captive skunks (Crowell et al. 1977; Ganley-Leal et al. 2007; Elhensheri et al. 2012).

Aleutian disease is caused by a parvovirus and, although more common in mink and ferrets, has been reported to cause severe nephritis in skunks (Allender et al. 2008). A related skunk amdoparvovirus has been shown to be widespread in one survey of wild skunks in Canada but pathological changes were only seen in a small proportion of infected animals (Canuti et al. 2017).

Diagnosis and management of renal disease in skunks reflects that of more familiar species, and treatment is based upon feline protocols and dosing regimens. It would be prudent to test for Aleutian disease and leptospirosis in cases of acute renal failure.

4.7.9 Intestinal Disease

Inappropriate diet, dietary change (including weaning), over-feeding, coliform overgrowth, endoparasitism, and rotavirus are postulated factors in development of diarrhoea in striped skunks (Evans 1984; Dragoo 2009). Common ferret intestinal diseases such as *Helicobacter mustelae*, enteric coronavirus, and inflammatory bowel disease are not reported in the skunk. Dietary modification and supportive therapy of fluid administration and domestic carnivore probiotic supplements is sufficient for mild cases of diarrhoea. Faecal parasitology is carried out routinely for these patients and microbiology or tests for specific viral pathogens may be necessary for severe or chronic cases.

Rectal prolapse is a possible sequel to enteritis, or associated with anal sphincter damage in surgically de-scented animals (Capello 2006). The prolapse needs to be replaced and secured, typically with a purse string suture placed around the anus to preserve the integrity of the soft tissues. Analgesia and antibiotic therapy are likely to be required if tissues are inflamed or traumatised. It is critical that the underlying cause is treated concurrently or the prolapse will invariably recur.

4.7.10 Respiratory Disease

Infectious respiratory disease appears uncommon in skunks, with occasional opportunistic infection seen in debilitated animals and few reports of primary infection. *Streptococcus equisimilis* has been found to cause pneumonia and meningoencephalitis in striped skunks (Hwang et al. 2002). Histoplasmosis has been reported as a cause of lung lesions in skunks in North America (Woolf and Gremillion-Smith 1985). Striped skunks are susceptible to some infection with some influenza A viruses and they can shed the virus through oral and nasal routes (Root et al. 2014).

4.7.11 Endoparasites

Most endoparasites are diagnosed on faecal screening, using both wet preparation and faecal flotation techniques.

Toxocara canis can infect skunks. If skunks are kept with dogs regular deworming may be advisable. Fenbendazole appears to be safe and effective at dog doses. Milbemycin has also been used successfully (Kubiak 2016).

Baylisascaris species (*B. procyonis* and *B. columnaris*) are nematodes with zoonotic potential, associated with encephalitis in humans due to migrating larvae. In a recent survey, 25% of captive skunks in Europe tested positive for *Baylisascaris* (d'Ovidio et al. 2017). *B. procyonis* is more pathogenic but rarer in skunks. *B. columnaris* has been recently reported in the UK (Mitchell et al. 2014). Faecal screening and parasite species identification in imported animals is imperative. It has been recommended that fenbendazole should be given at least twice a year or even monthly to at risk skunks to reduce the risk of shedding *Baylisascaris* eggs (Delaney 2014). There is no treatment for infected humans.

Imported animals may have a host of other helminths such as lung flukes and lungworms. Most of these can be treated with fenbendazole (Dragoo 2009).

Coccidia are especially seen in young animals and can cause diarrhoea. Treatment options include sulphadimethoxine (Dragoo 2009) or trimethaprim sulphamethoxazole.

Toxoplasma gondii infection has been seen in skunks (Wissink-Argilaga and Pellett 2014; Chitty 2015). As with other species it is due to ingesting oocysts found in infected cat faeces, or tissue cysts from intermediate hosts (e.g. rodents). Clinical signs can vary but include pyrexia and lymphadenopathy. Splenomegaly, myocarditis, pneumonitis, hepatitis, and encephalitis may be present (Diters and Nielsen 1978). Diagnosis is based on paired serology demonstrating a rising titre, or presence of tachyzoites in tissue samples. Preventing access to cat faeces and adequate rodent control will help to prevent the disease. Treatment can be attempted with clindamycin but prognosis is poor (Kubiak 2016).

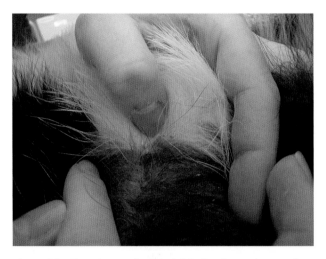

Figure 4.8 Hyperkeratosis with visible flea faeces in a cat flea infestation in a colony of skunks.

4.7.12 Ectoparasites

Skunks are susceptible to the cat flea *Ctenocephalides felis* (Figure 4.8). Routine preventative treatment is not needed but in cases of infestation, fipronil spray is effective (Rust 2005).

Ticks can also be encountered (especially in wild or imported animals) and may be treated with fipronil (Dragoo 2009).

Sarcoptic mange is common especially in young or stressed individuals (Chitty 2015). Signs include a pruritic papular rash, often found on the ventrum. A diagnosis is made on skin scrapes and treatment is with ivermectin.

4.8 Preventative Health Measures

4.8.1 Vaccinations

Skunks are susceptible to canine distemper virus, infectious canine hepatitis virus, and rabies virus (Diters and Nielsen 1978; Burcham et al. 2010). They are also likely to be susceptible to *Leptospirosis* (Crowell et al. 1977; Barker et al. 1983). Clinical signs for these infections are similar to those seen in dogs.

Vaccines licensed for dogs against these diseases have been used in skunks, but are not licensed and their efficacy is not documented, though vaccinated skunks were observed to survive a distemper outbreak that caused high mortality in unvaccinated animals (Kubiak M., pers. comm.). At-risk animals (i.e. those that come into contact with dogs or wildlife) should be vaccinated. It is advisable to contact vaccine manufactures when considering skunk vaccinations as some vaccinal viruses are attenuated in ferret cell lines and may be of higher potential for reversion to virulence in skunks.

Vaccinating skunks travelling to rabies endemic areas against rabies virus should be considered. Wild skunks are an important wildlife vector for rabies (Blanton et al. 2007) and there has been widespread oral vaccination of wild skunks against rabies. Studies show that this oral vaccination is effective (Brown et al. 2014). Currently no data exists on safety and efficacy of injectable rabies vaccinations.

Feline vaccinations do not appear to be necessary in skunks. There are no reported cases of feline herpes or feline calicivirus infections in skunks and it is unlikely that feline vaccines would protect against the skunk specific herpes or caliciviruses. Feline Panleukopaenia infections have been recorded in serological studies of skunks but no cases of disease were found following challenge studies (Barker et al. 1983).

4.8.2 Deworming

Regular deworming or faecal monitoring is recommended in young animals, imported animals, or those kept with other animals that may have endoparasites. Fenbendazole appears safe and effective. Kubiak (2016) has also used milbemycin and praziquantel at feline doses successfully.

4.9 Neutering Technique

Both male and female skunks can be neutered. Reasons for neutering include contraception, reducing general body odour (although it does not affect anal gland secretions or ejection), and reducing male aggression. Orchidectomy should be carried out before six months old to reduce the risk of aggression. Unlike ferrets, neutering does not appear to predispose to adrenal disease (Chitty 2015).

Ovariohysterectomy in skunks is recommended before their first season (i.e. during their first winter) as more abdominal fat will be encountered as they mature, compromising surgical access.

Surgical techniques for neutering are similar to those used in dogs. Absorbable suture material is used for the ligations and sutures. It is also recommended that opiates and non-steroidal anti-inflammatories (NSAIDs) are used in the premedication and NSAIDs are used post operatively as well. Reducing pain will also reduce the risk of the skunk traumatising the wound.

Orchidectomy: a ventral midline incision is made cranial to the scrotum. Testes are manipulated through the incision and the vessels ligated. It may be prudent to close the tunic if an open castration technique is chosen to reduce potential risk of herniation through the inguinal canal

(Figure 4.9). The skin should be closed using an intradermal suture pattern and/or surgical glue (Krupka 2003).

Ovariohysterectomy: A 2.5 cm incision is made between the umbilicus and the pubis. A large amount of peritoneal fluid can often be found within the abdomen and this is considered normal. The uterus and ovaries are identified and exteriorised using gentle traction. The ovarian pedicles are isolated and ligated. The body of the uterus is ligated at the level of the cervix and the uterus and ovaries are removed. The body wall is closed in three 3 layers, with the linea alba and subcuticular soft tissues sutured separately and the skin closed using intradermal sutures (Figure 4.10) (Krupka 2003).

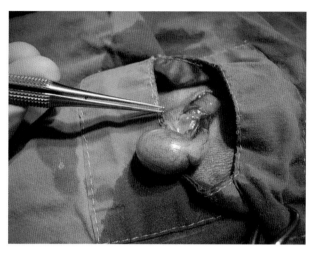

Figure 4.9 Exteriorisation of the testis during castration to expose vessels for ligation. If an open technique is used it is advisable to close the tunic after orchidectomy.

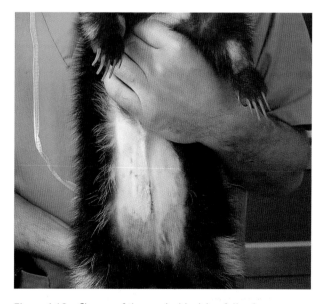

Figure 4.10 Closure of the surgical incision following ovariohysterectomy using a combination of intradermal absorbable sutures and tissue glue.

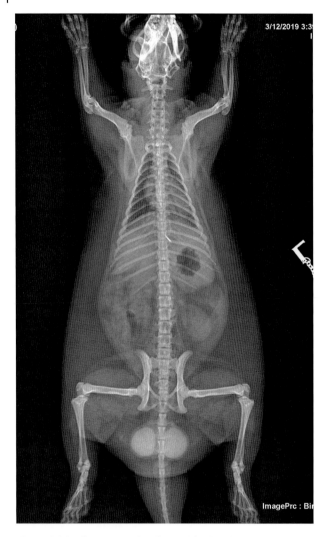

Figure 4.11 Dorsoventral radiographic view. Note the size and opacity of the scent glands.

Deslorelin implants have been used in skunks although response has not been fully evaluated yet (Chitty 2015). It is likely that they would be effective in males and females. Current guidelines suggest that, following an initial stimulation phase, a 4.7 mg implant should stop a female cycling for a minimum of six months and a 9.4 mg implant at least 12 months (Cowl 2017). Megestrol acetate tablets have been used to suppress the initial stimulation phase in similar species. It may be advisable to start this protocol a month before spring when skunks would normally come into season (Cowl 2017).

4.10 Radiographic Imaging

Routine views for survey radiographs may include right lateral and dorsoventral thoracic views and right lateral and ventrodorsal abdominal views. Anatomy reflects that of domestic mammals and clinicians familiar with cats, dogs, and ferrets should feel comfortable interpreting skunk radiographs (Figures 4.11 and 4.12).

Metabolic bone disease, fractures (Figure 4.13), and cardiomegaly are amongst the most common findings on radiography.

4.11 Formulary

Medicating skunks is usually simple; skunks are quite accepting of medication in food or syringing palatable liquids orally. However, there are no licensed drugs for skunks, and there are few pharmacokinetic and pharmacodynamic studies. Many doses are anecdotal, or extrapolated from feline or ferret dosing regimens.

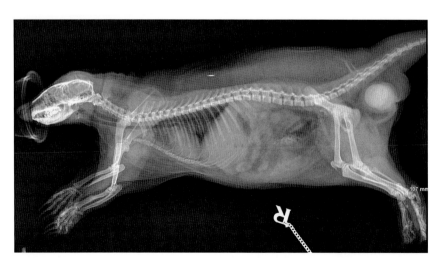

Figure 4.12 Laterolateral radiographic view.

Figure 4.13 Right lateral abdominal radiograph. Note the excess fat seen in this obese individual, demineralised bones due to metabolic bone disease and a displaced femoral fracture.

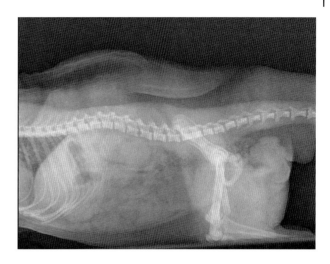

Formulary of medications

Medication	Dose	Dosing interval	Comments
Analgesics and anaesthetics			
Isoflurane	5% induction, 2–3% maintenance		(Brown 1993; Chitty 2015)
Propofol	25 mg/kg IV		Induction, ferret dose (Evans 1998)
Ketamine	11 mg/kg IM		Sedation for minor procedures (Kramer and Lennox 2003)
Ketamine (K)/ Medetomidine(M)	(K)5 mg/kg + (M)0.08 mg/kg IM		For general anaesthesia (Evans 1998). Medetomidine can be reversed with atipamezole at 5 times the dose (in mg) of medetomidine
Ketamine (K)/ midazolam (M)	(K) 5–10 mg/kg + (M) 0.25–0.5 mg/kg IM		For general anaesthesia (Morrisey 2009)
Meloxicam	0.2 mg/kg PO, SC, IM	q24h	For analgesia (Hoppes 2010). Monitor liver and kidney values
Buprenorphine	0.01–0.03 mg/kg SC, IM, IV	q8–12hrs	For analgesia (Marini and Fox 1998)
Antiparasitics			
Ivermectin	0.2–0.5 mg/kg SC	q14d ×3 treatments	To treat sarcoptic mange and other mites (Hillyer and Brown 1994; Wissink-Argilaga and Pellett 2014; Chitty 2015)
Fenbendazole	50 mg/kg PO	q24h for 5 days	To treat nematodes (Kramer and Lennox 2003; Wissink-Argilaga and Pellett 2014; Chitty 2015) and prevent *Baylisascaris* shedding (Delaney 2014)
Milbemycin(M) + Praziquantel(P)	2 mg/kg(M) + 5 mg/kg(P) PO		Anthelminthic (Kubiak 2016)
Fipronil spray	7.5–15 mg/kg sprayed over body (based on canine dose)		To treat fleas and ticks (Wissink-Argilaga and Pellett 2014; Chitty 2015)
Sulphadimethoxine	50 mg/kg PO, then 25 mg/kg	q24h ×9days	To treat Coccidia (Besch-Williford 1987; Dragoo 2009)
Trimethaprim Sulphamethoxazole	15–30 mg/kg PO	q12h	Treatment of bacterial and coccidial infections (Hillyer and Brown 1994)
Clindamycin	12.5 mg/kg PO	q12h	To treat toxoplasmosis (Brown 1999).

(Continued)

(Continued)

Medication	Dose	Dosing interval	Comments
Antibiotics			
Amoxicillin/clavulanic acid	12.5 mg/kg PO	q12h	(Brown 1999)
Clindamycin	5.5 mg/kg PO	q12h	For bacterial infections (Brown 1999)
Enrofloxacin	5–10 mg/kg PO,SC,IM	q12h	(Brown 1999)
Metronidazole	15–20 mg/kg PO	q12h	(Brown 1993)
Trimethaprim Sulphamethoxazole	15–30 mg/kg PO	q12h	(Hillyer and Brown 1994)
Other drugs that have been safely used in Skunks			
Frusemide	1–4 mg/kg PO, SC, IM, IV	q8–12h	Diuretic (Brown 1999; Chitty 2015)
Pimobendan	0.625–1.25 mg/kg PO	q12h	For cardiac disease (Kraus and Morrisey 2012; Chitty 2015)
Deslorelin implants	4.7 mg SC or 9.4 mg SC		For medical contraception (Cowl 2017).
Megestrol acetate	2 mg/kg PO	Q24h for 7 days before and 8 days after Deslorelin implantation	For short-term medical contraception (Cowl 2017).

References

Aldrich, T.B. (1896). A chemical study of the secretion of the anal glands of *Mephitis mephitiga* (common skunk), with remarks on the physiological properties of this secretion. *The Journal of Experimental Medicine* 1 (2): 323.

Aleksiuk, M. and Stewart, A.P. (1977). Food intake, weight changes and activity of confined striped skunks (*Mephitis mephitis*) in winter. *American Midland Naturalist*: 331–342.

Allender, M.C., Schumacher, J., Thomas, K.V. et al. (2008). Infection with Aleutian disease virus-like virus in a captive striped skunk. *Journal of the American Veterinary Medical Association* 232 (5): 742–746.

Barker, I., Povey, I., and Voigt, D. (1983). Response of mink, skunk, red fox and raccoon to inoculation with mink virus enteritis, feline panleukopenia and canine parvovirus and prevalence of antibody to parvovirus in wild carnivores in Ontario. *Canadian Journal of Comparative Medicine* 47: 188–197.

Benato, L., Wack, A., Cerveny, S. et al. (2014). Survey of cardiac pathologies in captive striped skunk (*Mephitis mephitis*). *Journal of Zoo and Wildlife Medicine* 45 (2): 321–327.

Besch-Williford, C. (1987). Biology and medicine of the ferret. *The Veterinary Clinics of North America. Small Animal Practice* 17: 1155–1183.

Bixler, A. and Gittleman, J. (2000). Variation in home range and use of habitat in the striped skunk (*Mephitis mephitis*). *Journal of Zoology* 251: 525–533.

Blanton, J., Hanlon, C., and Rupprecht, C. (2007). Rabies surveillance in the United States during 2006. *Journal of the American Veterinary Medical Association* 231 (4): 540–556.

Brown, S. (1993). Ferrets. In: *A Practitioners Guide to Rabbits and Ferrets* (eds. J. Jenkins and S. Brown), 43–111. Lakewood, CO: American Animal Hospital Association.

Brown, S. (1999). Ferret dosages. In: *Exotic Formulary* (eds. N. Antinoff, L. Bauk and T. Boyer), 43–61. Lakewood, CO: American Animal Hospital Association.

Brown, L.J., Rosatte, R.C., Fehlner-Gardiner, C. et al. (2014). Oral vaccination and protection of striped skunks (*Mephitis mephitis*) against rabies using ONRAB®. *Vaccine* 32 (29): 3675–3679.

Burcham, G., Ramos-Vara, J., and Vemulapalli, R. (2010). Systemic sarcocystosis in a striped skink (*Mephitis mephitis*). *Veterinary Pathology* 47 (3): 560–564.

Canuti, M., Doyle, H.E., P Britton, A. et al. (2017). Full genetic characterization and epidemiology of a novel amdoparvovirus in striped skunk (*Mephitis mephitis*). *Emerging Microbes & Infections* 6 (1): 1–8.

Capello, V. (2006). Sacculectomy in the pet ferret and skunk. *Exotic DVM* 8 (2): 15–24.

Chitty, J. (2015). Skunks: general care and health concerns. *Companion Animal* 20 (8): 472–478.

Cowl, V. (2017). EGZAC guidelines for small carnivores (Procyonidae, Herpestidae/Eupleridae, Mustelidae,

Viverridae, Mephitidae, Ailuridae). http://www.egzac.org/home/viewdocument?filename=Small%20carnivores%20taxon%20sheet%202017.pdf (accessed 27 November 2017).

Crowell, W., Stuart, B., and Adams, W. (1977). Renal lesions in striped skunk (*Mephitis mephitis*) from Louisiana. *Journal of Wildlife Diseases* 13 (3): 300–303.

Delaney, C. (2014). Pet Virginia opossums and skunks. *Journal of Exotic Pet Medicine* 23 (4): 317–326.

Diehl, K., Hull, R., Morton, D. et al. (2001). A good practice guide to the administration of substances and removal of blood, including routes and volumes. *Journal of Applied Toxicology* 21 (1): 15–23.

Diters, R. and Nielsen, S. (1978). Toxoplasmosis, distemper and herpesvirus infection in a skunk (*Mephitis mephitis*). *Journal of Wildlife Diseases* 14 (1): 132–136.

d'Ovidio, D., Pantchev, N., Noviello, E. et al. (2017). Survey of *Baylisascaris* spp. in captive striped skunks (*Mephitis mephitis*) in some European areas. *Parasitology Research* 116: 483–486.

Dragoo, J. (1982). Family mephitidae(skunks). In: *Handbook of the Mammals of the World. Vol. 1 Carnivores* (eds. D.E. Wilson and R.A. Mittemeier), 532–553. Barcelona, Spain: Lynx Edicions.

Dragoo, J. (2009). Nutrition and behaviour of striped skunks. *The Veterinary Clinics of North America. Exotic Animal Practice* 12: 313–326.

Elhensheri, M., Linke, R., Blankenburg, A. et al. (2012). Idiopathic systemic AA-amyloidosis in a skunk (*Mephitis mephitis*). *Journal of Zoo and Wildlife Medicine* 43 (1): 181–185.

Evans, R. (1984). Rotavirus-associated diarrhea in young raccoons (*Procyon lotor*), striped skunk (*Mephitis mephitis*) and red foxes (*Vulpes vulpes*). *Journal of Wildlife Diseases* 20 (2): 79–85.

Evans, A. (1998). Anesthesia of ferrets. *Seminars in Avian and Exotic Pet Medicine* 7: 48–52.

Ganley-Leal, L., Brown, C., Tulman, E. et al. (2007). Suppurative polyarthritis in striped skunks (*Mephitis mephitis*) from Cape Cod, Massachusetts: detection of mycoplasma DNA. *Journal of Zoo and Wildlife Medicine* 38: 388–399.

Greenwood, R., Newton, W., Pearson, G. et al. (1997). Population and movement characteristics of radio collared striped skunks in North Dakota during an epizootic of rabies. *Journal of Wildlife Diseases* 33 (2): 226–241.

Heatley, J.J. (2007). Small Exotic Mammal Cardiovascular disease. In: *Proceedings of the 28th Annual Association of Avian Veterinary Conference and Expo with Association of Exotic Mammal Veterinarians, Providence, USA* (eds. H. Bowles and E. Bergman), 69–79. Bedford, TX: Association of Avian Veterinarians.

Heatley, J. (2009). Cardiovascular anatomy, physiology, and disease of rodents and small exotic mammals. *The Veterinary Clinics of North America. Exotic Animal Practice* 12: 99–114.

Hillyer, E. and Brown, S. (1994). Ferrets. In: *Saunders Manual of Exotic Animal Practice* (eds. S. Birchard and R. Sherding), 1317–1344. Philadelphia: WB Saunders.

Hoppes, S.M. (2010). The senior ferret (*Mustela putorius furo*). *Veterinary Clinics: Exotic Animal Practice* 13 (1): 107–122.

Hwang, Y., Wobeser, G., Lariviere, S. et al. (2002). *Streptococcus equisimilis* infection in striped skunks (*Mephitis mephitis*) in Saskatchewan. *Journal of Wildlife Diseases* 38 (3): 641–643.

Johnson-Delaney, C. (1996). Exotic carnivores. In: *Exotic Companion Medicine Handbook* (eds. L. Harrison and C. Johnson-Delaney), 1–42. Lake Worth, FL: Wingers Publishing Incorporated.

Kim, S.M., Oh, Y., Oh, S.H. et al. (2016). Primary diffuse malignant peritoneal mesothelioma in a striped skunk (*Mephitis mephitis*). *Journal of Veterinary Medical Science* 78 (3): 485–487.

Kramer, M. and Lennox, A. (2003). What veterinarians need to know about skunks. *Exotic DVM* 5: 36–39.

Kraus, M. and Morrisey, J. (2012). Cardiovascular and other diseases. In: *Ferrets, Rabbits and Rodents: Clinical Medicine and Surgery*, 3e (eds. K. Quesenberry and J. Carpenter), 62–77. St. Louis, MO: Saunders/Elsevier.

Krauss, M., Benato, L., Wack, A. et al. (2014). Intervertebral disk disease in 3 striped skunks (*Mephitis mephitis*). *Veterinary Surgery* 43: 589–592.

Krupka, F. (2003). Review of neutering procedures in skunks. *Exotic DVM* 5: 8–10.

Kubiak, M. (2016). Skunk Medicine and Surgery. *Veterinary Times* (4 July): 46–48.

Lariviere, S. and Messier, F. (1998). Spatial organization of a prairie striped skunk population during the waterfowl nesting season. *Journal of Wildlife Management* 62 (1): 199–204.

Liptovszky, M., Kerekes, Z., Perge, E. et al. (2017). Mediastinal lymphoma and chylothorax in a striped skunk (*Mephitis mephitis*). *Journal of Zoo and Wildlife Medicine* 48 (2): 598–601.

Marcilla, M.G., Bosmans, T., Hellebuyck, T. et al. (2010). Anesthetic and analgesic management of a striped skunk (*Mephitis mephitis*) undergoing a laminectomy for cauda equine compression. *Vlaams Diergeneeskd Tijdschr* 79: 395–399.

Marini, R.P. and Fox, J.G. (1998). *Anesthesia, Surgery, and Biomethodology. Biology and diseases of the Ferret*, 2e, 449–484. Baltimore: Williams & Wilkins.

Miller, R., Turk, J., Wells, S. et al. (1985). Carcinoma of type II pneumocytes in a striped skunk. *Veterinary Pathology* 22: 644–645.

Mitchell, S., Anscombe, J., and Wessels, J. (2014). Disease risks from raccoons and skunks. *Veterinary Record* 174: 510–511.

Morrisey, J. (2009). Ferrets: therapeutics. In: *BSAVA Manual of Rodents and Ferrets* (eds. E. Keeble and A. Meredith), 237–244. Gloucester, UK: BSAVA.

Munday, J., Fairchild, S., and Brown, C. (2004). Retroperitoneal Teratoma in a skunk (*Mephitis mephitis*). *Journal of Zoo and Wildlife Medicine* 35 (3): 406–408.

Nowak, R.M. (1999). *Walker's Mammals of the World*, 6e. Baltimore, MD: Johns Hopkins University Press.

Pang, V.F., Lee, C.H., Chiou, M.T. et al. (1998). Biliary cystadenoma in a striped skunk (*Mephitis mephitis*). *Journal of Veterinary Diagnostic Investigation* 10 (4): 357–360.

Reilly, J.S. (2001). *Euthanasia of Animals used for Scientific Purposes*, 2e. Adelaide: Australia and New Zealand Council for the Care of Animals in Research and Training, Adelaide University.

Rivera, S. (2003). Other species seeing in practice. In: *Exotic Animal Medicine for the Veterinary Technician* (eds. B. Ballard and R. Cheek), 263–272. Ames. IA): Blackwell Publishing.

Root, J., Shriner, S., Bentler, K. et al. (2014). Extended viral shedding of a low pathogenic avian influenza virus by a striped skunk (*Mephitis mephitis*). *PLoS ONE* 9 (1): e70639. https://doi.org/10.1371/journal.pone.0070639.

Rust, M. (2005). Advances in the control of *Ctenocephalides felis* (cat flea) on cats and dogs. *Trends in Parasitology* 21 (5): 232–236.

Ryan, C., Hughes, P., and Howard, E. (1985). American trypanosomiasis (Chagas' disease) in a striped skunk. *Journal of Wildlife Diseases* 21: 175–176.

Schneider, R. (2003). Hypocalcemia in a skunk. *Exotic DVM* 5: 5–6.

Schoemaker, N. (2010). Ferrets, skunks and otters. In: *BSAVA Manual of Exotic Pets*, 5e (eds. A. Meredith and C. Johnson-Delaney), 127–138. Gloucester: BSAVA.

Smith, D. and Barker, I. (1983). Four cases of Hodgkin's disease in striped skunks (*Mephitis mephitis*). *Veterinary Pathology* 20: 223–229.

Summa, N., Eshar, D., Reynolds, D. et al. (2015). Successful diagnosis and treatment of bilateral perineal hernias in a skunk (*Mephitis mephitis*). *Journal of Zoo and Wildlife Medicine* 46 (3): 575–579.

Thatcher, E. (1980). Veterinary care of ferrets, raccoons and skunks. *Iowa State University Veterinarian* 42 (1): 9.

Wade-Smith, J., Richmond, M., Mead, R. et al. (1980). Hormonal and gestational evidence for delayed implantation in the striped skunk, *Mephitis mephitis*. *General and Comparative Endocrinology* 42 (4): 509–515.

Wissink-Argilaga, N. and Pellett, S. (2014). Guide to husbandry and common diseases in degus and skunks. *Veterinary Times* 44 (38): 16–19.

Wood, W., Sollers, B., Dragoo, G. et al. (2002). Volatile components in defensive spray of the hooded skunk, Mephitis macroura. *Journal of Chemical Ecology* 28 (9): 865–870.

Woolf, A. and Gremillion-Smith, C. (1985). Histoplasmosis in a striped skunk (*Mephitis mephitis* Schreber) from southern Illinois. *Journal of Wildlife Diseases* 21 (4): 441–443.

5

Degus
Marie Kubiak

5.1 Introduction

Degus (*Octodon degus*) are a medium sized rodent classi-fied as part of the Hystricomorph family, along with guinea pigs, chinchillas, and porcupines. They originate from semiarid scrubland habitats in mountainous areas of northern and central Chile, where wild populations are currently widely distributed and not considered to be under threat. Unlike most rodents, degus are diurnal and combined with their ready habituation to regular handling, inquisitive nature, and ability to be trained they can make entertaining pets. They have been kept widely in laboratory settings for investigation into diabetes mellitus, Alzheimers, circadian rhythm disruption, and cataract formation due to similarities to humans in these aspects. Degus biological parameters are included in Table 5.1.

5.2 Husbandry

Degus are social animals, living in groups of 5–10 animals consisting of related females and 1–3 males (Fulk 1976). Small single-sex groups, or groups of females and neutered males are recommended in captivity to allow social interac-tion but to avoid unwanted breeding. Keeping an individual in solitary isolation causes a variety of maladaptive abnormal behaviours and should be avoided (Colonnello et al. 2011).

Laboratory animals are housed in cages of $20 \times 20 \times 8''$ for a pair (Lee 2004) but this is a bare minimum and far larger pet cages are readily available and allow natural behaviours to be exhibited. Degus will use space given and owners should be encouraged to give cages with a floor space (as single or multilevel structures) of at least six square feet for groups of two to five animals (Figure 5.1).

In the wild, their natural habitat combines a complex system of underground tunnels with paths above ground (Vásquez 1997). Substrate should be at least 6 inches deep to allow primitive burrow formation. It is important that no heavy structures are supported solely by substrate as these may cause tunnel collapse. A sand and soil mix-ture allows for burrowing but is difficult to keep clean and of sufficient humidity to maintain tunnels, so often wood shavings and cardboard pellets are used with pipes placed within the substrate to mimic tunnels. Pine shav-ings have been found to cause skin irritation so are best avoided (Lee 2004).

Degus can be kept at room temperature with no supple-mentary heating necessary. Excessively high temperatures (>25 °C) lead to alteration of behaviour with animals retreating under substrate and demonstrating nocturnal patterns of activity.

Degus are herbivorous and adapted to the moderate pro-tein, low sugar, and exceptionally high fibre diet available in their natural habitat. In the wild, they feed on grasses, seeds, leaves, and branches of shrubs (Bozinovic et al. 1997; Gutiérrez and Bozinovic 1998). They have limited ability to modulate digestive performance in the face of increases in protein or carbohydrate content (Sabat and Bozinovic 2008) and have a well-developed caecum for fermentation of fibrous plant materials. They exhibit coprophagy, with up to 38% of the faeces re-ingested to enable absorption of the nutrients liberated by caecal fer-mentation (Hommel 2012). Captive diets should comprise a pelleted ration specifically formulated for degus, small quantities of leafy vegetables or weeds and ad lib good quality hay. Root vegetables and fruits, or other sources of simple carbohydrates, should be avoided due to this spe-cies' propensity to develop derangements of blood glucose. Food intake has been found to be 25–70 g of dry matter per kilogramme of bodyweight with the greater extent eaten when hay was the predominant food item (Hommel 2012).

Degus are able conserve water as an adaptation to a dry conditions, with highly concentrated urine and low faecal water losses resulting in lower fluid requirements than for

Handbook of Exotic Pet Medicine, First Edition. Edited by Marie Kubiak.
© 2021 John Wiley & Sons Ltd. Published 2021 by John Wiley & Sons Ltd.
Companion website: www.wiley.com/go/kubiak/exotic_pet_medicine

Table 5.1 Biological parameters.

Body weight	200–300 g (males slightly larger)
Lifespan	6–10 years
Body temperature (°C)	38.1–39.5
Respiratory rate (/min)	100–200
Heart rate (/min)	250–300
Sexual maturity	from 3 months
Gestation (days)	87–95
Litter size	Range: 1–10, mean: 8

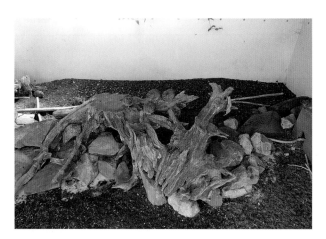

Figure 5.1 Degus are sociable, active animals and providing large, multi-level enclosures will enable normal behaviours.

rodents from temperate climes (Hagen et al. 2014). During drought, renal expression of aquaporin APQ-2 increases, leading to seasonal variation in urine concentration (Bozinovic et al. 2003). When water is freely available, urine produced is more dilute. Water should be provided ad libitum and can be offered in either bowls or sipper bottles (Wolf et al. 2008; Hagen et al. 2014). Some authors recommend acidifying drinking water for laboratory animals less than three months of age due to a reported susceptibility to *Pseudomonas* but this does not appear to be a significant concern for pet degus (Lee 2004).

Degus demonstrate a cognitive capacity higher than is reported for other rodents and small mammals. They can be trained to use tools, recognise colours, and learn new behaviours (Tokimoto and Okanoya 2004; Okanoya et al. 2008; Ardiles et al. 2013). As such, enrichment activities should be made available to captive degus to maintain mental stimulation. These include wheels, puzzle feeders, burrowing opportunities, branches for climbing and chewing, and sand baths. Conversely, degus shouldn't be exposed to constant light, loud or persistent noises, and excessive stimuli as this is considered detrimental (Longley 2009).

Ultraviolet (UV) light is rarely provided for pet degus but is used for laboratory animals. Given the ability of degus to see light of wavelengths within the UV spectrum, and the potential for UV-B light to aid in maintenance of calcium homeostasis, provision of UV light should be considered for this species (Jacobs et al. 2003). Lights should be positioned above the animals, outside the cage, and replaced when output begins to decline – either routinely based on manufacturer recommendations, or based on regular measurements of output using a UV-B metre. All wiring should be external to the cage and out of reach to prevent chewing and risk of electrocution.

5.3 Reproduction

Females tend to breed once a year in the wild during the rainy season and can breed up to four times a year in captivity, though this is not recommended. Although they can be fertile from three months of age (and one report suggests a case of conception prior to three months of age [Mancinelli et al. 2013]), in the wild animals typically mature around nine months of age when the breeding season begins. The oestrus cycle is 18–21 days and a post-partum oestrus is frequently observed in captivity though conception at this oestrus cycle is only around 50% (Palacios and Lee 2013). Gestation is longer than for other similarly sized rodents, lasting 87–95 days and a litter of 6–10 pups are born, though first litters tend to be smaller with only four to six pups (Lee 2004). Pups are precocious and are born fully furred, active and with open eyes, but remain in the nest site for two weeks. Females in a social group will share a nest to rear their litters together (Ebensperger et al. 2004; Ardiles et al. 2013). Solid food is taken from 1 to 2 weeks and weaning occurs at 4–5 weeks when pups weigh 60–80 g (Reynolds and Wright 1979; Lee 2004). Pups should be reared in small groups and not isolated as this can result in forming of fear response to humans and conspecifics, and failure of normal behaviours to develop (Palacios and Lee 2013).

5.4 Clinical Evaluation

5.4.1 History-Taking

History collection should include a full husbandry review as well as the specifics of the presenting complaint. Diet and group structure are the areas of management most commonly found to be implicated in clinical abnormalities.

5.4.2 Handling

Degus that are regularly handled are tolerant of human contact and will allow gentle restraint for examination with few animals demonstrating active aggression towards handlers. Restraining docile degus with one hand around the thorax and the body resting on an arm or the chest of the handler will allow a basic examination with minimal stress to the animal. Placing the second and third fingers either side of the neck with the hand wrapping round the thorax will allow better restraint for dental evaluation and auscultation (Figure 5.2). Degus can move quickly and jump, so firmer restraint is needed for more nervous animals. Wrapping them in a towel facilitates catching animals, allows for better restraint and some protection from bites. The tail skin can slough if grasped firmly so any restraint of the tail should be avoided.

Restraining degus by grasping the skin fold over the scruff is possible but is rarely appropriate.

5.4.3 Sex Determination

Degus are not sexually dimorphic, so genital examination is needed to determine sex. Males show a longer anogenital distance of approximately 1 cm with only anal and genital

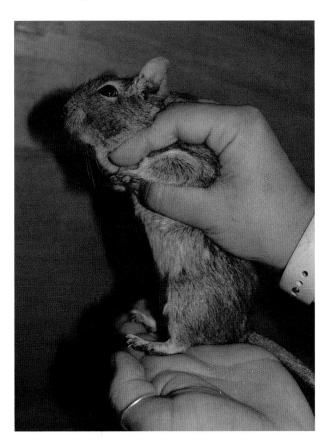

Figure 5.2 Restraint of a degu for examination.

orifices (Figure 5.3). The genital orifice is a raised preputial papilla from which a penis can be extruded and testes may palpable within a poorly defined, caudally placed scrotum though they can be withdrawn to an intraabdominal position. Females have an anogenital distance of less than 3 mm, with an anal orifice and the separate vaginal and urinary orifices in close association. The urethral papilla is pronounced in females and can be mistaken for the preputial papilla (Figure 5.4) (Mancinelli et al. 2013).

5.4.4 Clinical Examination

Clinical examination is carried out in as for other small rodents. An assistant is needed to hold the patient to perform evaluation of the mouth and eyes. A small otoscope cone can enable basic assessment of the cheek teeth but lateral spurs, caries, and minor changes are easily missed and proper evaluation requires anaesthesia.

Particularly important parts of the examination are intraoral evaluation, assessing fur for areas of alopecia and ophthalmic examination to identify any lenticular

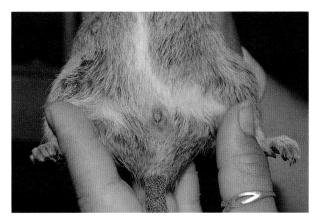

Figure 5.3 Male degu, note the lack of a clear scrotum. The testes are often palpable caudolateral to the prepuce but can be withdrawn into the abdomen.

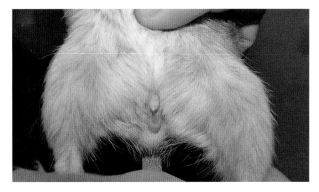

Figure 5.4 Female degu, note the pronounced urethral papilla but short anogenital distance compared to the male (Figure 5.3).

changes. It is prudent to weigh animals at each visit and to carry out a simple assessment of body condition. It is useful for owners to keep records that document weight changes of individuals.

5.5 Basic Techniques

5.5.1 Sample Collection

Blood samples are often difficult to obtain from small rodents due to difficulties in adequate restraint and the small size of blood vessels. Blood sampling from the cranial vena cava under isoflurane anaesthesia has been described, and allows for collection of relatively large volumes of blood (Jekl et al. 2005). A 23–25G needle with 1 ml syringe, or an insulin syringe is used. The technique involves placing the patient in dorsal recumbency and inserting the needle just cranial to the first rib and approximately 5 mm lateral to the midline, angled towards the contralateral hind leg (Jekl et al. 2005). Negative pressure is applied to the syringe and the needle slowly advanced until blood begins to flow into the hub. Up to 1 ml can be collected from this site in an adult animal, though sample size should not exceed 0.5% of patient weight. Digital pressure is applied for 30–60 seconds afterwards. It has been found to be a safe technique with no serious complications (Jekl et al. 2011b).

The femoral and cephalic veins can be used for small samples (<0.2 ml) but are more challenging due to small vein diameter. The jugular vein has also been described as an option (Johnson-Delaney 2006) but is difficult to access due to the short, thick neck in this species. Tail veins are not advised for sampling due to the potential for degloving injury on restraint (Bament 2013).

5.5.2 Nutritional Support

Owners can provide familiar or favourite items from the hospitalised patient's normal diet, to support voluntary feeding, and this can be supplemented by providing ad lib degu-specific concentrate and good quality hay, as well as small quantities of leafy greens.

An energy intake of 550–650 kJ/kg bodyweight has been shown to be appropriate for adults to maintain weight and this acts as a guide for nutritional requirements, though these often increase in sick animals (Hommel 2012). Nutritional support for anorexic animals typically consists of syringe feeding of a commercial herbivore diet to provide appropriate energy intake. Feeds of 3–5 ml every 3–4 hours are possible in adult degus and amounts fed are modified based on twice daily weight monitoring. Nasogastric feeding tubes are rarely used due to the necessarily small tube size preventing feeding of high fibre food, and poor patient tolerance.

5.5.3 Fluid Therapy

Fluid intake in degus has been demonstrated to be approximately 120 ml/kg/day under non-drought conditions (Cortes et al. 1988) and isotonic fluid solutions available for domestic mammals are suitable in degus. Nutritional support in debilitated animals will contribute significantly towards fluid replacement.

Where additional fluid support is needed, the subcutaneous route is used most commonly and the interscapular region is typically used though the flanks are also potential sites (Johnson-Delaney 2006). Recommended maximum volumes to be administered subcutaneously are 20 ml/kg at a maximum of 5 ml per site, but this can be repeated once absorption is complete. Intravenous catheters are difficult to place and maintain due to patient size and interference so intraosseous fluid therapy is used as an alternative in critical patients where more aggressive rehydration is necessary. The proximal tibia is the most common placement site used and constant infusion using a syringe driver is recommended.

5.5.4 Anaesthesia

Inhalational anaesthesia with isoflurane alone is commonly used due to ready availability and fast induction and recovery times. However, isoflurane is aversive to degus and restraint for mask induction can be stressful. Use of sevoflurane, pre-medication to reduce induction duration and stress, or preferably induction with injectable agents is recommended. Various combinations are highlighted in the formulary. Volatile agents can then be used to maintain anaesthesia. Halothane is to be avoided due to reported liver failure in this species (Lee 2004).

Oxygen should be administered to all sedated or anaesthetised patients and this is usually achieved by a nasal mask. Although endotracheal intubation provides a secure airway, the presence of a palatopharyngeal arch of soft tissue rostral to the glottis prevents intubation by standard techniques. Insertion of a 1.5 mm endotracheal tube under endoscopic visualisation of the glottis is possible but technically challenging.

5.5.5 Euthanasia

Anaesthesia followed by intracardiac injection of 100–200 mg/kg pentobarbitone is preferred, but intraperitoneal injection of 200–500 mg/kg pentobarbitone can also be used in an unconscious animal. Injection of intracardiac or intraperitoneal pentobarbitone in a conscious animal should be avoided.

5.5.6 Hospitalisation Requirements

Owners should be encouraged to bring in housing for hospitalised patients to maintain familiarity. Where this is not possible, degus can be housed short-term in basic rodent cages, but these should be assessed and confirmed to be secure prior to each use. Companions should be hospitalised with the patient to avoid isolation and to maintain the bond between animals. Hides or other cage furniture from home can be incorporated into the hospital cage. Substrate of hay or cardboard pellets works well in a hospital situation and cardboard boxes make good disposable hide areas.

Degus should be housed away from predatory animals such as cats, dogs, ferrets, snakes, and birds of prey.

5.6 Common Medical and Surgical Conditions

5.6.1 Dental Disease

Degu have the dental formula 1/1 0/0 1/1/3/3 and all teeth are of aradicular elodont type, meaning that there is no defined root and all teeth are continuously erupting (Woods and Boraker 1975; Jekl et al. 2011a). As with other rodents, there is a large diastema between the rostrally placed incisors and the premolars and molars (cheek teeth) and the two regions function separately with only incisors or cheek teeth in occlusion at a given time (Mans and Jekl 2016). Each molar occlusal surface is loosely shaped as a figure of eight, resulting in the genus name of 'Octodon'. The maxillary cheek teeth angle buccally, and the mandibular cheek teeth lingually, resulting spurs forming laterally and medially respectively in cases of overgrowth. Elongation of apices happens early in the process of dental disease and results in palpable elongation of protruding apices of the mandibular cheek teeth, and impingement of maxillary apices on the nasal cavity.

Dental changes are the most common pathology seen in pet degus, with one report finding 60% of all degus examined demonstrated dental abnormalities (Jekl et al. 2011a). The definitive cause of such widespread problems is unclear, though a high phosphorus diet, or reduced calcium: phosphorus ratio has been shown to result in dental abnormalities in this species (Jekl et al. 2011c). Additional factors postulated to contribute are insufficient dental wear, calcium or Vitamin D deficiency, or renally induced hyperparathyroidism (Gumpenberger et al. 2012).

Degus are selective feeders in the wild, prioritising nutritious young leaves available during the growing season and relying on increases in food intake and digestive time seen when digestibility of available food declines in drought periods (Bozinovic et al. 1997; Gutiérrez and Bozinovic

1998). In captivity they will actively select concentrates, grain, and sweet foods over fibrous browse and hay, resulting in reduced dental wear (Jekl et al. 2011a). If preferred foods are available consistently then progressive overgrowth of cheek teeth will result, followed by secondary overgrowth of the incisors.

5.6.1.1 Clinical Appraisal of Dental Disease

Dental disease commonly results in reduced food intake, weight loss, poor coat condition, epiphora and drooling, and in some cases dyspnoea may also be a presenting complaint (Jekl et al. 2016). Animals of all ages can be affected, though prevalence of dental disease increases with age (Jekl et al. 2011c). On clinical examination there may be evident incisor elongation, moist perioral dermatitis due to excess salivation or bony swellings along the ventral mandible (Figure 5.5). An otoscope-assisted dental examination can give some information on cheek tooth coronal changes but the small size of the oral cavity means that subtle changes are difficult to identify and up to 50% of changes may be overlooked (Jekl et al. 2008a).

Management of patients should focus on the secondary consequences as well as the suspected dental disease. Assist feeding, fluid therapy, and pain relief often need initiating after preliminary assessment to stabilise the patient prior to anaesthesia for diagnostics and intervention. Once stabilised and assessment has been completed, treatment should focus on improving the patient's welfare and allowing self-feeding and pain management. If a satisfactory level of welfare is unlikely to be achieved in future then euthanasia should be recommended. In cases where treatment is likely to restore a good quality of life to the patient, owners should be made aware of the likelihood of recurrence of pathology.

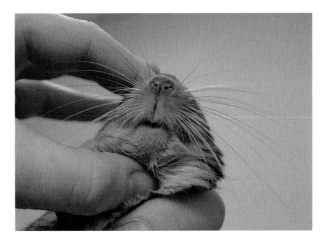

Figure 5.5 Palpation of the mandible should be carried out on every clinical examination as cheek tooth apices are commonly elongated in cases of dental disease.

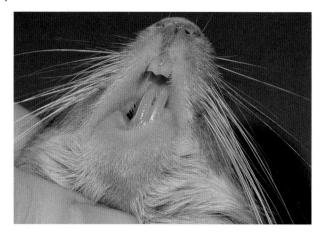

Figure 5.6 Normal appearance to degu incisors, note the yellow-orange pigmentation and sharp tips to each tooth.

5.6.1.2 Incisor Pathology

The incisors are a yellow-orange colour on the labial aspect and should have a smooth outer surface and a sharp tip (Figure 5.6). Normal occlusion results in the maxillary incisors sitting rostral to the mandibular incisors. A haired skin fold on the inner aspect of the lips is present on each side and sits behind the incisors when the jaw is in a resting position.

Elongation of the incisors is typically secondary to altered jaw position associated with cheek tooth elongation, and is the most common pathology noted, though traumatic fractures and dysplasia (secondary to dietary mineral deficiency or repeated trauma such as cage bar chewing) are occasionally seen (Mans and Jekl 2016). For incisor crown reduction, a dental burr or cutting disc can be used, but soft tissues should be retracted and protected using a spatula or other device. Sedation or anaesthesia is needed in these small patients to minimise patient distress and allow the procedure to be carried out properly. Incisor extractions are rarely appropriate, but may be needed in cases of periapical infection, abscessation, or early elodontoma formation (Mans and Jekl 2016). Large gauge (15–17G) hypodermic needles can be bent to the curvature of the tooth and used as luxators. The needle is passed along the length of the incisor on all surfaces to sever the periodontal ligament and once loosened gentle traction applied along the line of curvature of the tooth will enable removal. Care must be taken as iatrogenic fracture can result from excessive force. All incisors should be removed during the procedure to avoid the need for repeat treatments to reduce the length of the remaining incisors.

5.6.1.3 Cheek Tooth Pathology

Anaesthesia is necessary for complete examination of the cheek teeth. A small rodent handheld gag aids with maintaining an open mouth and cheek dilators are needed to retract soft tissues sufficiently to assess the clinical crowns. A flat bladed metal spatula helps with retraction of the tongue and other soft tissues during examination and is useful for passing along the buccal aspect of the maxillary cheek teeth to pick up on small spurs embedded in the buccal mucosa (Mans and Jekl 2016). Soft tissue ulceration, dental caries, resorptive lesions (and associated secondary fractures of the crown), food and hair impaction, and purulent discharge may be identified as well as the commonly seen elongated crowns and spur formation. The value of intraoral examination can be enhanced with the use of an endoscope as the illumination and magnification markedly increase visibility of lesions (Mans and Jekl 2016).

Cheek tooth malocclusion has been reported to be the most common dental abnormality in degus, accounting for 42% of dental disease in one review (Long 2012). Reduction of clinical crown height and removal of any associated spurs is best achieved with a low speed dental burr, ideally with a guard to protect soft tissues but in small individuals the guard may be too large to fit in the oral cavity. Extractions are uncommonly required and an intraoral approach is only possible for teeth that are already loose. Mandibular cheek teeth are easier to remove and an external approach is typically used. The skin is incised, soft tissues bluntly dissected (avoiding vessels and nerves) until the mandible is visualised. The overlying bone on the lateral and ventral aspect of the lower half of the reserve crown is removed with a fine drill or sharp scalpel, and the periodontal attachments are severed using a small scalpel or needle. Traction is then used, from the apex, to remove the tooth. For maxillary cheek teeth, a partial ostectomy of the zygomatic arch is needed for access and the procedure is technically challenging.

Caries can be managed by removing the abnormal enamel with a ball-tipped burr and the ongoing eruption of the tooth will allow a normal crown to move into occlusion over time (Mans and Jekl 2016). Facial abscessation appears an uncommon consequence of dental disease in degus (Long 2012; Mans and Jekl 2016).

5.6.1.4 Elodontoma

Elodontomas have been reported in this species (Jekl et al. 2008b) and are likely an underdiagnosed phenomenon. These proliferative accumulations of odontogenic tissue develop at the apices of elodont teeth resulting in damage to surrounding structures and displacement of the clinical and reserve crowns. Maxillary incisor or premolar involvement can result in progressive obstruction of the nasal passage and respiratory compromise. Attempted curative treatment is by surgical removal of the elodontoma and associated tooth but this is a technically challenging surgery and anaesthesia is often complicated by dyspnoea associated with nasal obstruction. Surgery involves removal of the overlying nasal or mandibular bone to access the elodontoma and enable complete removal. Dorsal rhinotomy, lateral rhinotomy, and transpalatal intraoral approach are options for maxillary incisor elodontomas (Mancinelli and Capello 2016). Approach chosen will depend on size and localisation of the lesion in the individual animal.

5.6.2 Skin Disease

Abnormalities of the skin or fur are frequently seen. Barbering or overgrooming (of self, or of companions) as a coping behaviour, related to psychological stress or pain is a common finding. Common factors in barbering are social isolation, lack of foraging opportunity, or a dysfunctional social group (Jekl et al. 2011c). In self-barbering cases the limbs and paws are most commonly affected, but in conspecific overgrooming the flanks and rump tend to be targeted (Figure 5.7). Dermatophytosis has been reported as an unusual cause of alopecia in degus (Jekl et al. 2011c) and it is assumed that, as with other hystricomorph rodents, *Trichophyton mentagrophytes* is the most common pathogen. It is worth noting that this species of dermatophyte does not fluoresce under a Wood's light and is a potential zoonosis (Donnelly et al. 2000). Lesions demonstrate broken hairs and hyperkeratosis, and are most frequently seen on the face. Primary bacterial or ectoparasitic dermatitis appears unusual (Jekl et al. 2011c) though *Demodex* and *Ornithonyssus bacoti* mites have both been reported in degus (Longley 2009; Jekl et al. 2011c). *O. bacoti* was noted to transfer to owners and cause skin lesions.

For cases of alopecia, a thorough husbandry review and clinical examination are necessary to identify causative factors, alongside microscopy of hair plucks and skin scrapes, with fungal culture carried out if there is clinical suspicion of dermatophytosis.

Conspecific injury is relatively common and secondary bacterial abscessation is sometimes seen, so antibiotic prophylaxis should be considered in bites that extend beyond the epidermis. Tail slip associated with improper handling or direct trauma to the tail is seen occasionally and necessitates tail amputation (Figures 5.8 and 5.9).

5.6.3 Hyperglycaemia and Cataract Formation

Degus demonstrate a reduced insulin receptor binding affinity and insulin activity equating to only 1–10% of that of non-hystricomorph mammals. Higher numbers of insulin receptors and higher circulating insulin levels help maintain blood glucose levels within similar ranges as those seen in domestic mammals and wild degus living on a low carbohydrate, high fibre diet rarely develop hyperglycaemia (Opazo et al. 2004). However, animals maintained

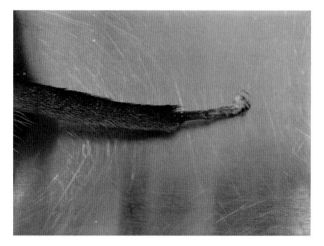

Figure 5.8 Degloving tail injury due to inappropriate handling.

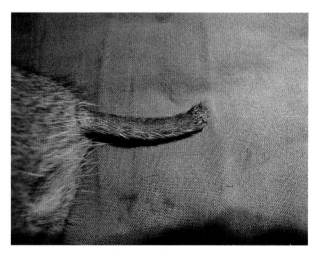

Figure 5.9 Appearance of tail after partial amputation. Note the intradermal sutures used to minimise patient interference.

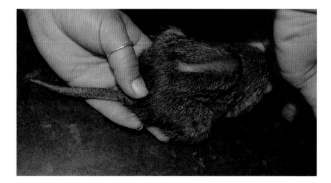

Figure 5.7 Alopecia due to over-grooming (barbering) by a companion.

in captivity with higher dietary carbohydrate levels, particularly presence of simple sugars, frequently develop episodic hyperglycaemia which is often incorrectly attributed to diabetes mellitus (Jekl et al. 2011c). It is believed that the inappropriate captive diet with the inherent reduced insulin activity gives a strong predisposition towards hyperglycaemia (Ardiles et al. 2013). Treatment in the majority of cases does not involve insulin as this is not a true diabetic status and dietary modification is the mainstay of therapy. Confoundingly, a diet high in sugar was fed to one population of degus over several weeks and resulted in neither cataracts nor glucosuria (Hommel 2012) suggesting that other factors are necessary to induce disease. Pancreatic pathology, including dietary-related pancreatitis, cytomegalovirus infection, and islet amyloidosis, is recognised as a common finding in degus and may influence individual susceptibility to hyperglycaemia (Fox and Murphy 1979; Spear et al. 1984; Westermark et al. 1990). Where pancreatic damage has been sustained, insulin therapy may be indicated if hyperglycaemia persists despite dietary correction but information on dosing is scant.

Degus demonstrate increased aldose reductase activity within the lens resulting in rapid accumulation of sorbitol during hyperglycaemia (Ardiles et al. 2013). The resulting osmotic changes cause movement of fluid into the lens, lens fibre degeneration, epithelial apoptosis, and cataract formation (Figure 5.10) (Pollreisz and Schmidt-Erfurth 2010). In one review, 13% of degus demonstrated cataracts on examination and secondary complications such as lens

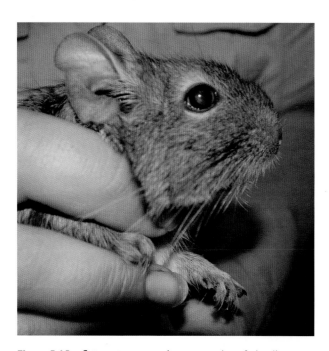

Figure 5.10 Cataract presence in a young degu fed a diet including high-sugar fruits.

luxation and uveitis were also seen (Jekl et al. 2011c). Cataracts are only noted after the period of hyperglycaemia and the only treatment option available is surgical removal but phacoemulsification techniques are limited by patient size. Treatment using an aldose reductase inhibitor has been shown to prevent cataract formation in degus (Datiles and Fukui 1989) and may be appropriate for degus with pancreatic pathology, but providing an appropriate diet remains the best way to avoid cataract formation.

5.6.4 Neoplasia

Neoplasia appears uncommon in degus with only scant case reports available. Wadsworth et al. (1982) state that hepatocellular carcinomas are relatively common but this is not reflected elsewhere with only two hepatomas, and two hepatocellular carcinomas reported (Murphy et al. 1980). Unfortunately many neoplasms have only been identified post-mortem due to the advanced stage of progression and these include a metastatic bronchoalveolar carcinoma, co-presentation of a transitional cell carcinoma and choristoma affecting one kidney (Anderson et al. 1990; Lester et al. 2005). Reproductive-tract tumours appear more common in females, with a uterine angioleiomyoma, vaginal leiyomyoma, and vaginal leiyomyosarcoma reported (Jakab et al. 2010; Skoric et al. 2010; Jekl et al. 2011a). A range of dermal tumours have been reported as isolated cases and include melanoma, myxosarcoma, and malignant histiocytoma (Jekl et al. 2011a). Further reports include a soft tissue sarcoma believed to be induced by a microchip, an oral fibrosarcoma, an abdominal lipoma, and a splenic haemangioma (Murphy et al. 1980; Pessier et al. 1999; Mans and Jekl 2016). Elodontomas have also been reported in degus (Jekl et al. 2008b) but these are a pseudoneoplastic condition and are discussed under dental pathology.

5.6.5 Renal Disease

Renal disease is common, with four cases reported in 300 animals in one review, and 13 cases in 68 animals in a post-mortem review (Cadillac et al. 2003; Jekl et al. 2011a). Causes are diverse and include nephrosis, pyelonephritis, glomerulonephritis, and chronic renal failure (Murphy et al. 1980; Cadillac et al. 2003). Unilateral polycystic renal changes with concurrent contralateral renal hypertrophy and interstitial nephritis have also been described in a single case report (Cadillac et al. 2003). On high calcium diets, degus excrete the excess renally so disease associated with urolith formation and crystalline 'sludge' would be expected as in other species that excrete calcium in a similar fashion, but these processes appear rare in degus.

5.6.6 Gastrointestinal Disease

As with other herbivores, an inappropriate diet, or insufficient fibre intake can result in ileus, gaseous bloat, soft faeces, and lack of ingestion of caecotrophs. Primary gastrointestinal disease appears rare. Treatment reflects that seen in rabbits and guinea pigs with assist feeding of a high fibre product, prokinetics, fluid therapy, and supportive care. As with all hind gut fermenters, only a limited number of antibiotics are suitable to be given orally in degus, and inappropriate medication can result in a severe enterotoxaemia.

5.6.7 Reproductive Pathology

Obstructive dystocia is relatively common due to large foetal size and requires caesarean section. This is carried out as for other mammals though the small size does make the surgery more challenging. Prolonged parturition carries a risk of subsequent haemometra and pyometra and ovariohysterectomy may be indicated in dystocia cases (Jekl et al. 2011a).

Penile prolapse is more common in hystricomorph rodents than other mammals and 12 cases in degus were reported by Jekl et al. (2011a). This syndrome is often attributed to accumulation of fur or other debris around the penile base preventing retraction, though trauma or infection may also be contributing factors. Surgical management of a recurrent case by debriding the preputial mucosa and apposing the edges of a section of the circumference to narrow the orifice has been described (Carrasco and Abou-Zahr 2015). This author has had success using a wedge resection as an alternative technique to narrow the preputial orifice.

5.6.8 Alzheimers-Like Disease

Older degus develop similar amyloid deposits within blood vessels and brain tissue as those seen in humans with Alzheimer's disease, and appear to develop similar cognitive deficits, anxiety, and altered circadian rhythms (Inestrosa et al. 2005; Castro-Fuentes and Socas-Pérez 2013). Significant amounts of amyloid-β-peptide deposits were found in blood vessel walls of three year old degus, and within the hippocampus of six year old degus (van Groen et al. 2011). Altered cognitive function in elderly degus is likely to relate to this phenomenon but therapeutic options are lacking currently.

5.6.9 Miscellaneous Conditions

Rhinitis is seen rarely as a primary process, but is often seen secondary to elodontoma or otitis media (Jekl et al. 2011a). Radiographs help with ascertaining the underlying pathology. Otitis media may also present with torticollis helping identify the primary site of infection.

Wild degus have been reported to be asymptomatic reservoirs of infection for *Trypanosoma cruzi*, the causative bacterium of Chagas disease (Campos et al. 2007).

5.7 Preventative Health Measures

Clinical endoparasitism appears very rare so the benefits of faecal screening in apparently healthy animals are negligible (Ward 2009). Even in animals with diarrhoea, one study found no evidence of endoparasites (Jekl et al. 2011a). As such routine testing of degus is not advisable and clinical examination (including dental assessment) and husbandry review on an annual basis is likely to be of greater benefit than laboratory evaluations.

5.7.1 Neutering Technique

Ovariohysterectomy is rarely carried out as a routine procedure in degus but has been described in management of pathology of the female reproductive tract. A ventral midline incision from the umbilicus to a point at the level of the centre of the ileal wings has been described for spaying a degu with foetal retention (Mancinelli et al. 2013). The intestinal tract is voluminous and gentle retraction of the caecum using moistened sterile cotton buds helps identify the uterus. The procedure is then carried out as for domestic mammals though use of ligating clips facilitates secure haemostasis of the ovarian pedicle and reduces surgical time. The cervix can be ligated with a transfixing ligature and all ligation sites should be carefully checked for haemorrhage prior to closure of the body wall, subcutaneous tissues and skin in three layers (Mancinelli et al. 2013). An intradermal pattern is preferred for the skin to limit patient interference with wound integrity.

Bilateral preputial incisions are most commonly used for castration. Gentle pressure on the caudal abdomen moves the testes into an inguinal position and incisions are made over each testis. Adipose tissue may be abundant and careful dissection is needed to visualise the testis. Once identified it can be exteriorised, the gubernaculum manually broken down and a closed technique used for castration. This technique has been associated with penile displacement in one case (Powers et al. 2008) but gentle tissue handling and incising directly over the testis should avoid this complication. Alternatively an abdominal approach can be utilised, with a single midline abdominal incision to access both testes within the abdomen. The caudal attachments are bluntly dissected and testes can be exteriorised and the spermatic cord ligated. The abdomen is closed in three layers as for ovariohysterectomy.

5.8 Radiographic Imaging

In all but collapsed animals sedation is needed for radiographic imaging.

The most common reason for imaging in practice is to assess dentition. Computed tomography is ideal for complete evaluation but radiography is more readily available. A series of radiographs, comprising laterolateral, right and left lateral oblique, and dorsoventral views is needed to evaluate incisors and cheek teeth adequately though superimposition of anatomic structures may still hamper identification of subtle lesions. A rostrocaudal view can be used to give further information on the nasal cavities, temporomandibular joint, and bullae (Mans and Jekl 2016). Imaging is imperative in any cases of dental disease to assess apical changes, to enable an accurate prognosis and to detect secondary changes such as elodontoma and apical infection.

Standard survey radiographs comprise right lateral thoracic and abdominal views and these give greater detail than dorsoventral views. For renal assessment, the gastrointestinal tract often overlies the kidneys and radiologically distinct lesions are uncommon so ultrasound is preferred (Reese and Hein 2009). Hyperechogenic areas on renal ultrasound have been correlated with nephrocalcinosis in degus (Gumpenberger et al. 2012).

Formulary

Medication	Dose	Dosing interval	Additional comments
Anaesthesia			
Buprenorphine	0.06 mg/kg IM		Given together as single injection, reversal of medetomidine with 0.5 mg/kg atipamezole
Midazolam	0.5 mg/kg IM		
Medetomidine	0.1 mg/kg IM		
Isoflurane	2–3% for maintenance		
Buprenorphine	0.03 mg/kg SC		Buprenorphine given 5 mins before midazolam and ketamine
Midazolam	1 mg/kg IM		
Ketamine	5 mg/kg IM		
Isoflurane	5% to induce, 2–3% for maintenance		(Calvo Carrasco and Abou-Zahr 2015)
Medetomidine	0.1–0.15 mg/kg IM		Reversed with atipamezole 0.5–0.75 mg/kg
Ketamine	5–7 mg/kg IM		(Gumpenberger et al. 2012)
Isoflurane	5% to induce, 1.5–3% for maintenance		Can cause breathholding (Record and Hargett Jr 1989)
Analgesia			
Buprenorphine	0.05–0.1 mg/kg SC	q6h	(Smith and Burgmann 1997)
Butorphanol	0.4–2.0 mg/kg SC	q 8–12 h	
Meloxicam	0.1–0.2 mg/kg PO, SC	q24h	
Carprofen	1–4 mg/kg PO	q12–24 h	(Johnson-Delaney 2006)
Antibiotics			
Long-acting penicillin G, benzathine/procaine combination	50 000 IU/kg SC	q3–5d	(Mans and Jekl 2006)
Enrofloxacin	10 mg/kg PO, IM, SC	q12–24 h	(Mans and Jekl 2016) Injections diluted 1:1 with saline to reduce potential for injection site necrosis
Metronidazole	10–20 mg/kg SC PO	q12h	(Morrisey and Carpenter 2012)
Doxycycline	2.5 mg/kg PO	q12h	(Johnson-Delaney 2008)
Trimethoprim/Sulfa	30 mg/kg PO	q12h	(Mans and Jekl 2006)

(Continued)

Medication	Dose	Dosing interval	Additional comments
Antiparasitics			
Fenbendazole	20–50 mg/kg PO	q 24 hr x 3 days; repeat in 14 days	For nematodes and cestodes
Ivermectin	0.2 mg/kg PO, SC	repeat in 14 days	For ectoparasites
Miscellaneous			
Ranitidine	5 mg/kg SC, IM, PO	q12h	Prokinetic of choice
Insulin (as Caninsulin)	1 U/animal SC	q24h	Based on chinchilla dose, can be gradually increased to effect. Should only be considered where hyperglycaemia persists on a suitable diet.

References

Anderson, W.I., Steinberg, H., and King, J.M. (1990). Bronchioloalveolar carcinoma with renal and hepatic metastases in a degu (*Octodon degus*). *Journal of Wildlife Diseases* 26 (1): 129–131.

Ardiles, A.O., Ewer, J., Acosta, M.L. et al. (2013). *Octodon degus* (Molina 1782): a model in comparative biology and biomedicine. *Cold Spring Harbor Protocols* 4: 312–318.

Bament, W. (2013). A VN's guide to degus: origins, natural behaviour, social activity and housing. VN Times, January 1.

Bozinovic, F., Gallardo, P.A., Visser, G.H. et al. (2003). Seasonal acclimatization in water flux rate, urine osmolality and kidney water channels in free-living degus: molecular mechanisms, physiological processes and ecological implications. *Journal of Experimental Biology* 206: 2959–2966.

Bozinovic, F., Novoa, F.F., and Sabat, P. (1997). Feeding and digesting fiber and tannins by an herbivorous rodent, *Octodon degus* (Rodentia: Caviomorpha). *Comparative Biochemistry and Physiology Part A: Physiology* 118 (3): 625–630.

Cadillac, J.M., Rush, H.G., and Sigler, R.E. (2003). Polycystic and chronic kidney disease in a young degu (*Octodon degus*). *Journal of the American Association for Laboratory Animal Science* 42 (2): 43–45.

Campos, R., Botto-Mahan, C., Ortiz, S. et al. (2007). *Trypanosoma cruzi* detection in blood by xenodiagnosis and polymerase chain reaction in the wild rodent *Octodon degus*. *The American Journal of Tropical Medicine and Hygiene* 76 (2): 324–326.

Carrasco, D.C. and Abou-Zahr, T. (2015). Surgical narrowing of the preputial orifice for treatment of recurrent penile prolapse in a degu (*Octodon degus*). *Veterinary Record Case Reports* 3 (1): e000223.

Castro-Fuentes, R. and Socas-Pérez, R. (2013). *Octodon degus*: a strong attractor for Alzheimer research. *Basic and Clinical Neuroscience* 4 (1): 91.

Colonnello, V., Iacobucci, P., Fuchs, T. et al. (2011). *Octodon degus*. A useful animal model for social-affective neuroscience research: basic description of separation distress, social attachments and play. *Neuroscience & Biobehavioral Reviews* 35 (9): 1854–1863.

Cortes, A., Zuleta, C., and Rosenmann, M. (1988). Comparative water economy of sympatric rodents in a Chilean semi-arid habitat. *Comparative Biochemistry and Physiology Part A: Physiology* 91 (4): 711–714.

Datiles, M.B. and Fukui, H. (1989). Cataract prevention in diabetic *Octodon degus* with Pfizer's sorbinil. *Current Eye Research* 8 (3): 233–237.

Donnelly, T.M., Rush, E.M., and Lackner, P.A. (2000). Ringworm in small exotic pets. *Seminars in Avian and Exotic Pet Medicine* 9 (2): 82–93.

Ebensperger, L.A., Hurtado, M.J., Soto-Gamboa, M. et al. (2004). Communal nesting and kinship in degus (*Octodon degus*). *Naturwissenschaften* 91 (8): 391–395.

Fox, J.G. and Murphy, J.C. (1979). Cytomegalic virus-associated insulitis in diabetic *Octodon degus*. *Veterinary Pathology* 16 (5): 625–628.

Fulk, G.W. (1976). Notes on the activity, reproduction, and social behavior of *Octodon degus*. *Journal of Mammalogy* 57 (3): 495–505.

van Groen, T., Kadish, I., Popović, N. et al. (2011). Age-related brain pathology in *Octodon degu*: blood vessel, white matter and Alzheimer-like pathology. *Neurobiology of Aging* 32 (9): 1651–1661.

Gumpenberger, M., Jeklova, E., Skoric, M. et al. (2012). Impact of a high-phosphorus diet on the sonographic and

CT appearance of kidneys in degus, and possible concurrence with dental problems. *Veterinary Record-English Edition* 170 (6): 153.

Gutiérrez, J.R. and Bozinovic, F. (1998). Diet selection in captivity by a generalist herbivorous rodent (*Octodon degus*) from the Chilean coastal desert. *Journal of Arid Environments* 39 (4): 601–607.

Hagen, K., Clauss, M., and Hatt, J.M. (2014). Drinking preferences in chinchillas (*Chinchilla laniger*), degus (*Octodon degu*) and guinea pigs (*Cavia porcellus*). *Journal of Animal Physiology and Animal Nutrition* 98 (5): 942–947.

Hommel, D. (2012). Untersuchungen an Degus (Octodon degus) zur Futter-und Wasseraufnahme sowie zur Verdaulichkeit von Nährstoffen bei Angebot unterschiedlicher Futtermittel. Doctoral dissertation. Bibliothek der Tierärztlichen Hochschule Hannover.

Inestrosa, N.C., Reyes, A.E., Chacon, M.A. et al. (2005). Human-like rodent amyloid-beta-peptide determines Alzheimer pathology in aged wild-type Octodon degu. *Neurobiology of Aging* 26: 1023–1028.

Jacobs, G.H., Calderone, J.B., Fenwick, J.A. et al. (2003). Visual adaptations in a diurnal rodent, *Octodon degus*. *Journal of Comparative Physiology A* 189 (5): 347–361.

Jakab, C., Rusvai, M., Biró, N. et al. (2010). Claudin-5-positive angioleiomyoma in the uterus of a degu (*Octodon degus*). *Acta Veterinaria Hungarica* 58 (3): 331–340.

Jekl, V., Hauptman, K., Jeklova, E. et al. (2005). Blood sampling from the cranial vena cava in the Norway rat (*Rattus norvegicus*). *Laboratory Animals* 39 (2): 236–239.

Jekl, V., Hauptman, K., and Knotek, Z. (2008a). Quantitative and qualitative assessments of intraoral lesions in 180 small herbivorous mammals. *The Veterinary Record* 162 (14): 442–449.

Jekl, V., Hauptman, K., Skoric, M. et al. (2008b). Elodontoma in a degu (*Octodon degus*). *Journal of Exotic Pet Medicine* 17 (3): 216–220.

Jekl, V., Gumpenberger, M., Jeklova, E. et al. (2011a). Impact of pelleted diets with different mineral compositions on the crown size of mandibular cheek teeth and mandibular relative density in degus (*Octodon degus*). *The Veterinary Record* 168 (24): 641.

Jekl, V., Hauptman, K., Jeklova, E. et al. (2011b). Selected haematological and plasma chemistry parameters in juvenile and adult degus (*Octodon degus*). *Veterinary Record-English Edition* 169 (3): 71.

Jekl, V., Hauptman, K., and Knotek, Z. (2011c). Diseases in pet degus: a retrospective study in 300 animals. *Journal of Small Animal Practice* 52 (2): 107–112.

Jekl, V., Zikmund, T., and Hauptman, K. (2016). Dyspnea in a degu (*Octodon degu*) associated with maxillary cheek teeth elongation. *Journal of Exotic Pet Medicine* 25 (2): 128–132.

Johnson-Delaney, C.A. (2006). Common procedures in hedgehogs, prairie dogs, exotic rodents, and companion marsupials. *Veterinary Clinics: Exotic Animal Practice* 9 (2): 415–435.

Johnson-Delaney, C.A. (2008). *Exotic Companion Medicine Handbook*. Lake Worth, FL: Zoological Education Network. Inc.

Lee, T.M. (2004). *Octodon degus*: a diurnal, social, and long-lived rodent. *ILAR Journal* 45 (1): 14–24.

Lester, P.A., Rush, H.G., and Sigler, R.E. (2005). Renal transitional cell carcinoma and choristoma in a degu (*Octodon degus*). *Journal of the American Association for Laboratory Animal Science* 44 (3): 41–44.

Long, C.V. (2012). Common dental disorders of the degu (*Octodon degus*). *Journal of Veterinary Dentistry* 29 (3): 158–165.

Longley, L. (2009). Rodents: dermatoses. In: *BSAVA Manual of Rodents and Ferrets*, 2e (eds. M. Keeble and M.A. Meredith), 107–122. Gloucester, UK: BSAVA.

Mancinelli, E. and Capello, V. (2016). Anatomy and disorders of the oral cavity of rat-like and squirrel-like rodents. *The Veterinary Clinics of North America. Exotic Animal Practice* 19 (3): 871–900.

Mancinelli, E., Eatwell, K., and Meredith, A. (2013). Successful management of a case of pregnancy failure in a degu (*Octodon degus*). *Journal of Exotic Pet Medicine* 22 (3): 293–300.

Mans, C. and Jekl, V. (2016). Anatomy and disorders of the oral cavity of chinchillas and degus. *Veterinary Clinics: Exotic Animal Practice* 19 (3): 843–869.

Morrisey, J.K. and Carpenter, J.W. (2012). Formulary. In: *Ferrets, Rabbits, and Rodents: Clinical Medicine and Surgery*, 3e (eds. K.E. Quesenbery and J.W. Carpenter), 566–575. St Louis: Elsevier.

Murphy, J.C., Corwell, T.P., Hewes, K.M. et al. (1980). Spontaneous lesions in the degu. In: *The Comparative Pathology of Zoo Animals* (eds. R.J. Montali and G. Migaki), 437–444. Washington, DC: Smithsonian Institution Press.

Okanoya, K., Tokimoto, N., Kumazawa, N. et al. (2008). Tool-use training in a species of rodent: the emergence of an optimal motor strategy and functional understanding. *PLoS One* 3: 1860.

Opazo, J.C., Soto-Gamboa, M., and Bozinovic, F. (2004). Blood glucose concentration in caviomorph rodents. *Comparative Biochemistry and Physiology Part A: Molecular & Integrative Physiology* 137 (1): 57–64.

Palacios, A.G. and Lee, T.M. (2013). Husbandry and breeding in the *Octodon degu* (Molina 1782). *Cold Spring Harbor Protocols* 2013 (4): 350–353.

Pessier, A.P., Stalis, I.H., and Sutherland-Smith, M. (1999). Soft tissue sarcomas associated with identification microchip implants in two small zoo animals. *Proceedings of the American Association of Zoo Veterinarians, Annual Meeting* 1999: 139–140.

Pollreisz, A. and Schmidt-Erfurth, U. (2010). Diabetic cataract – pathogenesis, epidemiology and treatment. *Journal of Ophthalmology* 2010: 608751.

Powers, M.Y., Campbell, B.G., and Finch, N.P. (2008). Preputial damage and lateral penile displacement during castration in a degu. *Journal of the American Veterinary Medical Association* 232 (7): 1013–1015.

Record, J.W. and Hargett Jr, C.E. (1989). Isoflurane Anesthesia in the Octodon degus (No. USAARL-89-23). Fort Rucker, AL: Army Aeromedical Research Laboratory.

Reese, S. and Hein, E. (2009). Abdomen. In: *Atlas der bildgebenden Diagnostik bei Heimtieren* (eds. M.E. Krautwald-Junghanns, M. Pees, S. Reese, et al.), 176–183. Hanover: Schlutersche Verlagsgesellschaft.

Reynolds, T.J. and Wright, J.W. (1979). Early postnatal physical and behavioural development of degus (*Octodon degus*). *Laboratory Animals* 13 (2): 93–100.

Sabat, P. and Bozinovic, F. (2008). Do changes in dietary chemistry during ontogeny affect digestive performance in adults of the herbivorous rodent *Octodon degus*? *Comparative Biochemistry and Physiology Part A: Molecular & Integrative Physiology* 151 (3): 455–460.

Skoric, M., Fictum, P., Jekl, V. et al. (2010). Vaginal leiomyosarcoma in a degu (*Octodon degus*): a case report. *Veterinární Medicína* 55 (8): 409–412.

Smith, D.A. and Burgmann, P.M. (1997). Formulary. In: *Ferrets, Rabbits and Rodents. Clinical Medicine and Surgery* (eds. E.V. Hillyer and K.E. Quesenberry), 392–404. Philadelphia: WB Saunders.

Spear, G.S., Caple, M.V., and Sutherland, L.R. (1984). The pancreas in the degu. *Experimental and Molecular Pathology* 40 (3): 295–310.

Tokimoto, N. and Okanoya, K. (2004). Spontaneous construction of "Chinese boxes" by Degus (Octodon degu): a rudiment of recursive intelligence? *Japanese Psychological Research* 46: 255–261.

Vásquez, R.A. (1997). Vigilance and social foraging in *Octodon degus* (Rodentia: Octodontidae) in central Chile. *Revista Chilena de Historia Natural* 70: 557–563.

Wadsworth, P.F., Jones, D.M., and Pugsley, S.L. (1982). Primary hepatic neoplasia in some captive wild mammals. *The Journal of Zoo Animal Medicine* 13 (1): 29–32.

Ward, M.L. (2009). Rodents: digestive system disorders. In: *BSAVA Manual of Rodents and Ferrets*, 2e (eds. M. Keeble and M.A. Meredith), 123–141. Gloucester, UK: BSAVA.

Westermark, P., Engström, U., Johnson, K.H. et al. (1990). Islet amyloid polypeptide: pinpointing amino acid residues linked to amyloid fibril formation. *Proceedings of the National Academy of Sciences* 87 (13): 5036–5040.

Wolf, P., Bucher, L., Zumbrock, B. et al. (2008). Daten zur Wasseraufnahme bei Kleinsäugern und deren Bedeutung für die Heimtierhaltung. *Kleintierpraxis* 7 (4): 217–223.

Woods, C.A. and Boraker, D.K. (1975). Octodon degus. *Mammalian Species* 67: 1–5.

6

Mongolian Gerbils
Marie Kubiak

6.1 Introduction

Mongolian gerbils (*Meriones unguiculatus*) originate from dry sandy grasslands of China, Mongolia, and Russia but are well established as companion animals worldwide (Figure 6.1). Duprasi, or fat-tail girds, (*Pachyuromys duprasi*) are also found in the gerbil subfamily and have broadly similar care, but this species is less frequently encountered. Mongolian gerbils' biological parameters are included in Table 6.1.

6.2 Husbandry

Gerbils are complex, social animals and stereotypies such as compulsive digging and cage bar chewing have been widely reported in laboratory gerbils. Lack of space, insufficient enrichment, lack of tunnelling opportunity, and poor cage design are highlighted as contributing factors and these deficiencies are also commonly present for pet animals (Figure 6.2) (Waiblinger and Konig 2004; Moons et al. 2012).

Gerbils live in mixed-sex family groups varying in size from 2 to 15 individuals that inhabit a defined territory (Zhou and Zhong 1989). In captivity, single-sex pairs or small groups, or groups of females and neutered males are recommended to allow normal social interactions to develop but to avoid unwanted breeding. Animals are best introduced at a young age, and keeping siblings together from weaning is ideal. It is important to use a neutral cage if introducing animals, as fighting and fatalities are more common in animals placed into an established territory (Norris and Adams 1972).

In the wild, they are active on the surface year round, but use underground burrows as nesting and retreat sites (Winkelmann and Getz 1962). Substrate is important in allowing captive gerbils to demonstrate normal digging behaviour. The creation of a network of interlinking tunnels and chambers provides ongoing stimulation, safe retreat from perceived threats and defined areas for food storage and nesting (Brunner 1993). Substrate should cover the entire base of the tank and be as deep as is feasible, ideally 70 cm or more. Soil, sand, paper or wood shaving substrates can be used, but where substrate isn't stable enough to retain tunnels, provision of artificial opaque burrows is necessary to avoid development of stereotypical behaviours (Wiedenmayer 1997). Tubes will need checking periodically as gerbils will chew at edges and may damage their structural integrity or create sharp points. Additional enrichment such as solid wheels, branches for chewing and cardboard boxes for hides and destruction will encourage activity and a range of behaviours (Figure 6.3).

The enclosure provided needs to retain substrate and resist chewing so glass tanks are commonly used, but ventilation can result in excessively high humidity or poor hygiene. A minimum floor area of 90 × 30 cm is advisable but larger areas should be provided where possible. Gerbils are arid adapted and produce dry faecal pellets and very little urine, resulting in enclosures only requiring cleaning out on a weekly basis.

Gerbils are best kept at 18–22 °C, so may need additional heating in colder climates. Sand baths should be provided to enable normal grooming and scent marking, and commercially available chinchilla sand is suitable.

The diet of wild gerbils is predominantly grass seeds for the majority of the year, but gerbils will readily feed on leaves and plant stems when these become abundant in the summer (Bannikov 1954; Pei et al. 2001). They will hoard seeds when these are numerous, and store them underground for winter when food is scarce. In captivity, dry pelleted diets for granivorous small mammals are available and are preferable to seed mixes. High protein (18–20%) and low fat (<4%) pelleted diets designed for gerbils, or other small granivorous rodents, alongside small quantities

Handbook of Exotic Pet Medicine, First Edition. Edited by Marie Kubiak.
© 2021 John Wiley & Sons Ltd. Published 2021 by John Wiley & Sons Ltd.
Companion website: www.wiley.com/go/kubiak/exotic_pet_medicine

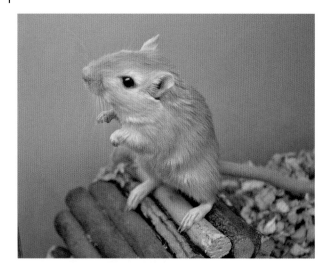

Figure 6.1   Standard agouti colouration of Mongolian gerbil.

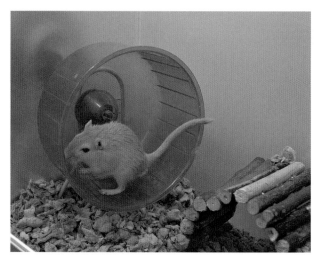

Figure 6.3   Gerbils will often readily use exercise wheels – Solid plastic wheels are preferred over fenestrated or wire wheels to avoided limb or tail injuries.

Table 6.1   Biological parameters.

	Female	Male
Adult weight	60–100 g	80–110 g
Longevity	2–4 years	2–4 years
Body temperature	38–39 °C	38–39 °C
Heart rate	160–480 /min	160–480 /min
Respiratory rate	75–125 /min	75–125 /min
Oestrus cycle	4–7 days	
Gestation	24–26 days[a]	
Litter size	1–7 (usually 4–6)	
Sexual maturity	70–84 days	63–84 days

[a] Implantation can be delayed resulting in an apparent increase in gestation length beyond the standard range.

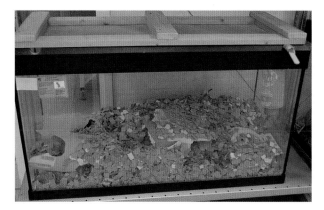

Figure 6.2   Traditional gerbil enclosures such as this one lack sufficient space, substrate depth and complexity to allow exhibition of normal behaviours.

of vegetables provided daily is ideal. The dry pellets can be scattered over the substrate to encourage foraging behaviour. Calorific requirements for this species approximate 40 kcal per 100 g bodyweight (Kanarek et al. 1977), and typically this equates to an intake of 8–10 g/per 100 g bodyweight daily (Benevenga et al. 1995). Coprophagy is not seen frequently in gerbils on a balanced diet.

Water intake in gerbils with free access is 4–7 ml/100 g per day but water deprivation is tolerated, with an initial weight reduction of up to 15% bodyweight, then stabilisation at this level using water obtained from nutrition alone with no apparent adverse effect (Winkelmann and Getz 1962; Harriman 1969). Ad lib water should be provided for captive gerbils.

6.3   Reproduction

Gerbils breed in spring and summer in the wild, producing two litters a year, but can breed year round in captivity. Crowding of animals or water deprivation suppresses reproductive potential (Hull et al. 1974; Yahr and Kessler 1975). Gerbils are often monogamous and will commonly form stable pairs within larger groups, however maintaining a single pair appears the most successful strategy for breeding (Hull et al. 1974; Liu et al. 2009). Females are polyoestrus spontaneous ovulators and also demonstrate a post-partum oestrus. Litter size tends to be 3–4, and mortality is reportedly higher in single pup litters (Elwood and Broom 1978). Juveniles remain with the family group, supporting their mother with care of new pups and show suppression of sexual maturity whilst remaining within the family group (Salo and French 1989). The breeding male aids in pup care, predominantly with nest building, grooming, social stimulation, and maintaining nest temperatures (Ahroon and Fidura 1976).

Gerbils are able to delay implantation of blastocysts when lactating, so gestation length can increase with the longest reported gestation being 48 days in a female nursing an exceptionally large litter of nine pups (Norris and Adams 1981).

6.4 Clinical Evaluation

6.4.1 History-Taking

Anamnesis is carried out in the same way as for other small mammals but should include detailed discussion of husbandry as well as social grouping and observed behaviours. Asking owners to bring in photographs of cages can aid in assessing cage suitability.

6.4.2 Handling

Gerbils are rarely aggressive but are easily startled and can move at speed. Gently picking up animals around the thorax with a paper towel or thin cloth aids in efficient capture and restraint whilst minimising potential for bites. Cupping docile individuals in a hand, or placing the second and third fingers either side of the neck with the hand wrapping round the body will allow examination. Scruff restraint can be utilised but is rarely necessary and is stressful for the patient. The tail should not be handled or used for restraint as degloving injuries can occur.

6.4.3 Sex Determination

Male gerbils have a markedly longer anogenital distance and mature males have a well-developed scrotum with large testes (Figure 6.4). The scrotum is pigmented in the gerbil and a well-developed ventral midline sebaceous scent gland is present. Females have a short anogenital distance, four pairs of mammary glands and a less pronounced ventral scent gland (Figure 6.5).

6.4.4 Clinical Examination

Observation of the gerbil in its cage should be carried out prior to handling. Demeanour, interaction with any other animals, coat and skin appearance, respiratory rate and effort, body condition, and response to a novel environment may be evaluated remotely.

Clinical examination may be limited in fractious animals. Gentle but firm restraint in a small cloth can enable visual

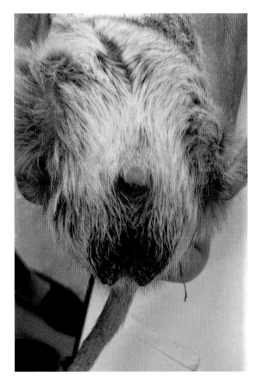

Figure 6.4 Male gerbil, note the prominent papilla and pigmented scrotum (*Source:* Photo courtesy of Jackie Clarke-Williams).

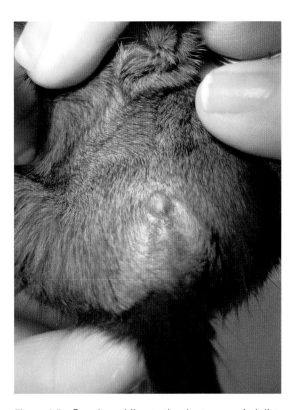

Figure 6.5 Female gerbil, note the short anogenital distance and presence of a urethral papilla that can be mistaken for a male prepuce.

evaluation of external surfaces, palpation, auscultation, and a basic orthopaedic examination. Commonly detected lesions include fur loss, masses present on abdominal palpation or scent gland evaluation, and inflammation around the nares.

6.5 Basic Techniques

6.5.1 Sample Collection

Urine can be obtained by housing the animal in a plastic container without substrate, voluntary voiding when an animal is restrained or on gentle palpation of the bladder, or by cystocentesis under anaesthesia. However, in gerbils, urine is passed in very small volumes hampering collection of adequate quantities. Small amounts of glucose may be present physiologically as a consequence of stress.

Faecal pellets are often passed in response to handling, or these can be retrieved from the latrine area of the enclosure.

Blood samples are often difficult to obtain from small rodents, due to difficulties in adequate restraint and small size of blood vessels and anaesthesia is typically needed to immobilise the patient for this procedure. The lateral tail veins in gerbils are small, and so samples are generally collected from the cranial vena cava or jugular veins under anaesthesia. Up to 1 ml/100 g body weight can be collected in a healthy animal, though acceptable sample size should be reduced by 50% in a debilitated patient.

For vena cava access, a 23–25G needle with 1 ml syringe or an insulin syringe is used. The anaesthetised patient is placed in dorsal recumbency and the needle is inserted 5–10 mm lateral to the manubrium, cranial to the clavicle and the first rib. The needle is advanced caudomedially, towards the contralateral hind leg. Negative pressure is applied to the syringe and the needle slowly advanced until blood begins to flow into the hub. Potential complications include venous laceration, inadvertent arterial puncture and intrathoracic haemorrhage though the procedure appears safe in animals with normal clotting capabilities and a gentle technique.

The jugular veins are accessed blind under anaesthesia, and are located on each side of the neck in a shallow groove running from the caudal border of the mandible to the thoracic inlet.

The femoral and saphenous veins can be used for small samples (<0.2 ml) and samples should be collected in capillary tubes following puncture (Hem et al. 1998; Perez-Garcia et al. 2003).

6.5.2 Nutritional Support

Nutritional support of anorexic patients is crucial to prevent gastrointestinal hypomotility. A baseline maintenance requirement energy intake of 33.2–36.4 kcal/100 g bodyweight has been identified in adult gerbils and this acts as a guide for nutritional requirements, though these often increase by 100% in sick animals (Harriman 1969; Wade and Bartness 1984). Nutritional support for anorexic animals typically consists of syringe feeding of a commercial herbivore/granivore diet to provide appropriate energy intake. Feeds of up 3 ml every 3–4 hours are possible in adult gerbils and amounts fed are modified based on twice daily weight monitoring. Nasogastric feeding tubes are rarely used due to poor patient tolerance of the external tubing, difficulties with maintaining patency of narrow tubes, and irritation at the nares.

6.5.3 Fluid Therapy

Fluids should be warmed to the body temperature of the patient before administration and fluids used in domestic species are suitable for use in rodents. Fluid deficits can be calculated based on weight loss or dehydration level but both of these may be hard to determine accurately and subjective estimation based on clinical appearance, including skin turgor, sunken eyes, and mucous membrane desiccation is commonly applied alongside monitoring of weight changes. Maintenance requirements in gerbils are 40–70 ml/kg/day (Johnson et al. 2016). These should be provided alongside replacement of losses.

For animals with 10% or more dehydration, fluids should be provided into the circulation if possible. Due to difficulties of venous access, intraosseous routes are typically used. Intraosseous catheters are most commonly placed in the tibial crest or the greater trochanter of the femur, under general anaesthesia and with ongoing analgesia. Constant infusion can be used but repeated bolus administration may be more practical in mobile patients.

The interscapular region is typically used for subcutaneous fluid administration in animals with less than 10% dehydration. Recommended maximum volume to be administered is 5 ml, but this can be repeated once absorption is complete.

6.5.4 Anaesthesia

Pre-anaesthetic fasting is not mandatory and indeed is often contraindicated in small rodents, however a brief period of 30 minutes food withdrawal prior to induction means that the oral cavity is clear of food debris. Inhalational anaesthesia with isoflurane alone is commonly used due to ready availability and fast induction and

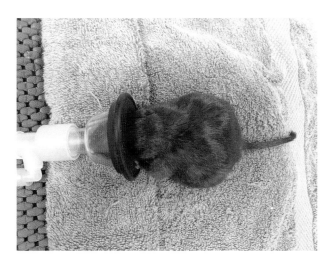

Figure 6.6 Pre-medication allows for rapid, calm induction of anaesthesia using volatile agents by face mask, with minimal restraint.

recovery times but restraint and administration of an irritant gaseous agent can be stressful for the patient. Manual restraint can be avoided by using a small animal face mask as an induction chamber, and sevoflurane and other less aversive volatile agents can be used instead of isoflurane to reduce negative effects. Where possible pre-medication is recommended to reduce induction duration and stress (Figure 6.6). Pre-medication will also aid in providing analgesia and to achieve a more predictable plane of anaesthesia for surgical procedures. Administration of injectable sedatives alone is unreliable in this species so a combination of injectable agent and volatile agent is preferred (Flecknell et al. 1983). Various combinations are highlighted in the formulary.

Oxygen should be administered to all sedated or anaesthetised patients and this is usually achieved by a nasal mask. Endotracheal intubation is possible but is technically challenging and narrows the effective airway significantly, necessitating ventilation (intermittently or continuously) to avoid occlusion of the tube by secretions.

Analgesia should be provided where any potential for pain exists to improve welfare, facilitate healing, and prevent self-trauma. Extrapolation of doses used in other small mammals is necessary as published data on analgesic agent doses and efficacy in this species is lacking.

6.5.5 Euthanasia

Anaesthesia followed by intracardiac injection of 100–200 mg/kg pentobarbitone is preferred, but intraperitoneal injection of 200–500 mg/kg pentobarbitone can also be used in an unconscious or anaesthetised animal. Injection of intracardiac or intraperitoneal pentobarbitone in a conscious

animal should be avoided. An overdose of inhalant anaesthesia is an alternative but can be prolonged. Physical trauma or carbon dioxide inhalation methods should be avoided.

6.5.6 Hospitalisation Requirements

Gerbils with bonds to conspecifics should be hospitalised with their partner/group. Although it is possible to separate bonded gerbils for up to 15 days without aggression on reintroduction (Norris and Adams 1972), it remains important to minimise stress experienced by the patient by providing a familiar companion and social stimulation. The home cage should be brought in if this is possible, to minimise disruption to the patient but in many cases cage size will hamper transport or housing within a hospital situation.

Alternatively basic rodent cages can be used in the hospital, with deep substrate, hide, food, and water provided. It is important to ensure cages are secure and escape is not possible. Providing an accessible opaque chamber within the substrate will reduce stress and aid regular capture of animals for assessment or treatment.

6.6 Common Medical and Surgical Conditions

6.6.1 Seizures

Spontaneous seizures are recognised as a phenomenon in the some gerbil strains. There appears to be an inherited predisposition which results in novel stimuli inducing seizures. Seizures are more common in predisposed gerbils that have been isolated from normal social contact and stimuli (Berg et al. 1975). Twitching of the ears and whiskers is followed by a tonic–clonic seizure which lasts for approximately 30 seconds (Thiessen et al. 1968). Central amines appear to be involved as manipulation of levels allows alteration of seizure frequency and severity (Cox and Lomax 1976). Seizures can be controlled medically using diphenyl hydantoin or reserpine (Thiessen et al. 1968). Most are managed simply by habituation to their environment and avoiding excessive excitation with a view to reducing rather than eliminating the seizures due to the lack of associated negative consequences. Due to inheritance, breeding from gerbils demonstrating seizure activity should be discouraged.

6.6.2 Neoplasia

Neoplasia appears common in gerbils, though the published literature provides contrasting estimates of incidence, from 1.6–38% (Meckley and Zwicker 1979; Rowe et al. 1974).

This variability may reflect differing study populations as neoplasia tends to occur in animals over two years of age, and more commonly affects female gerbils (Chen et al. 1992; Rembert et al. 2000). The skin, ovary and adrenal gland are the most common sites affected (Vincent et al. 1979).

The ventral scent gland within the skin is particularly commonly affected, with ulcerated, raised lesions seen grossly (Figures 6.7 and 6.8). Presentation is typically due to haemorrhage or focused grooming of the affected area noted by owners. Pathology is likely related to androgen-associated increased activity of the gland, with neoplasia occurring almost exclusively in mature males. Surgical removal is advisable in cases of scent gland masses or ulceration. An elliptical incision of the surrounding skin, with at least 2 mm margins around the gland is advised and histology of the removed gland is essential for identifying responsible pathology and determining prognosis (Deutschland et al. 2011). Squamous cell carcinoma, papilloma, benign hyperplasia, epithelioma, and poorly differentiated carcinomas have all been reported (Meckley and Zwicker 1979; Jackson et al. 1996; Deutschland et al. 2011). Surgical excision is curative in most cases, though recurrence and metastasis of malignant tumours has been identified. Where scent gland lesions are seen in young animals, these tend to be benign adenomas (Deutschland et al. 2011).

Other neoplasms involving the skin are less common and include poorly differentiated carcinomas, melanomas (commonly affecting the ear, foot, or tail base), sebaceous gland carcinoma, salivary gland carcinoma and squamous cell carcinoma (usually affecting the pinna) (Raflo and Diamond 1980; Toyoda et al. 2011; Fenton et al. 2016).

Reproductive tract neoplasia appears prevalent in female gerbils over two years of age, with ovarian tumours particularly common and comprising 60% of neoplasms in one study (Meckley and Zwicker 1979). Ovarian tumours include granulosa and theca cell tumours, leiomyoma, teratoma, papillary cystadenoma, and interstitial cell tumours (Figure 6.9). Uterine hemangiopericytoma, leiomyoma, and leiomyosarcoma have also been reported in gerbils (Rowe et al. 1974; Vincent and Ash 1978; Meckley and Zwicker 1979; Hong et al. 2009; Kubiak et al. 2015).

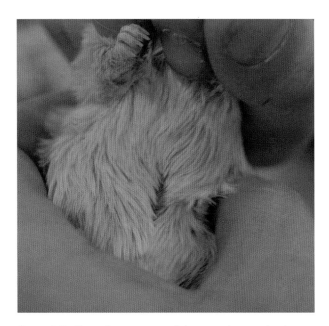

Figure 6.7 Normal appearance of the ventral scent gland.

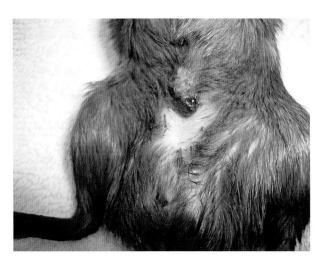

Figure 6.8 Ventral scent gland adenocarcinoma.

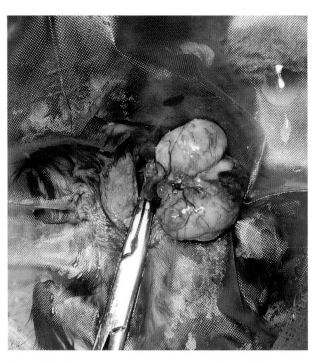

Figure 6.9 Ovariectomy to remove an interstitial cell tumour.

Helicobacter pylori has been shown to induce severe gastritis and gastric adenocarcinomas in experimentally infected gerbils but natural infection has not been reported (Watanabe et al. 1998).

A wide range of other neoplasms have been reported infrequently, commonly as single case reports and these include intracranial, adrenal, caecal, hepatic, and renal neoplasms, and one case of osteosarcoma (Vincent and Ash 1978; Meckley and Zwicker 1979; Guzmán-Silva et al. 1988; Salyards et al. 2013). Round cell neoplasms are uncommon with a single case each of cutaneous B cell lymphoma, leukemic lymphoblastic lymphoma and multifocal histiocytic sarcoma reported (Chen et al. 1992; Rembert et al. 2000; Su et al. 2001).

6.6.3 Alopecia

Ectoparasites are rare in gerbils but *Demodex meroni* and *Acarus farris* have been associated with clinical disease (Meredith 2010).

Barbering by a companion is common under stress conditions, resulting in broken or absent hairs. In these cases, removal of stressors and providing sufficient space and substrate for animals may help.

6.6.4 Nasal Dermatitis

The periocular Harderian gland opens onto the nictitating membrane and excretes porphyrins and pheromones for marking, contributes to the ocular tear film, produces lipids for thermoregulation, and is postulated to play a role in immune response and social grooming (Arrington and Ammerman 1969). However, excess accumulation of secretions is associated with facial dermatitis (Farrar et al. 1988). During periods of stress glandular activity increases and progressive alopecia and dermatitis develop in response to contact with the irritant secretions. Lesions start on the nose as secretions drain to the nares, and progress to contact sites of the face, forepaws, and abdomen. Secondary self-trauma and infection, particularly with Staphylococcal bacteria, are common and can be debilitating. High humidity, overcrowding, inappropriate substrate and lack of a dust bath have been postulated as significant contributing factors (Meredith 2010). Environmental corrections alongside systemic antibiotics for secondary infections are often sufficient to resolve lesions but severe cases may be associated with significant mortality.

6.6.5 Cholesteatoma

Aural cholesteatomas appear common in adult gerbils, with one study identifying 32 cases in 70 ears examined (Chole et al. 1981). These benign keratinised epithelial growths originate from the tympanic membrane or distal ear canal and expand to invade the middle ear causing progressive erosion of surrounding bone (Olszewska et al. 2004). Otitis may be a factor in cholesteatoma growth but bacterial flora present within cholesteatomas generally reflect normal flora of the ear suggesting infection is unlikely to cause these lesions (Fulghum and Chole 1985). Foreign material in the ear canal can act as an inducing factor but aetiopathogenesis remains poorly understood. Gerbils with cholesteatoma commonly present with a head tilt, aural discomfort, facial paralysis or discharge from the affected ear. Medical management with non-steroidal anti-inflammatories (and antimicrobials where indicated) can improve discomfort from secondary tissue inflammation but resolution is unlikely as the causative cholesteatomas are progressive and poorly accessible for surgical removal.

6.6.6 Renal Disease

Renal pathology is acknowledged to be common in gerbils though supporting information in the literature is scant. One retrospective study of a laboratory colony of gerbils identified a high level of chronic renal pathology in aged animals with interstitial necrosis, tubular necrosis, glomerulonephropathy, glomerulonephrosis, glomerular and tubular amyloidosis, hydronephrosis, nephrocalcinosis, pyelonephritis, and renal neoplasia all noted (Bingel 1995). Diagnosis of renal disease is similar to that of domestic species. Clinical signs include polyuria, polydipsia, dehydration, weight loss, reduced activity, and loss of appetite (Figure 6.10). A consistently low urine-specific gravity (<1.015) with increased serum urea (>31.3 mg/dl) and creatinine (>1.4 mg/dl) levels in a dehydrated animal is strongly indicative of renal compromise (Johnson-Delaney 1998; Jenkins 2008). Proteinuria and hypoalbuminaemia are also commonly found. Urine culture can be used to identify infectious contributors to disease. Treatment of renal disease

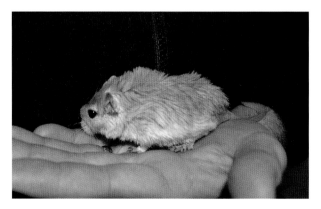

Figure 6.10 Weight loss, poor coat condition and lethargy in a gerbil with chronic renal failure. Polyuria was also noted and azotaemia was found on blood analysis.

is similar to other species though medication is used off licence with no pharmacokinetic or pharmacodynamic data.

6.6.7 Reproductive Disease

The incidence of ovarian cysts has been reported to be 47% in gerbils aged over 400 days (Norris and Adams 1972) and 73% in gerbils of 600–900 days of age (Adams 1970). Whilst unilateral ovarian cysts are more common, bilateral cysts are reported to occur in 33% of cases (Norris and Adams 1972). Cysts can be identified on abdominal palpation, with smooth spherical masses of 1 to 50 mm diameter present in the craniodorsal abdomen (Figure 6.11). Reproductive capabilities may be affected with litter size reduced, but affected animals typically present for abdominal swelling, discomfort, reduced activity, or dyspnoea. Confirmation is simple via ultrasound examination and percutaneous drainage can be carried out under sedation for short-term relief (and to facilitate surgery) but cysts tend to refill quickly (Lewis 2003). Ovariohysterectomy is the treatment of choice and is described under neutering.

6.6.8 Tail Injury

Gerbils should not be handled or restrained by the tail as the thin skin can separate from the underlying muscle and leave a painful bare tail which will dessicate and become necrotic. Tail slip necessitates amputation and this is carried out as for other mammals.

6.7 Preventative Health Measures

The pinworm *Dentostomella translucida* is present in apparently healthy gerbils but may have some effects on growth and immunocompetence. Faecal flotation identifies the ovoid eggs and fenbendazole is used for treatment (Wilkerson et al. 2001).

Infections with dwarf tapeworms, *Hymenolepis diminuta* and *Hymenolepis nana*, are reported in pet gerbils as causes of dehydration and mucoid diarrhoea (Vincent et al. 1975). *H. nana* has a direct life cycle and is potentially zoonotic, though is uncommon in temperate climes (Baily and Garcia 2014).

Faecal parasitology of new animals is recommended prior to introduction into a household.

6.7.1 Neutering Technique

Neutering of females is rarely carried out as a routine procedure. Surgery is typically planned in response to

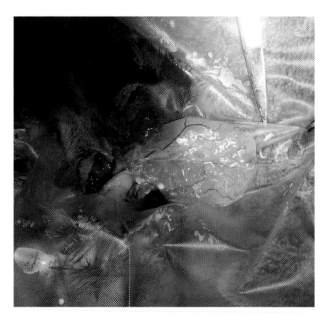

Figure 6.11 Unilateral ovarian cyst measuring 4 cm diameter, drained to facilitate exteriorisation for ovariectomy.

pathology such as ovarian cysts or neoplasia (Figures 6.9 and 6.11). A ventral paramedian incision is used to avoid the scent gland. The intestinal tract is displaced using moistened sterile cotton buds, and the uterine horns are identified. The procedure is carried out as for domestic mammals though ovarian access is limited by patient size, voluminous intestinal tract, and the short length of the ovarian pedicle. Use of small ligating clips is preferred over traditional ligation for haemostasis of the ovarian pedicle and this reduces surgical time and incision size. The cervix can be ligated with an encircling or transfixing ligature and all ligation sites should be carefully checked for haemorrhage prior to closure. The incision is closed with the body wall, subcutaneous tissues, and skin sutured as three separate layers (Olson and Bruce 1986). An intradermal pattern is preferred for the skin to limit patient interference with the wound post-operatively.

Routine neutering of males is uncommonly carried out but may be used to prevent breeding in a mixed sex group. An incision is made longitudinally over the tip of each testis and an open or closed technique can be used for castration. The author prefers a modified open technique. Here the tunic is also incised, the testicle exteriorised and a ligature placed around both the ductus deferens and pampiniform plexus, but not including the more proximal fat pad. The testicle is sharply dissected, the ligated stump and fat pad are then replaced into the scrotum, reducing potential for herniation. The tunic is closed using a cruciate suture of absorbable material and the scrotal skin closed with tissue glue or fine intradermal sutures.

6.8 Radiographic Imaging

Due to small patient size, high resolution or mammography film is preferred but detail may still be insufficient due to the rapid respiratory rate creating movement blur. Dental radiography units can also be used. Correct positioning of patients can be challenging due to their size. Rotation is common, and artefactual torsion of the vertebrae and superimposition of structures may result (Klaphake 2006).

Ultrasound is invaluable for confirming presence of ovarian cysts and guiding drainage for temporary relief.

Formulary

Medication	Dose	Dosing interval	Additional comments
Anaesthesia			
Medetomidine, Buprenorphine and Midazolam	0.1 mg/kg SC/IM (Me)		Used by the author for sedation, can be extended to surgical anaesthesia using volatile agents via face mask
	0.06 mg/kg SC/IM (Bu)		
	0.5 mg/kg SC/IM (Mi)		
Isoflurane	5% to induce, 1–3% for maintenance		Useful for critically ill patients, sevoflurane preferred where available
Medetomidine and Ketamine	0.5 mg/kg (Me) SC and 75 mg/kg (K) SC		(Johnson-Delaney 1999)
Fentanyl, fluanisone and midazolam	0.095 mg/kg (Fe); 3 mg/kg (Fl), 2 mg/kg (Mi) respectively SC		Fentanyl combinations may cause respiratory depression necessitating reversal with 0.1 mg/kg naloxone. Published doses of this combination used experimentally in gerbils for prolonged anaesthesia (Flecknell and Mitchell 1984) are higher than those stated here, but should be used with caution.
Analgesia			
Buprenorphine	0.1–0.2 mg/kg SC	q8h	(Harkness and Wagner 1995)
Butorphanol	1–5 mg/kg SC	q4h	(Heard 1993)
Meloxicam	0.2–1 mg/kg PO, SC	q24h	Based on doses for other rodents, no species-specific dose (Flecknell 2001; Deutschland et al. 2011)
Ketoprofen	5 mg/kg SC	q24h	(Pollock 2002)
Carprofen	5 mg/kg SC	q24h	(Pollock 2002)
Antibiotics			
Enrofloxacin	5–10 mg/kg IM, PO, SC	q12-24 h	Injections diluted 1:1 with saline to reduce potential for injection site necrosis (Adamcak and Otten, 2000; Morrisey and Carpenter 2004)
Trimethoprim-sulfa	30 mg/kg PO, SC	q12-24 h	(Rosskopf 2003)
Doxycycline	2.5 mg/kg PO	q12h	(Rosskopf 2003)
Gentamicin	10 mg/l drinking water or applied topically		For nasal dermatitis therapy (Donnelly 1997)

Dihydrostreptomycin and streptomycin are toxic in gerbils and should be avoided (Morris 1995)

Medication	Dose	Dosing interval	Additional comments
Antiparasitics			
Fenbendazole	20 mg/kg PO	q24h for 7 days	To treat Dentostomella infection (Wilkerson et al. 2001)
Amitraz	100 ppm topically	3–6 times at 2 wk intervals	For demodecosis (Meredith 2010)
Ivermectin	0.2–0.4 mg/kg PO, SC, topically	repeat at 14 and 28 days	For mite infestations (Meredith 2010)

References

Adamcak, A. and Otten, B. (2000). Rodent therapeutics. *Veterinary Clinics of North America: Exotic Animal Practice* 3 (1): 221–237.

Adams, C.E. (1970). Ageing and reproduction in the female mammal with particular reference to the rabbit. *Journal of Reproduction and Fertility* 12: 1–16.

Ahroon, J.K. and Fidura, F.G. (1976). The influence of the male on maternal behaviour in the Mongolian gerbil (*Meriones unguiculatus*). *Animal Behaviour* 24: 372–375.

Arrington, L.R. and Ammerman, C.B. (1969). Water requirements of gerbils. *Laboratory Animal Care* 19: 503–505.

Baily, G. and Garcia, H.H. (2014). Other cestode infections: intestinal cestodes, cysticercosis, other larval cestode infections. In: Manson's Tropical Infectious Diseases, 23e (eds. J.R. Farrar and P. Manson), 820–832. Philadelphia: W.B. Saunders.

Bannikov, A.G. (1954). The places inhabited and natural history of *Meriones unguiculatus*. In: Mammals of the Mongolian Peoples Republic, 410–415. Moscow: USSR Academy of Sciences.

Benevenga, N.J., Calvert, C., Eckhert, C.D. et al. (1995). Nutrient requirements of the gerbil. In: Nutrient Requirements of Laboratory Animals, 140–143. Washington, DC: National Academy Press.

Berg, R.A., Shanin, R.D., and Hull, E.M. (1975). Early isolation in the gerbil (*Meriones unguiculatus*): behavioral and physiological effects. *Physiological Psychology* 3 (1): 35–38.

Bingel, S.A. (1995). Pathologic findings in an aging Mongolian gerbil (*Meriones unguiculatus*) colony. *Laboratory Animal Science* 45: 597–600.

Brunner, C. (1993). The digging behaviour in the Mongolian Gerbil (Meriones unguiculatus) in a semi-natural enclosure. Masters thesis. Zoologisches Institut, Universität Zürich, Switzerland.

Chen, H.C., Slone, T.W. Jr., and Frith, C.H. (1992). Histiocytic sarcoma in an aging gerbil. *Toxicologic Pathology* 20 (2): 260–263.

Chole, R.A., Henry, K.R., and McGinn, M.D. (1981). Cholesteatoma: spontaneous occurrence in the Mongolian gerbil *Meriones unguiculatis*. *Otology and Neurotology* 2 (3): 204–210.

Cox, B. and Lomax, P. (1976). Brain amines and spontaneous epileptic seizures in the Mongolian gerbil. *Pharmacology Biochemistry and Behavior* 4 (3): 263–267.

Deutschland, M., Denk, D., Skerritt, G. et al. (2011). Surgical excision and morphological evaluation of altered abdominal scent glands in Mongolian gerbils (*Meriones unguiculatus*). *Veterinary Record* 169 (24): 636.

Donnelly, T. (1997). Nasal lesions in gerbils. *Laboratory Animals* (February): 17–18.

Elwood, R.W. and Broom, D.M. (1978). The influence of litter size and parental behaviour on the development of Mongolian gerbil pups. *Animal Behaviour* 26: 438–454.

Farrar, P.L., Opsomer, M.J., Kocen, J.A. et al. (1988). Experimental nasal dermatitis in the Mongolian gerbil: effect of bilateral Harderian gland adenectomy on development of facial lesions. *Laboratory Animal Science* 38 (1): 72–76.

Fenton, H., Forzán, M.J., Desmarchelier, M. et al. (2016). Poorly differentiated cutaneous carcinoma of non-sebaceous origin in a 3-year-old Mongolian gerbil (*Meriones unguiculatus*). *The Canadian Veterinary Journal* 57 (1): 80.

Flecknell, P.A. (2001). Analgesia of small mammals. *The Veterinary Clinics of North America. Exotic Animal Practice* 4: 47–56.

Flecknell, P.A. and Mitchell, M. (1984). Midazolam and fentanyl-fluanisone: assessment of anaesthetic effects in laboratory rodents and rabbits. *Laboratory Animals* 18 (2): 143–146.

Flecknell, P.A., John, M., Mitchell, M. et al. (1983). Injectable anaesthetic techniques in 2 species of gerbil (*Meriones libycus* and *Meriones unguiculatus*). *Laboratory Animals* 17 (2): 118–122.

Fulghum, R.S. and Chole, R.A. (1985). Bacterial flora in spontaneously occurring aural cholesteatomas in Mongolian gerbils. *Infection and Immunity* 50 (3): 678–681.

Guzmán-Silva, M.A., Rossi, M.I.D., and Guimarães, J.S.P. (1988). Craniopharyngioma in the Mongolian gerbil (*Meriones unguiculatus*): case report. *Laboratory Animals* 22 (4): 365–368.

Harkness, J.E. and Wagner, J.E. (1995). The Biology and Medicine of Rabbits and Rodents, 4e. York, PA: Williams and Wilkins.

Harriman, A.E. (1969). Food and water requirements of Mongolian gerbils as determined through self-selection of diet. *American Midland Naturalist* 82 (1): 149–156.

Heard, D. (1993). Principles and techniques of analgesia and anaesthesia for exotic practice. *Veterinary Clinics of North America: Small Animal Practice* 23: 1301–1327.

Hem, A., Smith, A.J., and Solberg, P. (1998). Saphenous vein puncture for blood sampling of the mouse, rat, hamster, gerbil, guineapig, ferret and mink. *Laboratory Animals* 32 (4): 364–368.

Hong, S., Lee, H.A., Song, J. et al. (2009). A spontaneous uterine Leiomyosarcoma in an aged Mongolian gerbil (*Meriones unguiculatus*). *Laboratory Animal Research* 25 (1): 65–67.

Hull, E.M., Chapin, E., and Kastaniotis, C. (1974). Effects of crowding and intermittent isolation on gerbils (*Meriones unguiculatus*). *Physiology and Behavior* 13 (6): 723–727.

Jackson, T.A., Heath, L.A., Hulin, M.S. et al. (1996). Squamous cell carcinoma of the midventral abdominal pad in three gerbils. *Journal of the American Veterinary Medical Association* 209 (4): 789–791.

Jenkins, J.R. (2008). Rodent diagnostic testing. *Journal of Exotic Pet Medicine* 17 (1): 16–25.

Johnson, J.G., Brandao, J., Perry, S.M. et al. (2016). Urinary system. In: Current Therapy in Exotic Pet Practice (eds. M.A. Mitchell and T.N. Tully Jr.), 536. St. Louis, MO: Elsevier Health Sciences.

Johnson-Delaney, C.A. (1998). Diseases of the urinary system of commonly kept rodents: diagnosis and treatment. *Seminars in Avian and Exotic Pet Medicine* 7 (2): 81–88.

Johnson-Delaney, C.A. (1999). Post-operative care of small mammals. *Exotic DVM* 1 (5): 19–21.

Kanarek, R.B., Ogilby, J.D., and Mayer, J. (1977). Effects of dietary caloric density on feeding behavior in Mongolian gerbils (*Meriones unguiculatus*). *Physiology and Behavior* 19 (4): 497–501.

Klaphake, E. (2006). Common rodent procedures. *Veterinary Clinics of North America: Exotic Animal Practice* 9 (2): 389–413.

Kubiak, M., Jayson, S.L., and Denk, D. (2015). Ovarian interstitial cell tumour in a Mongolian gerbil (*Meriones unguiculatus*). *Veterinary Record Case Reports* 3 (1): e000182.

Lewis, W. (2003). Cystic ovaries in gerbils. *Exotic DVM* 5 (1): 12–13.

Liu, W., Wang, G., Wang, Y. et al. (2009). Population ecology of wild Mongolian gerbils *Meriones unguiculatus*. *Journal of Mammalogy* 90 (4): 832–840.

Meckley, P.E. and Zwicker, G.M. (1979). Naturally-occurring neoplasms in the Mongolian gerbil, *Meriones unguiculatus*. *Laboratory Animals* 13 (3): 203–206.

Meredith, A. (2010). Skin diseases of rodents. *In Practice* 32 (1): 16.

Moons, C.P., Breugelmans, S., Cassiman, N. et al. (2012). The effect of different working definitions on behavioral research involving stereotypies in Mongolian gerbils (*Meriones unguiculatus*). *Journal of the American Association for Laboratory Animal Science* 51 (2): 170–176.

Morris, T.H. (1995). Antibiotic therapeutics in laboratory animals. *Laboratory Animals* 29 (1): 16–36.

Morrisey, J.K. and Carpenter, J.W. (2004). Formulary. In: Ferrets, Rabbits and Rodents: Clinical Medicine and Surgery, 2e (eds. K.E. Quesenberry and J.W. Carpenter), 436–444. St. Louis: WB Saunders.

Norris, M.L. and Adams, C.E. (1972). Incidence of cystic ovaries and reproductive performance in the Mongolian gerbil, *Meriones unguiculatus*. *Laboratory Animals* 6 (3): 337–342.

Norris, M.L. and Adams, C.E. (1981). Mating post partum and length of gestation in the Mongolian gerbil (*Meriones unguiculatus*). *Laboratory Animals* 15 (2): 189–191.

Olson, M.E. and Bruce, J. (1986). Ovariectomy, ovariohysterectomy and orchidectomy in rodents and rabbits. *The Canadian Veterinary Journal* 27 (12): 523.

Olszewska, E., Wagner, M., Bernal-Sprekelsen, M. et al. (2004). Etiopathogenesis of cholesteatoma. *European Archives of Oto-Rhino-Laryngology and Head and Neck* 261 (1): 6–24.

Pei, Y.X., Wang, D.H., and Hume, I.D. (2001). Effects of dietary fibre on digesta passage, nutrient digestibility, and gastrointestinal tract morphology in the granivorous Mongolian gerbil (*Meriones unguiculatus*). *Physiological and Biochemical Zoology* 74 (5): 742–749.

Perez-Garcia, C.C., Pena-Penabad, M., Cano-Rabano, M.J. et al. (2003). A simple procedure to perform intravenous injections in the Mongolian gerbil (*Meriones unguiculatus*). *Laboratory Animals* 37 (1): 68–71.

Pollock, C. (2002). Post-operative management of the exotic animal patient. *The Veterinary Clinics of North America. Exotic Animal Practice* 5: 183–212.

Raflo, C.P. and Diamond, S.S. (1980). Metastatic squamous-cell carcinoma in a gerbil (*Meriones unguiculatus*). *Laboratory Animals* 14 (3): 237–239.

Rembert, M.S., Coleman, S.U., Klei, T.R. et al. (2000). Neoplastic mass in an experimental Mongolian gerbil. *Journal of the American Association for Laboratory Animal Science* 39 (3): 34–36.

Rosskopf, W.J. (2003). Drug dosages for small rodents. Proceedings of the Atlantic Coast Veterinary Conference. Atlantic City. Atlantic Coast Veterinary Conference, Springfield, NJ.

Rowe, S.E., Simmons, J.L., Ringler, D.H. et al. (1974). Spontaneous neoplasms in aging Gerbillinae. A summary of forty-four neoplasms. *Veterinary Pathology* 11 (1): 38–51.

Salo, A.L. and French, J.A. (1989). Early experience, reproductive success, and development of parental behaviour in Mongolian gerbils. *Animal Behaviour* 38 (4): 693–702.

Salyards, G.W., Blas-Machado, U., Mishra, S. et al. (2013). Spontaneous osteoblastic osteosarcoma in a Mongolian gerbil (*Meriones unguiculatus*). *Comparative Medicine* 63 (1): 62–66.

Su, Y.C., Wang, M.H., and Wu, M.F. (2001). Cutaneous B cell lymphoma in a Mongolian gerbil (*Meriones unguiculatus*). *Journal of the American Association for Laboratory Animal Science* 40 (5): 53–56.

Thiessen, D.D., Lindzey, G., and Friend, H.C. (1968). Spontaneous seizures in the Mongolian gerbil (*Meriones unguiculatus*). *Psychonomic Science* 11 (7): 227–228.

Toyoda, T., Tsukamoto, T., Cho, Y.M. et al. (2011). Undifferentiated sarcoma of the salivary gland in a Mongolian gerbil (*Meriones unguiculatus*). *Journal of Toxicologic Pathology* 24 (3): 173–177.

Vincent, A.L. and Ash, L.R. (1978). Further observations on spontaneous neoplasms in the Mongolian gerbil, *Meriones unguiculatus*. *Laboratory Animal Science* 28 (3): 297–300.

Vincent, A.L., Porter, D.D., and Ash, L.R. (1975). Spontaneous lesions and parasites of the Mongolian gerbil, *Meriones unguiculatus*. *Laboratory Animal Science* 25 (6): 711–722.

Vincent, A.L., Rodrick, G.E., and Sodeman, W.A. Jr. (1979). The pathology of the Mongolian gerbil (*Meriones unguiculatus*): a review. *Laboratory Animal Science* 29 (5): 645–651.

Wade, G.N. and Bartness, T.J. (1984). Effects of photoperiod and gonadectomy on food intake, body weight, and body composition in Siberian hamsters. *American Journal of Physiology. Regulatory, Integrative and Comparative Physiology* 246 (1): R26–R30.

Waiblinger, E. and Konig, B. (2004). Refinement of gerbil housing and husbandry in the laboratory. *ATLA, Alternatives to Laboratory Animals* 32: 163–169.

Watanabe, T., Tada, M., Nagai, H. et al. (1998). *Helicobacter pylori* infection induces gastric cancer in Mongolian gerbils. *Gastroenterology* 115 (3): 642–648.

Wiedenmayer, C. (1997). Causation of the ontogenetic development of stereotypic digging in gerbils. *Animal Behaviour* 53 (3): 461–470.

Wilkerson, J.D., Brooks, D.L., Derby, M. et al. (2001). Comparison of practical treatment methods to eradicate pinworm (*Dentostomella translucida*) infections from Mongolian gerbils (*Meroines unguiculatus*). *Journal of the American Association for Laboratory Animal Science* 40 (5): 31–36.

Winkelmann, J.R. and Getz, L.L. (1962). Water balance in the Mongolian gerbil. *Journal of Mammalogy* 43 (2): 150–154.

Yahr, P. and Kessler, S. (1975). Suppression of reproduction in water-deprived Mongolian gerbils (*Meriones unguiculatus*). *Biology of Reproduction* 12 (2): 249–254.

Zhou, Q. and Zhong, W. (1989). Ecology and social behaviour of Mongolian gerbils, *Meriones unguiculatus*, at Xilinhot, Inner Mongolia, China. *Animal Behaviour* 37: 11–27.

7

Hamsters

Marie Kubiak

7.1 Introduction

Hamsters are commonly kept as children's pets and although there are approximately 24 different species, only five are established pets. Of these the Syrian or golden hamster (*Mesocricetus auratus*) and dwarf hamsters (*Phodopus sungorus, Phodopus campbelli* and *Phodopus roborowskii*) are popular whereas the Chinese hamster (*Cricetulus griseus*) is less frequently kept (Kondo et al. 2008). Biological parameters for these species are included in Table 7.1 and visual differentiation of species is detailed in Table 7.2.

The majority of published information relates to the Syrian hamster with extrapolation of findings across species and this is reflected in the content of this chapter. Where known differences exist in other species this is highlighted.

7.2 Husbandry

These small rodent species are often kept as children's pets and although small and unobtrusive, they have more complex management than is often appreciated.

Syrian and Chinese hamsters are solitary and adults should not be kept in groups. Dwarf hamsters are more social and can be kept in small groups, and housing same sex siblings from weaning tends to work well. Unrelated animals can be introduced by housing in an adjacent enclosure and swapping bedding to familiarise scents prior to introduction, but this is often unsuccessful and fighting frequently results on mixing animals.

All common species are nocturnal, so cages should not be placed in busy household areas that are likely to disrupt their daytime resting. A huge variety of hamster cages are available in pet shops, and the cage chosen should be appropriate for the species of hamster – for example dwarf species may be able to escape between cage bars that would

be suitable for a Syrian hamster. Cages should be as large as is possible as these are very active, inquisitive species that naturally inhabit large territories. Evidence suggests that a floor area of at least $1\,m^2$ is needed avoid welfare compromise, with hamsters in smaller cages showing abnormal behaviours (Fischer et al. 2007). These include cage bar chewing, as well as frequently climbing and utilising the walls and roof of the enclosure since floor space is insufficient. Climbing and burrowing opportunities, and exercise wheels are readily accepted by hamsters, as are exercise balls for use outside of the cage, but all enrichment devices must be safe and secure. Hamsters also appreciate sand baths and these can aid in grooming as well as enrichment (Fischer et al. 2007).

Separate toilet, sleeping, and feeding areas should be provided, and multilevel cages allow for good separation of these regions. The sleeping area is usually a solid or fabric enclosed area, filled with paper or natural cloth-based substrate. Use of synthetic or loose fibres as substrate risks entanglement injury to limbs or digits, or impaction of cheek pouches (Keeble 2009). The main enclosure can be filled with fine paper or wood shaving substrate and chosen latrine areas are well defined enabling easy daily cleaning of the chosen area. Wild Syrian hamsters live in subterranean burrow systems 0.5 m below the ground and substrate is an area often neglected in captivity. Lack of sufficient substrate appears to be associated with welfare compromise, demonstrated as stereotypies, aggression, and reduced food intake (Hauzenberger et al. 2006). Provision of deep substrate (over 40 cm depth) results in burrows similar to those created in the wild and more natural behaviours (Hauzenberger et al. 2006). This may be a challenge to achieve with typical cages but in most interconnected systems a chamber can be added that can be filled with substrate, or the cage base replaced by a deep plastic or glass tank filled with substrate.

Handbook of Exotic Pet Medicine, First Edition. Edited by Marie Kubiak.
© 2021 John Wiley & Sons Ltd. Published 2021 by John Wiley & Sons Ltd.
Companion website: www.wiley.com/go/kubiak/exotic_pet_medicine

Table 7.1 Biological parameters of commonly kept hamster species (NR = no reported value).

	Syrian hamster	Campbell's hamster	Roborowski hamster	Siberian/ Djungarian hamster	Chinese hamster
Adult weight (g)	100–180	20–35	20–25	25–45	30–45
Longevity (years)	2–2.5	1.5–2	3–3.5	1.5–2	2–2.5
Body temperature (°C)	37–38	NR	NR	NR	37–38
Heart rate (/min)	275–450	NR	NR	NR	275–425
Respiratory rate (/min)	60–250	NR	NR	NR	70–180
Oestrus cycle (days)	4	4	4–6	4	4–5
Gestation (days)	15–18	18–20	20–22	18–25	18–21
Litter size	3–12 (typically 4–6)	1–9 (7–8)	3–9 (6)	1–9 (4–6)	(4–6)
Sexual maturity	40–70 days (female) 70–100 days (male)	from 30 days, typically 60 days for females	from 30 days	from 30 days	from 30 days

Table 7.2 Visual differentiation of hamster species.

	Size	Colour of normal variety (mutations vary)	Dorsal stripe	Scent glands	Distinctive features
Syrian hamster (*Mesocricetus auratus*) (Figure 7.1)	Large	Golden brown	Absent	Paired flank glands	Much larger than dwarf species
Campbells hamster (*Phodopus campbelli*)	Small	Grey brown, pale grey ventrum	Present	Ventral abdominal gland	Smaller ears than Djungarian, do not turn white in winter
Roborovski hamster (*Phodopus roborowskii*) (Figure 7.2)	Small	Sandy brown	Absent	Ventral abdominal gland	White spots above eyes
Russian/Siberian/Djungarian/ winter white hamster (*Phodopus sungorus*) (Figure 7.3)	Small	Grey brown, white ventrum	Present	Ventral abdominal gland	Dark spot on head, 0.5–1.5 cm tail. May turn grey/white in winter
Chinese hamster (*Cricetulus griseus*)	Small	Brown	Present	Ventral abdominal gland	Longer, thinner body shape, 3–4 cm prehensile tail

Hamsters cope well at room temperatures but most species will exhibit torpor if kept below 5 °C (Sonoyama et al. 2009). This torpor is an adaptation to cold conditions, and is interspersed with sporadic activity where normal body temperature is re-established and feeding occurs using stashed food. Syrian hamsters show approximately four day cycles of inactivity followed by a short period of activity, whereas Djungorian hamsters have a shorter torpor period of four to eight hours and photoperiod and food availability appear a bigger stimulus than reduced temperature (Ruf et al. 1991; Sonoyama et al. 2009). When presented with a non-responsive hamster, torpor is a differential and so rectal temperature measurement is important to differentiate physiological changes in activity from advanced illness. Siberian hamsters in torpor typically have a temperature of less than 25 °C (Heldmaier and Steinlechner 1981). True hibernation with prolonged inactivity is not seen in hamsters.

Hamsters feed on seeds, fruits, grasses, leaves, and insects but can tolerate reductions in protein availability due to foregut fermentation in their partially compartmentalised stomach (Grant 2014). Hindgut fermentation also occurs and coprophagy is common, to maximise the nutritional benefits of hindgut microbe activity (Benevenga et al. 1995; Grant 2014). Syrian hamsters will eat 10–14 g of food daily and this is best provided as a pelleted hamster diet with small quantities of fresh high-fibre, low-sugar vegetables (Grant 2014). Muesli type mixtures result in selective feeding and an imbalanced diet. Food is taken into the extensive cheek pouches and is eaten once the hamster has retreated to a safe enclosed area. Hamsters will also hoard food so substrate should be kept dry and food stashes checked daily for evidence of spoilage. Providing non-toxic, clean branches helps with incisor wear, provides enrichment and gives an additional source of fibre.

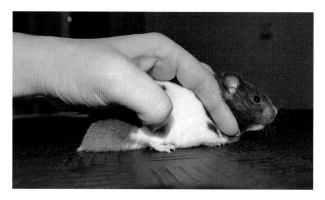

Figure 7.1 Syrian hamster restrained on table prior to examination.

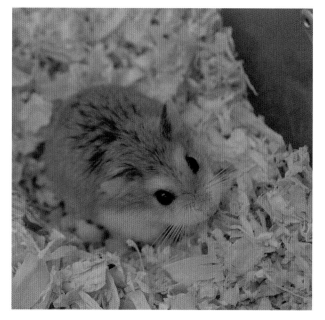

Figure 7.2 Roborovski hamster with characteristic pale fur over eyes.

Syrian hamsters drink 5–15 ml of water per 100 g bodyweight daily, with females drinking significantly more than males (Fitts and St. Dennis 1981). Other hamster species appear to show less variation in intake between the sexes (Thompson 1971). Free access to water should be provided, from a sipper bottle that is cleaned and checked daily.

7.3 Reproduction

Hamsters are spontaneous ovulators, with a defined breeding season. They respond to photoperiod, with long days inducing reproductive activity in wild individuals and breeding occurring in Spring and Summer (Pévet 1988). The 8–22 hours oestrus commonly occurs overnight so introducing the female to the male in the evening for four consecutive nights gives a good chance of successful breeding. If aggression is seen the female should be removed, but when in oestrus the female is receptive to the male and they can be left together to mate. There is no delayed implantation in hamsters (Pratt and Lisk 1989). The female will create the nest and rear the pups without male involvement. Interference with the nest, including for cleaning, should be avoided for the first two weeks after birth as cannibalism of neonates may result from disturbance. Juveniles will wean at two to three weeks and sexes should be separated before sexual maturity to prevent inbreeding.

7.4 Clinical Evaluation

7.4.1 History-Taking

Anamnesis is carried out in the same way as for other small mammals but should include detailed discussion of husbandry and diet. Owners will often transport the animal in all or part of the home cage, allowing assessment of suitability of the set-up. Where this is not possible, owners should be encouraged to bring photographs of the enclosure provided.

7.4.2 Handling

Hamster temperament varies, and those that are not regularly handled and socialised may resent being restrained. All hamster species can inflict painful bites with their incisor teeth. Syrian hamsters are more likely to react aggressively if disturbed when asleep so should be gently roused before handling. Picking up animals by encircling the thorax with a paper towel or thin cloth allows for gentle handling whilst giving some protection against bites. Placing the second and third fingers either side of the neck with the hand wrapping round the body will allow for restraint and examination (Figure 7.1). Scruff restraint should be avoided as this risks exophthalmos in the hamster, but if absolutely necessary the large quantity of loose skin along the neck and back should be gripped to enable secure restraint (Orcutt 2005).

7.4.3 Sex Determination

Females have a short anogenital distance and six or seven paired mammary glands (Figure 7.4). Males have a longer anogenital distance and testes are large and caudally located (Figure 7.5). It is not uncommon for owners to present animals for evaluation due to misinterpretation of testes as abnormal masses.

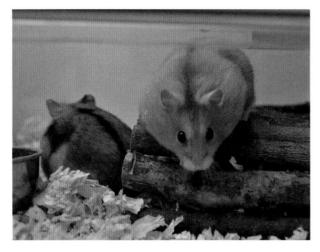

Figure 7.3 Russian hamster, note the prominent dorsal stripe.

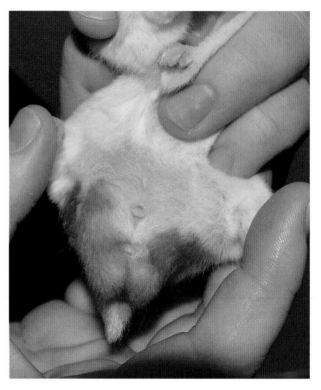

Figure 7.5 Male Syrian hamster with longer anogenital distance and prominent testes.

7.5 Basic Techniques

7.5.1 Sample Collection

Urine can be obtained by housing the animal in a plastic container without substrate, or is often voided when an animal is restrained or the bladder is palpated. Where collection requires a sterile sample, anaesthesia and cystocentesis is necessary, preferably under ultrasound guidance. Urine specific gravity in the hamster is 1.050–1.060 and low-moderate amounts of protein are present in normal hamster urine (Jenkins 2008; Hoefer and Latney 2009). Small amounts of glucose may be present physiologically as a consequence of stress.

Faecal pellets are often passed in response to handling, or these can be retrieved from the latrine area of the enclosure.

For blood sample collection, the jugular vein and cranial vena cava can be accessed under anaesthesia, though the jugular is harder to access due to the short, thick neck and presence of cheek pouches. For vena cava access, a 23–25G needle with 1 ml syringe, or insulin syringe is used. The anaesthetised patient is placed in dorsal recumbency and the needle is inserted 3–5 mm lateral to the manubrium, cranial to the clavicle and the first rib, and angled caudomedially towards the contralateral hind leg. Negative pressure is applied to the syringe and the needle

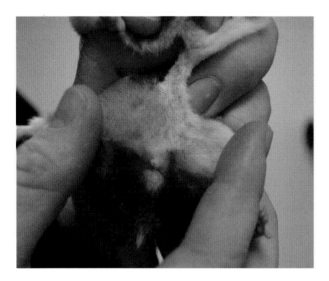

Figure 7.4 Female Syrian hamster, note the short anogenital distance.

7.4.4 Clinical Examination

Observation of the hamster in its cage should be carried out prior to handling. Demeanour, coat and skin condition, respiratory rate and effort, body condition, presence of cyanosis, and response to a novel environment may be evaluated remotely. However, it is not unusual for hamsters presented in the daytime to be asleep, limiting observational assessment.

Clinical examination may be limited in poorly socialised or painful animals as they will resent restraint. A thorough visual evaluation of external surfaces, incisors, abdominal palpation, auscultation, and a basic orthopaedic examination should be carried out where possible.

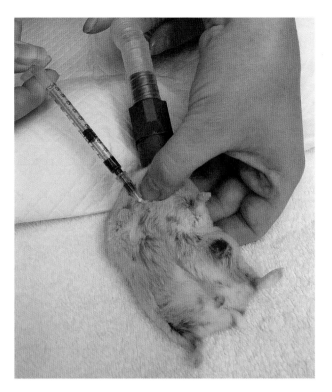

Figure 7.6 Blood sample collection from the vena cava in an anaesthetised Russian hamster with a soft tissue mass.

slowly advanced until blood begins to flow into the hub (Figure 7.6). Up to 1 ml/100 g body weight can be collected from this site in a healthy animal, though in a debilitated patient this should be reduced to 0.5 ml/100 g bodyweight. Potential complications include venous laceration, inadvertent arterial puncture and intrathoracic haemorrhage though the procedure appears safe in animals with normal clotting capabilities and a gentle technique.

7.5.2 Nutritional Support

Nutritional support of anorexic patients is crucial to prevent gastrointestinal hypomotility and secondary metabolic consequences of inadequate nutrition. A daily energy intake of 40–50 kcal/100 g in Siberian hamsters acts as a guide for nutritional requirements, though these increase in sick animals (Wade and Bartness 1984). Nutritional support for anorexic animals typically consists of syringe feeding of a commercial herbivore or granivore liquid diet, or blended pellet slurry to provide appropriate energy intake. Feeds of up 2.5 ml every 3–4 hours are possible in Syrian hamsters and amounts fed are modified based on twice daily weight monitoring.

7.5.3 Fluid Therapy

Fluids must be warmed to the body temperature of the patient before administration to prevent cooling of the patient, and fluids used in domestic species are suitable for use in rodents. Fluid deficits can be calculated based on weight loss or dehydration level but both of these may be hard to determine accurately. Subjective estimation of percentage dehydration based on clinical appearance, including skin turgor, sunken eyes, and mucous membrane desiccation is commonly applied. Maintenance requirements in hamsters are 75–100 ml/kg/day, and should be provided alongside replacement of losses (Lichtenberger 2007).

For animals with 10% or more dehydration, fluids should be provided into the circulation if possible. Due to difficulties of venous access, intraosseous routes are typically used. Intraosseous catheters are most commonly placed in the tibial crest under general anaesthesia (Capello 2003). Constant infusion can be used in critical or anaesthetised patients but repeated small bolus administration may be more practical in mobile patients, alongside analgesia.

The interscapular region is typically used for subcutaneous fluid administration in animals with less than 10% dehydration though is important not to inject laterally as the cheek pouches extend to the level of the shoulder. Recommended maximum volume to be administered is 5 ml (2.5 ml in dwarf hamsters), and this can be repeated once absorption is complete. The flanks can also be used for subcutaneous fluid administration.

7.5.4 Anaesthesia

Pre-anaesthetic fasting is not mandatory and indeed is contraindicated in small rodents, however a brief period of 20 minutes food withdrawal prior to induction means that the oral cavity is clear of food debris. Hamsters may still retain food in their cheek pouches however and this should be cleared promptly after induction. Inhalational anaesthesia with isoflurane alone is commonly used due to ready availability and fast induction and recovery times but restraint and administration of an irritant gaseous agent can be stressful for the patient. Manual restraint can be avoided by using a small clear plastic box or a small animal face mask as an induction chamber (Figure 7.7), and sevoflurane and other less aversive volatile agents can be used instead of isoflurane to reduce negative effects. Where possible pre-medication is recommended to reduce induction duration and stress, to provide analgesia, and to achieve a more predictable plane of anaesthesia for surgical procedures. Various combinations are highlighted in the formulary.

Oxygen should be administered to all sedated or anaesthetised patients and this is usually achieved by a nasal or facial mask. Endotracheal intubation is possible and commercial kits are available for intubation of laboratory rodents. However, it is technically challenging and narrows the effective airway significantly, necessitating ventilation

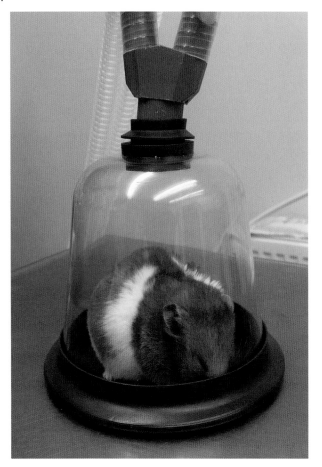

Figure 7.7 Induction of anaesthesia in a Syrian hamster using sevoflurane and a canine facemask as an induction chamber.

(intermittently or continuously) to avoid occlusion of the tube by secretions, and impedes access to the oral cavity for dental procedures.

7.5.5 Euthanasia

Anaesthesia followed by intracardiac injection of 100–200 mg/kg pentobarbitone is preferred, with a left lateral approach, and injection caudal to the axilla where the cardiac pulse is palpable (Figure 7.8). Alternatively an intraperitoneal injection of 200–500 mg/kg pentobarbitone can also be used in an unconscious animal. Injection of intracardiac or intraperitoneal pentobarbitone in a conscious animal should be avoided. Physical trauma or use of carbon dioxide is not appropriate.

7.5.6 Hospitalisation Requirements

Hamsters should be maintained in their own cage where possible or, for multi-chamber cages, the segment with sleeping area can be separated to be used as a smaller temporary enclosure.

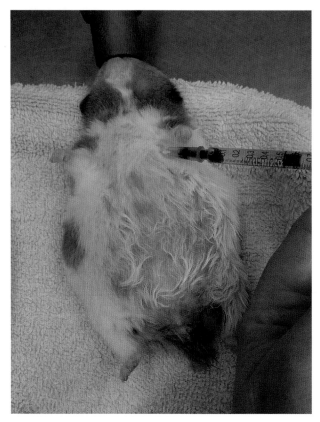

Figure 7.8 Euthanasia of a Syrian hamster using pentobarbitone via the intracardiac route.

Alternatively basic rodent cages can be used in the hospital, with substrate, hide, food and water provided. It is important to ensure these are secure and escape is not possible. Small cardboard boxes make good hide areas that can be disposed of after use.

7.6 Common Medical and Surgical Conditions

7.6.1 Neoplasia

There is significant species variation in incidence and predominating type of neoplasms.

In Syrian hamsters neoplasia is uncommon with a reported incidence of 3.7%, and tumours are primarily seen in animals over 2 years of age (Kirkman and Algard 1968).

Adrenocortical neoplasms are the most common neoplastic pathology in Syrian hamsters, with adenomas predominating over carcinomas (Greenacre 2004; McInnes et al. 2013). Clinical signs are common and this syndrome is discussed under endocrine diseases. Spontaneous cutaneous lymphoma is the second most common neoplasm in adult Syrian hamsters, and presents with alopecia, exfoliative dermatitis, skin thickening, dermal nodules and often concurrent debilitation. Examination of impression smears from open lesions or skin biopsies confirms diagnosis. Palliative therapy with corticosteroids can reduce symptoms temporarily. Occasionally multicentric lymphoma is seen in adults, with the thymus, lymph nodes, spleen, liver, and other sites involved (Brown and Donnelly 2012). Cases are often presented late in the disease process when euthanasia is the only remaining option.

Hamster papova virus (HaPV) can cause outbreaks of lymphoma in young hamsters with high morbidity in naïve populations. Animals develop palpable abdominal masses, enlarged lymph nodes or weight loss and prognosis is grave (Brown and Donnelly 2012). Established endemic infection in colonies, or infection in adult hamsters, tends to result in benign trichoepitheliomas instead of lymphoma.

Thyroidal neoplasia is common in hamsters with an incidence of 1.5–7% but most neoplasms are clinically benign (Pour et al. 1976; Collins 2008). Adenomas are most prevalent and may be associated with iodine deficiency (Follis 1959; Harkness et al. 2013). Thyroidectomy has been evaluated but post-operative mortality is high.

Melanomas of pigmented skin are common and are more frequently diagnosed in male hamsters. The head, back, and scent glands are often affected (Longley 2009).

Reproductive tract tumours are most frequently unilateral thecal or granulosa cell tumours, though vaginal papillomas are also seen commonly (Greenacre 2004).

A wide variety of other neoplasms have been reported in small numbers in Syrian hamsters, commonly affecting the skin, so biopsy is always recommended for masses to make a diagnosis and determine prognosis.

Russian hamsters appear more commonly affected by neoplasia, with incidence five times higher than is seen in Syrian hamsters (Kondo et al. 2008). Geriatric animals, over 18 months of age, are more frequently affected. Skin neoplasms predominate, particularly papillomas, mastocytomas, squamous cell carcinomas, and basal cell tumours, and mammary neoplasms are also seen (Pogosianz 1975; Nishizumi et al. 2000; Kondo et al. 2008).

The Chinese hamster is reportedly predisposed to uterine adenocarcinomas (Lipman and Foltz 1995).

7.6.2 Alopecia and Dermatitis

Alopecia is a common presentation, particularly in older hamsters and can have a variety of causes. The normal hairless scent glands may be misidentified as alopecia by owners, particularly in males in breeding season when they become more prominent.

Syrian hamsters commonly carry *Demodex criceti* or *Demodex aurati* asymptomatically, but immunosuppression can result in clinical disease with scaling and alopecia. Sarcoptic and notoedric mange have also been reported in the Syrian hamster as a cause of crusting, pruritic dermatitis and dermatophytosis is infrequently seen (Donnelly et al. 2000).

Endocrine diseases such as adrenal pathology and hypothyroidism may cause alopecia, as can cutaneous lymphoma. Mild patchy coat thinning is also seen in geriatric hamsters. Unusually in rodents, barbering is not a well-recognised cause of fur loss.

Due to a multitude of causes resulting in similar presentation, investigation is necessary to make a diagnosis. Skin scrapes may be obtained in the conscious, restrained hamster and if these fail to identify cause then general anaesthesia for blood sample collection to investigate endocrine factors and to collect a skin biopsy is indicated.

7.6.3 Ocular Disease

Exophthalmos is common in hamsters, associated with trauma or occasionally inappropriate restraint. Replacement is carried out under anaesthesia, following lavage of the globe with warmed isotonic fluids and application of lubrication. The globe is then manipulated back into the orbit by elevating the lids around the proptosed globe and applying gentle pressure. Tarsorraphy may be indicated if the globe prolapses again, or enucleation if the eye is non-vital, traumatised, or cannot be replaced into the orbit (Orcutt 2005).

Ocular discharge is a common sign in hamsters but is more commonly associated with dehydration and increased viscosity of ocular secretions rather than localised inflammation or infection.

7.6.4 Dental Disease

The hamster dental formula is 1/1 0/0 0/0 3/3. The incisor teeth are open rooted and constantly growing, but molar teeth have closed roots.

The lower incisors are approximately three times as long as the upper incisors and are not rigidly fixed in position, enabling some movement (Figure 7.9). Trimming should only be carried out where there is identifiable overgrowth or deviation and requires use of a dental burr or cutting disc, under anaesthesia. Clipping incisors is not appropriate as this often results in sharp edges, longitudinal fractures and exacerbation of pathology.

Fractures to the incisor teeth may result from hamsters being dropped, from cage bar-biting or as a consequence of malocclusion (Pellett and Mancinelli 2017). Often no treatment is necessary, but if one incisor is lost and the adjacent

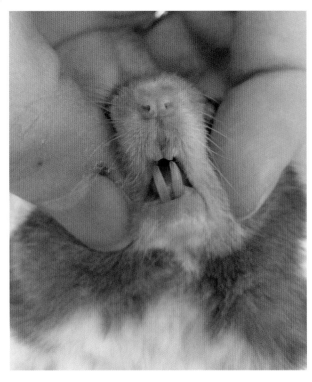

Figure 7.9 Normal appearance of hamster incisors, note the longer crowns of the mandibular incisors.

one is unsupported, reducing the height of the remaining incisor may avoid subsequent development of malocclusion.

Incisor malocclusion is more commonly seen in maxillary incisors with resulting increased curvature or lateral displacement of crowns. Penetration of the hard palate or facial skin may follow in chronic, untreated cases. Regular length reduction of the abnormal incisor teeth is necessary under anaesthesia. Incisor extraction can be carried out but may be unsuccessful as the angle of curvature of the reserve crown prevents severing of the periodontal ligaments along the full length complicating extraction of an entire tooth with germinal pulp.

Caries may develop on molar teeth. Factors postulated include a diet high in sugar, genetic susceptibility, mineral deficiency, and oral microflora with particular emphasis on *Streptococcus mutans* presence (Keyes and Fitzgerald 1962). The focus is on prevention, with correct diet and avoiding breeding severely affected animals. Antibiotic therapy may be used in colonies where caries are a common pathology and an infectious aetiology is suspected.

7.6.5 Cheek Pouch Impaction

Dried food or bedding materials may impact within pouches and this can be removed by everting the pouches under anaesthesia and gently flushing debris away.

Infection or dental pathology are common predisposing factors and a thorough examination of the oral cavity and teeth should be carried out.

Occasionally eversion of the cheek pouch can follow impaction or infection, in these cases the pouch should be checked for areas of necrosis and debrided and repaired if indicated. The pouch is then placed back in the correct anatomical position and a cruciate suture placed through the skin and pouch to anchor the pouch for 10–14 days (Bennett 2012). Amputation of the pouch can be carried out if tissues are devitalised, or neoplasia is present. For this procedure, the cheek pouch is entirely everted and clamped across the base prior to removal of the pouch mucosa. The resulting wound edges are apposed and closed with simple interrupted sutures (Capello 2003).

7.6.6 Respiratory Disease

Streptococcus pneumoniae has been reported as a cause of respiratory disease (Renshaw et al. 1975). Infection may present as sneezing, nasal or ocular discharge, dyspnoea, or non-specific signs of anorexia and lethargy. Presence of gram-positive diplococci on cytology of nasal or ocular discharge is strongly supportive but culture is recommended to confirm diagnosis (Orcutt 2005). *Staphylococcus, Klebsiella, Bordetella,* and *Salmonella* have also been identified (Innes et al. 1956; Goodman 2004). Treatment includes oxygen therapy, broad-spectrum antibiotic treatment, nutritional support, and nebulisation.

Pasteurella multocida and *Pasteurella pneumotropica* can cause respiratory disease as well as subcutaneous abscess formation (Harkness and Wagner 1995). Antibiotic therapy rarely eliminates the causative bacteria but episodic treatment may manage symptoms.

Hamsters are susceptible to Sendai virus but clinical disease is mild or asymptomatic (Percy et al. 2007). Cardiomyopathy and atrial thrombosis are common in older hamsters and may also present with severe dyspnoea (Langan et al. 2000; Donnelly 2004).

7.6.7 Cardiac Disease

Hypertrophic cardiomyopathy, dilative cardiomyopathy, and atherosclerosis have been recognised in Syrian hamsters and appear common in individuals over 18 months of age (Orcutt 2005; Schmidt and Reavill 2007).

An autosomal recessive inheritable cardiomyopathy is also recognised in Syrian hamsters of the 14.6 line, associated with progressive ventricular dilation from 60 to 120 days of age (Schmidt and Reavill 2007). In animals of the 15.0 line a familial myopathy is present which results in congestive heart failure. In these individuals creatinine phosphokinase is markedly elevated at 30 days of age and from 55 days of age lingual myolysis is also present – evident as white dots of 1–5 mm diameter on the underside of the tongue (Homburger 1979). Infectious myocarditis has been reported with a wide variety of experimental infections, including *Borrelia burgdorferi*, but lesions associated with naturally occurring infections appear rare (Goodman et al. 1991; Schmidt and Reavill 2007).

Overt clinical signs develop when congestive heart failure results, when lethargy, generalised oedema, dyspnoea, tachycardia, cyanosis, and anorexia may be noted. Owners may not readily identify changes and so hamsters tend to present late in the course of disease, resulting in a guarded prognosis. Ultrasonography is recommended to confirm disease and provide information on primary cause, but presumptive treatment using diuretics and high inspired oxygen concentrations is advisable prior to sedation or prolonged restraint. Treatment is based on medications available for domestic pets, and doses are often extrapolated from laboratory studies in hamster strains with predisposition to cardiac disease and response may vary in pet animals with spontaneous cardiac disease.

Atrial thrombosis is a condition predominantly seen in older females, with acute dyspnoea or sudden death seen (Langan et al. 2000). At post-mortem examination, pale adherent plaques of thrombi are seen in the left atrium or auricle (Percy et al. 2007).

7.6.8 Abdominal Cysts

Polycystic disease is present in up to 15% of Syrian hamsters and patients may show discomfort, lethargy, or abdominal distension (Kaup et al. 1990). The liver is most frequently affected, and cysts can range from 2.5–30 mm in diameter (Somvanshi et al. 1987). Ultrasonography confirms diagnosis and fluid can be drained with ultrasound guidance but cysts tend to refill within one month.

7.6.9 Renal Disease

Spontaneous amyloidosis is noted to occur in hamsters over 12 months in age and amyloid deposition and glomerulosclerosis have been hypothesised to occur in hamsters of any age as a secondary consequence of chronic antigenic stimulation (Gleiser et al. 1971; Crowell and Votava 1975). The resulting proteinuria can cause in hypoalbuminaemia, peripheral oedema, ascites, pleural effusion, lethargy, and loss of body condition.

Diagnosis of renal disease is similar as for domestic species. Clinical signs include polyuria, polydipsia, dehydration and weight loss, reduced activity, and loss of appetite. The clinical parameters assessed in suspected renal disease are shown in Table 7.3. Urinalysis confirms significant pro-

Table 7.3 Clinical parameters assessed in suspected renal disease.

Parameter	Reference range
Urine output	5.1–8.4 ml/day
Urine specific gravity	1.014–1.060
Serum urea	2.0–4.3 mmol/l
Serum creatinine	35.4–88.4 umol/l
PCV	45–50%

teinuria, and biochemistry shows hypoalbuminaemia, azotaemia, and increased creatinine (Johnson-Delaney 1998; Jenkins 2008). Urine protein:creatinine ratio assessment is complicated by excretion of protein in the urine of normal hamsters. Urine culture can be used to identify infectious contributors to disease. Treatment of renal disease is similar to other species though medication is used off licence with no pharmacokinetic or pharmacodynamics data.

7.6.10 Reproductive Disease

Pyometra is commonly suspected in hamsters but in most cases it is misinterpretation of the normal profuse white discharge that occurs on day 3 of oestrus. True pyometra is rare. Cytology of exudate and abdominal ultrasonography should differentiate physiological and pathological discharge. If pyomera is confirmed then ovariohysterectomy is the treatment of choice. Aglepristone has been used successfully as medical treatment of one case of confirmed pyometra, alongside systemic antibiotics (Pisu et al. 2012).

Ectopic pregnancy with foetal degeneration was reported at a level of 4.5% of breeding females in one laboratory colony of Russian hamsters (Buckley and Caine 1979). The main symptom seen was failure of normal breeding, however peritonitis was identified in 37.5% of these cases.

7.6.11 Endocrine Disease

Clinical hyperadrenocorticism is common in Syrian hamsters (Orr 2009). Laboratory animals over two years of age have a 40% incidence of hyperplastic or neoplastic change in the adrenal glands, and the teddy bear variety of Syrian hamster appears predisposed (Figure 7.10) (Bauck et al. 1984; Tanaka et al. 1991). Elevated cortisol and corticosterone results in a non-pruritic symmetrical alopecia, polyuria, polydipsia, skin thinning and hyperpigmentation, and abdominal distension (Longley 2009). Elevation of serum cortisol (reference range 13.8–27.6 nmol/l) and alkaline phosphatase (50–186 IU/l), or identification of enlarged adrenal glands on abdominal

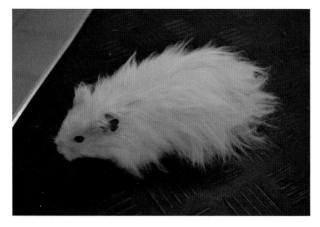

Figure 7.10 Teddy bear variety of Syrian hamster, predisposed to hyperadrenocorticism.

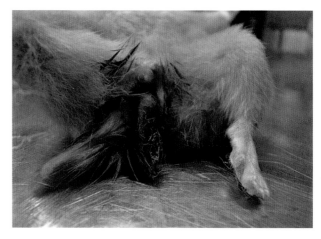

Figure 7.11 Colonic prolapse in a Syrian hamster with enteritis.

ultrasound examination, are strongly supportive of adrenal disease (Orcutt 2005; Suckow et al. 2012). An elevated urinary cortisol:creatinine ratio may support diagnosis, with values of >20 (ug:g/ml) suggested to be abnormal (Martinho 2006). Prognosis is poor, with lack of response to therapy used in domestic species.

Hypothyroidism has been described in hamsters with clinical signs of alopecia, hyperpigmentation and thickening of the skin, and lethargy (Keeble 2001). The serum total thyroxine reference range is 38–90 nmol/l but may be depressed by other factors such as reduced daylight hours, low temperatures, concurrent disease, and in geriatric hamsters (Mayer and Donnelly 2012; Thorson 2014). Methimazole therapy can be used but other more common diseases such as adrenal pathology should be ruled out first.

Spontaneous diabetes mellitus has been reported in specific lines of Chinese hamsters and clinical presentation reflects disease in domestic mammals. Diarrhoea, delayed intestinal transit time and steatorrhea may be seen in addition to polyuria (up to 75 ml/day) and polydipsia (Diani et al. 1979; Gerritsen 1982). In diabetic hamsters, non-fasting glucose levels are consistently above 16.65 mmol/l and urinary glucose loss can reach 3 g/day (Gerritsen 1982; Orr 2009). Dietary changes to reduce sugar and fat content are the mainstay of therapy but insulin has also been used (Goodman 2002).

7.6.12 Diarrhoea

A syndrome of 'wet tail', or juvenile diarrhoea is well recognised in hamsters aged one to three months particularly after a stressor such as weaning or a change of environment. The causative bacterium is *Lawsonia intracellularis* which disrupts enterocyte absorption, causing diarrhoea and electrolyte derangements (McOrist et al. 1995; Vannucci et al. 2010). Liquid diarrhoea, staining of

peri-anal fur, anorexia, lethargy and dehydration are commonly seen. In some cases, intussusception or secondary prolapse of the colon occurs (Figure 7.11). Euthanasia is warranted for haemorrhagic diarrhoea or where enteric prolapse occurs, especially if necrosis or dessication compromise prolapsed tissue integrity. Coeliotomy for reduction and resection of a prolapse has been described but prognosis is poor (Capello 2003). Treatment of early cases involves assist feeding, parenteral fluid therapy, oral antibiotics, and thermal support but prognosis is poor and death often results within 48 hours (Frisk and Wagner 1977).

Clostridium difficile, Clostridium piliforme, Escherichia coli, Campylobacter, Salmonella, Proteus spp. and many other bacteria may be associated with diarrhoea in adult animals. Treatment is broadly similar as for wet tail but prognosis is improved.

Use of inappropriate antibiotics can cause a potentially fatal enterotoxaemia in hamsters. Penicillins, first generation cephalosporins, bacitracin, lincomycin, clindamycin, erythromycin, and vancomycin should be avoided (Orcutt 2005).

7.6.13 Musculoskeletal Disease

Conspecific traumatic injuries tend to be superficial in hamsters requiring little intervention.

Occasionally fractures are seen due to animals being dropped or limbs trapped in cage bars, with tibial fractures most common. Hamsters tolerate external coaption poorly but internal fixation using hypodermic needles or Kirschner wires used as intramedullary pins can work well where applicable (Capello 2003). Many reasonably aligned fractures will heal with just analgesia and confinement to a small cage with smooth sides to prevent climbing (McLaughlin and Strunk 2016) Amputation of limbs is often necessary for comminuted, open fractures.

7.7 Preventative Health Measures

The pinworm *Dentostomella translucida* is present in apparently healthy Syrian hamsters but may have some effects on growth and immunocompetence. Faecal flotation identifies the ovoid eggs and fenbendazole is likely to clear infection (Wilkerson et al. 2001). Faecal parasitology of new animals is recommended prior to introduction into a household.

7.7.1 Neutering Technique

Neutering of females is rarely carried out as a routine procedure. Surgery is typically planned in response to reproductive pathology such as ovarian cysts, pyometra or neoplasia of the reproductive tract (Capello 2003). A midline ventral abdominal incision is made and the voluminous, sacculated caecum is retracted using moistened sterile cotton buds. The uterine horns are identified and tracked back to the ovaries. Ovarian access is limited by patient size, intestinal tract volume, and the short length of the pedicle. Use of small ligating clips is preferred over traditional ligation for haemostasis of the ovarian pedicle. The cervix can be ligated with an encircling or transfixing ligature and all ligation sites should be carefully checked for haemorrhage prior to closure of the body wall, subcutaneous tissues, and skin in three layers. An intradermal pattern using 5–0 absorbable monofilament material is preferred for the skin to limit patient interference with the wound post-operatively (Capello 2003).

Routine neutering of males is uncommonly carried out as testicular pathology is rare, though epididymal abscessation and a scrotal sarcoma have been described (Capello 2003). Where necessary, an incision is made longitudinally at the tip of each testis and an open or closed technique can be used for castration. The author prefers a modified open technique. Here the tunic is also incised, the testicle exteriorised and a ligature placed around both the ductus deferens and pampiniform plexus. The testicle is sharply dissected and ligature and fat pad replaced into the scrotum, reducing potential for herniation. The tunic is then closed using a cruciate suture of absorbable material, and the scrotal skin closed with tissue glue.

7.8 Radiographic Imaging

Due to small patient size, high resolution or mammography film is preferred but detail may still be insufficient due to the rapid respiratory rate creating movement blur. Dental radiography units can also be used. The cheek pouches should be emptied prior to assessing the neck and cranial thorax radiographically as superimpostition of food

material results in a loss of diagnostic detail (Figure 7.12). The standard views taken for survey radiographs are laterolateral and either ventrodorsal or dorsoventral (Figures 7.13 and 7.14).

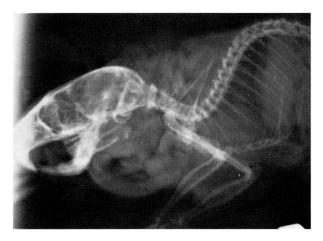

Figure 7.12 Lateral radiograph of head and thorax, note the soft tissue opacities of cheek pouches.

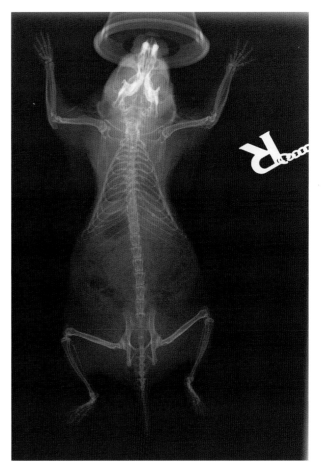

Figure 7.13 Dorsoventral radiograph of a Syrian hamster. *Source:* Courtesy of Manor vets.

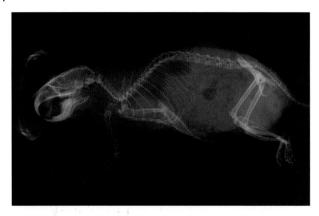

Figure 7.14 Laterolateral radiograph of a Syrian hamster.
Source: Courtesy of Manor vets.

Little information is published on imaging in hamsters, with focus on experimental techniques for laboratory animals that are not applicable to diagnostic procedures. Contrast studies using barium have demonstrated gastrointestinal transit time to be 90–340 minutes in Chinese hamsters, with gastric emptying demonstrated to take 150–270 minutes (Diani et al. 1979).

Ultrasound examination can be valuable in assessing abdominal and ovarian cysts, pyometra, and palpable masses but typically requires anaesthesia for diagnostic images.

Formulary

Medication	Dose	Dosing interval	Additional comments
Anaesthesia			
Ketamine	50–100 mg/kg		Used in combination in Syrian hamsters, lower end of ketamine dose range for Djungarian hamsters (Curl and Peters 1983; Curl 1988). Intraperitoneal dose reported but SC or IM routes preferred
Xylazine	10 mg/kg		
Ketamine	75–90 mg/kg IM		
Medetomidine	0.1–0.5 mg/kg IM		(Johnson-Delaney 1999)
Isoflurane	5% to induce, 1–3% for maintenance		(Carpenter 2012)
Analgesia			
Buprenorphine	0.5 mg/kg SC	q8h	(Harkness 1993)
Butorphanol	1–5 mg/kg SC	q4h	(Heard 1993)
Meloxicam	0.5–1 mg/kg PO, SC	q24h	(Mayer 2013)
Tramadol	5–10 mg/kg PO, SC	q12–24h	(Mayer 2013)
Antibiotics			
Trimethoprim/ Sulfa	15–30 mg/kg PO, SC	q12h	(Rosskopf 2003)
Enrofloxacin	5–20 mg/kg PO, SC, IM	q12h	(Adamcak and Otten 2000)
Chloramphenicol	30–50 mg/kg IM, SC, PO	q8–12h	For *Lawsonia* enteritis (Carpenter 2012)
Neomycin	0.5 mg/ml drinking water		For *Lawsonia* enteritis (Anderson 1994)
Penicillin, cephlosporin, aminoglycoside, tetracycline and lincosamide antibiotics all have high mortality when given orally (Morris 1995)			
Antiparasitics			
Fenbendazole	20 mg/kg PO	sid for 7d	(Wilkerson et al. 2001)
Ivermectin	0.2–0.4 mg/kg SC, topical	q7d for demodecosis, q14d for sarcoptic mange	(Carpenter 2012)
Amitraz	100 ppm topically	3–6 times at 2 week intervals	Based on gerbil dose (Meredith 2010)
Metronidazole	70 mg/kg PO	q8h	For intestinal flagellates (Adamcak and Otten 2000)

(Continued)

Medication	Dose	Dosing interval	Additional comments
Miscellaneous			
Aglepristone	20 mg/kg sc	Four doses, on day 1, 2, 8, and 15	Protocol used successfully in one case of pyometra, alongside antibiotics (Pisu et al. 2012)
Metapyrone	8 mg PO	sid for 1 month	Successful in one case of hyperadrenocorticism (Bauck et al. 1984)
Ketoconazole	5 mg/kg PO	q12h for 1 month	Appears ineffective in hyperadrenocorticism (Brown and Donnelly 2012)
Methimazole	0.5 mg/kg PO	q12–24hrs	Extrapolated from guinea pig dose, taper up to effect (Mayer et al. 2010)
Hydroxyzine Insulin	2 U/animal SC	to effect	(Carpenter 2012)
Enalapril	0.5–1 mg/kg PO	q24h	For volume overload with congestive heart failure (Mayer 2013). Doses as high as 25 mg/kg, in combination with 10 mg/kg losartan, to delay onset of cardiac disease in laboratory strains with hereditary cardiomyopathy (Crespo et al. 2008).
Carvedilol	1 mg/kg PO	q24h	(Inoue et al. 2003) Beta blocker used to counter sympathetic response to cardiac failure, increasing cardiac function and reducing symptoms in human patients (Packer et al. 1996).
Furosemide	0.3–4 mg/kg PO, SC	q12–24 h	Diuretic used in congestive heart failure (Mayer 2013)
Pimobendan	0.2–0.4 mg/kg PO	q12h	Positive inotrope for dilated cardiomyopathy (Mitchell et al. 2008)

References

Adamcak, A. and Otten, B. (2000). Rodent therapeutics. *The Veterinary Clinics of North America. Exotic Animal Practice* 3 (1): 221–237.

Anderson, N.L. (1994). Basic husbandry and medicine of pocket pets. In: *Saunders Manual of Small Animal Practice* (eds. S.J. Birchard and R.G. Sherding), 1363–1389. Philadelphia: WB Saunders CO.

Bauck, L.B., Orr, J.P., and Lawrence, K.H. (1984). Hyperadrenocorticism in three teddy bear hamsters. *The Canadian Veterinary Journal* 25 (6): 247.

Benevenga, N.J., Calvert, C., Eckhert, C.D. et al. (1995). *Nutrient Requirements of Laboratory Animals*, 125–139. Washington, DC: National Academy Press.

Bennett, R.A. (2012). Soft tissue surgery. In: *Ferrets, Rabbits and Rodents. Clinical Medicine and Surgery*, 3e (eds. K.E. Quesenberry and J.W. Carpenter), 373–391. St Louis, MO: Elsevier Saunders.

Brown, C. and Donnelly, T.M. (2012). Disease problems of small rodents. In: *Ferrets, Rabbits and Rodents. Clinical Medicine and Surgery*, 3e (eds. K.E. Quesenberry

and J.W. Carpenter), 354–372. St Louis, MO: Elsevier Saunders.

Buckley, P. and Caine, A. (1979). A high incidence of abdominal pregnancy in the Djungarian hamster (*Phodopus sungorus*). *Journal of Reproduction and Fertility* 56 (2): 679–682.

Capello, V. (2003). Surgical techniques in pet hamsters. *Exotic DVM* 5 (3): 32–37.

Carpenter, J.C. (2012). Formulary. In: *Ferrets, Rabbits and Rodents. Clinical Medicine and Surgery*, 3e (eds. K.E. Quesenberry and J.W. Carpenter), 566–575. St Louis, MO: Elsevier Saunders.

Collins, B.R. (2008). Endocrine diseases of rodents. *The Veterinary Clinics of North America. Exotic Animal Practice* 11 (1): 153–162.

Crespo, M.J., Cruz, N., Altieri, P.I. et al. (2008). Enalapril and losartan are more effective than carvedilol in preventing dilated cardiomyopathy in the Syrian cardiomyopathic hamster. *Journal of Cardiovascular Pharmacology and Therapeutics* 13 (3): 199–206.

Crowell, W.A. and Votava, C.L. (1975). Amyloidosis induced in hamsters by a filarid parasite (*Dipetalonema viteae*). *Veterinary Pathology* 12 (3): 178–185.

Curl, J.L. (1988). Ketamine-xylazine anaesthesia in the Djungarian hamster (*Phodopus sungorus*). *Laboratory Animals* 22 (4): 309–312.

Curl, J.L. and Peters, L.L. (1983). Ketamine hydrochloride and xylazine hydrochloride anaesthesia in the golden hamster (*Mesocricetus auratus*). *Laboratory Animals* 17 (4): 290–293.

Diani, A.R., Grogan, D.M., Yates, M.E. et al. (1979). Radiologic abnormalities and autonomic neuropathology in the digestive tract of the ketonuric diabetic Chinese hamster. *Diabetologia* 17 (1): 33–40.

Donnelly, T.M. (2004). Disease problems of small rodents. In: *Ferrets, Rabbits and Rodents. Clinical Medicine and Surgery*, 2e (eds. K.E. Quesenberry and J.W. Carpenter), 299–315. St. Louis, MO: Saunders, Elsevier.

Donnelly, T.M., Rush, E.M., and Lackner, P.A. (2000). Ringworm in small exotic pets. *Seminars in Avian and Exotic Pet Medicine* 9 (2): 82–93.

Fischer, K., Gebhardt-Henrich, S.G., and Steiger, A. (2007). Behaviour of golden hamsters (*Mesocricetus auratus*) kept in four different cage sizes. *Animal Welfare* 16 (1): 85.

Fitts, D.A. and St. Dennis, C. (1981). Ethanol and dextrose preferences in hamsters. *Journal of Studies on Alcohol* 42: 901–907.

Follis, R.H. Jr. (1959). Experimental colloid goiter in the hamster. *Proceedings of the Society for Experimental Biology and Medicine* 100 (1): 203–206.

Frisk, C.S. and Wagner, J.E. (1977). Hamster enteritis: a review. *Laboratory Animals* 11 (2): 79–85.

Gerritsen, G.C. (1982). The Chinese hamster as a model for the study of diabetes mellitus. *Diabetes* 31 (Supplement 1): 14–23.

Gleiser, C.A., Van Hoosier, G.L., Sheldon, W.G. et al. (1971). Amyloidosis and renal paramyloid in a closed hamster colony. *Laboratory Animal Science* 21 (2): 197–202.

Goodman, G. (2002). Hamsters. In: *BSAVA Manual of Exotic Pets*, 4e (eds. A. Meredith and S. Redrobe), 26–33. Quedgeley, UK: British Small Animal Veterinary Association.

Goodman, G. (2004). Infectious respiratory disease in rodents. *In Practice* 26 (4): 200–205.

Goodman, J.L., Jurkovich, P., Kodner, C. et al. (1991). Persistent cardiac and urinary tract infections with *Borrelia burgdorferi* in experimentally infected Syrian hamsters. *Journal of Clinical Microbiology* 29 (5): 894–896.

Grant, K. (2014). Rodent nutrition: digestive comparisons of 4 common rodent species. *The Veterinary Clinics of North America. Exotic Animal Practice* 17 (3): 471–483.

Greenacre, C.B. (2004). Spontaneous tumors of small mammals. *Veterinary Clinics: Exotic Animal Practice* 7 (3): 627–651.

Harkness, J.E. (1993). *A practitioner's guide to domestic rodents*. Denver, CO: American Animal Hospital Association.

Harkness, J.E. and Wagner, J.E. (1995). Specific diseases and conditions. In: *The Biology and Medicine of Rabbits and Rodents*, 4e (eds. J.E. Harkness and J.E. Wagner), 171–322. York, PA: Williams and Wilkins.

Harkness, J.E., Turner, P.V., VandeWoude, S. et al. (2013). Specific diseases and conditions. In: *Harkness and Wagner's Biology and Medicine of Rabbits and Rodents*, 5e (eds. J.E. Harkness, P.V. Turner, S. VandeWoude, et al.), 249–396. Ames, IA: Wiley-Blackwell.

Hauzenberger, A.R., Gebhardt-Henrich, S.G., and Steiger, A. (2006). The influence of bedding depth on behaviour in golden hamsters (*Mesocricetus auratus*). *Applied Animal Behaviour Science* 100 (3): 280–294.

Heard, D.J. (1993). Principles and techniques of anesthesia and analgesia for exotic practice. *Veterinary Clinics of North America: Small Animal Practice* 23 (6): 1301–1327.

Heldmaier, G. and Steinlechner, S. (1981). Seasonal pattern and energetics of short daily torpor in the Djungarian hamster, *Phodopus sungorus*. *Oecologia* 48 (2): 265–270.

Hoefer, H. and Latney, L. (2009). Rodents: urogenital and reproductive system disorders. In: *BSAVA Manual of Rodents and Ferrets* (eds. E. Keeble and A. Meredith), 150–160. Gloucester: British Small Animal Veterinary Association.

Homburger, F. (1979). Myopathy of hamster dystrophy: history and morphologic aspects. *Annals of the New York Academy of Sciences* 317 (1): 2–17.

Innes, J.R.M., Wilson, C., and Ross, M.A. (1956). Epizootic *Salmonella enteritidis* infection causing septic pulmonary phlebothrombosis in hamsters. *The Journal of Infectious Diseases* 98 (2): 133–141.

Inoue, A., Yamashina, S., and Yamazaki, J. (2003). The effect of β-blocker on hamster model BIO 53.58 with dilated cardiomyopathy determined using 123 I-MIBG myocardial scintigraphy. *Annals of Nuclear Medicine* 17 (8): 677–683.

Jenkins, J.R. (2008). Rodent diagnostic testing. *Journal of Exotic Pet Medicine* 17 (1): 16–25.

Johnson-Delaney, C.A. (1998). Diseases of the urinary system of commonly kept rodents: diagnosis and treatment. *Seminars in Avian and Exotic Pet Medicine* 7 (2): 81–88.

Johnson-Delaney, C.A. (1999). Post-operative care of small mammals. *Exotic DVM* 1 (5): 19–21.

Kaup, F.J., Konstýř, I., and Drommer, W. (1990). Characteristic of spontaneous intraperitoneal cysts in golden hamsters and European hamsters. *Experimental Pathology* 40 (4): 205–212.

Keeble, E. (2001). Endocrine diseases in small mammals. *In Practice* 23 (10): 570–585.

Keeble, E. (2009). Rodents: biology and husbandry. In: *BSAVA Manual of Rodents ets* (eds. E. Keeble and A. Meredith), 9. Gloucester: British Small Animal Veterinary Association.

Keyes, P.H. and Fitzgerald, R.J. (1962). Dental caries in the Syrian hamster—IX. *Archives of Oral Biology* 7 (3): 267–277.

Kirkman, H. and Algard, F.T. (1968). Spontaneous and nonviral-induced neoplasms. In: *The Golden Hamster: Its Biology and Use in Medical Research* (eds. H. Hoffman, R. Robinson and P. Magalhaes), 227–240. Ames, IA: Iowa State University Press.

Kondo, H., Onuma, M., Shibuya, H. et al. (2008). Spontaneous tumors in domestic hamsters. *Veterinary Pathology* 45 (5): 674–680.

Langan, G.P., Lohmiller, J.J., Swing, S.P. et al. (2000). Respiratory diseases of rodents and rabbits. *Veterinary Clinics: Small Animal Practice* 30 (6): 1309–1335.

Lichtenberger, M. (2007). Shock and cardiopulmonary-cerebral resuscitation in small mammals and birds. *The Veterinary Clinics of North America. Exotic Animal Practice* 10 (2): 275–291.

Lipman, N.S. and Foltz, C. (1995). Hamsters. In: *Handbook for Rodent and Rabbit Medicine* (eds. K. Laber-Laird, M.M. Swindle and P. Flecknell), 65–82. New York: Pergamon.

Longley, L. (2009). Rodents: dermatoses. In: *BSAVA Manual of Rodents and Ferrets* (eds. E. Keeble and A. Meredith), 107–122. Gloucester: BSAVA.

Martinho, F. (2006). Suspected case of hyperadrenocorticism in a golden hamster (*Mesocricetus auratus*). *The Veterinary Clinics of North America. Exotic Animal Practice* 9 (3): 717–721.

Mayer, J. (2013). Rodents. In: *Exotic Animal Formulary*, 4e (eds. J.W. Carpenter and C. Marion), 477–516. St. Louis, MO: Elsevier Saunders.

Mayer, J. and Donnelly, T. (2012). Laboratory tests: thyroid hormones. In: *Clinical Veterinary Advisor. Birds and Exotic Pets*, 648–649. St Louis (MO): Saunders Elsevier.

Mayer, J., Wagner, R., and Taeymans, O. (2010). Advanced diagnostic approaches and current management of thyroid pathologies in Guinea pigs. *Veterinary Clinics: Exotic Animal Practice* 13 (3): 509–523.

McInnes, E.F., Ernst, H., and Germann, P.G. (2013). Spontaneous neoplastic lesions in control Syrian hamsters in 6-, 12-, and 24-month short-term and carcinogenicity studies. *Toxicologic Pathology* 41 (1): 86–97.

McLaughlin, A. and Strunk, A. (2016). Common emergencies in small rodents, hedgehogs, and sugar gliders. *The Veterinary Clinics of North America. Exotic Animal Practice* 19 (2): 465–499.

McOrist, S., Gebhart, C.J., Boid, R. et al. (1995). Characterization of *Lawsonia intracellularis* gen. nov., sp. nov., the obligately intracellular bacterium of porcine proliferative enteropathy. *International Journal of Systematic and Evolutionary Microbiology* 45 (4): 820–825.

Meredith, A. (2010). Skin diseases of rodents. *In Practice* 32 (1): 16–21.

Mitchell, E.B., Zehnder, A.M., Hsu, A. et al. (2008). Pimobendan: treatment of heart failure in small mammals. Proceedings of the Association of Exotic Mammal Veterinarians meeting, Savannah, Georgia: 71–79.

Morris, T.H. (1995). Antibiotic therapeutics in laboratory animals. *Laboratory Animals* 29 (1): 16–36.

Nishizumi, K., Fujiwara, K., and Hasegawa, A. (2000). Cutaneous mastocytomas in Djungarian hamsters. *Experimental Animals* 49 (2): 127–130.

Orcutt, C.J. (2005). Common hamster diseases and treatment. Proceedings of the North American Veterinary Conference 8–12 January 2005, Orlando, FL: 1358–1360.

Orr, H. (2009). Rodents: neoplastic and endocrine disease. In: *BSAVA Manual of Rodents and Ferrets* (eds. E. Keeble and A. Meredith), 181–192. Gloucester: BSAVA.

Packer, M., Bristow, M.R., Cohn, J.N. et al. (1996). The effect of carvedilol on morbidity and mortality in patients with chronic heart failure. *New England Journal of Medicine* 334 (21): 1349–1355.

Pellett, S. and Mancinelli, E. (2017). Veterinary care of hamsters. Part 2: diagnostics, diseases. *Companion Animal* 22 (12): 743–749.

Percy, D.H., Barthold, S.W., and Griffey, S.M. (2007). *Pathology of Laboratory Rodents and Rabbits*, 226–283. Ames, IA: Blackwell.

Pévet, P. (1988). The role of the pineal gland in the photoperiodic control of reproduction in different hamster species. *Reproduction Nutrition Développement* 28 (2B): 443–458.

Pisu, M.C., Andolfatto, A., and Veronesi, M.C. (2012). Pyometra in a six-month-old nulliparous golden hamster (*Mesocricetus auratus*) treated with aglepristone. *Veterinary Quarterly* 32 (3–4): 179–181.

Pogosianz, H.E. (1975). Djungarian hamster – a suitable tool for cancer research and cytogenetic studies. *Journal of the National Cancer Institute* 54 (3): 659–664.

Pour, P., Mohr, U., Althoff, J. et al. (1976). Spontaneous tumors and common diseases in two colonies of Syrian hamsters. III. Urogenital system and endocrine glands 2. *Journal of the National Cancer Institute* 56 (5): 949–961.

Pratt, N.C. and Lisk, R.D. (1989). Effects of social stress during early pregnancy on litter size and sex ratio in the golden hamster (*Mesocricetus auratus*). *Journal of Reproduction and Fertility* 87 (2): 763–769.

Renshaw, H.W., Van Hoosier, G.L. Jr., and Amend, N.K. (1975). A survey of naturally occurring diseases of the Syrian hamster. *Laboratory Animals* 9 (3): 179–191.

Rosskopf, W.J. (2003). Drug dosages for small rodents. Proceedings of the Atlantic Coast Veterinary Conference. Atlantic City, NJ. http://www.vin.com/Members/Proceedings/Proceedings.plx?CID=ACVC2003&PID=4996&Category=809&O=VIN (accessed 26 June 2019).

Ruf, T., Klingenspor, M., Preis, H. et al. (1991). Daily torpor in the Djungarian hamster (*Phodopus sungorus*): interactions with food intake, activity, and social behaviour. *Journal of Comparative Physiology B: Biochemical, Systemic, and Environmental Physiology* 160 (6): 609–615.

Schmidt, R.E. and Reavill, D.R. (2007). Cardiovascular disease in hamsters: review and retrospective study. *Journal of Exotic Pet Medicine* 16 (1): 49–51.

Somvanshi, R., Iyer, P.K.R., Biswas, J.C. et al. (1987). Polycystic liver disease in golden hamsters. *Journal of Comparative Pathology* 97 (5): 615–618.

Sonoyama, K., Fujiwara, R., Takemura, N. et al. (2009). Response of gut microbiota to fasting and hibernation in Syrian hamsters. *Applied and Environmental Microbiology* 75 (20): 6451–6456.

Suckow, M.A., Stevens, K.A., and Wilson, R.P. (2012). *The Laboratory Rabbit, Guinea Pig, Hamster, and Other Rodents*. Oxford: Academic Press.

Tanaka, A., Hisanaga, A., and Ishinishi, N. (1991). The frequency of spontaneously-occurring neoplasms in the male Syrian golden hamster. *Veterinary and Human Toxicology* 33 (4): 318–321.

Thompson, R. (1971). The water consumption and drinking habits of a few species and strains of laboratory animals. *Institute of Animal Technology* 22: 29–36.

Thorson, L. (2014). Thyroid diseases in rodent species. *Veterinary Clinics: Exotic Animal Practice* 17 (1): 51–67.

Vannucci, F.A., Borges, E.L., de Oliveira, J.S.V. et al. (2010). Intestinal absorption and histomorphometry of Syrian hamsters (*Mesocricetus auratus*) experimentally infected with *Lawsonia intracellularis*. *Veterinary Microbiology* 145 (3–4): 286–291.

Wade, G.N. and Bartness, T.J. (1984). Effects of photoperiod and gonadectomy on food intake, body weight, and body composition in Siberian hamsters. *American Journal of Physiology. Regulatory, Integrative and Comparative Physiology* 246 (1): R26–R30.

Wilkerson, J.D., Brooks, D.L., Derby, M. et al. (2001). Comparison of practical treatment methods to eradicate pinworm (*Dentostomella translucida*) infections from Mongolian gerbils (*Meroines unguiculatus*). *Journal of the American Association for Laboratory Animal Science* 40 (5): 31–36.

8

Rats
Richard Saunders

The Brown Rat (*Rattus norvegicus*), also known as the Common, Norway or Norwegian Rat, is frequently kept as a companion animal and this chapter will focus solely on this species. The Black Rat (*Rattus rattus*), also known as the house, ship, or roof rat is not commonly kept as a domestic pet, and does not adapt well to captivity. More exotic species are rarely seen, such as the Giant Gambian Pouched Rat (*Cricetomys gambianus*) and kangaroo rats (*Dipodomys* spp.) but these are outside the scope of this chapter. Biological parameters for the Brown Rat are given in Table 8.1.

The Brown Rat originated in Asia, and subsequently spread to Europe, Africa, and the Americas along human trade routes, on ships. It is now found almost everywhere in the world, with the exception of Antarctica and a number of islands, some of which it has been deliberately eradicated from for conservation purposes. (Puckett et al. 2016). Their ubiquity and status as unwanted pests, led to the popularity of organised rat catching by specially bred and trained dogs, and, as a result, the breeding of rats for the sport. Different colour varieties produced were bred and domesticated, and became pets, famous owners include Beatrix Potter (Potter 1926), Clint Eastwood, and Theodore Roosevelt. Rats have also been used as laboratory subjects since the 1800s (Krinke 2000) and breeding specific strains or lines has become a huge industry. Some have made it into the pet trade and the genetic selection for laboratory studies has lead to specific disease patterns within the different strains (Mac Kenzie and Garner 1973). From these beginnings, we now have a huge range of colour varieties, many different breeds, and some different body types (Table 8.2).

8.1 Husbandry

It is important that rats have enough space in their cages. Commercially sold 'starter kit' cages are often inappropriately small. The minimum suggested cage size for two rats is 72 cm × 36 cm × 44 cm, provided this area is not overcrowded with toys and allows room to run and hide but larger cage sizes are preferred. A multi-levelled cage is ideal, particularly for energetic young females (Lawlor 1990, 2002). When choosing a cage, it is also important to take the doors and any other access areas into consideration; a simple under hook cage door will be swiftly deciphered by the intelligent rat.

Cage bars spaced 1 cm apart will be suitable for any rat over the age of three weeks. Bars spaced 2.5 cm apart will be suitable for bucks, but does and juveniles may be able to escape. Cage bars come in a variety of coatings, the most suitable of which is enamelled. This is highly durable and unlikely to chip even under repeated nibbling. Galvanised bars are also an excellent option; although harder to clean than enamelled bars they are unlikely to rust. Rust and corrosion are particularly problematic if the rat is prone to urinating on the bars. If the bars require re-coating, non-toxic paints or enamel sprays can be used. Plastic coating is not suitable, as it will be gnawed and ingested. Cage levels are generally made from either wood or plastic and may be removable or fixed to the bars. Wood is potentially softer and thermally neutral but is more difficult to keep clean. Rats should be able to move easily between different levels, this is particularly important for older rats with reduced mobility. Ramps should be of solid, non-slip material, not too steep, wide enough to avoid falls and with horizontal ridges to provide grip.

A latrine area should be provided: normally a flat rock, brick, or piece of slate which encourages rats to urinate in one place and is also helpful for keeping nails short. Rats may be litter trained, either to defaecate in a box or a specific area of the cage. It is most helpful to fill this area with a different type of bedding and add some of their droppings so they can differentiate this from the rest of the cage.

Handbook of Exotic Pet Medicine, First Edition. Edited by Marie Kubiak.
© 2021 John Wiley & Sons Ltd. Published 2021 by John Wiley & Sons Ltd.
Companion website: www.wiley.com/go/kubiak/exotic_pet_medicine

Table 8.1 Biological parameters.

Parameter	Value
Gestation	19–23 days
Life expectancy	2–3.5 years
Oestrus cycle	4–5 days
Duration of oestrus	10–20 hours
Young per litter	8–18
Size of young at birth	4–6 g
Age when eyes open	12–15 days
Weaning age	17–21 days
Sexual maturity	6–8 weeks
Pairs of mammary glands	6
Body temperature	35.9–37.5 °C
Heart Rate	330–480 beats per minute
Respiratory Rate	85–130
Dental formula	1/1 0/0 0/0 3/3

Rats' incisor teeth grow continually throughout their lives, and it is vital they are given the opportunity to gnaw, for behavioural reasons. Wood, branches, and specially formulated rat chew blocks are all excellent choices and will help keep the rat entertained. If a rat is constantly chewing on the bars of their cage, this can be taken as a sign of frustration or boredom; the rats will appreciate more time being handled, free-roaming or, if this is not available, further enrichment within their cage environment.

Cages with wire bottoms are to be avoided as although they allow waste food, faeces and urine to fall through, they are a causative factor in pododermatitis (bumblefoot). Wood chip, cat litter, shavings, and sawdust are controversial substrates as they are absorbent and often scented, naturally or artificially, helping to cover the smell of urine, but generate dust that can irritate the delicate rat respiratory system, and may mask ammonia accumulation. Dust extracted shavings and woodchip are preferred but softwood varieties may still contain irritating and potentially toxic resins. These can cause respiratory tract irritation, and have been known to cause elevations in liver enzymes in laboratory situations (Schoental 1973). Bedding specifically designed and sold for rats is preferred. Commercial paper based products can be soft and absorbent. Shredded waste paper can be useful for burrowing or hiding food. Newspaper, tissue or kitchen paper can be added to the cage, as the rat will enjoy shredding the material and adding it to their sleeping area or nest box. Paper must be regularly changed as it will quickly absorb urine. Cloth is another alternative, with the added bonus that it can be washed and re-used but any cloth that unravels easily must be avoided as long threads will quickly get tangled and may

cause injury. Fleece is an ideal choice, especially in colder months. Rats will chew material items over time, and they will require frequent washing and replacement.

Hammocks and soft material cubes are a popular choice for sleeping areas as they can be washed, and multi-levelled hammocks allow rats to choose their own sleeping area. However, chewing can result in limited longevity of these items. Plastic sleeping tubs or tunnels are easily washed but will need plenty of shredded cloth or paper for the rat to fill them with before they are comfortable (Figure 8.1).

Rats are highly intelligent and require a substantial amount of enrichment within their cage to ensure they are not bored. Alexander et al. (1978) demonstrated that with sufficient cage enrichment, rats would choose to drink plain water over morphine water whilst rats in an empty cage would consistently choose narcotics. Toys should be made out of plastic or wood, the former is easier to clean but may be chewed through, the latter may be more durable but will absorb a lot of the rats' scent marking and potentially urine. Removing some of the cage levels and replacing them with ropes, tunnels and hammocks will make climbing the cage much more of a challenge and keep rats active. Simple puzzles, such as hiding treats in egg boxes or twists of paper are cheap but effective ways of keeping rats entertained. Food can be used in multiple ways, for example dropping frozen peas into a small tub of earth or water for the rats to find is an easy way of keeping them happy and cool on a warm day. A hard-boiled egg still in its shell is a nutritious treat and a puzzle all in one! Switching round the toys and levels in the cage after cleaning will help keep rats on their toes and they will enjoy discovering all the new areas of their homes. There is a fine balance, however, and cages should not be completely changed, especially with regard to bedding, to maintain some feeling of a consistent environment. Ideally, rats should spend at least an hour outside their cage a day, interacting with their owners and free-roaming. As many human living spaces are unsuitable for free roaming, due to wires or electric appliances, owners may choose to cordon off a safe area in which their rat can free-roam. With frequent handling, rats make affectionate pets and can even be taught simple tricks.

Rats are highly social animals and are best kept in pairs or small groups. Generally speaking these should be single sex to avoid unwanted pregnancies, but neutered males can live alongside entire or neutered females. When introducing any new rat into an established group, the 'carrier method' is advised. The carrier cage will be a small, neutral space that should not carry the scent of any of the rats. The rats are placed in the cage with two separate water sources for a short period of time. Harmless but strongly smelling material such as vanilla essence or coconut oil can be

Table 8.2   Coat and body type variations seen in captive rats.

Coat colouration	Description
Self-colour	Single coat colour. Includes Pink/Red-Eyed Whites, Champagne, Black-Eyed Whites, British/American Blue, Chocolate, Black (not to be confused with the Black Rat, *Rattus rattus*), Russian Blue and many more. These colours may fade or change noticeably as the rat ages.
Berkshire	white chest and belly
Irish	a white triangle at the thoracic inlet
Hooded	these have a darker coloured head, extending down the dorsal midline, of variable width
Variegated	randomly patterned in 2 colours
Capped	a darker head only
Essex	a single colour, darker at the head end and lightening towards the tail
Badger	a dark body, white face and other patches over the body
Chinchilla	dark grey dorsally, white ventrally
Roan	white and dark grey hairs intermingled
Siamese	white or cream body with dark patch on nose and near base of tail
Coat type	
Normal	Full coat
Rex	These lack guard hairs and have curled whiskers
Hairless or Sphinx	There are gradations of hairlessness from short, brittle fur which breaks easily, through to totally bald rats, with no body hair whatsoever, including whiskers. Whilst hairless or 'Sphinx' rats are popular with some owners, as well as causing problems with thermoregulation, this is depriving the animal of an important sense organ, and could be considered to be a deliberately induced genetic deformity with significant welfare concerns. For this reason, Sphinx rats are banned from National Fancy Rat Society (NFRS) UK shows and breeders' lists.
Body type	
Normal	Morphologically identical to wild rats
Tailless rats	These rats possess a genetic abnormality leading to a rounded, smooth rump, and no evidence of a tail. Such rats have impaired balance and thermoregulation. A number of rats bred to tailless parents will have either an incomplete tail, or spinal defects. Tailless rats are banned from NFRS associations.
Dumbo	These rats have their ears set lower and more laterally on the skull compared to the more dorsal position in standard rats. There is no definitive evidence either way on whether this variety is more likely to develop health problems associated with this anatomical feature, but it is worth noting that in the quest to breed a specific variety of animal, there is less emphasis on breeding from healthy animals or those with good temperaments, and in-breeding may be over-utilised to in order to breed suitable animals.

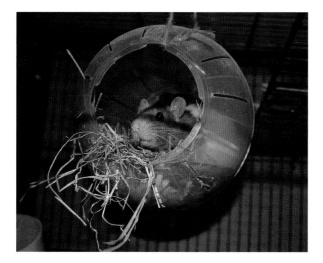

Figure 8.1   Rats will readily use hides at height. Plastic is easily cleaned but may be chewed so requires regular checks.

rubbed around the rats' tail, nose and genitals to encourage mutual grooming. A small amount of fighting is normal with both genders, but drawing blood is a sign of aggression and introductions should be halted, and the rats separated until the wounds heal. If the small carrier cage introduction is successful, the rats can be moved to a larger space for a longer period of time, until they are ready to move into a proper cage together. Rat groups have a hierarchy, and the dominant rat is likely to make their presence known by fighting or attempting to mate with their cage-mates.

A new rat will often seem shy until they are fully adjusted to their new surroundings. To encourage the rat, the owners' fingers can be dipped in yoghurt, coconut oil, or vanilla essence. Once the rat seems comfortable licking from the fingers, the owner can move on to offering solid treats until the rat is confident enough around them to be removed from the cage. Generally speaking, rats can spend up to three hours out of the cage without defecating; new rats may need to be potty trained as they may excrete after being out of the cage for only a few minutes. To do this, the rat should be placed swiftly back in the cage at the first sign of faeces, and the droppings placed alongside them in the cage. They will adjust to this system within a few weeks.

Rats are generalist, opportunistic omnivores (Suckow et al. 2006). Whilst this means that they can survive on almost anything, it does not mean that they do not develop nutritionally induced diseases if incorrectly fed. Considerable research has gone into developing balanced diets for laboratory rats and commercially available complete pelleted diets are the best option, supplemented by small pieces of fruit or vegetables and dog biscuits. 'Muesli mix' type diets allow selective feeding for favoured high fat items over the complete pelleted components. Treats such as biscuits and chocolate may lead to obesity and dental caries, and should be avoided in favour of small pieces of dog treats. A balanced diet should be 12–18% protein for maintenance (18–25% for pregnant and lactating females) and 5% fat, and may contain animal protein sources as well as vegetable protein sources. Rats are not at significant risk of gastrointestinal stasis, and their nutritional needs are simpler and easier to fulfil than herbivorous rodents. There is no specific fibre requirement for rats, but lower levels will lead to decreased gastrointestinal transit time and loose faeces (Suckow et al. 2006). Rats' sense of taste is exceptionally good, especially at detecting new and potentially dangerous food items in this neophobic species. A single poor experience is enough to deter them from eating that food item again (Garcia et al. 1974).

Using standard commercial rat foods, suggested dietary intakes are 15 g of food per rat each day for growing rats or maintenance of adult rats, 15–20 g/day during pregnancy and 30–40 g/rat/day during lactation (NRC 1995). Rats generally eat to meet energy requirements and so ad-lib feeding is generally acceptable in unneutered groups with all individuals of normal weight, especially if they obtain sufficient exercise and are not geriatric (over 20 months of age). If any start gaining weight above a Body Condition Score (BCS) of 5/9 (ZIMS 2017) then restricted food intake (or separated feeding) is necessary. If one or two individuals develop a significantly higher BCS than the group as whole, there may be social or health concerns that need addressing.

Food may be provided in bowls (several, to avoid one rat dominating food), or scattered/hidden, to encourage positive behaviours. Rats may cache food, though not to the same degree as gerbils and hamsters. Rats have highly developed hearing, with a wide range of frequencies detectable (200 Hz to 90 kHz) (Fay 1988) and rats are particularly sensitive to ultrasound. For this reason, rats should be fed in ceramic bowls rather than metal, to avoid generation of ultrasonic frequency sounds.

Water is rarely provided in bowls, as they rapidly become soiled. Water drinkers are attached to the cage, ensuring all individuals can reach at least one. Rats may chew plastic attachment points or the bottles themselves, thus depriving themselves of water. Average water consumption is 100 ml/kg/day, on a totally dry diet (Wade et al. 2002).

8.2 Reproduction

Rats are prolific breeders, with a pair of rats able to produce 800–1000 descendants in one year (Almeida et al. 2013). Females are polyoestrous, with spontaneous ovulation and a post-partum oestrus. The vaginal opening is separate from the urethral opening and is only open for oestrus and parturition (Clark and Price 1981). After mating the copulatory plug formed by male's accessory sex gland secretions seals the vaginal opening for 12–24 hours.

Two or three days before the doe is due she should be moved to a separate carrier or single level cage and provided with a nestbox (a small cardboard box of plastic tube) and abundant bedding material, such as paper or tissue. Pre-partum she will shred this material and create a large nest space in which she can give birth and safely cover the young. Young are altricial, described as 'pinkies', with closed eyes and no fur at all. Dystocia and other periparturient problems are very rare given their small size, although vaginal and sometimes uterine prolapse are reported.

The young should stay in the birth cage undisturbed for three weeks, when they can be moved into a larger cage. At five weeks the young will be weaned and sexually mature and must be separated from the mother into single sex groups to avoid in-breeding. Note the importance of narrower cage bars at this point, or young may escape.

8.3 Clinical Evaluation

8.3.1 History-Taking

Taking a full history is vital with rats, as husbandry methods can vary widely between owners, and poor husbandry is often present and may lead to problems. The animal is totally dependent on the limited environment available to it, and awareness of ideal husbandry is lower in rodent owners than those of more commonly kept pets. The substrate, cage construction, and layout should be described, ideally with the aid of photos. The placement of the cage with regard to ventilation, sunlight, and sources of heat or fans, should be noted. The owner should be asked for cleaning frequency and materials used.

The age, sex, and reproductive history should be obtained, along with any familial history of disease. Details of previous homes, and the length of time in the current location should be established. The health status of any cagemates, living, or recently dead, should be ascertained.

The diet of the animal, both currently and historically, is important. Ideally, samples should be brought in, as 'Rat food' is variable in composition and quality. Method of provision, which animals share it, and any changes in appetite should be noted, along with water source and intake. Any changes in urine or faecal output, such as altered consistency or odour, should be identified.

The owner may need careful questioning regarding mobility. Whilst some rats have a history of visibly reduced mobility and/or exercise tolerance, more subtle changes such as avoidance of higher cage levels may be identifiable. Any time out of the cage means that possible sources of injury should be elucidated, e.g. gnawing through electrical cables.

8.3.2 Sex Determination

Sex determination is far easier in rats than in many rodent species. Males and females can be distinguished from birth if necessary, with a much shorter anogenital distance in does (Figures 8.2 and 8.3). At two to three weeks the female can be distinguished from the male by the dark dots on her underbelly which will develop into teats. From the age of five weeks the males' distinctive testicles will be visible.

8.3.3 Handling

Docile rats may simply be approached slowly and cupped in the hands, allowed to walk onto the hand or forearm from the owners, or picked up with the hand under the body and the thumb on top. This grip can be modified to place a forefinger under the mandible to prevent being bitten, if necessary, or reversed, with the thumb under the mandible and the hand on the dorsum. Scruffing rats is not effective or comfortable and should not be performed.

Less friendly rats may be picked up by the base of the tail, and permitted to take their weight on and grip with, their foreclaws resting on an arm. This works best with long sleeves.

Aggressive rats should be moved directly from their box, e.g. via tubes, nestboxes, or hammocks, into a gaseous anaesthesia induction chamber. Examination under anaesthesia is often beneficial for a full clinical examination, especially involving an intraoral, intra-aural, or ocular exam, or if samples are required.

Physical restraint devices have been developed for use in laboratory settings, but in inexperienced hands are best avoided.

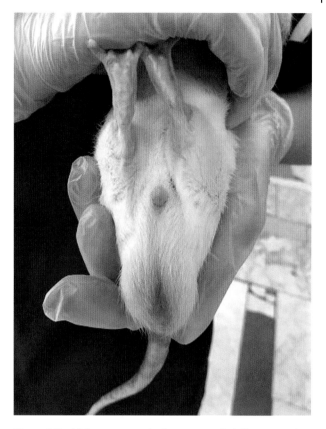

Figure 8.2 Male rat – note the long anogenital distance and single genital and urethral orifice (*Source:* Photo courtesy of Sarah Pellett).

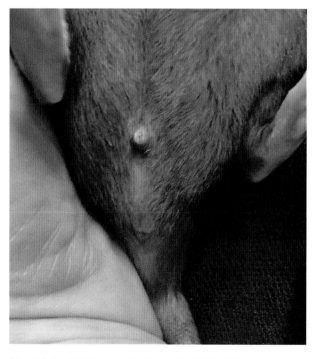

Figure 8.3 Female rat with short anogenital distance and urethral papilla and vaginal orifice in close association.

8.3.4 Clinical Examination

Observation prior to handling is generally advised, as behaviour may change after handling. Lethargic animals will appear livelier and escape attempts may make assessment of demeanour and measurement of respiratory rate, depth, and pattern more difficult. Mobility can be judged most effectively in a cage with a wide variety of climbing furniture. Rats should not be loose in the room, off the table, as a healthy rat will be challenging to catch.

After observation, the rat should be restrained for examination. The head is easily examined without restraint, and any abnormalities of the eyes (a variable degree of bulging is often seen due to stress), ears, and nose noted. Chromodacryorrhoea (porphyrin production from the eyes or nose), is common in rats, denoting stress and/or disease, especially upper respiratory tract disease. The rest of the body may be examined with minimal restraint. The skin of the dorsum, especially over the scapulae, is the most common area for mite infestation and other skin diseases.

Abdominal palpation and thoracic auscultation should be carried out. Examination of the mammary glands is important in females, but all skin should be examined, rolling it between the fingers to detect masses. The author rarely takes the rectal temperature of rats other than under anaesthesia or if presented collapsed or with a suspicion of either hypo or hyperthermia. If this is needed, a flexible, well lubricated digital thermometer, with a fast recording time is preferred.

Oral examination is best performed last, as it is the most stressful part. The incisors may be seen easily, by everting the lips evenly. Whilst an otoscope may be used conscious to examine the molars, visibility is limited. If dental disease is suspected, a more complete view can be obtained under brief volatile agent anaesthesia, using either an otoscope, or opening the mouth using purpose designed instruments.

Bodyweight and condition should be determined. Rats normally stand on scales long enough to directly obtain a weight. If not, a small carry box can be used to confine them, and its weight deducted from the total afterwards. BCS is determined on a 1–5 or 1–9 scale, based on the ease of palpation of the ribs, spine and hips, and the amount of intra-abdominal fat present.

8.4 Basic Techniques

8.4.1 Sampling

8.4.1.1 Blood Sampling

General anaesthesia greatly facilitates vascular access. Blood volume in rats is 5.5–7 ml/100 g bodyweight and 10% of this (i.e. 0.55–0.7 ml/100 g) can be collected, assuming no significant bruising at the site (Parasuraman et al. 2010).

For very small samples, for a blood smear, manual haematocrit, or blood glucose estimation, a lancet may be used on the marginal ear vein, but volumes are minimal. For larger samples, the femoral vein may be accessed, especially in rats of normal to underweight body condition. The rat is placed in dorsal recumbency and the leg abducted to access the medial thigh. A palpable femoral pulse identifies the femoral artery, and a 25–27 g needle is advanced blindly towards this, accessing the more superficial vein first. If the artery is entered, gentle but firm pressure is applied for two minutes to avoid a haematoma. The jugular or cranial vena cava (CVC) may also be used. (Figure 8.4) The jugular is straightforward in underweight rats where it may be visualised, but more challenging in those with more subcutaneous fat. The CVC is perhaps the most reliable site for sampling, as in other species such as degus and gerbils, especially for volumes greater than 0.5 ml, and sampling is described in Chapter 6.

The tail of the rat has lateral veins in the '3 o'clock' and '9 o'clock' positions. These can be accessed at the furred base of the tail, where they can be seen, or approximately

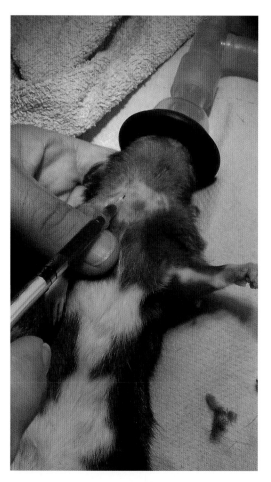

Figure 8.4 Jugular blood sample collection in the anaesthetised rat.

half way down the tail as a blind approach. This may be carried out conscious more easily than the other techniques. Applying local anaesthetic cream and warming the tail prior to sampling may increase success with this site (Parasuraman et al. 2010).

Anticoagulant choice is dependent on testing required. If sample volume is small, heparin anticoagulant often preserves samples adequately for both biochemistry and haematology.

8.4.1.2 Urine

Rats may void their bladder on the examination table or on anaesthetic induction. Alternatively, the anaesthetised rat may have its bladder expressed via manual pressure. Catheterisation is possible although the male urethra is usually too small for standard catheters. The female's separate urethral aperture makes catheterisation relatively straightforward. Cystocentesis, either manually or ultrasound guided, is the preferred technique where the bladder can be identified.

8.4.1.3 Faeces

Rats usually void faeces when examined or anaesthetised. Fresh faeces can often be collected from the transport cage.

8.4.1.4 Skin Sampling

Fur plucks and skin scrapes may be taken for microscopy and fungal (dermatophyte) culture conscious or under anaesthesia.

8.4.2 Nutritional Support

Calorie intake in healthy adult rats is 70–80 kcal/day (Corwin 2004) though requirements can increase in sick animals. Purpose designed liquid diets for exotic patients are preferred for assist feeding, with combination of herbivore and carnivore products, or use of pre-formed omnivore diets. These may be supplied via syringe, free choice, or by gavage feeding. Syringe feeding of palatable foods is generally tolerated well. Gavage administration may be a suitable method where a brief, stressful intervention is deemed better than prolonged and repeated attempts to hand feed a reluctant rat. Pharyngostomy tubes have been used in laboratory settings, but are not often used in pet rats. They are largely unnecessary, invasive, and difficult to maintain and prevent interference.

8.4.3 Fluid Therapy

Maintenance fluid requirements are 80–100 ml/kg/day and standard crystalloids or dextrose containing solutions are suitable (Klaphake 2006). All anorexic and debilitated rats should be considered as dehydrated with deficits replaced over 48 hours. Fluids should be warmed to the rats' normal body temperature prior to administration. Routes for fluid therapy are described in Table 8.3.

8.4.4 Anaesthesia

General anaesthesia is required for restraint, to reduce the stress associated with non-painful procedures, and for more invasive procedures including surgery. Anaesthesia is considered a higher risk in rats (2.01% mortality rate) compared to cats (0.24%) and dogs (0.17%) (Brodbelt et al. 2008). Amongst the reasons suggested to account for this are that rats have a very high surface-area to volume ratio predisposing to perioperative hypothermia, they have fewer easily accessible veins for venous catheterisation and endotracheal intubation is much more technically demanding than in cats and dogs. A significant number of rats presenting for anaesthesia also have pre-existing respiratory disease such as Mycoplasmosis. Rats cannot vomit, and have a rapid metabolic rate so pre-operative starvation should be avoided.

Unless specifically contra-indicated then pain relief should be pre-emptive, to reduce maintenance anaesthesia doses and to prevent 'wind up' potentiation of pain. In rats, multimodal analgesia, for example using opioids, non-steroidal anti-inflammatory drugs (NSAIDS), and local analgesia together, has a synergistic effect, and avoids overdependence on one agent. As well as the welfare issues, pain may prevent a rat from eating, slowing its recovery and encouraging it to self-traumatise lesions or surgical incisions, increasing the risk of perioperative infections, wound dehiscence, and other complications (Lichtenberger and Ko 2007).

Drug combinations may be given by intramuscular or subcutaneous injection, which is technically simple but cannot be given incrementally to effect. Intravenous induction agents can be delivered to effect but are technically challenging. Volatile agents can be used, and these minimise handling, are straightforward to deliver and can be delivered to effect, but involve a stressful induction phase, and cause environmental contamination. A compromise is to use injectable sedation, and then induce to effect, and maintain, with a volatile agent.

The volatile agents of choice are generally isoflurane or sevoflurane. No significant difference is seen in induction time between these two agents but isoflurane is aversive and may cause mucous membrane irritation during induction (Cesarovic et al. 2010; Khan et al. 2014). The minimum alveolar concentration (MAC) of sevoflurane is 2.29% in adult rats and 2.68% in juvenile rats, and a MAC of 1.85% has been reported for isoflurane in mice

Table 8.3 Fluid therapy routes.

Fluid route	Site	Volume to be given	Pros	Cons
Subcutaneous	Over the ribs or flanks and between the scapulae	No more than 5 ml per site	Rats have loose, mobile skin, with sufficient space for relatively large volumes of fluids (Figure 8.5)	SC fluids are not absorbed rapidly, especially with the poor tissue perfusion seen in shock, so are only suitable for gradual rehydration of non-critical patients. Uptake may be accelerated by adding hyaluronidase
Intraperitoneal	Hold the rat in dorsal recumbency, and place the needle in the caudal left or right quadrant of the abdomen (Figure 8.6)	Up to 15 ml	Well-established for rats in laboratory settings and has a more rapid uptake than the SC route.	It is possible to perforate the bladder or bowel. Avoiding moving the needle once in place, and aspirating before injection minimises this risk. Only non-irritant isotonic crystalloids may be given via this route.
Intravenous	The lateral tail vein is the most practical, using a 26–24 g cannula.	Large volumes can be infused over time.	Rapid rehydration possible.	Technically more challenging. A tourniquet placed at the base of the tail and gentle warming of the tail assist with vasodilation and venous access.
Intraosseous	Proximal humerus and femur	Large volumes can be infused over time.	Allows for rapid rehydration of critical patients without the need for venous access. Hypodermic needles can be used.	Anaesthesia required for aseptic catheter placement. Needles may be occluded by bone after placement and require replacing. Complications include iatrogenic fracture or introduction of infection.

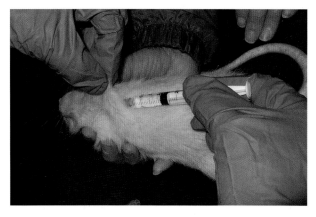

Figure 8.5   Subcutaneous injection in the rat.

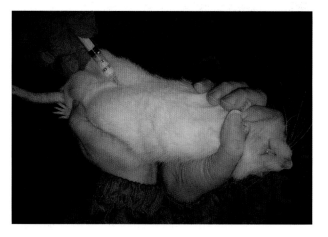

Figure 8.6   Intraperitoneal injection in the rat.

(Kashimoto et al. 1997; Cesarovic et al. 2010). Both agents cause respiratory depression and monitoring of oxygenation during anaesthesia is essential (Cesarovic et al. 2010). Concerns have been raised with sevoflurane as rats are capable of producing higher levels of a nephrotoxic metabolite than other species (Sheffels et al. 2004; Kharasch et al. 2005). However, in clinical settings nephrotoxicity appears unlikely (Kharasch et al. 2005). Neurodegeneration has been reported in newborn rats following the use of a number of anaesthetic agents, including sevoflurane, but the significance in older rats is unknown (Bercker et al. 2009).

Endotracheal intubation is challenging in the rat. Whilst carried out routinely in the laboratory setting, it requires practice and the very small tubes used are prone to kinking or becoming obstructed with mucus. An intranasal cannula may be placed to deliver oxygen and volatile agents. Facemasks may be constructed from syringe barrels or similar materials, but commercially available small masks with a more secure fit, and coaxial scavenging systems are preferred.

Prevention of hypothermia is vital by insulating the patient and providing supplementary heating. Reducing losses is achieved by minimising removal of insulating fur, warming surgical skin preparations and avoiding those which significantly cool the skin through evaporation. The body temperature should be monitored throughout the anaesthesia and recovery periods.

The eyes are protuberant and must be well protected with ophthalmic lubricants regularly as they do not blink effectively under anaesthesia. This also makes a blink unhelpful to assess depth of anaesthesia, and eye position does not alter significantly. Anaesthetic depth may be assessed by changes to respiratory and heart rates. Response to a tail pinch is lost at a medium depth, prior to a toe pinch at deeper planes. Any monitoring must have respiratory and cardiac monitoring capable of measuring the high rates for this species and pulse oximetry is advisable to monitor oxygenation with probes attached to the tongue, foot, or tail base.

8.4.4.1 Surgical Principles

Even small absolute amounts of blood loss can be an issue. Loss of 20% of the circulating blood volume is potentially fatal, equating to 5 ml for a 250 g rat. Magnification helps with surgical precision and minimises tissue trauma and blood loss. Radiosurgery can aid in haemostasis but care must be taken with these small patients to avoid collateral damage as the current passes through the body.

Respiration should not be impaired by placing instruments on the thorax.

Wound closure is a challenge in rats, as they are capable of opening up almost any surgical wound. Pre-emptive and ongoing multimodal analgesia are the key to keeping rats comfortable and minimising interference but closure technique can also have effects. Small diameter atraumatic monofilament suture material (maximum 1.5 metric), on swaged on needles minimises tissue trauma and thus wound interference. Intradermal or subcuticular patterns hide the suture line from the rat, reducing the risk of it being gnawed through, but not preventing it completely. Stainless steel wire and staples have been used for wound closure. Rats can get either of these out by traumatising the skin, but the latter are a quick method to re-close wounds that have been opened, at which point extra steps are needed to protect them. Skin glue is useful, but has limitations. It may be applied rapidly in the anaesthetised or conscious patient (although the exothermic reaction of it hardening can generate heat and pain), but has no significant strength holding, and is therefore best for adhering adjoining skin already closed with intradermal or subcuticular sutures. Excessive amounts can cause thermal pain and damage, and overlapping or untidy closures can increase the rat's determination to groom it off.

Dressings are generally not protective, although bodywraps can be highly effective (Figure 8.7). Aversive sprays are ineffective. Elizabethan collars are effective, but difficult

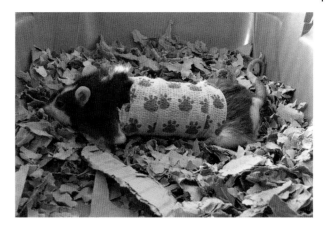

Figure 8.7 Use of a bandage body wrap to protect wounds.

to fit on rats: If they are too loose, they easily slip over the small head, and if too tight, can cause feeding difficulties, dyspnoea, and skin trauma as the rat tries to scratch them off. Trimming the incisor teeth to prevent gnawing may lead to incisor malformation, and difficulty prehending food, and is not recommended. Chemical sedation, using opioids and benzodiazepines for several days post operatively, may be needed in severe cases to prevent self-trauma. Analgesia should be reviewed in any case of self-trauma.

8.4.5 Euthanasia

Euthanasia is best carried out by intravenous or intracardiac barbiturate overdose under anaesthesia. Alternative routes, such as intraosseous, may be used, but intraperitoneal injection is slow to take effect and potentially irritant to the peritoneal cavity.

8.4.6 Hospitalisation Requirements

Rats should ideally be kept separate from predator species, away from their sight, sound and smell. Where possible hospitalised rats should be kept in their social group. Though in some cases they may need to be separated to monitor food intake and prevent wound interference by conspecifics, ideally visual and olfactory contact with companions should still be maintained. Cage fronts must be small enough to prevent escape, or the rat(s) should be hospitalised in their own cage within the kennel. Supplementary heating may be needed if the animal is hypothermic, in recovery from anaesthesia, or the room itself is cold, but unprotected wires may be chewed through by rats. Cooling and ventilation may be needed in hot and/or humid weather, especially in rats with respiratory disease.

Bedding may be replaced, temporarily, postoperatively by plain paper to show up blood loss, or soft artificial sheepskin style products to provide a comfortable, warm bed.

Owners should be encouraged to bring in the rat's usual diet to provide familiar food items and encourage self-feeding, even is diet is less than ideal.

8.5 Common Medical and Surgical Conditions

8.5.1 Neoplasia

Tumour types commonly seen in rats include mammary fibroadenoma, lipoma, lymphoma, pituitary chromophore adenoma, and Zymbals gland tumour (Figures 8.8 and 8.9) (Chandra et al. 1992; Harleman et al. 2012).

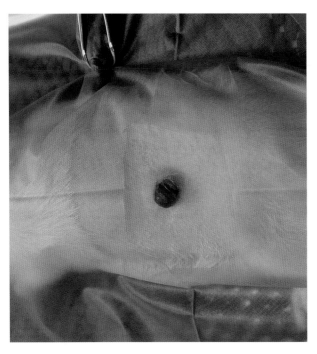

Figure 8.8 Dermal lymphoma in a pet rat.

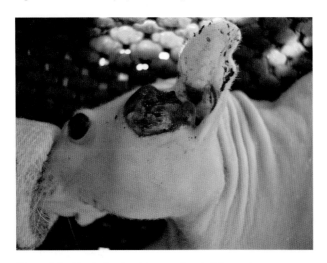

Figure 8.9 Zymbals gland tumour in a hairless rat.

The mammary glands are the most common site for tumour development in the female rat. Fibroadenomas are most common, comprising 80–90% mammary neoplasms, with adenocarcinomas less common (Greenacre and Gibbons 2011). Fibroadenomas develop under hormonal influences, with ovariectomy/ovariohysterectomy (OVH) at or before 90 days being preventative (Hotchkiss 1995). Male incidence in one study was shown to be 0.5%, compared to 33% in a comparable group of females (Barsoum et al. 1984). The prevalence of pituitary neoplasia is not significantly different between pet rats with or without mammary fibroadenoma, suggesting that mammary fibroadenoma is spontaneous rather than induced (Vergneau-Grosset et al. 2016). Mammary tissue extends from the level of the scapula, to the inguinal region, along the lateral and ventral body wall (O'Malley 2005). Surgical excision at an early stage is generally straightforward (Figure 8.10) but if delayed becomes more complicated with large, ulcerated or infiltrating growths. It is important to note that new tumours may develop de novo after previous tumours have been surgically removed, and this is not local spread. Rats appear to interfere post-operatively most with surgery of the most caudal mammary gland, possibly through discomfort, or it being the easiest to reach, even with a collar on. Neutering at the same time as the first tumour develops, can prevent others developing if carried out early enough. After that, repeat surgeries are required, although prevention can be attempted with husbandry or medical techniques.

A significant reduction in food energy intake reduces the incidence of mammary tumours (Tucker 1979), but this is unlikely to be practical long-term with pet rats. Tamoxifen is used in human mammary gland carcinoma treatment but is ineffective for fibroadenomas and induces hepatic neoplasia in rats (Keeble 2001). Cabergoline has been dem-

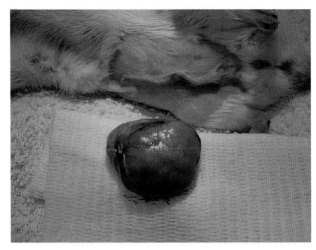

Figure 8.10 Excision of a mammary fibroadenoma, note the typical smooth, encapsulated appearance.

onstrated as more effective than bromcriptine, and has been used for suppression of development of mammary tumours (Eguchi et al. 1995; Mayer et al. 2011).

Pituitary tumours also occur in older rats of both sexes, with intact non-breeding females more commonly affected and neutering before 90 days of age effective at reducing incidence (Trouillas et al. 1982). Clinical signs include a head tilt, ataxia, and a general slowing down in activity and diagnosis is typically presumptive by exclusion of differentials, and treatment is palliative.

The sebaceous Zymbals gland is present at the base of the external ear and carcinomas occur occasionally, ulcerating onto the skin, and becoming locally invasive (Figure 8.9) (Rudmann et al. 2012). Surgery may be curative if carried out before significant local spread occurs.

8.5.2 Respiratory Infections and Chromodacryorrhoea/Porphyria

Rats may have, solely or in conjunction, a number of infectious respiratory tract pathogens present. *Mycoplasma pulmonis, Filobacterium rodentium* (previously known as Cilia-associated respiratory bacillus), *Corynebacterium kutscheri, Klebsiella pneumoniae*, sialodacryoadenitis virus (SDAV) and Sendai virus are all common in rats, with mycoplasma and SDAV the most frequent pathogens. As well as increased porphyrin secretion, clinically affected rats present with increased respiratory sounds and effort, reduced appetite, weight loss, open mouth breathing, and an unkempt coat. (NRC 1991).

Diagnosis of respiratory disease is readily made by history and clinical examination, but pathogens can only be identified with specific testing, using culture, polymerase chain reaction (PCR), and enzyme-linked immunosorbent assay (ELISA) techniques. This is rarely carried out in pet rats due to the difficulty of obtaining a representative sample in small rodents ante-mortem, the ubiquity of *M. pulmonis* and the fact that presumptive treatment is generally preferred. Testing in breeding colonies and other large groups in an outbreak situation may be more practical and useful. Thoracic radiography can be helpful in identifying focal abscessation and extent of pathology to determine prognosis as disease is often more severe than clinical status would indicate (Figure 8.11).

Treatment of bacterial pathogens is possible and, even where viral disease is present, it is hoped that antibacterial treatment will improve the rat's clinical status by management of co-infections. The choice of antibiotic(s) should be determined by culture and sensitivity ideally, or empirically based on suspected pathogens present. Best practice guidelines (BVA 2017) suggest the avoidance of fluoroquinolones as first line treatments. Any drug selected must

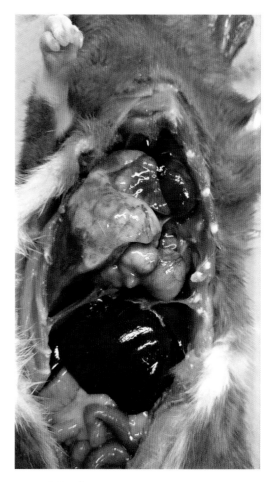

Figure 8.11 Post-mortem assessment of extensive pulmonary abscessation in rat with chronic mycoplasmosis.

have good patient compliance to enable it to be given effectively. For this reason human paediatric generics, which are highly palatable liquids, may be the only practical option, especially where they have a suitable spectrum (e.g. azithromycin for mycoplasma, sulphonamides for susceptible bacterial infections). Rats have a shorter intestinal tract, with no need for bacterial fermentation of cellulose, and are therefore relatively unaffected by oral broad spectrum antimicrobials which can cause fatal dysbiosis in herbivorous rodents. They can therefore safely be given oral penicillins, lincosamides, and cephalosporins.

Adjunctive treatment is important. Anti-inflammatories reduce discomfort, and clinical improvement results from the reduction in inflammation and associated widening of the airways. Given the presence of a mixed pathogen load, some of which may not be treatable, NSAIDs are the most commonly used. Steroids may help in severe dyspnoea or palliation of terminal cases, but should be used for the minimum time possible, with care. Bronchodilators symptomatically improve breathing, as well as making it easier for the rat to expel material from the lungs, and work synergistically with corticosteroids. (Sathe et al. 2015; Nagakumar and Rao 2019). Acetylcysteine reduces the viscosity of thicker mucus and purulent material to assist its removal. Sildenafil has been shown to attenuate mucus production and airway constriction in experimental rat models (Wang et al. 2009).

Nebulisation delivers a fine mist of liquid (typically isotonic saline, with or without medication) into the respiratory tract. There is some controversy around how far the fine particles are able to travel down the respiratory tract, and this depends on the particle size and electrostatic charge, and turbulence within the respiratory tract. Portable nebulisers are readily available but not all create consistently small particles of 3–5 μm to treat lower respiratory tract disease. For upper respiratory tract infections, the particle size is less crucial.

Nebulising saline alone helps to moisten, dilute, and expel purulent exudate. Antibiotics are commonly added, for example aminoglycosides, which are often effective against respiratory tract disease organisms, but which may cause adverse reactions when given parenterally. Disinfectants, such as quaternary ammonium and biguanide compounds (F10, Health and Hygiene, SA) may be helpful in treating bacterial, fungal, and viral pathogens. Bronchodilators may assist antibiotic therapy by widening the airway, encouraging expulsion of material and increasing antibiotic penetration to the alveolus.

Cleaning and nursing care is also important. Crusted material around the nares impedes breathing and causes discomfort. Patients may need hand feeding if appetite is reduced by general debility and a diminished sense of smell.

Environmental conditions can affect respiratory tract health profoundly. Damp, poorly ventilated areas with high levels of irritant particulate materials and high ammonia levels trigger or exacerbate respiratory tract disease. Ammonia, in particular, causes damage to the defence mechanisms of the respiratory tract, slowing the mucociliary elevator and destroying cilia. Environmental improvements must go hand in hand with prevention or medical treatment. Inspired air quality can be improved by using barred cages rather than glass, providing hammocks to allow sleeping off the floor and by reducing ammonia levels with frequent bedding changes.

Prognosis depends on the presence or absence of any pathogens which cannot be treated (resistant bacteria, or viral agents), the general health of the patient, any environmental constraints, owner compliance, and the presence or absence of irreversible respiratory tract damage from chronic or recurrent infections. Early aggressive treatment of respiratory tract disease is advisable, both at the start,

and with any flare-ups of infection. Treatment failure, especially after repeated bouts, leading to chronic, irreversible changes, is common and many cases will eventually progress to an intractable state.

As well as providing optimal husbandry from acquisition, sourcing animals of high health status helps to avoid bringing in problems. As a minimum, any animals with clinical signs should be rejected, and, ideally, pre-import testing performed to detect, and guide treatment where necessary. However, *M. pulmonis* is considered ubiquitous in the pet rat population and a single negative PCR test should not be considered definitive.

Rats produce a red, porphyrin-rich secretion from the Harderian glands associated with the eyes. When produced in greater than normal quantities (with stress and disease, especially respiratory tract disease), or when it is not cleaned away by the rat (e.g. with pain or general debility) or conspecifics (with altered social interaction), it accumulates around nose, and particularly the eyes (Williams 2002). Whilst it does not typically result in the sore nasal planum seen in gerbils, it is often a marker of significant disease or welfare problems, with the most common cause being *M. pulmonis* (Young and Hill 1974).

8.5.3 Cardiac Disease

Congestive heart failure is seen in older rats, with either hypertrophic or dilated cardiomyopathy being potentially present. Clinical signs vary, with sudden death, or a slow progressive or intermittent decline in activity, reduced weight and appetite, and possible respiratory signs that can be difficult to differentiate from primary respiratory tract disease. Treatment is as for other species, with supportive care, oxygen therapy if collapsed, diuretics, angiotensin-converting-enzyme (ACE) inhibitors and/or pimobendan as required (Sweet et al. 1987).

8.5.4 Renal Disease

The most common renal disorder in rats is a chronic, gradually progressive nephropathy typically starting to affect rats from one year of age (Ijpelaar et al. 2008). Clinical signs include weight loss, muscle wasting, and inappetence. On investigation, azotaemia, proteinuria, isosthenuria, and elevated urine protein:creatinine ratios may be noted. On radiography, there may be calcification of the renal parenchyma, gastric mucosa, and great vessels. Management is by providing a low protein diet and ensuring ad-lib water is always available. Therapeutic options, such as ACE-inhibitors, phosphate binders, and telmisartan have not been evaluated in this species.

Renal calcification may also occur in nephrocalcinosis, typically seen in entire female rats, and similarly, management with ad lib drinking water, supplementary fluids where required, and a low protein diet, is possible (Hoefer and Latney 2009).

Hydronephrosis is a genetic linked disorder in some strains and is usually an incidental finding but may, in some cases, predispose to urolithiasis and secondary problems. (O'Donoghue and Wilson 1977). Ascending renal infections are also seen, which typically involve *Escherichia coli, Proteus, Pseudomonas,* or *Klebsiella.*

8.5.5 Skin Conditions

Primary bacterial dermatitis is rare. It is usually secondary to self-trauma, bites, or, in pododermatitis, to multiple factors (Meredith 2006).

Ulcerative dermatitis, especially over the neck and shoulders, may be associated with *Staphlococcus aureus*. A range of other bacteria can be associated with local abscesses, pyodermas and pododermatitis, including *C. kutscheri*. Rats may be treated with appropriate systemic and topical antimicrobial treatment, NSAIDS, and clipping of the claws to minimise self-trauma. Maropitant has been used as a modifier of Substance P, reducing the itch-scratch cycle, in ulcerative dermatitis susceptible mice to good effect, and may be considered for intractable cases in rats. (Williams-Fritze et al. 2011).

Fungal disease (most commonly *Trichophyton mentagrophytes*) is rare, and almost always asymptomatic where encountered (Donnelley 2018).

Behavioural skin disease is seen, with individuals fighting, causing small wounds which may become infected, or barbering, where one dominant individual trims the fur of subordinates, typically over the face and head. Barbering damage is usually in symmetrical patterns, with hairs cut down to the skin but very rarely damaging the skin itself.

Older entire males develop thickened, yellowish skin with a greasy yellow secretion and thinning of the coat (Figure 8.12). Their thicker skin may make them more prone to developing constricting rings of skin round the tail, in low humidity conditions (<40% relative humidity), but is otherwise asymptomatic (Donnelley 2018).

8.5.5.1 Pododermatitis

Pododermatitis or bumblefoot is a multifactorial condition affecting the weight-bearing pads primarily of the hind feet. It presents initially as erythema of the plantar/palmar surfaces, with development to ulceration, swelling, bacterial infection and abscessation, and finally osteomyelitis.

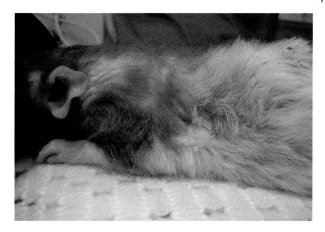

Figure 8.12 Coat thinning and skin changes common to geriatric male rats.

Poor substrate and floor surface hygiene are risk factors, with totally smooth, wire, abrasive, splintered, wet, or dirty flooring all potential causes. Obese animals and those with poor mobility who sit in one place constantly are at high risk. Treatment is challenging. In the earliest stages, weight loss, treatment of any musculoskeletal disorders, and provision of suitable clean, gently irregular, dry flooring is sufficient (Mecklenburg et al. 2013). In advanced cases surgical debridement and long courses of antimicrobials, together with judicious use of local dressings to protect the tissues, may be effective. Dressings may not be well tolerated, can constrict blood flow to the distal foot, and may worsen the condition by localising pressure on the lesion. Euthanasia is often required for advanced cases (Meredith 2006), particularly where osteomyelitis is established and radiography is prudent for to aid determination of prognosis prior to initiating intensive and protracted treatment.

8.5.5.2 Ectoparasites

Fur mites (*Radfordia ensifera*) are a common initiating cause of self-trauma around the neck, ears, and shoulders. Ear mites (*Notoedres muris*) mainly cause irritation and self-trauma of the pinnae. Mites may be seen on microscopy of skin scrapes or biopsies. Lice (*Polyplax spinulosa*) may be seen (Figure 8.13), especially if the rat is immune suppressed or from an environment of poor hygiene (Uhlíř and Volf 1992). Treatment is with avermectins.

Pinworms (*Syphacia obvelata* and *Syphacia muris*) cause pruritus and self-trauma to the tail base and perineal region. Their eggs may be detected using adhesive acetate strips applied to the area, and then examined under a microscope.

(a)

(b)

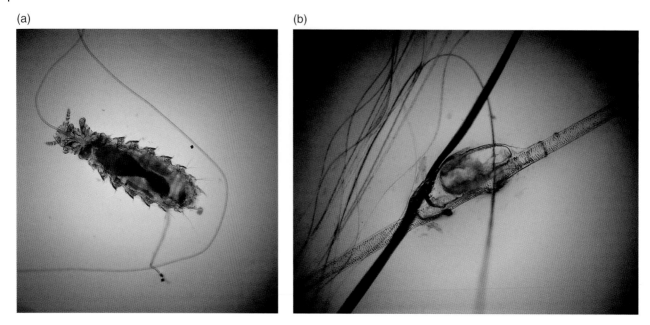

Figure 8.13 (a) *Polyplax spinulosa* louse on a hair pluck sample. (b) *Polyplax spinulosa* egg on a hair pluck sample.

Even in cases of negative findings, it is worth considering antiparasitic treatment as a trial therapy in suspect cases of dermatitis, as false negatives are possible (Meredith 2006).

8.5.5.3 Gastrointestinal Disease

Gastrointestinal problems are uncommon in rats. Changes of diet can lead to transient diarrhoea, but not the life threatening dysbiosis that occurs in herbivorous rodents. Supportive treatment of nutritional and fluid support is usually all that is required, but antibiotic therapy, probiotics, or transfaunation using faeces from a healthy rat can be considered in more severe cases.

Tyzzers disease (*Clostridium piliforme*) may affect weanling rats, resulting in potentially fatal diarrhoea. Treatment, with tetracyclines, may be considered, but elimination of the organism is challenging (Motzel and Riley 1992).

Heavy burdens of either of the cestodes *Hymenolepis nana* or *Hymenolepis dimunita* may cause weight loss and death. *H. nana* is usually asymptomatic (CDC 2019), however euthanasia should be considered due to zoonotic potential.

Systemic infections with *C. kutscheri* may result in fatal hepatitis (Barthold and Brownstein 1988).

8.5.5.4 Dental Disease

Congenital dental disease is very rare in rats, and most problems arising with the teeth are acquired through trauma and, less commonly, infection, diet, or neoplasia (Boehmer 2015).

Incisors: The incisors grow continuously throughout life. There is a very mobile mandibular symphysis, meaning that when palpated and manipulated, the lower jaw can move with significant separation of the lower incisors from one another at the tips. The incisor apices extend back to the level of the first molar (Boehmer 2015). Incisor fracture is common, either from falls or pulling at the bars. A fracture of one or more incisors means that the opposing incisor(s) overgrow. The maxillary incisors, if not occluding with the mandibular ones, describe a complete circle and ultimately penetrate the roof of the mouth. The opposite situation occurs less commonly, and leads to the lower incisors protruding, but rarely impinging on soft tissues (Jekl 2009).

In most cases, trimming incisors which are overgrowing due to an absent apposing tooth is sufficient as once the apposing tooth regrows, they will come back into alignment. If there is permanent malocclusion removal can be carried out. The extremely long reserve crown of the mandibular incisors, and the laxity of the mandibular symphysis, means that removal of one incisor with trimming the adjacent one prior to removal of the second incisor four weeks later is preferred. This helps avoid an unstable mandibular symphysis by permitting remodelling in between. (Sato 2005)

Other incisor lesions are rare, but may include neoplasia or osteomyelitis of the periapical tissues.

8.5.5.5 Cheek Teeth

The molars are closed rooted, not continually growing throughout life, and therefore do not malocclude. They are, however, subject to dental caries (the second molar is most commonly affected), fracture, or abscessation. Affected teeth may be extracted, after dental radiography to determine any bone involvement (Jekl 2009).

8.5.6 Neurological Disease

M. pulmonis and *Streptococcus pneumoniae* may cause otitis media or interna in rats, arising from the upper respiratory tract and translocating up the Eustachian tube. This can lead to a head tilt, and severe ataxia and depression in more serious cases (Hollamby 2009).

Pituitary neoplasia is not uncommon especially in nulliparous entire females and, as with mammary tumours, is correlated with high planes of nutrition. The tumour development causes gradually progressive neurological signs, including head tilt, reduced activity, and obtundation. Euthanasia is generally required at the obtunded stage (Orr 2009).

A tailless variety of rat has been selectively bred. Uncommonly, associated spinal and hindlimb defects can result in deformed hindlimbs and pelvis, or neurological conditions affecting mobility, bladder and bowel function, and with no treatment options, affected animals are likely to require euthanasia (Royer 1998).

8.5.7 Musculoskeletal Disease

Osteoarthritis may occur as a degenerative/ageing change or less commonly secondary to trauma or infection such as penetrating injury or chronic pododermatitis (Hollamby 2009). Any primary infectious factors should be treated and the long-term mobility limitations addressed. A single, or low-level cage, is more suitable for affected rats, and ramps should be solid, with adequate grip, and not too steep. Medical treatment options include NSAIDS or corticosteroids and other analgesic agents such as tramadol, gabapentin, or amantadine (Philips et al. 2017).

A spontaneous degenerative radiculoneuropathy occurs in lab rats, and may occur in similarly aged (approximately 18 months onwards) pet rats. Progressive demyelination of the spinal cord and peripheral nerves leads to paresis and paralysis of the hindlimbs (Gilmore 1972). Known collo-

quially as hind-leg degeneration (HLD), this greatly reduces their agility. Management is similar to that for chronic osteoarthritis and is purely palliative.

8.5.8 Zoonoses

Streptobacillus moniliformis, *Salmonella enteritidis*, and *Salmonella tymphimurium* may be carried by rats, either subclinically, or causing diarrhoea, with or without melaena. *S. moniliformis* is the causal organism of rat bite fever, a zoonotic condition spread by bites or ingestion of urine or faeces via contaminated food (Himsworth et al. 2013).

Leptospirosis is common in wild rats, but is not considered a significant risk in indoor pet rats, unless their food is contaminated with wild rat urine (Strand et al. 2019).

Yersinia pseudotuberculosis and *Campylobacter spp* have been isolated from wild British rodents (Pocock et al. 2001; Kageyama et al. 2002), and could be present in pet rodents if their environment or food are contaminated with rodent faeces.

After six cases of acute renal injury caused by hantaviruses contracted from rat exposure were recorded in the UK, a sero-surveillance study was conducted. 32.9% of specialist pet fancy rat owners recruited to the study tested positive for hantavirus antibodies, showing previous exposure to hantavirus (Public Health England 2014).

Whilst not strictly speaking a zoonosis, an allergy to rodent dander or urine is possible. Typically, these are seen in laboratory workers exposed to multiple rats, but may occur in owners of companion rats. Owners may request nail clipping in rats due to the small scratches their claws can inflict on skin which can become quite inflamed and visible in affected people.

8.6 Preventative Health Care

Nail trimming may be carried out if necessary, but rats with normal foot anatomy only tend to develop overlong claws if the substrates are poorly abrasive and no climbing options are provided. Acquired foot lesions such as bumblefoot or fractures changing the relative angle of claw to substrate may lead to overlong claws, which can get snagged and broken. Trimming claws unnecessarily may lead to reluctance to climb until they have regrown.

Teeth do not require any routine prophylactic care, apart from provision of suitable gnawing substrates.

8.6.1 Neutering

Neutering may be carried out for reproductive control in mixed sex groups, for reduction of aggression between males in the presence of females, and for physical health reasons. Male reproductive health problems are rare, but neutering (either ovariectomy or OVH) in females significantly reduces the frequency of uterine diseases, mammary gland tumours (from 47% to 4%), and pituitary adenomas (from 66% to 4%) (Hotchkiss 1995).

8.6.1.1 Castration

In males, it is rare that anything other than bilateral orchiectomy (castration) is carried out. The testicles are large, with an open inguinal ring. A large fat pad in the caudal abdomen and another associated with the epididymis prevent spontaneous herniation. There are a number of possible techniques:

Intra-abdominal castration may be performed. It has the advantage of not creating a wound in the dependent areas of the scrotum, which are prone to contamination, and avoids opening the vaginal tunic. However, the potential risks of wound interference with this site include eventration and death. If this option is selected, a midline approach is made, cranial to the penis. The testicles are located, exteriorised in turn, and the spermatic cord and blood vessels are clamped, ligated and transected together. A suture material which dissolves by hydrolysis is used (e.g. polyglactin, poliglecaprone, or polydioxanone) and should be of the smallest diameter reasonably possible (e.g. 1–1.5 metric). The abdominal wall should be closed separately to the skin. A continuous pattern is quicker, but if the rat chews through any part of the suture line, the entire wound closure becomes undone, with potentially fatal consequences. The skin should be closed with a continuous subcuticular pattern and the knot buried (Richardson and Flecknell 2006).

Alternatively, parallel longitudinal incision(s) may be made on either side of the ventral aspect of the scrotum or a single transverse incision at the tip of the scrotum. The former is a more familiar approach for most practitioners, but the latter keeps the incision from contact with the ground. A closed technique with preservation of the fat pads should be used to avoid herniation of abdominal contents into the scrotum afterwards. Where a transfixing ligature is placed, polydioxanone or poliglicaprone are preferred over polyglactin, to avoid tissue microtrauma as the suture is drawn through tissues (Richardson and Flecknell 2006). If the vaginal tunic is incised, an open technique may be performed, followed by closure of the inguinal ring or very proximal tunic. Scrotal wounds are under no tension and may be closed using sutures (intradermal or subcuticular sutures are difficult to place in the very fine scrotal skin) or surgical adhesive.

8.6.1.2 Ovariohysterectomy (OVH)

A standard midline approach is used to carry out a total OVH, preventing reproductive behaviour, or addressing pathology of the genital tract. The procedure is comparable to OVH in other species, though patient size makes surgery more challenging.

OVH carries a significant risk of wound interference by the rat, and the ventral position of an incision directly into the abdominal cavity carries a significant risk of fatal complications including intestinal dehiscence. Ovariectomy is often preferred where the uterus has no pathology. Suture material choice is as for castration.

8.6.1.3 Ovariectomy

There is relatively less trauma with this technique, as the uterus is not removed. (Steele and Bennett 2011). A smaller single dorsal (or dual flank skin incisions) is made, rather than a midline ventral incision, The dorsal skin incision is made at the level midway between the last rib and the greater trochanter of the hip, and the skin slipped ventrally to position it over the mid flank. The offset muscle incisions have the advantage of preventing abdominal viscera exposure if skin wounds are traumatised. Sharp incision of the muscle is carried out to allow exteriorisation of the ovary. The ovary is ligated or clips applied prior to removal. The incision is then manipulated to the other side and the process repeated. The skin incision on the dorsum is closed in two layers. Alternatively flank skin incisions may be made directly over the muscle incisions, but this incision overlap allows gnawing by the rat directly over the body cavity incisions.

8.7 Radiographic Imaging

Survey radiographs typically comprise right lateral radiographic (Figure 8.14) and dorsoventral (Figure 8.15) views. Radiography is well described and follows the same principles as in other species. High-detail digital systems should be used as obtaining good contrast at such small body sizes is otherwise challenging.

Good positioning is vital, with porous adhesive tape used to position the anaesthetised animal for orthogonal views. In the lateral view, the forelimbs are extended fully to avoid superimposition of the triceps over the cranial thorax. In this view, particularly with obese rats, the forelimbs and

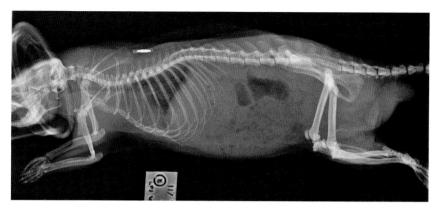

Figure 8.14 Right lateral survey radiograph.

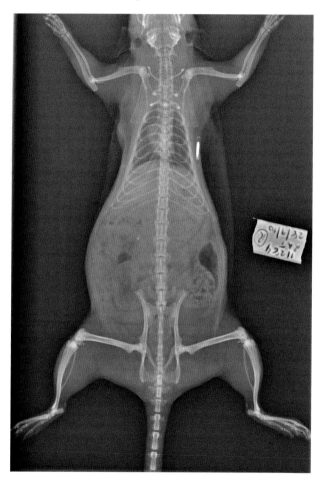

Figure 8.15 Dorsoventral survey radiograph.

In the ventrodorsal view this can cause difficulty breathing, so is best kept to a minimal duration. Avoidance of rotation is vital in these views, to avoid artefactual appearances of masses in the thorax in particular.

Thoracic lesions (pneumonia, pulmonary abscessation) are common in rats. It can be challenging to obtain inspiratory views, due to the fast respiratory rate, and difficulty of intubation (Krautwald-Junghanns et al. 2010). Abdominal views are more straightforward to evaluate than in the herbivorous rodents as the GI tract is simpler, the abdomen is narrower, and rats usually have sufficient intra-abdominal fat for excellent contrast (Tully 2009).

8.7.1 CT/MRI

More advanced imaging is ideal if possible, but requires relatively high resolution machines, with 'slices' of no more than 1 mm. It is particularly appropriate for imaging of the skull (including dentition and ears) and spine. Large pituitary masses may be diagnosed by MRI, but image quality is often insufficient in these small patients.

8.7.2 Ultrasound

Ultrasound examination is limited by the small patient size, but may be utilised for echocardiography, identification of thoracic abscessation, or abdominal examination (Heatley 2009).

hindlimbs should be separated from one another by radiolucent material to avoid the upper body rotating ventrally.

In the ventrodorsal or dorsoventral view, the limbs should be taped down symmetrically away from the body.

Acknowledgement

I'd like to thank Jasmine Woods for her assistance on the husbandry section of this chapter.

Formulary

Drug	Dose	Interval	Comments
Analgesic and anti-inflammatory drugs			
Amantidine	3–5 mg/kg PO	q12–24h	(Suckow et al. 2012)
Acetaminophen	200 mg/kg PO	prn	(Im et al. 2012)
Aspirin	50–150 mg/kg PO	q4–8 h	(Jablonski and Howden 2002)
Betamethasone	0.1 mg/kg SC	q24h	(Hedley 2019)
	Otic: 4 drops of polypharmaceutical solution	q12h;	
	Ocular: 1 drop of ophthalmic solution	q6–8h;	
	Skin: Apply cream	q8–12h.	
Buprenorphine	0.5 mg/kg po	q6–12h;	(Jablonski and Howden 2002;
	0.01–0.05 mg/kg IM, SC, IV	q6–12h;	Curtin et al. 2009)
Butorphanol	2 mg/kg (1–5 mg/kg) IM, SC, IV	q4h	(Gades et al. 2000)
Carprofen	5 mg/kg total daily dose, IM, SC, IV, PO	q24h	(Zegre Cannon et al. 2011)
Fluticasone	50–250 µg/rat by inhalation	q12–24h	(Hedley 2019)
Gabapentin	30 mg/kg PO	q8h.	(Coderre et al. 2005)
Meloxicam	1–2 mg/kg PO, SC	Q12–24h	(Nunamaker et al. 2018)
Morphine	1.7–5.6 mg/kg IM, SC	q2–4h;	(Morgan et al. 2012)
Tramadol	12.5 mg/kg	prn	(Zegre Cannon et al. 2011)
Anaesthesia			
Acepromazine	0.5–2.5 mg/kg IM, SC, PO		The higher doses should only be given orally
Atipamezole	Five times the previous medetomidine dose or ten times previous dexmedetomidine dose in milligrammes, SC, IM	Single dose	(Jang et al. 2009)
Atropine	0.05–0.1 mg/kg IM, SC	Pre-anaesthetic for reduction of salivation	(Olson et al. 1994)
Alfaxan	20 mg/kg IM 2–5 mg/kg IV, IP		(Lau et al. 2013)
Glycopyrolide	50 µg/kg IM, SC	Pre-anaesthetic for reduction of salivation	(Olson et al. 1994)
Diazepam or midazolam	1–2.5 mg/kg IM, SC. Midazolam or water soluble diazepam can also be given IV or IP	Prn	Used in conjunction with ketamine or fentanyl
Isoflurane	Up to 5% in oxygen induction; 1.5–2.0% maintenance.		(Richardson and Flecknell 2008)
Sevoflurane	Up to 8% in oxygen, 3–5% maintenance		(Richardson and Flecknell 2008)
Ketamine	50–100 mg/kg IM, SC as a sole agent for immobilisation		Poor muscle relaxation and not advised as a sole agent (Melo et al. 2016)
Ketamine/ Medetomidine	75 mg/kg/0.5 mg/kg IP		Anaesthesia (Richardson and Flecknell 2008)
Medetomidine	0.030–0.10 mg/kg, SC, IM		Sedation (Richardson and Flecknell 2008)
Dexmedetomidine	0.015–0.05 mg/kg, SC, IM		Sedation (Richardson and Flecknell 2008)
Propofol	7.5–10 mg/kg IV		Sedation (Richardson and Flecknell 2008)
Alfaxan and midazolam	midazolam at 0.5 mg/kg IM, followed by alfaxalone at 2–3 mg/kg IM		Midazolam often combined with an opioid for superior sedation (Lennox 2015)

(Continued)

Drug	Dose	Interval	Comments
Anaesthetic emergencies			
Atropine	0.05–0.1 mg/kg IM, SC	Pre-anaesthetic for mitigation of bradycardia.	(Olson et al. 1994)
Adrenaline	0.04–0.4 mg/kg IC, IV, IO, IM, SC	prn	For cardiac arrest (Chen et al. 2010)
Antimicrobials			
Amikacin	5–15 mg/kg IV, IM, SC	q8–12 h	Concurrent fluid therapy advised, especially if hydration status poor or uncertain.
	10 mg in 10 ml water for injection nebulised	q6–12h	(Mehta et al. 2018)
Amoxycillin	100–150 mg/kg IM, SC	q12h.	(Melo et al. 2016a)
Amoxycillin/ clavulanate	50 mg/kg (as amoxicillin) IM, SC, PO	q12h.	(Woodnutt and Berry 1999)
Ampicillin	50–100 mg/kg IM, SC,PO	q12h.	(Ritzerfeld 1979)
Azithromycin	50 mg/kg PO	q12h for 14 days.	(Deshmukh and Tamboli 2013)
Carbenacillin	50–100 mg/kg PO	q12h	(English et al. 1972)
Cephalexin	15–33 mg/kg IM, SC	q12h.	(English et al. 1972) (Flecknell 2016)
Clindamycin	25 mg/kg PO	q12h	(Gisby et al. 1994)
	50 mg/kg PO	q24h	
Chloramphenicol	50 mg/kg IM, PO	q12h	(Meyer and Mans 2018)
	0.5 mg/ml in drinking water		
Ciprofloxacin	20–40 mg/kg PO	q12–24h	(Rajasekaran et al. 2006)
Doxycycline	2.5–5 mg/kg PO	q12h	(Mayer and Mans 2018)
Enrofloxacin	5–25 mg/kg PO, SC	q12–24h	(Flecknell 2016)
	10 mg/kg enrofloxacin plus 5 mg/kg doxycycline in combination PO	q12h	(Adamcak and Otten 2000)
Erythromycin	18–25 mg/kg PO	q12–24h	(Adamcak and Otten 2000)
Gentamycin	2–5 mg/kg IM, SC	q8–24h	(Adamcak and Otten 2000)
Itraconazole	2.5–10.0 mg/kg PO	q24h	(European medicines Agency 2014)
Marbofloxacin	5 mg/kg SC, PO	q24h	(Chauhan et al. 2017)
Metronidazole	10–40 mg/kg PO	q12h–24h	(Adamcak and Otten 2000)
Oxytetracycline	60 mg/kg IM, SC	q3d	Using the 10% injectable preparation (anecdotal)
	10–20 mg/kg PO	q8h	(Adamcak and Otten 2000)
Terbinafine	15–80 mg/kg PO	q24h × 4–6 weeks	(Walzer and Ashbaugh 2002)
Tylosin	10 mg/kg PO, IM, SC	q12h	(Adamcak and Otten 2000)
TMPS	48–96 mg/kg PO, IM, SC	q24h	(Adamcak and Otten 2000)

(Continued)

(Continued)

Drug	Dose	Interval	Comments
Parasiticides			
Amitraz	0.007% solution (1.4 ml Aludex in 1000 ml water) topically	q14d for 3–6 treatments	Demodecosis (Adamcak and Otten 2000)
Fenbendazole	20–50 mg/kg PO	q24h for 5 consecutive days.	(Adamcak and Otten 2000)
Fipronil	7.5 mg/kg topically	Repeat q30–60d.	(Diaz 2005)
Imidocloprid	10–20 mg/kg topically	q30d	(Bhardwaj et al. 2010)
Ivermectin	0.2–0.5 mg/kg SC, PO, topical	q7–14 d	(Adamcak and Otten 2000)
Selamectin	6 mg/kg topically	monthly	(DiGeronimo 2016)
Miscellaneous			
Aluminium hydroxide	2.4–9.6 g/kg PO	q24h	For management of CRF (Sanai et al. 1991)
Acetylcysteine	50 mg diluted in water or saline for nebulisation	q6–12 hours for 10–30 minutes	Removal of purulent material (Mata et al. 2003)
	1–2 ml of a 20% solution for otic lavage	q12–24 h	
Aglepristone	10 mg/kg SC 24 hours apart	Days 11 and 12 after mating (mid-pregnancy)	Pregnancy termination (Gogny and Fiéni 2016)
Amitryptilline	10 mg/kg PO	q24h	Self-mutilation and analgesia (Esser and Sawynok 1999)
Atenolol	0.2–5 mg/kg PO	q24hrs	Congestive heart failure (Shen et al. 2005)
Benazepril	0.5–1.0 mg/kg PO	q24h	Protein losing nephropathy (Mudagal et al. 2011)
Bromhexine	0.3 mg/rat PO	q24h	Enhances antibiotic uptake in the tissues of the lower respiratory tract (Boothe 2000)
Cabergoline	0.6 mg/kg PO	q72h	(Eguchi et al. 1995; Mayer et al. 2011)
Chitosan	200 mg/kg PO	q24h	Prevention of paracetamol related (and potentially other aetiology) hepatotoxicity (Ozcelik et al. 2014)
	165–825 mg/kg PO	q24h	Renal failure treatment (Chou et al. 2015)
Chlorpheniramine	0.6 mg/kg PO	q24	Allergic reactions, anaphylaxis (Adamcak and Otten 2000)
Ciclosporin	10 mg/kg PO	q24h	Sebaceous adenitis (Wassef et al. 1985)
Cimetidine	5–10 mg/kg PO, SC, IM, IV	q6–12 h	(Mojaverian et al. 1985)
Delmadinone acetate	1 mg/rat SC	Single injection, repeat if required in 3–4 weeks	Assessment of the effects of castration, prior to decision to surgically castrate (anecdotal)
Deslorelin	4.7 mg implant SC	Unknown, approx. 1 year	Reduction of fertility, reproductive behaviours, and, by extrapolation, reduction of mammary tumours (the latter has not been proven) (Risi 2014)

(Continued)

Drug	Dose	Interval	Comments
Diazepam	2–5 mg/kg IM	prn	Sedative, anxiolytic, pruritic seizures (Adamcak and Otten 2000)
Fluoxetine	10 mg/kg PO	q24h	Behavioural modification (Ariel et al. 2017)
Furosemide	5–10 mg/kg SC, IM, IV	q12 h	(Adamcak and Otten 2000)
Imidapril	protein-losing nephropathy at 2.0 mg/kg PO	q24h	(Ogiku et al. 1993)
Insulin	1–3 iu/rat SC	q12h	Diabetes control (Adamcak and Otten 2000)
Metoclopramide	0.2–1 mg/kg PO, SC, IM	q12h	Anti-emetic (Adamcak and Otten 2000)
Pimobendan	0.5–1.0 mg/kg PO	q12h	(Iwasaki et al. 1999)
Salbutamol	100 μg (micrograms)/rat by inhalation	q4–6h	(Hedley 2019; Phillips et al. 2017)
Sildenafil	5 mg/kg PO	q24	Respiratory tract disease (Sun et al. 2012)
Terbutaline	5 mg/kg PO	q12h	(Zanasi et al. 2017)

References

Adamcak, A. and Otten, B. (2000). Rodent therapeutics. *The Veterinary Clinics of North America. Exotic Animal Practice* 3 (1): 221–237.

Alexander, B.K., Coambs, R.B., and Hadaway, F. (1978). The effect of housing and gender on morphine self-administration in rats. *Psychopharmacology* 58 (2): 175–179.

Almeida, A., Corrigan, R., and Sarno, R. (2013). The economic impact of commensal rodents on small businesses in Manhattan's Chinatown: trends and possible causes. *Suburban Sustainability* 1 (1): 2.

Ariel, L., Inbar, S., Edut, S. et al. (2017). Fluoxetine treatment is effective in a rat model of childhood-induced post-traumatic stress disorder. *Translational Psychiatry* 7 (11): 1260.

Barsoum, N.J., Gough, A.W., Sturgess, J.M. et al. (1984). Morphologic features and incidence of spontaneous hyperplastic and neoplastic mammary gland lesions in Wistar rats. *Toxicologic Pathology* 12 (1): 26–38.

Barthold, S.W. and Brownstein, D.G. (1988). The effect of selected viruses on *Corynebacterium kutscheri* infection in rats. *Laboratory Animal Science* 38 (5): 580–583.

Bercker, S., Bert, B., Bittigau, P. et al. (2009). Neurodegeneration in newborn rats following propofol and sevoflurane anesthesia. *Neurotoxicity Research* 16 (2): 140–147.

Bhardwaj, S., Srivastava, M.K., Kapoor, U. et al. (2010). A 90 days oral toxicity of imidacloprid in female rats: morphological, biochemical and histopathological evaluations. *Food and Chemical Toxicology* 48 (5): 1185–1190.

Boehmer, E. (2015). *Dentistry in Rabbits and Rodents*, 21–34. Oxford: Wiley Blackwell.

Boothe, D.M. (2000). Drugs affecting the respiratory system. *The Veterinary Clinics of North America. Exotic Animal Practice* 3 (2): 371–394.

Brodbelt, D.C., Blissitt, K.J., Hammond, R.A. et al. (2008). The risk of death: the confidential enquiry into perioperative small animal fatalities. *Veterinary Anaesthesia and Analgesia* 35 (5): 365–373.

BVA (2017). Responsible use of antimicrobials in veterinary practice. https://www.bva.co.uk/take-action/our-policies/responsible-use-of-antimicrobials (accessed 26 December 2019).

CDC (Centers for Disease Control and Pevention) (2019). Parasites – Hymenolepiasis FAQ. https://www.cdc.gov/parasites/hymenolepis/faqs.html (accessed 27 June 2019).

Cesarovic, N., Nicholls, F., Rettich, A. et al. (2010). Isoflurane and sevoflurane provide equally effective anaesthesia in laboratory mice. *Laboratory Animals* 44 (4): 329–336.

Chandra, M., Riley, M.G., and Johnson, D.E. (1992). Spontaneous neoplasms in aged Sprague-Dawley rats. *Archives of Toxicology* 66 (7): 496–502.

Chauhan, V.B., Modi, C.M., Patel, U.D. et al. (2017). Safety profile of marbofloxacin following repeated intramuscular administration alone and piperine pretreated rats. *Annals of Phytomedicine* 6 (2): 88–92.

Chen, M.H., Lu, J.Y., Xie, L. et al. (2010). What is the optimal dose of epinephrine during cardiopulmonary resuscitation in a rat model? *The American Journal of Emergency Medicine* 28 (3): 284–290.

Chou, C.K., Li, Y.C., Chen, S.M. et al. (2015). Chitosan prevents gentamicin-induced nephrotoxicity via a carbonyl stress-dependent pathway. *BioMed Research International* 2015: 675714.

Clark, B.R. and Price, E.O. (1981). Sexual maturation and fecundity of wild and domestic Norway rats (Rattus norvegicus). *Reproduction* 63 (1): 215–220.

Coderre, T.J., Kumar, N., Lefebvre, C.D. et al. (2005). Evidence that gabapentin reduces neuropathic pain by inhibiting the spinal release of glutamate. *Journal of Neurochemistry* 94 (4): 1131–1139.

Corwin, R.L. (2004). Binge-type eating induced by limited access in rats does not require energy restriction on the previous day. *Appetite* 42 (2): 139–142.

Curtin, L.I., Grakowsky, J.A., Suarez, M. et al. (2009). Evaluation of buprenorphine in a postoperative pain model in rats. *Comparative Medicine* 59 (1): 60–71.

Deshmukh, J.B. and Tamboli, S.B. (2013). Study of CNS effects of macrolide antibiotics: an experimental study. *Journal of Evolution of Medical and Dental Sciences* 2 (7): 653–657.

Diaz, S.L. (2005). Efficacy of fipronil in the treatment of pediculosis in laboratory rats. *Laboratory Animals* 39 (3): 331–335.

DiGeronimo, M. (2016). Therapeutic review. *Journal of Exotic Pet Medicine* 25: 80–83.

Donnelley, T. (2018). Mice and rats as pets. MSD Veterinary Manual. https://www.msdvetmanual.com/exotic-and-laboratory-animals/rodents/mice-and-rats-as-pets (accessed 20 June 2019).

Eguchi, K., Kawamoto, K., Uozumi, T. et al. (1995). Effect of cabergoline, a dopamine agonist, on estrogen-induced rat pituitary tumors: in vitro culture studies. *Endocrine Journal* 42 (3): 413–420.

English, A.R., Retsema, J.A., Ray, V.A. et al. (1972). Carbenicillin indanyl sodium, an orally active derivative of carbenicillin. *Antimicrobial Agents and Chemotherapy* 1 (3): 185–191.

Esser, M.J. and Sawynok, J. (1999). Acute amitriptyline in a rat model of neuropathic pain: differential symptom and route effects. *Pain* 80 (3): 643–653.

European medicines Agency (2014). CVMP assessment report for Fungitraxx (EMEA/V/C/002722/0000). https://www.ema.europa.eu/en (accessed 5 July 2019).

Fay, R.R. (1988). *Hearing in Vertebrates: A Psychophysics Databook*. Winnetka IL: Hill-Fay Associates.

Flecknell, P.A. (2016). Analgesia and post-operative care. In: *Laboratory Animal Anaesthesia*, 4e, 141–192. Boston: Academic Press.

Gades, N.M., Danneman, P.J., Wixson, S.K. et al. (2000). The magnitude and duration of the analgesic effect of morphine, butorphanol, and buprenorphine in rats and mice. *Journal of the American Association for Laboratory Animal Science* 39 (2): 8–13.

Garcia, J., Hankins, W.G., and Rusiniak, K.W. (1974). Behavioral regulation of the milieu interne in man and rat. *Science* 185 (4154): 824–831.

Gilmore, S.A. (1972). Spinal nerve root degeneration in aging laboratory rats: a light microscopic study. *The Anatomical Record* 174 (2): 251–257.

Gisby, J., Beale, A.S., Bryant, J.E. et al. (1994). Staphylococcal osteomyelitis – a comparison of co-amoxiclav with clindamycin and flucloxacillin in an experimental rat model. *Journal of Antimicrobial Chemotherapy* 34 (5): 755–764.

Gogny, A. and Fiéni, F. (2016). Aglepristone: a review on its clinical use in animals. *Theriogenology* 85 (4): 555–566.

Greenacre, C. and Gibbons, P. (2011). Mammary tumours in small mammals. Lefeber Vet https://lafeber.com/vet/mammary-tumors-in-small-mammals (accessed 20 June 2019).

Harleman, J.H., Hargreaves, A., Andersson, H. et al. (2012). A review of the incidence and coincidence of uterine and mammary tumors in Wistar and Sprague-Dawley rats based on the RITA database and the role of prolactin. *Toxicologic Pathology* 40 (6): 926–930.

Heatley, J.J. (2009). Cardiovascular anatomy, physiology, and disease of rodents and small exotic mammals. *The Veterinary Clinics of North America. Exotic Animal Practice* 12 (1): 99–113.

Hedley, J. (2019). *British Small Animal Veterinary Association Small Animal Formulary*, 10e, part B. Gloucester, UK: BSAVA.

Himsworth, C.G., Parsons, K.L., Jardine, C. et al. (2013). Rats, cities, people, and pathogens: a systematic review and narrative synthesis of literature regarding the ecology of rat-associated zoonoses in urban centers. *Vector Borne and Zoonotic Diseases* 13 (6): 349–359.

Hoefer, H. and Latney, L.T. (2009). Rodents: urogenital and reproductive system disorders. In: *BSAVA Manual of Rodents and Ferrets* (eds. E. Keeble and A. Meredith), 150–160. Cheltenham, UK: BSAVA Publications.

Hollamby, S. (2009). Rodents: neuromuscular and musculoskeletal disorders. In: *BSAVA Manual of Rodents and Ferrets* (eds. E. Keeble and A. Meredith), 161–168. Cheltenham, UK: BSAVA Publications.

Hotchkiss, C.E. (1995). Effect of surgical removal of subcutaneous tumors on survival of rats. *Journal of the American Veterinary Medical Association* 206 (10): 1575–1579.

Ijpelaar, D.H., Schulz, A., Aben, J. et al. (2008). Genetic predisposition for glomerulonephritis-induced glomerulosclerosis in rats is linked to chromosome 1. *Physiological Genomics* 35 (2): 173–181.

Im, K.S., Jung, H.J., Kim, J.B. et al. (2012). The antinociceptive effect of acetaminophen in a rat model of neuropathic pain. *The Kaohsiung Journal of Medical Sciences* 28 (5): 251–258.

Iwasaki, A., Matsumori, A., Yamada, T. et al. (1999). Pimobendan inhibits the production of proinflammatory cytokines and gene expression of inducible nitric oxide synthase in a murine model of viral myocarditis. *Journal of the American College of Cardiology* 33 (5): 1400–1407.

Jablonski, P. and Howden, B.O. (2002). Oral buprenorphine and aspirin analgesia in rats undergoing liver transplantation. *Laboratory Animals* 36 (2): 134–143.

Jang, H.S., Choi, H.S., Lee, S.H. et al. (2009). Evaluation of the anaesthetic effects of medetomidine and ketamine in rats and their reversal with atipamezole. *Veterinary Anaesthesia and Analgesia* 36 (4): 319–327.

Jekl, V. (2009). Rodents: dentistry. In: *BSAVA Manual of Rodents and Ferrets* (eds. E. Keeble and A. Meredith), 86–95. Cheltenham, UK: BSAVA Publications.

Kageyama, T., Ogasawara, A., Fukuhara, R. et al. (2002). Yersinia pseudotuberculosis infection in breeding monkeys: detection and analysis of strain diversity by PCR. *Journal of Medical Primatology* 31 (3): 129–135.

Kashimoto, S., Furuya, A., Nonaka, A. et al. (1997). The minimum alveolar concentration of sevoflurane in rats. *European Journal of Anaesthesiology* 14 (4): 359–361.

Keeble, E. (2001). Endocrine diseases in small mammals. *In Practice* 23 (10): 570–585.

Khan, K.S., Hayes, I., and Buggy, D.J. (2014). Pharmacology of anaesthetic agents II: inhalation anaesthetic agents. *Continuing Education in Anaesthesia, Critical Care and Pain* 14 (3): 106–111.

Kharasch, E.D., Schroeder, J.L., Sheffels, P. et al. (2005). Influence of sevoflurane on the metabolism and renal effects of compound A in rats. *Anesthesiology* 103 (6): 1183–1188.

Klaphake, E. (2006). Common rodent procedures. *The veterinary clinics of North America. Exotic animal practice* 9 (2): 389–413.

Krautwald-Junghanns, M.E., Pees, M., and Reese, S. (2010). *Diagnostic Imaging of Exotic Pets: Vogel–Kleins Auger–Reptilien*, 143–299. Hannover, Germany: Schlutersche.

Krinke, G.J. (2000). History, strains and models. In: *The Laboratory Rat (Handbook of Experimental Animals)* (eds. G.R. Bullock and T. Bunton), 3–16. London: Academic Press.

Lau, C., Ranasinghe, M.G., Shiels, I. et al. (2013). Plasma pharmacokinetics of alfaxalone after a single intraperitoneal or intravenous injection of Alfaxan® in rats. *Journal of Veterinary Pharmacology and Therapeutics* 36 (5): 516–520.

Lawlor, M. (1990). The size of rodent cages. In: *Guidelines for the Well-Being of Rodents in Research* (ed. H.N. Guttman), 19–27. Bethesda: Scientist Centre for Animal Welfare.

Lawlor, M.M. (2002). Comfortable quarters for rats in research institutions. In: *Comfortable Quarters for Laboratory Animals*, 9e (eds. V. Reinhardt and A. Reinhardt), 26–32. New York: Animal Welfare Institute.

Lennox, A. (2015). Introducing Alfaxalone into Exotic Companion Mammal Practice. Proceedings of AEMV Conference, San Antonio, Texas, 29 August to 2 September 2015. Association of Avian Veterinarians. https://www.vin.com/members/cms/project/defaultadv1.aspx?id=7184780&pid=13815& (accessed 20 June 2019).

Lichtenberger, M. and Ko, J. (2007). Anesthesia and analgesia for small mammals and birds. *The Veterinary Clinics of North America. Exotic Animal Practice* 10 (2): 293–315.

Mac Kenzie, W.F. and Garner, F.M. (1973). Comparison of neoplasms in six sources of rats. *Journal of the National Cancer Institute* 50 (5): 1243–1257.

Mata, M., Ruiz, A., Cerda, M. et al. (2003). Oral N-acetylcysteine reduces bleomycin-induced lung damage and mucin Muc5ac expression in rats. *European Respiratory Journal* 22 (6): 900–905.

Mayer, J. and Mans, C. (2018). Rodents. In: *Exotic Animal Formulary*, 5e (eds. J.W. Carpenter and C.J. Marion), 459–493. St. Louis, MO: Elsevier.

Mayer, J., Sato, A., Kiupel, M. et al. (2011). Extralabel use of cabergoline in the treatment of a pituitary adenoma in a rat. *Journal of the American Veterinary Medical Association* 239 (5): 656–660.

Mecklenburg, L., Kusewitt, D., Kolly, C. et al. (2013). Proliferative and non-proliferative lesions of the rat and mouse integument. *Journal of Toxicologic Pathology* 26 (3_Suppl): 27S–57S.

Mehta, S., Lamarche, I., Adier, C. et al. (2018). Pulmonary pharmacokinetics of amikacin and cefoxitin after nebulization in rats 28th European Congress of Clinical Microbiology and Infectious Diseases, Madrid, Spain.

Melo, A., Leite-Almeida, H., Ferreira, C. et al. (2016). Exposure to ketamine anesthesia affects rat impulsive behavior. *Frontiers in Behavioral Neuroscience* 10: 226.

Meredith, A. (2006). Skin disease and treatment of rats. In: *Skin Diseases of Exotic Pets* (ed. S. Paterson), 312–324. Oxford: Blackwell Publishing.

Mojaverian, P., Rocci, M.L., Saccar, C.L. et al. (1985). Cimetidine versus famotidine: the effect on the pharmacokinetics of theophylline in rats. *European Journal of Drug Metabolism and Pharmacokinetics* 10 (2): 155–159.

Morgan, D., Mitzelfelt, J.D., Koerper, L.M. et al. (2012). Effects of morphine on thermal sensitivity in adult and aged rats. *The Journals of Gerontology Series A: Biomedical Sciences and Medical Sciences* 67 (7): 705–713.

Motzel, S.L. and Riley, L.K. (1992). Subclinical infection and transmission of Tyzzer's disease in rats. *Laboratory Animal Science* 42 (5): 439–443.

Mudagal, M., Patel, J., Nagalakshmi, N.C. et al. (2011). Renoprotective effects of combining ACE inhibitors and statins in experimental diabetic rats. *Daru: Journal of Faculty of Pharmacy, Tehran University of Medical Sciences* 19 (5): 322.

Nagakumar, P. and Rao, S. (2019). When is difficult asthma severe? *Paediatrics and Child Health* 29 (4): 161–166.

NRC (National Research Council [US]), Committee on Infectious Diseases of Mice and Rats (1991). *Infectious Diseases of Mice and Rats*. Washington, DC: National Academies Press (US).

NRC (National Research Council [US]) (1995). *Nutrient Requirements of Laboratory Animals*, 4e. Washington, DC: National Academies Press (US).

Nunamaker, E.A., Goldman, J.L., Adams, C.R. et al. (2018). Evaluation of analgesic efficacy of meloxicam and 2 formulations of buprenorphine after laparotomy in female Sprague–Dawley rats. *Journal of the American Association for Laboratory Animal Science* 57 (5): 498–507.

O'Donoghue, P.N. and Wilson, M.S. (1977). Hydronephrosis in male rats. *Laboratory Animals* 11 (3): 193–194.

Ogiku, N., Sumikawa, H., Minamide, S. et al. (1993). Influence of imidapril on abnormal biochemical parameters in salt-loaded stroke-prone spontaneously hypertensive rats (SHRSP). *Japanese Journal of Pharmacology* 61 (1): 69–73.

Olson, M.E., Vizzutti, D., Morck, D.W. et al. (1994). The parasympatholytic effects of atropine sulfate and glycopyrrolate in rats and rabbits. *Canadian Journal of Veterinary Research* 58 (4): 254.

O'Malley, B. (2005). *Clinical Anatomy and Physiology of Exotic Species. Structure and Function of Mammals, Birds, Reptiles and Amphibians*. Edinburgh: Elsevier.

Orr, H. (2009). Rodents: neoplastic and endocrine disease. In: *BSAVA Manual of Rodents and Ferrets* (eds. E. Keeble and A. Meredith), 181–192. Cheltenham, UK: BSAVA Publications.

Ozcelik, E., Uslu, S., Erkasap, N. et al. (2014). Protective effect of chitosan treatment against acetaminophen-induced hepatotoxicity. *The Kaohsiung Journal of Medical Sciences* 30 (6): 286–290.

Parasuraman, S., Raveendran, R., and Kesavan, R. (2010). Blood sample collection in small laboratory animals. *Journal of Pharmacology and Pharmacotherapeutics* 1 (2): 87.

Philips, B.H., Weisshaar, C.L., and Winkelstein, B.A. (2017). Use of the rat grimace scale to evaluate neuropathic pain in a model of cervical radiculopathy. *Comparative Medicine* 67 (1): 34–42.

Phillips, J.E., Zhang, X., and Johnston, J.A. (2017). Dry powder and nebulized aerosol inhalation of pharmaceuticals delivered to mice using a nose-only exposure system. *Journal of Visualized Experiments: JoVE* (122): e55454.

Pocock, M.J.O., Searle, J.B., Betts, W.B. et al. (2001). Patterns of infection by salmonella and Yersinia spp. in commensal house mouse (Mus musculus domesticus) populations. *Journal of Applied Microbiology* 90 (5): 755–760.

Potter, B. (1926). *The Tale of Samuel Whiskers*. London: Frederick Warne & Co.

Public Health England (2014). Hantavirus infection in people with contact with wild and pet rats in England. Preliminary results of a sero-surveillance study. London: PHE. https://assets.publishing.service.gov.uk/government/uploads/system/uploads/attachment_data/file/385205/Public_Health_England_Hantavirus_Sero-surveillance_study_Report_of_preliminary_results_final_version_180914.pdf (accessed 26 December 2019).

Puckett, E.E., Park, J., Combs, M. et al. (2016). Global population divergence and admixture of the brown rat (Rattus norvegicus). *Proceedings of the Royal Society B: Biological Sciences* 283 (1841): 20161762.

Rajasekaran, S.K., Lawless, U., and Kelly, J. (2006). A behavioural investigation of ciprofloxacin and ofloxacin in the rat. *The FASEB Journal* 20 (4): A679.

Richardson, C. and Flecknell, P. (2006). Routine neutering of rabbits and rodents. *In Practice* 28 (2): 70–79.

Richardson, C. and Flecknell, P. (2008). Rodents: anaesthesia and analgesia. In: *BSAVA Manual of Rodents and Ferrets* (eds. E. Keeble and A. Meredith), 63–72. Cheltenham, UK: BSAVA Publications.

Risi, E. (2014). Control of reproduction in ferrets, rabbits and rodents. *Reproduction in Domestic Animals* 49: 81–86.

Ritzerfeld, W. (1979). Efficacy of bacampicillin and ampicillin in experimental pyelonephritis in the rat. *Infection* 7 (5): S443–S445.

Royer, N. (1998). Trouble with tailless. http://www.afrma.org/taillesstrbl.htm (accessed 20 June 2019).

Rudmann, D., Cardiff, R., Chouinard, L. et al. (2012). Proliferative and nonproliferative lesions of the rat and mouse mammary, Zymbal's, preputial, and clitoral glands. *Toxicologic Pathology* 40 (6_suppl): 7S–39S.

Sanai, T., Okuda, S., Onoyama, K. et al. (1991). Effect of different doses of aluminium hydroxide on renal deterioration and nutritional state in experimental chronic renal failure. *Mineral and Electrolyte Metabolism* 17 (3): 160–165.

Sathe, N.A., Krishnaswami, S., Andrews, J. et al. (2015). Pharmacologic agents that promote airway clearance in hospitalized subjects: a systematic review. *Respiratory Care* 60 (7): 1061–1070.

Sato, D. (2005). Socket healing after rat mandibular incisor extraction. *Kokubyo Gakkai zasshi. The Journal of the Stomatological Society, Japan* 72 (1): 98–105.

Schoental, R. (1973). Carcinogenicity of wood shavings. *Laboratory Animals* 7 (1): 47–49.

Sheffels, P., Schroeder, J.L., Altuntas, T.G. et al. (2004). Role of cytochrome P4503A in cysteine S-conjugates sulfoxidation and the nephrotoxicity of the sevoflurane degradation product fluoromethyl-2, 2-difluoro-1-(trifluoromethyl) vinyl ether (Compound A) in rats. *Chemical Research in Toxicology* 17 (9): 1177–1189.

Shen, F.M., Xie, H.H., Ling, G. et al. (2005). Synergistic effects of atenolol and amlodipine for lowering and stabilizing blood pressure in 2K1C renovascular hypertensive rats 1. *Acta Pharmacologica Sinica* 26 (11): 1303–1308.

Steele, M.S. and Bennett, R.A. (2011). Clinical technique: dorsal ovariectomy in rodents. *Journal of Exotic Pet Medicine* 20 (3): 222–226.

Strand, T.M., Pineda, S., Backhans, A. et al. (2019). Detection of Leptospira in Urban Swedish Rats: Pest Control Interventions as a Promising Source of Rats Used for Surveillance. *Vector-Borne and Zoonotic Diseases* 19 (6): 414–420.

Suckow, M.A., Weisbroth, S.H., and Franklin, C.L. (eds.) (2006). *The Laboratory Rat*, 2e. San Diego, CA: Elsevier Academic Press.

Suckow, M.A., Stevens, K.A., and Wilson, R.P. (2012). *The Laboratory Rabbit, Guinea Pig, Hamster, and Other Rodents*. London: Academic Press.

Sun, C.K., Lin, Y.C., Yuen, C.M. et al. (2012). Enhanced protection against pulmonary hypertension with sildenafil and endothelial progenitor cell in rats. *International Journal of Cardiology* 162 (1): 45–58.

Sweet, C.S., Emmert, S.E., Stabilito, I.I. et al. (1987). Increased survival in rats with congestive heart failure treated with enalapril. *Journal of Cardiovascular Pharmacology* 10 (6): 636–642.

Trouillas, J., Girod, C., Claustrat, B. et al. (1982). Spontaneous pituitary tumors in the Wistar/Furth/Ico rat strain. An animal model of human prolactin adenoma. *The American Journal of Pathology* 109 (1): 57.

Tucker, M.J. (1979). The effect of long-term food restriction on tumours in rodents. *International Journal of Cancer* 23 (6): 803–807.

Tully, T.N. (2009). Mice and rats. In: *Manual of Exotic Pet Practice* (eds. M.A. Mitchell and T.N. Tully), 326–344. St. Louis, MO: W.B. Saunders.

Uhlíř, J. and Volf, P. (1992). Ivermectin: its effect on the immune system of rabbits and rats infested with ectoparasites. *Veterinary Immunology and Immunopathology* 34 (3–4): 325–336.

Vergneau-Grosset, C., Keel, M.K., Goldsmith, D. et al. (2016). Description of the prevalence, histologic characteristics, concomitant abnormalities, and outcomes of mammary gland tumors in companion rats (Rattus norvegicus): 100 cases (1990–2015). *Journal of the American Veterinary Medical Association* 249 (10): 1170–1179.

Wade, C.E., Miller, M.M., Baer, L.A. et al. (2002). Body mass, energy intake, and water consumption of rats and humans during space flight. *Nutrition* 18 (10): 829–836.

Walzer, P.D. and Ashbaugh, A. (2002). Use of terbinafine in mouse and rat models of Pneumocystis carinii pneumonia. *Antimicrobial Agents and Chemotherapy* 46 (2): 514–516.

Wang, T., Liu, Y., Chen, L. et al. (2009). Effect of sildenafil on acrolein-induced airway inflammation and mucus production in rats. *European Respiratory Journal* 33 (5): 1122–1132.

Wassef, R., Cohen, Z., and Langer, B. (1985). Pharmacokinetic profiles of cyclosporine in rats. Influence of route of administration and dosage. *Transplantation* 40 (5): 489–493.

Williams, D.L. (2002). Ocular disease in rats: a review. *Veterinary Ophthalmology* 5 (3): 183–191.

Williams-Fritze, M.J., Carlson Scholz, J.A., Zeiss, C. et al. (2011). Maropitant citrate for treatment of ulcerative dermatitis in mice with a C57BL/6 background. *Journal of the American Association for Laboratory Animal Science* 50 (2): 221–226.

Woodnutt, G. and Berry, V. (1999). Two pharmacodynamic models for assessing the efficacy of amoxicillin-clavulanate against experimental respiratory tract infections caused by strains of *Streptococcus pneumoniae*. *Antimicrobial Agents and Chemotherapy* 43 (1): 29–34.

Young, C. and Hill, A. (1974). Conjunctivitis in a colony of rats. *Laboratory Animals* 8 (3): 301–304.

Zanasi, A., Mazzolini, M., and Kantar, A. (2017). A reappraisal of the mucoactive activity and clinical efficacy of bromhexine. *Multidisciplinary Respiratory Medicine* 12 (1): 7.

Zegre Cannon, C., Kissling, G.E., Goulding, D.R. et al. (2011). Analgesic effects of tramadol, carprofen or multimodal analgesia in rats undergoing ventral laparotomy. *Lab Animal* 40 (3): 85.

ZIMS (2017). Zoological Information Management System. http://training.species360.org/Documents/ZIMShelp/ZIMSHELP-medical%20-%20body%20condition%20score.docx (accessed 20 June 2019).

9

Sugar Gliders
Marie Kubiak

9.1 Introduction

Sugar gliders (*Petaurus breviceps*) are small nocturnal marsupials that originate from the forests of Australia, Papua New Guinea, and Irian Jaya (Di Qual 2013). Standard colouration is grey-brown dorsum, pale ventrum, and striped appearance to the head, however multiple colour variations have been selectively bred (Figures 9.1 and 9.2). They are well established within the pet trade across Europe, Asia, and North America, with reports of captive specimens being held as pets as early as the 1830s (Gunn 1851). There are no restrictions on ownership or trade of captive bred sugar gliders in the UK but they are not permitted to be kept as pets in some states in Australia and the USA. Biological parameters for sugar gliders are given in Table 9.1.

There are seven sub species recognised though all are managed in a similar way in captivity:

Petaurus breviceps breviceps
Petaurus breviceps longicaudatus
Petaurus breviceps ariel
Petaurus breviceps flavidus
Petaurus breviceps tafa
Petaurus breviceps papuanus
Petaurus breviceps biacensis (Franklin 2005).

9.1.1 Husbandry

Sugar gliders are arboreal, active animals, with a weakly prehensile tail and a functional patagium (gliding membrane). They are able to climb, jump, walk, and glide and enclosures must allow sufficient space and suitable furniture to permit these behaviours. A large aviary with fine wire mesh (no larger than 1.5 cm gaps) is ideal with a minimum cage height of 1.8 m (Johnson-Delaney 2002a). Large zinc-free wire cages can suffice but available commercial cages are often of insufficient size to permit normal activity (Figure 9.3). A system of non-toxic branches should be secured inside the enclosure with the sleeping area placed close to the top. This sleeping area is typically a soft material pouch or a wooden hide box and should be large enough for the whole group to fit into. As a social species, sugar gliders should be kept in pairs or small groups but with no more than one adult male per enclosure (Booth 2000). In the wild, groups consists of a dominant male, subordinate males, and several females up to a maximum group size of 12 individuals (Booth 2003).

Substrate should be non-toxic and shredded paper, woodchip (excluding pine and cedar products), leaf litter, or corn cob can be used. Cloth or towelling with linear fibres should be avoided for substrate or sleeping areas as digit or limb entrapment can result from threads tangling around extremities.

Sugar gliders are best kept at 24–27 °C though they can tolerate short-term fluctuations above and below this range well. An ambient temperature of no less than 20 °C is recommended day and night, with a protected heat source providing a focal basking spot of 31 °C during the day. All heat sources should be controlled by a thermostat to regulate temperatures safely. Cold sugar gliders will develop a negative energy balance and then go into an unresponsive torpor. They are a nocturnal species adapted to obtaining Vitamin D from the diet rather than sunlight exposure so providing ultraviolet lighting is not considered of significant benefit (Johnson and Hemsley 2008).

Sugar gliders are opportunistic omnivores (Booth 2000). Their natural diet is a variety of small invertebrates (insects, spiders, worms), small mammals and birds, eggs, tree sap, gum, nectar, pollen, and flowers (Howard 1989; Gamble 2004). There is little fruit, vegetable, or grain intake in wild animals and this should be reflected in the captive diet. The recommended daily quantity of food is 25–35 g (Eshar 2016).

Handbook of Exotic Pet Medicine, First Edition. Edited by Marie Kubiak.
© 2021 John Wiley & Sons Ltd. Published 2021 by John Wiley & Sons Ltd.
Companion website: www.wiley.com/go/kubiak/exotic_pet_medicine

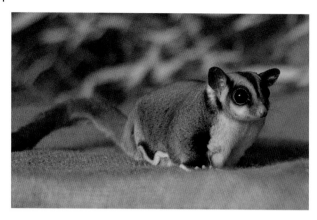

Figure 9.1 Standard coat appearance of a wild type sugar glider. Note this animal is obese. *Source:* photo courtesy of Helen Wolfy.

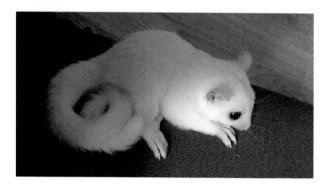

Figure 9.2 Various alternative colour variations have been selectively bred. *Source:* photo courtesy of Siobhan Caladine.

Table 9.1 Biological parameters for sugar gliders.

	Female	Male
Adult weight	95–135 g	115–160 g
Longevity	12–14 years	12–14 years
Body temperature	32 °C (cloacal) 35.8–36.6 °C (rectal)	32 °C (cloacal) 35.8–36.6 °C (rectal)
Heart rate	200–300/min	200–300/min
Respiratory rate	16–40/min	16–40/min
Sexual maturity	8–12 months	12–14 months

Recommendations are for 50% of the diet to comprise high protein food items (mineral/multivitamin supplemented insects, egg, small rodents, lean meat) and 50% sugars (nectar, acacia gum, gum arabic, commercial syrups) (Johnson 2004). Another option is to feed Leadbeater's mix (see Table 9.2) with a commercial insectivore/carnivore diet. Small amounts of fresh fruit and vegetables can be offered alongside the staple diet as treats. Food and water should be provided at height and cleaned and refreshed twice daily with the main food quantity provided in the evening to reflect the natural nocturnal feeding behaviour.

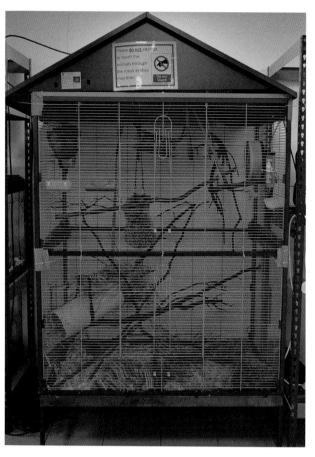

Figure 9.3 Commercial wire cages are cost effective housing options but size is typically insufficient to allow exhibition of a full range of behaviours.

Table 9.2 Recipe for Leadbeater's mix, a common addition to sugar glider diets. Once mixed this can be frozen in ice cube trays and aliquots thawed for daily use.

Honey	150 ml
Warm water	150 ml
Hardboiled egg with shell on, blended	1
High protein baby cereal	25 g
Multivitamin supplement	1 teaspoon

9.1.2 Breeding

Sugar gliders are marsupials and young undergo the majority of development within the female's pouch. Sexual maturity is reached at 8–12 months in females and 12–14 months in males. Adults will breed year round and can have 2–3 litters annually (Johnson-Delaney 2006). Gestation is only 15–17 days, with the foetuses (typically a litter of two) moving to the pouch after birth (Booth 2003). Dystocia is not a concern as young are very small (0.2 g in weight) when born. The neonate attaches to a teat within

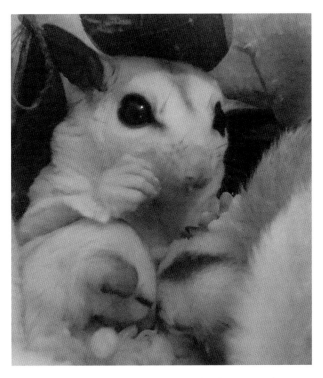

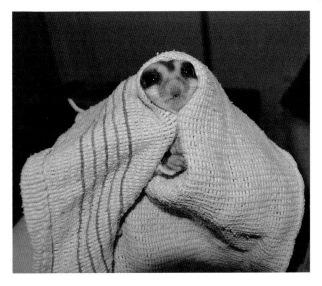

Figure 9.5   Sugar glider restraint in a small towel. The sharp nails will often grip on to fabric hindering examination.

Figure 9.4   Joeys feeding from the pouch prior to weaning. *Source:* photo courtesy of Siobhan Caladine.

the pouch and remains there for 70–74 days. Young continue to take milk until weaning at 110–120 days (Figure 9.4) but remain within the family group until maturity. Females may conceive at a post-partum oestrus but the blastocyst remains in diapause until the suckling joey is weaned (Johnson-Delaney 2002b).

9.2   Clinical Evaluation

9.2.1   History-Taking

Husbandry should be reviewed at the time of presentation to identify any potential factors in the development of clinical concerns. Recent changes to management, introduction of new animals, reproductive status, and details of the presenting condition are all pertinent.

9.2.2   Handling

Sugar gliders are rarely tame enough to tolerate handling and restraint for extensive examination but gently wrapping an individual in a small towel will allow for basic evaluation (Figure 9.5). Animals can and will bite on handling without restraint of the head and although bites and scratches are common they are typically minor (Di Qual 2013). Scruffing the glider, or encircling the neck with

thumb and forefinger results in better immobilisation but is considered stressful and examination should be carried out as quickly and efficiently as possible.

Sugar gliders will tend to grip firmly onto surrounding material and removal from towels or clothing requires gentle lifting of claws and may require restraint of feet by an assistant to avoid immediate reattachment.

9.2.3   Sex Determination

Marsupial mammals have a single cloacal orifice instead of the separate external urogenital and gastrointestinal tract terminations seen in placental mammals. Female sugar gliders have a pouch on the ventral abdomen (Figure 9.6). Males have more prominent scent glands (with the most prominent being the frontal gland on the forehead) and a pendulous scrotum on the ventral abdomen (Figures 9.7 and 9.8).

9.2.4   Clinical Examination

It is sensible to observe gliders prior to handling to determine resting respiratory rate, response to stimuli, and to visually assess external structures. This can be difficult as these animals are reclusive and are often presented hiding within a soft pouch.

Clinical examination is carried out in a similar fashion as for small rodents but restrained sugar gliders will often emit a low pitched growl, known as 'crabbing' hampering value of thoracic auscultation. For very fractious animals, examination may require general anaesthesia.

Particularly important parts of the examination are dental assessment, spinal and limb palpation for angular

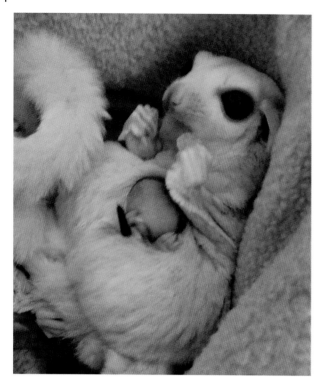

Figure 9.6 Female with joey present in pouch. *Source:* photo courtesy of Siobhan Caladine.

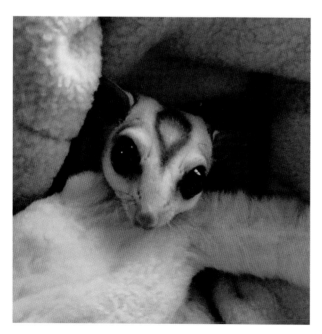

Figure 9.7 Male sugar glider with prominent scent gland. *Source:* photo courtesy of Siobhan Caladine.

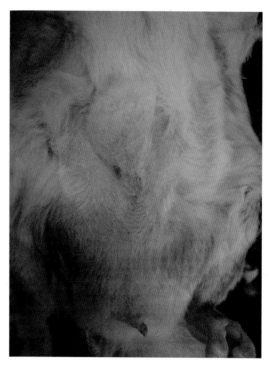

Figure 9.8 Ventral location of pendulous scrotum in a male sugar glider. Note the prepuce more caudally with forked penis.

deformities or traumatic injury, ophthalmic evaluation, vent examination, and assessment of skin, including that over the patagium. It is prudent to weigh animals at each visit and to carry out a basic assessment of body condition. It is useful for owners to keep records that document weight changes of individuals.

9.3 Basic Techniques

9.3.1 Sample Collection

Maximum blood sample volume able to be collected has been previously described as 1 ml per 100 g bodyweight (Ness and Johnson-Delaney 2012), but 0.5 ml per 100 g would be considered a more appropriate maximum sample for gliders of unknown or abnormal health. Anaesthesia is necessary for venepuncture in sugar gliders due to patient stress, difficulties in maintaining secure restraint, and small vessel size. Potential sample sites for obtaining up to 0.1 ml are the cephalic, lateral saphenous, femoral, ventral and lateral tail veins. Insulin syringes are most suitable for accessing these small blood vessels. For samples of up to 0.5 ml, the jugular veins or cranial vena cava are used (Evans and Souza 2010). The jugular veins are located on either side of the ventral neck, lateral to the trachea along a line from the point of shoulder to the ramus of the mandible (Ness and Johnson-Delaney 2012). For cranial vena cava sampling, the animal is placed in dorsal recumbency and the needle is inserted under the manubrium and angled approximately 30° laterally to blindly access the vessel (Figure 9.9).

Faeces should form pellets in sugar gliders and owners should be encouraged to bring samples to appointments, although animals will often pass faeces during transport or handling. Faecal flotation techniques to detect nematodes

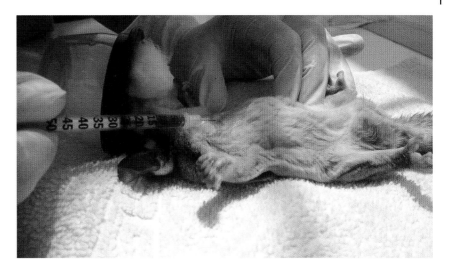

Figure 9.9 Cranial vena cava sample collection under anaesthesia. *Source:* photo courtesy of Sarah Pellett.

and cestodes should be recommended annually for healthy animals, and direct and flotation techniques should be used for animals with abnormal faecal appearance.

9.3.2 Nutritional Support

Maintenance nutritional requirements are 2.5% of body-weight (Johnson 2004) and sick animals often have markedly increased nutritional demands. Animals with feeding responses will often take insect prey above other food items and offering of gut-loaded, multivitamin supplemented insects will help maintain levels of macro and micro-nutrients. Nutritional support for anorexic animals typically consists of syringe feeding of a combination of nectarivore and insectivore liquid diets. Young, healthy male animals have been shown to require 100–150 kJ/day though it is expected that clinically unwell animals may have higher requirements (Dierenfeld et al. 2006). Amounts fed should be modified based on weight changes with twice daily weight monitoring routinely carried out.

9.3.3 Fluid Therapy

Fluid requirements are approximately 60 ml/kg/day and isotonic preparations available for domestic mammals are suitable in sugar gliders (Johnson 2004).

Animals with a functioning intestinal tract, able to self-feed or being assist fed will obtain the majority of their maintenance fluid requirements from food.

Where additional fluid support is needed, the subcutaneous route is used most commonly. Subcutaneous fluids can be administered in the interscapular region but when administered in large quantities, or absorption is slow, fluid deposits may pool in the gliding membrane and dermal necrosis is a possible consequence (Eshar 2016). Recommended maximum volumes to be administered subcutaneously are 10 ml/kg (Longley 2008) but this can be repeated once absorption is complete. Intravenous catheters are difficult to place and maintain due to patient size and interference so intraosseous fluid therapy is preferred for more aggressive rehydration of critical patients. The proximal tibia is the most common placement site though the proximal femur can also be used (Antinoff 1998; Longley 2008) but bone perforation and fractures are potential complications (Eshar 2016). For intraosseous fluid administration, constant infusion using a syringe driver is recommended.

9.3.4 Anaesthesia

Where possible, fasting for three to four hours prior to anaesthesia is advisable. Gliders can be restrained with the head in a small, fitted anaesthetic mask or in a small anaesthetic chamber for induction of anaesthesia using a volatile agent (Figure 9.10). Where volatile agents are used alone it is preferable to use sevoflurane over isoflurane due to the irritation of mucous membranes and adverse smell associated with isoflurane (Guedes et al. 2017). Premedication with butorphanol at 0.2 mg/kg or midazolam at 0.3 mg/kg can improve induction quality and reduce patient stress so is advisable (Pye 2001; Ness and Johnson-Delaney 2012). Other anaesthetic options are included in the formulary.

Tracheal diameter is markedly reduced with endotracheal tube placement so maintenance of anaesthesia is most commonly carried out using a facemask, or with intubation using a 1 mm endotracheal tube and intermittent positive pressure ventilation to maintain tube patency. Intubation can be challenging and is best achieved with a small, fine laryngoscope blade and with the head extended and tongue pulled forward to visualise the glottis.

Due to the small size of glider patients, hypothermia is a concern during anaesthesia and thermal support by way of heat pads, high ambient temperatures, or circulating hot air devices is necessary. During recovery a neonatal incubator can be useful for maintaining temperature.

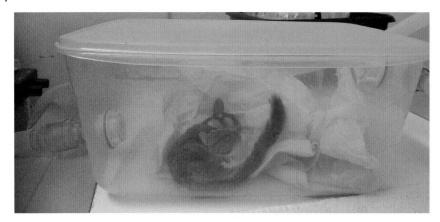

Figure 9.10 Use of an induction chamber to anaesthetise a sugar glider using sevoflurane in oxygen. *Source:* photo courtesy of Sarah Pellett.

9.3.5 Euthanasia

Intravenous (via the cranial vena cava) or intracardiac injection of pentobarbitone are appropriate methods of euthanasia but should be carried out under sedation or anaesthesia (Reilly 2001). Intraperitoneal injection is an alternative where venous access has failed in an anaesthetised animal.

9.3.6 Hospitalisation Requirements

It is helpful to encourage owners to provide a small cage and familiar food items for short periods of hospitalisation. Standard hospital cages for domestic mammals or birds are rarely secure enough to keep sugar gliders safely contained. Small gauge wire cages designed for small bird species are often adequate for security and for limited climbing opportunities. At least one hide area must be provided and soft fleece pouches are safe and can be washed and disinfected between patients. Sugar gliders should not be kept in the same ward as predatory species such as dogs or cats, and require quiet dim conditions and appropriate temperatures to minimise stress.

9.4 Common Medical and Surgical Conditions

9.4.1 Malnutrition

Inappropriate diet is common in pet gliders and is a significant factor in many cases presenting to veterinary surgeons (Eshar 2016). Malnutrition may present as non-specific signs such as weakness, lethargy, inappetance, dehydration, diarrhoea, hypothermia, or secondary infections or more easily identifiable changes such as cataracts, dental changes, pathological fractures, tremors, or weight loss. Diagnosis is achieved with dietary review and clinical examination in many cases.

Nutritional secondary hyperparathyroidism is well recognised in this species with dietary deficiency of calcium and vitamin D primarily responsible (Helmer and Lightfoot 2002). In most cases the calcium or Vitamin D deficiency results in weakness, progressive demineralisation of bones with associated fibrous osteodystrophy and pathological fractures (Figure 9.11), and seizures in advanced cases (Gamble 2004; Eshar 2016). Hind limb paralysis may result in some cases and radiography is necessary to assess extent and location of lesions and to determine prognosis. Increased demands will hasten onset of symptoms, with one case of hypocalcaemic tetany reported in a female sugar glider on an inappropriate diet (Nelson 2000). Supportive care, administration of calcium and vitamin supplementation, analgesia, and restriction of activity may result in resolution of mild–moderate cases. Where lesions are present that will result in long-term restriction of mobility, or pain cannot be managed, then euthanasia is advisable on welfare grounds.

Sugar gliders are reported to suffer from haemochromatosis (Iron storage disease), due to a higher iron diet being offered in captivity than is seen in wild counterparts and an abundance of vitamin C in the diet of fruit-fed individuals (Clauss and Paglia 2012). It appears an uncommon pathology in pet gliders but should be considered in cases with hepatomegaly and polycythaemia.

Obesity is common as a consequence of husbandry shortcomings (Figure 9.1). Common contributing factors being an excess of dietary fat, limited opportunity for activity due to enclosure size or design, or a sedentary lifestyle in animals kept in social isolation (Eshar 2016). Enclosure and diet improvements should be introduced to achieve a gradual weight loss.

Juvenile onset cataracts appear associated with diet, particularly an inappropriate formula composition, as seen in other marsupials (Johnson-Delaney 2002b).

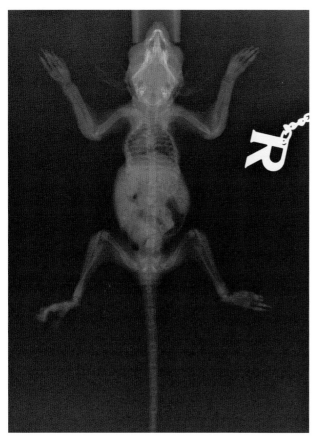

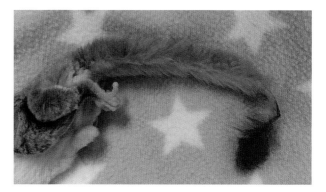

Figure 9.12　Tail tip injury following use of a fenestrated exercise wheel. Solid wheels are preferred to avoid limb or tail injury. Amputation was carried out in this glider.

Figure 9.11　NSHP in a juvenile glider, associated with intestinal stasis, poor bone mineralisation, deformities, and pathological fracture of the right femur. *Source:* Courtesy of Manor vets.

9.4.2　Traumatic Injury

Conspecific injury, self-trauma, and falls can result in wounds. These should be treated as for any other species with analgesia, cleaning, and repair as necessary. Patagial injuries larger than 5 mm should be sutured with fine absorbable suture with careful attention to ensure that the normal anatomy and skin integrity on either side of the gliding membrane is restored. Digital injuries relating to entrapment can occur in animals on inappropriate substrate and may necessitate amputation of one or more digits.

Tail injuries are occasionally seen, associated with bite injuries, falls or from inappropriate cage equipment (Figure 9.12). Amputation is prudent for many injuries as self-trauma is common.

9.4.3　Neoplasia

Neoplasia was identified as the most common diagnosis in fatalities in one survey, accounting for 17.8% of fatalities where a diagnosis was made (Di Qual 2013). Lymphoma

has been reported as common but published case reports are lacking (Booth 2003). Reported neoplasms are listed in Table 9.3.

A benign paracloacal gland cyst has been reported in a castrated male sugar glider, with presence of a fluctuant mass adjacent to the cloaca (Thomas et al. 2019). Surgical excision was curative.

9.4.4　Dental Disease

The dental formula is 3/2, 1/0, 3/3, 4/4 and all teeth are closed rooted (Johnson 2004). The incisors are long as an adaptation to gouging tree bark to obtain sap. These teeth do not grow continuously so trimming should be avoided.

Periodontal disease and caries can result from a high sugar diet (Booth 2000). Dental scaling can aid in management but often extractions are necessary due to the advanced nature of changes on presentation in many cases (Figure 9.13). Incisor extraction should be done only when absolutely necessary due to the presence of minimal supporting bone and risk of symphyseal fracture (Johnson 2004). A technique has been described to extract a damaged incisor, involving gingival reflection, severing of periodontal ligaments with a curved needle and flushing of the cavity with dilute chlorhexidine followed by instilling of a synthetic bone replacement and gingival closure with sutures (Ness and Johnson-Delaney 2012)

9.4.5　Respiratory Tract Disease

Respiratory infections are often multifactorial with chronic stress, malnutrition, inappropriate temperatures or humidity, and poor hygiene amongst the inciting influences. Bacterial pneumonia appears common and *Pasteurella multocida* has been reported as one cause (Ness and Booth 2004).

Table 9.3 Neoplasms reported in sugar gliders.

Neoplasm	Site	Age	Sex	References
Lymphosarcoma	Multiple subcutaneous masses	7 yrs	male	Gentz et al. (2003)
Lymphosarcoma		4 yrs (1), 8 yrs (1), 12 yrs (2)	male (3), female (1)	Hough et al. (1992), Gentz et al. (2003)
Lymphosarcoma/fibrosarcoma		11 yrs	male	Gentz et al. (2003)
Leukaemia	Splenic (4), unknown (1)	Adults (3), unknown (2)	male (3), unknown (2)	Canfield et al. (1990), Gentz et al. (2003)
Round cell neoplasm	Unknown	14 yrs	female	Sokol et al. (2017)
Hepatocellular carcinoma	Liver	14 yrs	female	Sokol et al. (2017)
Hepatocellular carcinoma	Liver	9 yrs	male	Sokol et al. (2017)
Transitional call carcinoma	Pericloacal	10 yrs	male	Marrow et al. (2010)
Carcinoma	Paracloacal gland	4 yrs	male	Chen et al. (2018)
Carcinoma	Mammary	9 yrs	female	Keller et al. (2014)
Carcinoma	Mammary	4 yrs (1), 6 yrs (1)	female (2)	Gentz et al. (2003)
Carcinoma	Liver and adrenal gland concurrently	15 yrs	female	Lindemann et al. (2016)
Carcinoma	Intestines	11 yrs	male	Gentz et al. (2003)
Adenocarcinoma	Mammary	9 yrs (1), unknown (1)	female (1), unknown (1)	Gentz et al. (2003), Churgin et al. (2015)
Adenocarcinoma	Chest gland	Unknown	unknown	Gentz et al. (2003)
Adenocarcinoma	Multifocal	Unknown	unknown	Gentz et al. (2003)
Adenocarcinoma	Abdominal	10 yrs	male	Gentz et al. (2003)
Adenocarcinoma	Duodenum	Unknown	male	Canfield et al. (1990)
Adenocarcinoma	Unknown	adult	female	Gentz et al. (2003)
Adenocarcinoma	lung	7 yrs	female	Gentz et al. (2003)
Adrenal cortical carcinoma	Adrenal gland	Adult	female	Gentz et al. (2003)
Phaeochromocytoma	Adrenal gland	5 yrs	female	Gentz et al. (2003)
Squamous cell carcinoma	Vagina	7 yrs	female	Gentz et al. (2003)
Fibrosarcoma		1 yr	male	Gentz et al. (2003)
Haemangiosarcoma	Skin of patagium	11 yrs	female	Rivas et al. (2014)
Sarcoma	Urinary bladder	3.5 yrs	female	Sokol et al. (2017)
Myxosarcoma		11 yrs	male	Gentz et al. (2003)
Spindle cell tumour	Unknown	11 yrs	male	Gentz et al. (2003)
Fibroma	Subcutaneous (2)	11 yrs., (1), Unknown (2)	male (1), unknown (2)	Canfield et al. (1990); Gentz et al. (2003)
Sebaceous epithelioma	Skin	4 yrs	male	Gentz et al. (2003)
Histiocytoma	Subcutaneous	7 yrs	female	Gentz et al. (2003)
Dysgerminoma		1 yr	female	Gentz et al. (2003)

Cardiac disease associated with malnutrition and sepsis has also been reported and may present in a similar fashion to infectious respiratory disease (Heatley 2009; Garner 2011). A similar approach to domestic species is taken. In cases with a high index of suspicion of primary or second-ary bacterial pneumonia empirical antibiotic therapy is used, alongside husbandry improvements and supportive care as needed. Where diagnosis is less certain, or response to empirical therapy is poor then further investigative techniques include radiography, echocardiography with a high

(a)

(b)

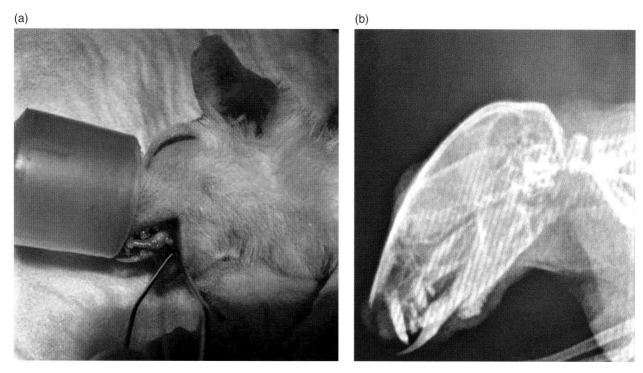

Figure 9.13 (a) Advanced dental disease with calculus, gingival regression and mandibular bone exposure. (b) Laterolateral radiograph of the same glider, demonstrating changes consistent with osteomyelitis. *Source:* Images courtesy of Siobhan Caladine.

frequency probe, and tracheal wash or bronchoalveolar lavage sample collection under anaesthesia.

Recently pulmonary hyalinosis was described in sugar gliders as an apparent cause of respiratory symptoms including dyspnoea and tachypnoea (Sokol et al. 2017). No clear cause of the lesions identified post-mortem was determined and severity of lesions did not correlate with age.

Fatal pulmonary haemorrhage has been reported in one sugar glider as a consequence of *Ophidascaris robertsi* infestation and nematodes were found within the heart (Agúndez et al. 2014). Cross-infection from wild-caught reptiles was presumed to be the source of the parasites.

Hyperthermia can also result in respiratory compromise (Eshar 2016).

9.4.6 Urinary Tract Disorders

Renal disease is thought to be relatively common with urinary tract obstruction, nephritis, pyelonephritis, and chronic renal failure reported (Johnson-Delaney 2002a). Urine samples may be passed on handling and even small volumes can be evaluated using human or domestic animal urinalysis strips, refractometry, and sediment microscopy. Specific gravity for this species ranges from 1.020 to 1.040 and a small amount of protein (up to 0.15 g/l) is considered normal (Brust and Pye 2012). Reference ranges for urine

protein:creatinine ratios have not been validated in this species but comparison with existing ranges for other small mammals may assist in following progression of disease. Biochemistry with evaluation of urea, creatinine, and phosphorus in particular may further assist diagnosis of acute or chronic renal disease.

9.4.7 Dermatological Disease

Gliders under chronic stress may develop abnormal coping behaviours such as self-trauma, overgrooming, aggression, and coprophagy (Johnson 2004). Common stressors include inappropriate social group (including social isolation), lack of cover in enclosures, or excessive human contact in animals that have not been habituated to handling (Ellis and Moris 2001). Animals with inappropriate diet may also develop fur chewing behaviours. Medical therapy has been reported with fluoxetine (Johnson 2004), but correction of husbandry and reduction of stress is the mainstay of management.

A case of self-mutilation associated with aberrant migration of intestinal nematodes has been reported but appears an uncommon presentation of endoparasitism (Johnson 2004).

Dermatophytosis can affect sugar gliders, and may present with pruritus, crusting, scaling, and alopecia (Marshall 2003). Treatment mirrors that of domestic species, with topical agents preferred where possible as accurate dosing with systemic agents can be complicated by the small patient size.

9.4.8 Gastrointestinal Disease

Acute enteritis and colitis are common in sugar gliders, with subsequent endotoxaemia resulting in neurological signs and death (Reavill 2014). Subacute cases may present with debilitation and diarrhoea. Inappropriate diet, parasitism (including protozoal causes), or primary bacterial enteritis may be inciting factors and specific microbes are rarely determined. Supportive care is crucial as many affected animals will be anorexic, dehydrated, and hypothermic on presentation. A thorough dietary review, faecal examination (both direct and flotation techniques), and faecal culture are advisable to determine cause where possible. *Clostridium piliforme* infection, Giardiasis, coccidiosis, *Plagiorchis* trematodes, Salmonellosis, and cryptosporidiosis have all been associated with gastrointestinal disease in captive sugar gliders (Johnson 2004; Reavill 2014). Salmonellosis is a potential zoonotic risk, with transfer of Salmonella from sugar gliders to humans resulting in clinical disease (Woodward et al. 1997). One survey found 15.4% of clinically healthy sugar gliders were shedding *Salmonella* spp. in faeces at the time of sampling, so hygiene precautions should be taken with all animals (Diana et al. 2016).

Chronic or severe enteritis can uncommonly result in a prolapse of cloacal or rectal tissue, complicated by poor muscle tone associated with nutritional secondary hyperparathyroidism (Johnson-Delaney 2000). The tissue should be cleaned and inspected for areas of necrosis or self-trauma under sedation or anaesthesia. If intact then application of a hypertonic sugar solution will help reduce oedema and aid replacement using lubricated cotton buds. Any areas of superficial necrosis require gentle debridement but where damage extends beyond the mucosa surgical resection should be considered prior to replacement. The vent aperture can be narrowed using a purse string suture but single interrupted sutures at the lateral extent on each side are preferred as the normal vent shape is maintained.

Gastric dilation and volvulus has been reported in two sugar gliders (Lennox and Reavill 2013). Presenting signs were acute debilitation and abdominal distension and diagnosis was made post-mortem. Cause was not determined.

9.4.9 Penile Prolapse

Males occasionally develop penile prolapse as a mating or self-injury, or as a rare complication of anaesthesia. Where possible, sedation or anaesthesia, lubrication and replacement of the penis into the cloaca should be attempted. However, where necrosis is present or is considered likely to result then partial penile amputation may be necessary. This species has a forked penis with the urethral opening located at the level of the bifurcation. This allows for simple amputation of the penile fork distal to the urethral opening without affecting urination and a urethral catheter should be placed to protect and highlight the urethral opening location during surgery (Miwa 2008). Urethrostomy following a proximal penile amputation has been carried out but is technically challenging and carries a poor prognosis (Johnson-Delaney 2000).

9.4.10 Ocular Disorders

As nocturnal prey animals, sugar gliders have large, laterally placed, protruding eyes which are prone to traumatic injury. Superficial corneal abrasions are treated with topical lubricants and antibiotic therapy. Retrobulbar abscesses as a consequence of bite wounds from conspecifics have been described with radiography to determine presence of osteomyelitis, surgical debridement of affected tissue, drain placement, systemic antibiotics, and analgesia suggested (Ness and Johnson-Delaney 2012).

Periocular swelling and death have been reported in a group of five sugar gliders associated with Trypanosomiasis presumed to be due to ingestion of insect vectors (Latas et al. 2004).

9.4.11 Toxoplasmosis

An outbreak of toxoplasmosis has been reported in a zoo colony of sugar gliders with individuals showing symptoms including anorexia, weight loss, weakness, seizures, and acute death. Post-mortem examination showed no gross lesions but protozoal tachyzoites were identified on histopathology in multiple organs. These were subsequently confirmed as *Toxoplasma gondii* on immunostaining. Administration of clindamycin was associated with no further cases in the remaining animals (Barrows 2006). Although toxoplasmosis is typically associated with contact with feline faeces, ingestion of infected insects or rodents, or contact with contaminated substrate may be potential routes of infection transfer. In other Australian marsupials, *T. gondii* also occurs as a recrudescent infection as well as the classic acute infection (Blyde 1993). For pre-mortem diagnosis, serology using assay of both IgM and IgG can be carried out.

9.4.12 Miscellaneous Infections

In one report, bacterial infections were diagnosed in 15% of the samples submitted to a pathology laboratory for this species (Garner 2011). These included dermatitis, sepsis, systemic and central nervous system (CNS) infection associated with Listeria and two cases of *C. piliforme*.

Listeria monocytogenes septicaemia has been reported in one sugar glider fed contaminated food (Nichols et al. 2015).

9.4.13 Neonatal Rejection

Distressed gliders may, rarely, discard young from the pouch – removing inciting stressors and returning the joey to the pouch may lead to acceptance but repeated rejection necessitates hand rearing or euthanasia. Pouch infections and over-breeding may also contribute to failure of joeys to thrive, necessitating intervention (Johnson-Delaney 2000).

Hand-rearing can be challenging and carries a poor prognosis, especially in early stages of pouch development (Woods 1999). An artificial pouch can be created from cloth and it is important to ensure no loose threads are present which could cause injury or be ingested (Doneley 2002). The pouch should be kept within a controlled temperature environment, such as an incubator or brooder at 34–35 °C for unfurred joeys, 32–34 °C for lightly furred animals and dropping to 28 °C when joeys are fully furred (Doneley 2002). Neonates require feeding every two to three hours initially and a protein and fat-enriched milk substitute low in lactose is advisable. For feeding, the joey should be restrained in dorsal recumbency and a syringe or bottle with an elongated, elastic teat used to replicate the maternal teat. Chemical free ointments such as lanolin should be applied to skin daily as neonates can develop skin dessication outside of the natural pouch conditions (Gamble 2004). Once mobile and furred joeys can start weaning and introduction to the family group may be considered. Diarrhoea, inhalation pneumonia, cataract formation, dermatitis, hypothermia, and hypoglycaemia are common ailments in hand-reared joeys (Doneley 2002).

9.5 Preventative Health Measures

An annual review of husbandry alongside physical examination is recommended with particular focus on body condition, dental health, and long bone structure. A faecal sample should be checked for evidence of parasites at the same time.

9.5.1 Neutering Technique

Ovariohysterectomy is rarely carried out as a routine procedure due to patient size and anatomy making this a technically demanding procedure with potential compli-

cations (Gamble 2004). Cases of reproductive tract pathology appear rare but would justify surgical intervention. A ventral paramedian incision is made to avoid the pouch, the skin retracted and the underlying muscle is incised along the linea alba, taking care not to involve the bladder which lies just underneath. The bladder is expressed, urine aspirated with a sterile syringe, or the bladder reflected to allow visualisation of the uterus. The technique is similar to that used for domestic species, with ligatures or vascular clips placed on the ovarian pedicles, and the two uteri are ligated at their junctions with the vaginas. Care should be taken not to ligate the ureters which are in close association with the vaginal canals (Johnson 2004).

Castration is relatively simple in males and is more frequently carried out to avoid unwanted breeding, or to allow males to cohabit peacefully. It should be noted that the peripenile swellings seen in this species are scent glands and should not be surgically excised. The testes of males are located at the level of the umbilicus and are prominent due to a pronounced scrotal sac and long pedicle. For castration, scrotal ablation is also carried out to avoid leaving a pendulous flap of skin. A circumferential incision is made around the stalk of the scrotum and transfixing ligatures are placed around each spermatic cord followed by sharp dissection to remove the testes (Newbury et al. 2005). The skin incision is closed with a single intradermal suture or tissue glue. Techniques using carbon dioxide laser or electrosurgery to sever the scrotal stalk have also been described (Morges et al. 2009; Malbrue et al. 2018). Use of local anaesthesia instilled into the spermatic cords pre-operatively may help prevent post-operative self-trauma and post-operative continuation of analgesia is important. Close monitoring is necessary during the anaesthesia recovery as self-injury from wound interference is not uncommon (Ellis and Moris 2001).

9.6 Radiographic Imaging

Radiography necessitates anaesthesia in all but the most debilitated animals. Whole body survey radiographs are commonly taken due to patient size and frequency of non-specific clinical signs (Figures 9.14 and 9.15). It is useful to reflect the patagium away from the body cavity or area of interest to improve diagnostic quality of radiographs (Ness and Johnson-Delaney 2012). If young are present in the pouch where possible they should be removed (if not attached to the teat) or shielded from the xray beam. Common radiographic findings include metabolic bone disease (Figure 9.11), dental pathology (Figure 9.13b), gastrointestinal distension and traumatic or pathological fractures.

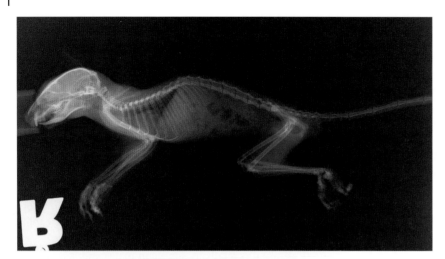

Figure 9.14 Right lateral radiograph of a sugar glider. *Source:* Courtesy of Manor vets.

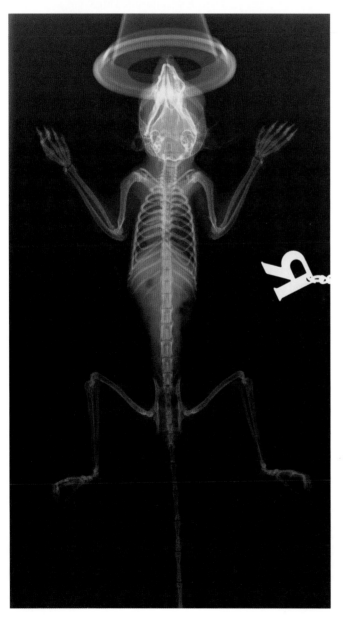

Figure 9.15 Ventrodorsal radiograph of a sugar glider. *Source:* Courtesy of Manor vets.

Formulary for sugar gliders

Medication	Dose[a]	Dosing interval	Additional comments
Anaesthesia			
Buprenorphine	0.03 mg/kg/ SC		30 mins prior to induction
Midazolam	0.3 mg/kg SC		30 mins prior to induction
Ketamine	2–3 mg/kg		
Medetomidine	0.05–0.1 mg/kg		(Ness and Johnson-Delaney 2012)
Isoflurane	5% to induce, 2–3% for maintenance		(Ness and Johnson-Delaney 2012)
Analgesia			
Buprenorphine	0.01–0.03 mg/kg PO, SC	q12h	(Ness and Johnson-Delaney 2012)
Butorphanol	0.5 mg/kg SC	q6-8h	(Newbury et al. 2005)
Meloxicam	0.1–0.2 mg/kg PO, SC	q24h	(Ness and Johnson-Delaney 2012)
Ketoprofen	1 mg/kg SC		(Newbury et al. 2005)
Carprofen	2 mg/kg bid PO		(Newbury et al. 2005)
Antibiotics			
Amoxicillin	30 mg/kg IM, PO	q24h	(Johnson 2004) Sugar gliders do utilise caecal fermentation but dysbiosis does not appear a concern with oral antibiotic therapy (Eshar 2016)
Enrofloxacin	5 mg/kg IM, PO, SC	q12–24h	Injections diluted 1 : 1 with saline to reduce potential for injection site necrosis (Johnson 2004; Ness and Johnson-Delaney 2012)
Metronidazole	25 mg/kg PO	q24h	(Ness and Johnson-Delaney 2012)
Trimethoprim/Sulfa	15 mg/kg PO	q12h	(Ness and Johnson-Delaney 2012)
Antiparasitics			
Fenbendazole	20–50 mg/kg PO	q 24 hr × 3 days; repeat in 14 days	For nematodes and cestodes
Ivermectin	0.2 mg/kg PO, SC	repeat in 14 days	For nematodes, ear mites
Selamectin	6–18 mg/kg topically	repeat monthly	For ectoparasites (Johnson 2004)
Clindamycin	12.5 mg/kg PO	q12h for 4 weeks	For toxoplasmosis (Barrows 2006)
Metronidazole	25 mg/kg PO	q24h	For enteric protozoa (Ness and Johnson-Delaney 2012)
Miscellaneous			
Calcium gluconate	100 mg/kg SC	q12h	Dilute to 10 mg/ml before injection, for acute management of hypocalcaemia (Johnson 2004)
Calcium gluconate and cholecalciferol	35 mg/kg and 25iu/kg PO	q24h	For chronic management of hypocalcaemia (NOAH 2004)
Fluoxetine	1 mg/kg PO	q12h	For behavioural abnormalities (Johnson 2004)
Enalapril	0.22–0.44 mg/kg PO	q24h	Cardiac disease (Ness and Johnson-Delaney 2012)
Furosemide	1–5 mg/kg PO	q6–12h	Diuretic (Ness and Johnson-Delaney 2012)

[a] Drug dosages are often extrapolated from placental mammals, but metabolic rate is estimated to be 45% lower for a sugar glider (Eshar 2016).

References

Agúndez, M.G., Rodríguez, J.E.V., Juan-Sallés, C. et al. (2014). First report of parasitism by *Ophidascaris robertsi* (nematoda) in a sugar glider (*Petaurus breviceps*, marsupialia). *Journal of Zoo and Wildlife Medicine* 45 (4): 984–986.

Antinoff, N. (1998). Small mammal critical care. *The Veterinary Clinics of North America. Exotic Animal Practice* 1: 153–175.

Barnes, M. (2002). Sugar gliders. In: *Hand-Rearing Wild and Domestic Mammals* (ed. L.J. Gage), 55–62. Ames: Iowa State Press.

Barrows, M. (2006). Toxoplasmosis in a colony of sugar gliders (*Petaurus breviceps*). *The Veterinary Clinics of North America. Exotic Animal Practice* 9 (3): 617–623.

Blyde, D. (1993). Common diseases and treatments in macropods. In: *Proceedings of the American Association of Zoo Veterinarians*, 168–170. St. Louis: The American Association of Zoo Veterinarians.

Booth, R.J. (2000). General husbandry and medical care of sugar gliders. In: *Kirk's Current Therapy of Small Animal XIII* (ed. J.D. Bonagura), 1157–1163. Philadelphia: WB Saunders.

Booth, R. (2003). Sugar gliders. *Seminars in Avian and Exotic Pet Medicine* 12 (4): 228–231.

Brust, D. and Pye, G. (2012). Sugar gliders. In: *Exotic Animal Formulary*, 4e (ed. J.W. Carpenter), 449. St. Louis: Elsevier.

Canfield, P.J., Hartley, W.J., and Reddacliff, G.L. (1990). Spontaneous proliferations in Australian marsupials – a survey and review. 2. Dasyurids and bandicoots. *Journal of Comparative Pathology* 103 (2): 147–158.

Chen, J.C., Yu, P.H., Liu, C.H. et al. (2018). Paracloacal gland carcinoma in a sugar glider (*Petaurus breviceps*). *Journal of Exotic Pet Medicine* 27 (1): 36–40.

Churgin, S.M., Deering, K.M., Wallace, R. et al. (2015). Metastatic mammary adenocarcinoma in a sugar glider (*Petaurus breviceps*). *Journal of Exotic Pet Medicine* 24 (4): 441–445.

Clauss, M. and Paglia, D.E. (2012). Iron storage disorders in captive wild mammals: the comparative evidence. *Journal of Zoo and Wildlife Medicine* 43 (3s): S6–S18.

Di Qual, A. (2013). The suitability of Sugar Gliders (Petaurus breviceps) as domestic companions: an analysis of survey data. MPhil thesis. (Biological Sciences Research) of the University of New South Wales. http://unsworks.unsw.edu.au/fapi/datastream/unsworks:11627/SOURCE01, (accessed 22 May 2019).

Diana, H.N., Saleha, A.A., Azlan, C.M. et al. (2016). Oral microbes of pet sugar gliders and detection of *Salmonella* in their faeces. *Journal Veterinar Malaysia* 28 (1): 24–25.

Dierenfeld, E.S., Thomas, D., and Ives, R. (2006). Comparison of commonly used diets on intake, digestion, growth, and health in captive sugar gliders (*Petaurus breviceps*). *Journal of Exotic Pet Medicine* 15 (3): 218–224.

Doneley, B. (2002). Hand-rearing orphan marsupials. *Exotic DVM* 4 (3): 79–82.

Ellis, C. and Moris, M. (2001). Skin diseases of rodents and small exotic mammals. *The Veterinary Clinics of North America. Exotic Animal Practice* 4: 493–542.

Eshar, D. (2016). Husbandry and medicine of the sugar glider. ISVMA Proceedings Oct 17, 2016, ASVMA. https://www.isvma.org/2016-convention-proceedings (accessed 22 May 2019).

Evans, E.E. and Souza, M.J. (2010). Advanced diagnostic approaches and current management of internal disorders of select species (rodents, sugar gliders, hedgehogs). *The Veterinary Clinics of North America. Exotic Animal Practice* 13 (3): 453–469.

Franklin, J. (2005). Natural history of the sugar glider (*Petaurus breviceps*). *Journal of Exotic Mammal Medicine and Surgery* 3 (2): 7–9.

Gamble, K.C. (2004). Marsupial care and husbandry. *The Veterinary Clinics of North America. Exotic Animal Practice* 7 (2): 283–298.

Garner, M.M. (2011). Diseases of pet hedgehogs, chinchillas, and sugar gliders. In: *Proceedings of the Association of Avian Veterinarians, Seattle, WA*, 351–359. Denver: AAV.

Gentz, E.J., Richard, M.J., Crawshaw, G. et al. (2003). Neoplasia in sugar gliders (*Petaurus breviceps*): thirty-three cases. In: *Proceedings of American Association of Zoo Veterinarians*, 132–134. Yulee, FL: AAZV.

Guedes, S.R., Valentim, A.M., and Antunes, L.M. (2017). Mice aversion to sevoflurane, isoflurane and carbon dioxide using an approach-avoidance task. *Applied Animal Behaviour Science* 189: 91–97.

Gunn, R.C. (1851). On the introduction and naturalisation of *Petaurus sciureus* in Tasmania. In: *Papers and Proceedings of the Royal Society of Tasmania*, vol. 1, 253–255. Hobart: Royal Society of Tasmania.

Heatley, J.J. (2009). Cardiovascular anatomy, physiology, and disease of rodents and small exotic mammals. *The Veterinary Clinics of North America. Exotic Animal Practice* 12 (1): 99–113.

Helmer, P.J. and Lightfoot, T.L. (2002). Small exotic mammal orthopedics. *The Veterinary Clinics of North America. Exotic Animal Practice* 5 (1): 169–182.

Hough, I., Reuter, R.E., Rahaley, R.S. et al. (1992). Cutaneous lymphosarcoma in a sugar glider. *Australian Veterinary Journal* 69 (4): 93–94.

Howard, J. (1989). Diet of *Petaurus breviceps* (Marsupialia: Petauridae) in a mosaic of coastal woodland and heath. *Australian Mammalogy* 12: 15–21.

Johnson, D. (2004). Sugar glider medicine and surgery. In: *Proceedings of Atlantic Coast Veterinary Conference, Atlantic City, New Jersey USA*. Atlantic City, NJ: Veterinary Information Network.

Johnson, R. and Hemsley, S. (2008). Gliders and possums. In: *Medicine of Australian Mammals* (eds. L. Vogelnest and R. Woods), 395–438. Collingwood, Victoria: CSIRO Publishing.

Johnson-Delaney, C. (2000). Medical update for sugar gliders. *ICE Proceedings* 2 (3): 91–93.

Johnson-Delaney, C.A. (2002a). Other small mammals. In: *Manual of Exotic Pets*, 4e (eds. A. Meredith and S. Redrobe), 102–115. Quedgeley, Gloucester: BSAVA.

Johnson-Delaney, C.A. (2002b). Reproductive medicine of companion marsupials. *The Veterinary Clinics of North America. Exotic Animal Practice* 5 (3): 537–553.

Johnson-Delaney, C.A. (2006). Practical marsupial medicine. In: *Proceedings of the Association of Avian Veterinarians. San Antonio, August, 6* (eds. J. Carpenter and E. Bergman), 51–60. Bedford, TX: Association of Avian Veterinarians.

Keller, K.A., Nevarez, J.G., Rodriguez, D. et al. (2014). Diagnosis and treatment of anaplastic mammary carcinoma in a sugar glider (*Petaurus breviceps*). *Journal of Exotic Pet Medicine* 23 (3): 277–282.

Latas, P., Reavill, D.R., and Nicholson, D. (2004). Trypanosoma infection in sugar gliders (Petaurus breviceps) and a hedgehog (Atelerix albiventris) from Texas. *Joint conference-American Association of Zoo Veterinarians* 2004: 183–184.

Lennox, A.M. and Reavill, D.R. (2013). Gastric dilatation and gastric dilatation with volvulus in two sugar gliders (*Petaurus breviceps*). In: *Proceedings of Association of Exotic Mammal Veterinarians*, 21–22. Indianapolis, IN: AEMV.

Lindemann, D.M., Carpenter, J.W., DeBey, B.M. et al. (2016). Concurrent adrenocortical carcinoma and hepatocellular carcinoma with hemosiderosis in a sugar glider (*Petaurus breviceps*). *Journal of Exotic Pet Medicine* 25 (2): 144–149.

Longley, L. (2008). *Anaesthesia of Exotic Pets*, 99–102. Edingurgh: Elsevier Saunders.

Malbrue, R.A., Arsuaga, C.B., Collins, T.A. et al. (2018). Scrotal stalk ablation and orchiectomy using electrosurgery in the male sugar glider (*Petaurus breviceps*) and histologic anatomy of the testes and associated scrotal structures. *Journal of Exotic Pet Medicine* 27 (2): 90–94.

Marrow, J.C., Carpenter, J.W., Lloyd, A. et al. (2010). A transitional cell carcinoma with squamous differentiation in a pericloacal mass in a sugar glider (*Petaurus breviceps*). *Journal of Exotic Pet Medicine* 19 (1): 92–95.

Marshall, K.L. (2003). Fungal diseases in small mammals: therapeutic trends and zoonotic considerations. *The Veterinary Clinics of North America. Exotic Animal Practice* 6 (2): 415–427.

Miwa, Y. (2008). Locating the urethral opening in a male sugar glider. *Exotic DVM* 10 (3): 4.

Morges, M.A., Grant, K.R., MacPhail, C.M. et al. (2009). A novel technique for orchiectomy and scrotal ablation in the sugar glider (*Petaurus breviceps*). *Journal of Zoo and Wildlife Medicine* 40 (1): 204–206.

Nelson, S. (2000). A presumed case of 'milk fever' hypocalcemia in a sugar glider. *Exotic DVM* 1 (6): 42.

Ness, R.D. and Booth, R. (2004). Sugar gliders. In: *Ferrets, Rabbits and Rodents: Clinical Medicine and Surgery*, 2e (eds. K. Quesenberry and J.W. Carpenter), 330–338. St Louis: Saunders.

Ness, R.D. and Johnson-Delaney, C. (2012). Sugar gliders. In: *Ferrets, Rabbits and Rodents: Clinical Medicine and Surgery*, 3e (eds. K. Quesenberry and J.W. Carpenter), 330–338. St. Louis: Saunders.

Newbury, S., Hanley, C.S., and Paul-Murphy, J. (2005). Sugar glider castration and scrotal ablation. *Exotic DVM* 7 (1): 27–30.

Nichols, M., Takacs, N., Ragsdale, J. et al. (2015). Listeria monocytogenes infection in a sugar glider (*Petaurus breviceps*) New Mexico, 2011. *Zoonoses and Public Health* 62 (4): 254–257.

NOAH (2004). Compendium, VetARK ZolcalD Datasheet. http://www.noahcompendium.co.uk/?id=-459124 (accessed 3 September 2017).

Pye, G. (2001). Marsupial, insectivore and chiropteran anesthesia. *The Veterinary Clinics of North America* 4 (1): 211–237.

Reavill, D. (2014). Pathology of the exotic companion mammal gastrointestinal system. *The Veterinary Clinics of North America. Exotic Animal Practice* 17 (2): 145–164.

Reilly, J.S. (ed.) (2001). *Euthanasia of animals used for scientific purposes*. Adelaide: Australian and New Zealand Council for the Care of Animals in Research and Teaching (ANZCCART).

Rivas, A.E., Pye, G.W., and Papendick, R. (2014). Dermal hemangiosarcoma in a sugar glider (*Petaurus breviceps*). *Journal of Exotic Pet Medicine* 23 (4): 384–388.

Sokol, S.A., Agnew, D.W., Lewis, A.D. et al. (2017). Pulmonary hyalinosis in captive sugar gliders (*Petaurus breviceps*). *Journal of Veterinary Diagnostic Investigation* 29 (5): 691–695.

Thomas, M., Parkinson, L., Shaw, G. et al. (2019). Paracloacal cyst in a sugar glider (*Petaurus breviceps*). *Journal of Exotic Pet Medicine* 29: 40–44.

Woods, R. (1999). Prevention of disease in hand-reared marsupials; Wildlife in Australia, Helathcare and Management. In: *Proceedings, Post-graduate Committee in Veterinary Science*, 455–490. Sydney: University of Sydney.

Woodward, D.L., Khakhria, R., and Johnson, W.M. (1997). Human salmonellosis associated with exotic pets. *Journal of Clinical Microbiology* 35 (11): 2786–2790.

10

Budgerigars and Cockatiels
Marie Kubiak

10.1 Introduction

Budgerigars (*Melopsittacus undulatus*) and cockatiels (*Nymphicus hollandicus*) are two small parrot species originating from inland Australia. Since their introduction to the UK in 1840, budgerigars have become the most commonly kept pet bird (Samour 2002). As with cockatiels, with the right care, they can make rewarding and long-lived pets. Although most parrot species are considered endangered, or at risk of becoming endangered, both budgies and cockatiels have stable wild populations and there are no restrictions on trade of captive bred animals (Kalmar et al. 2010). Biological parameters for budgerigars and cockatiels are given in Table 10.1.

10.1.1 Husbandry

The natural scenario for both species in the wild is large communal flocks, and so multianimal social groups in large enclosures are recommended for captive birds to enable normal behaviours to be exhibited. Budgies housed singly in small cages are less active, eat less and show more cautious behaviour than those in flocks (Nicol and Pope 1993). Budgerigars accustomed to other birds will generally accept new birds into their flock (Wyndham 1980b).

Cage size must be sufficient to allow birds to stretch their wings in each direction when perching, and be long enough to allow flight. Space requirements for a pair of budgies are a minimum of 0.5 m × 0.5 m with greater size enclosures (>1 m in length) preferred to allow sustained flight (Hawkins 2001). For birds of cockatiel-size, a minimum length of 2 m is necessary. The majority of commercially available cages are unacceptably undersized for permanent enclosures, and are only suitable for providing a feeding and sleeping base whilst allowing free access to a larger area (Figure 10.1). Large parrot cages can be of suitable dimensions but the bar widths are typically too large to confine birds within the cage. Cages made of wire mesh or horizontal bars allow natural climbing behaviour and good ventilation. Two layers of mesh with a gap in between should be used where cages or aviaries are adjacent, to prevent neighbouring birds injuring each other. Any metals used should be non-toxic, with galvanised or zinc powder coated metals avoided (unless electroplated). Cage flooring should be solid for cockatiels as they demonstrate an unusual running behaviour (Hawkins 2001).

Multiple perches should be placed in the cage at different levels. Uniform dowel-rod type perches should be avoided as birds using these will continuously bear weight on the same area of the foot, maintain a fixed position and be more prone to foot conditions. Perches such as non-toxic natural branches, or artificial equivalents, are preferred as weight-bearing area varies with the irregular surface provided and they provide chewing enrichment opportunities. Retreat areas should be available that allow a visual barrier between the bird and humans or other birds. For breeding animals nest boxes are necessary.

Budgerigars suffer high mortality at climatic extremes and their thermoneutral range is 22–35°C (Wyndham 1981; Buttemer et al. 1986). Indoor cages should not be placed where there are marked temperature fluctuations, and outdoor enclosures should have protection from adverse weather and ideally a protected heat source. Parrots require a defined day/night cycle with budgerigars requiring darkness for nine hours of undisturbed sleep so cages should be positioned in rooms that are not utilised by owners in the late evening (Ayala-Guerrero 1989).

All parrot species are highly intelligent and active and require enrichment and stimulation. Many enrichment options are available, but most are designed to appeal to owners rather than their birds. Climbing, foraging, and chewing enrichment should all be provided to stimulate

Handbook of Exotic Pet Medicine, First Edition. Edited by Marie Kubiak.
© 2021 John Wiley & Sons Ltd. Published 2021 by John Wiley & Sons Ltd.
Companion website: www.wiley.com/go/kubiak/exotic_pet_medicine

Table 10.1 Biological parameters for budgerigars and cockatiels

	Budgerigar	Cockatiel
Adult weight	26–29 g (wild type), 48–50 g (show type)	80–125 g
Lifespan	10–15 years	15–25 years
Sexual maturity	3.5–4 months	12–18 months (can be as early as 6 months)
Internal gestation period	8–10 days	8–12 days
Inter-egg hatching interval	2–3 days	2 days
Incubation period	13–21 days (typically 18–20)	18–21 days
Average clutch size	4–5	4–6
Age at fledging	30–40 days	32–38 days
Respiratory rate (/min)	60–75	40–50
Heart rate (bpm)	240–360	180–240

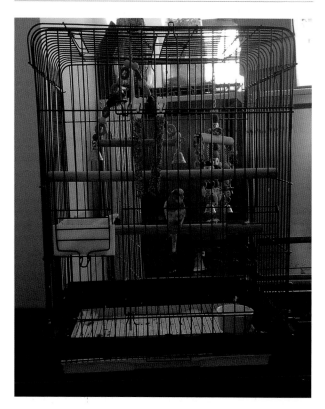

Figure 10.1 Typical cage provided for a pet budgerigar. The size is inadequate to allow sustained flight, additional access to a flight area is necessary.

birds throughout the day. Destruction of materials such as branches or untreated cardboard, providing climbing ropes and ladders, and scattering or hiding food are simple but effective measures alongside regular interaction with companions and a selection of toys or activity items.

Wild budgerigars feed on a variety of seasonally available seeds from grasses and shrubs, which are dehusked before swallowing (Wyndham 1980a). Intake is 8–12 g/d (Earle and Clarke 1991). Cockatiels prefer soft, young seeds over harder mature ones (Jones 1987). Commercial seed mixtures may be suitable for both species, when seeds provided are varied, seed quality and storage conditions are appropriate, and when additional supplementation is provided (Hawkins et al. 2001). When birds are moulting or rearing young, providing high protein seeds such as canary seed and hulled oats will meet the increased requirements (Earle and Clarke 1991; Koutsos et al. 2001a). For cockatiels, small amounts of greens and fresh fruit should also be provided and pelleted diets are a more nutritionally balanced alternative to seeds. Food should be available at all times.

In arid conditions budgies can survive on metabolised water alone but choose to drink when water is available (Koutsos et al. 2001a). In captivity, budgies drink 3–5 ml daily on a standard seed diet, and intake increases markedly in breeding birds. Cockatiels require 2–3 ml/day but will choose to drink an average of 13.6 ml/day when water is available ad lib (Wolf and Kamphues 1997).

10.1.2 Breeding

Budgies have a short breeding cycle and are able to rapidly increase numbers when conditions are favourable. Rainfall is a strong stimulating factor for onset of breeding and there is often a clear breeding season but captive budgies appear not to exhibit the cyclic gonadal development and regression seen in their wild counterparts (Wyndham 1981; del Hoyo et al. 1997). Cockatiels breed year round but long day length does encourage breeding (Myers et al. 1988).

Reproductive status of budgerigars is reinforced when paired birds are in close proximity to other breeding pairs, and cockatiels are reliant on regular interaction with their mate (Ficken et al. 1960; Shields et al. 1989). Both species naturally nest in cavities in trees and adapted branches can be provided, but artificial nest boxes are generally preferred for convenience. Artificial insemination has been successful in budgerigars and cockatiels but has not been used outside a research setting (Hänse et al. 2008; Neumann et al. 2013).

Female budgerigars remain on eggs to incubate them and are fed by the male through incubation and early chick rearing, but as nestlings develop the mother starts to leave the nest to obtain food to maintain the growing chicks (Stamps et al. 1987). Once fledged, juveniles are rarely fed by their parents but often develop supportive relationships with a sibling (Stamps et al. 1990). Male and female cockatiels

Table 10.2   Common symptoms of a sick bird.

Disinterested in surroundings	Partially closed eyes
Sitting on floor of cage	Fluffed up/untidy feathers (Figure 10.2)
Reduced weight or condition	Polyuria
Visible mass or swelling	Change in behaviour
Increased/decreased appetite	Increased/decreased drinking
Loose or abnormal faeces	Reduced activity
Loss or change of voice	Sleeping more
Altered perching (stance/chosen perch)	Altered balance (tail up/down)
Dyspnoea/tail bobbing	Audible breathing
Open beak breathing	Vomiting/regurgitating (Figure 10.3)
Wings extended/dropped	Holding on to cage bars with beak
Lameness/ataxia	Discharge from eyes/nose
Altered interactions with other birds	Spending more time in nest box

share incubation of eggs with the hen sitting on eggs at night, and the cock during the day (Brzezinski 2003).

Hand-rearing is to be discouraged as birds are deprived of the parental interaction that is necessary to develop normal social and sexual behaviours. Budgies reared in isolation exhibit abnormal vocalisation and behaviour, such as establishing pair bonds with inanimate objects (Farabaugh and Dooling 1996). Hand-reared male cockatiels are severely impaired in a breeding situation and hand-reared females tend to lay eggs outside nesting areas (Myers et al. 1988).

10.2   Clinical Evaluation

Prey species will mask any overt evidence of ill health and so on initial presentation these small bird species may appear in good health. However, as they acclimatise to unfamiliar surroundings and time elapses, subtle signs of illness may become evident. For this reason, it is prudent to observe the bird in its carrier initially and take a detailed history before a hands-on clinical examination as the bird's apparent status may change during this time. The common symptoms that may be seen on observation are listed in Table 10.2.

10.2.1   History-Taking

A thorough evaluation of husbandry is essential as in many cases husbandry is a primary factor in disease development. Diet (including any supplements), access outside the cage, access to metal objects, contact with any other bird, change in behaviour or droppings, and reproductive history are all important.

10.2.2   Handling

Before handling any birds, ensure that the room is secure with no hazards such as open windows or running fans.

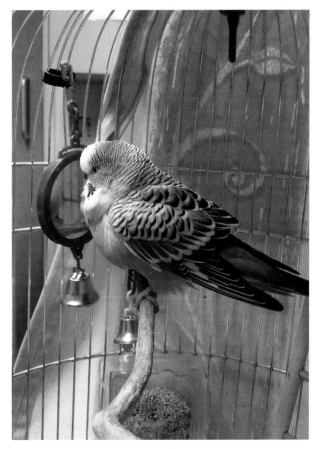

Figure 10.2   Fluffed up appearance to feathers in a budgerigar – a common, non-specific abnormality seen in clinically unwell small birds.

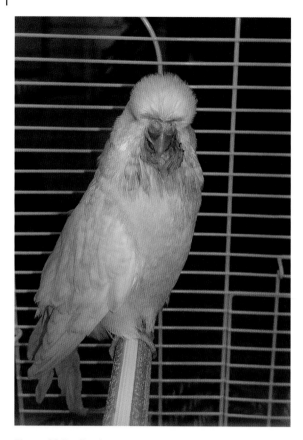

Figure 10.3 Food material around the mouth of a budgerigar consistent with dysphagia, vomition, or regurgitation.

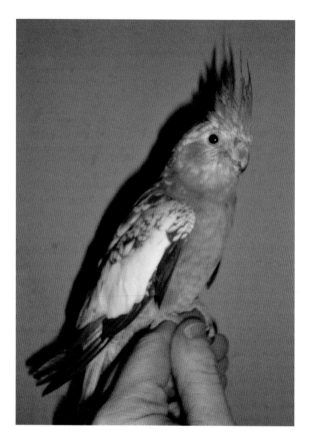

Figure 10.4 Imprinted cockatiel permitting handling with minimal restraint – note the toes being gently restrained by the thumb to prevent movement.

A small proportion of birds will voluntarily perch on an index finger and can then be gently restrained by trapping the toes with the thumb (Figure 10.4). If further restraint is needed the other hand is moved behind the bird to encircle the neck and body gently. In most cases birds are presented free-moving in cages and will require catching. Catching birds is easiest when they are in a small cage with minimal furniture, using a paper or thin cloth towel. Dim lights and approaching a stationary bird from behind, with the towel held open to wrap around the wings, aids in a fast, smooth capture. Once captured, the grip used should be encircling the neck with thumb or index finger and 3rd finger and the back gently cupped with the hand (Figure 10.5). The keel should never be included in restraint as this will severely limit respiratory function. Budgerigars can bite but lack the strength to cause injury, though cockatiels can bite firmly and penetrate soft tissues so a secure head restraint is necessary for handler safety.

10.2.3 Sex Determination

For most budgerigars, the cere (fleshy tissue surrounding the nostrils) allows sex determination. In females this is typically a brown colour with a roughened surface (though in

inactive females it can be white/pale blue), and in males it is bright blue and smooth (Figure 10.6). Juveniles of both sexes have barring of feathers over the head, a dark iris and a pale cere but reach adult colouration at three to six months. Some colour variants, such as albinos, do not follow the same pattern with males demonstrating a pink smooth cere.

Cockatiels from six to nine months can often be visually sexed. Juveniles and adult females have barring or dots on the underside of the tail feathers and a grey face with yellow patches around the eyes and beak. Males have solid colour to the tail feathers, a darker grey body and a predominantly yellow head. Clear differentiation is harder for colour dilute mutations and pieds and DNA sexing on plucked feathers or a blood sample is an option for confirmation of sex.

10.2.4 Clinical Examination

Handling should be limited to the minimum duration to avoid undue stress or hyperthermia. In healthy birds a restraint period of 1–2 minutes is typically tolerated and allows an efficient examination. In sick birds a very limited examination is required which should immediately cease if respiratory distress, unresponsiveness, or

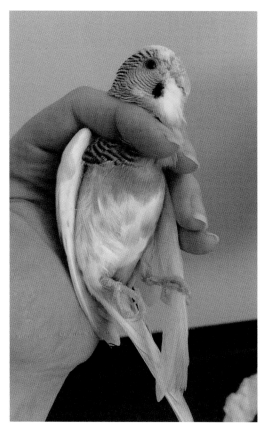

Figure 10.5 Gentle manual restraint of a budgerigar.

excessive agitation develop. In critically unwell birds examination should be deferred until the bird can be stabilised where possible. This typically comprises oxygen administration, warming, access to familiar food, and subsequent brief administration of fluids, glucose, or assist feeding at the time of evaluation.

In birds where examination is tolerated, systematic appraisal is carried out with assessment including in particular the eyes, oral cavity, plumage, body condition, wings, legs, feet, and coelomic palpation.

10.3 Basic Techniques

10.3.1 Medication Administration

Oral medications can be administered on food, syringed directly into the mouth, or by instilling medication into the crop. Crop tube placement is a simple method of administration for most species. If the handler is right handed the bird is restrained in the left hand. The blunt tipped metal tube is passed into the mouth on the bird's left side and advanced over the tongue and across the mouth to the bird's right side to avoid the glottis and slid down the oesophagus into the crop. The end of the tube should be palpated at the base of the neck and the glottis confirmed visibly clear of the tube before administering food.

Figure 10.6 (a) Female budgerigar with brown cere (unfeathered skin around nares). (b) Male budgerigar with blue cere.

(a)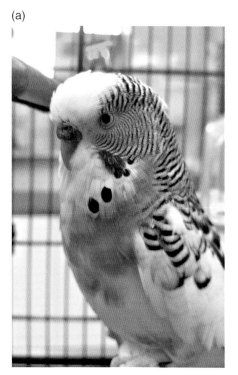

(b)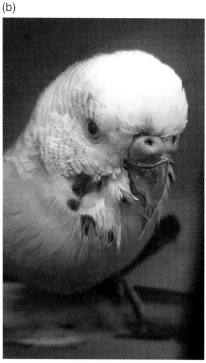

Injectable medications can be given into the pectoral muscles, or subcutaneously into the loose skin in the inguinal region or between the scapulae.

10.3.2 Sample Collection

Blood samples are easiest collected from the right jugular (Figure 10.7), though the smaller left jugular can also be used. An insulin syringe, or 1 ml syringe with 25G needle is used, and the needle is bent at a 30° angle to facilitate successful entry into the vein and avoid passing through the superficial vessel. The jugular vein is located in a featherless tract on the side of the neck and the feathers can be damped with water or surgical spirit to allow better visualisation. The jugular is gently compressed at the level of the thoracic inlet and the bird's neck is rotated until the vein lies directly over the cervical vertebral column. The needle is then inserted from caudal to cranial to collect the sample. After collection, pressure is applied to the venepuncture site for 30 seconds – if the puncture site is not over the vertebrae then reliable compression is difficult to achieve.

The medial metatarsal vein or superficial ulnar vein (Figure 10.8) are also options but are much smaller veins.

The nails can be clipped short to yield small volumes of blood in a conscious or anaesthetised bird, followed by chemical cautery with silver nitrate, potassium permanganate, or similar. These samples are likely to be contaminated with debris from the nail and osteocytes that may affect haematology values. This procedure is also painful and is best avoided.

10.3.3 Nutritional Support

Small birds require frequent feeds to maintain weight and nutritional status. If not feeding and maintaining weight, budgerigars and cockatiels should be assist fed every 3–4 hours. Hand rearing and critical care liquid foods for parrots are commercially available. Rough estimates of volumes per feed are 0.5–3 ml for budgerigars and 1–8 ml for cockatiels (de Matos and Morrisey 2005), but energy requirements can be calculated. Baseline calorific requirements for hospitalised birds are:

$$155 \times BW^{0.73} \text{ (BW = bodyweight in kg) (Koutsos et al. 2001a).}$$

Sick birds will typically require 1.5–2 × baseline requirements for maintenance of weight and metabolic processes.

Small birds should be weighed at least twice daily, ideally at similar times and prior to feeding/fluids. An accurate scale able to record variations of 0.1 g is necessary and feeding frequency and volume should be amended based on weight changes.

Where multiple treatments or assessments are to be carried out, feeding should be the last task in order to minimise handling post-feed and avoid increasing the risk of regurgitation.

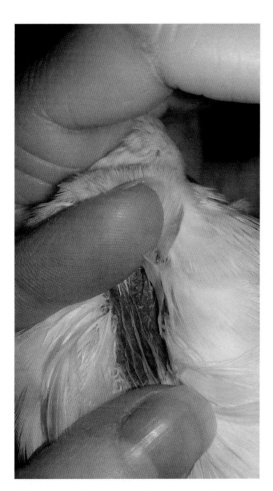

Figure 10.7 The jugular veins are located in apteria (featherless tracts) on the lateral neck and can be visualised through the thin skin.

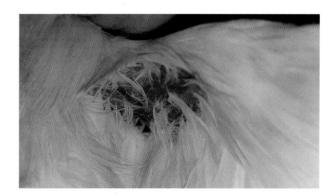

Figure 10.8 The superficial ulnar (or basilar) vein is small but easily identified running over the medial elbow (arrowheads). The more dorsal artery should be avoided.

10.3.4 Fluid Therapy

Intravenous catheters are challenging to place and maintain in small birds, though the right jugular vein can be used. The catheter is placed under anaesthesia and protected by a neck bandage to prevent patient interference, though clinician access is difficult at this site. An intraosseous catheter is more reliable and easier to access. Under anaesthesia and with analgesia, the carpus is flexed and a 25G hypodermic needle placed into the distal ulna using gentle pressure and rotation of the bevel to push through the bone. Once in the medullary cavity there should be no resistance to advancement. Flushing the needle confirms patency and position within the bone. If the needle is obstructed by a bone plug, withdrawal and placement of a fresh needle is necessary (de Matos and Morrisey 2005). The proximal tibiotarsus can also be used for IO catheter placement.

Maintenance requirements are estimated to be 50 ml/kg/day (de Matos and Morrisey 2005), but ongoing losses, fluid deficits, and fluid provided in food should be considered when calculating daily requirements.

10.3.5 Beak Trimming

Beak overgrowth is an indication of a health concern, with the common causes being hepatocutaneous syndrome, chronic malnutrition, hyperoestrogenism, and malocclusion secondary to trauma. Investigation and resolution of the underlying cause should be the primary focus. The beak can be corrected using a rotating sanding device (or a dental burr in an emergency situation).

10.3.6 Anaesthesia

Anaesthesia is generally induced and maintained by administering a volatile agent and oxygen using a face mask for short procedures but injectable protocols have also been described. Tracheal intubation is possible with 1–2 mm endotracheal tubes or modified intravenous cannulae, but will narrow the functional diameter of the upper airways and secretions can obstruct the tube. Intermittent positive pressure ventilation and close monitoring of tube patency is needed to avoid respiratory arrest.

10.3.7 Euthanasia

For small birds, administration of a gaseous anaesthetic followed by intravenous or intraperitoneal injection of pentobarbitone is recommended. Conscious intravenous injection of pentobarbitone can be carried out where birds are sufficiently subdued to permit this but intracoelomic injection should be avoided in conscious animals. Exposure to carbon dioxide is advised against due to aversive effects on birds and unreliable efficacy, and cervical dislocation is only appropriate for individuals competent with this technique and where no alternative method is available.

10.3.8 Hospitalisation Requirements

These birds are typically kept in small cages which can be brought to the clinic. If safe and suitable the bird can be admitted in its own cage for hospitalisation. If small birds are an expected part of the practice caseload it is prudent to have one or more basic hospitalisation cages available. These should be a minimum of $60 \times 60 \times 60$ cm with bars 1 cm apart, and contain perches, food and water supplies and a retreat area with visual barriers. Larger cages and extensive décor complicate efficient capture of birds for treatment and are not necessary for short-term hospitalisation.

Cages should be sited away from predators such as cats and dogs, in a quiet room.

10.4 Common Medical and Surgical Conditions

10.4.1 Collapsed Bird

Many birds present with non-specific signs of collapse, commonly associated with acute decompensation following chronic, masked disease. These cases are often critical with hypothermia, electrolyte abnormalities, hypoglycaemia, and dehydration present as secondary sequelae. They need immediate support for stabilisation before investigating the causative factors.

Provide a warm environment to minimise ongoing energy losses. Small avian species have high metabolic rates, a core temperature of 38–42°C, and anorexic or sick birds are prone to hypothermia. Environmental temperatures of 29–32°C assist in maintaining normothermia and humidity should be maintained at 50–60% to prevent dehydration (de Matos and Morrisey 2005). If birds are observed open beak breathing then temperatures should be reduced. Critical care incubators are ideal but should be secure and made from chew-resistant materials.

For hypovolaemic birds, administer crystalloid fluids at shock rates of 30–60 ml/kg over a 1 hour period (de Matos and Morrisey 2005) followed by ongoing fluid support for losses and maintenance.

Offer palatable food familiar to the bird, or assist feed if the bird is not feeding but alert and able to swallow. This procedure can often be delayed if fluids administered contain glucose.

Provide dim lighting and minimise handling and human presence where possible. Providing perches at the level the bird is at as well as using visual barriers will reduce stress. Avoid placing enclosures at floor level, place them on tables or within higher level cages.

For birds with acute/severe respiratory distress, provide 100% oxygen and assess response over 1–2 minutes. Exposure to 100% oxygen for a prolonged period causes pulmonary congestion and oedema in budgerigars (Jaensch et al. 2001) so periods of less than 3 hours at 100% oxygen, or use of 40–50% oxygen is advisable. Placement of an air sac tube should be considered if signs are consistent with upper respiratory occlusion.

10.4.2 Flock Mortality Investigation

Breeders may seek advice for mass mortality events in their flock. Table 10.3 lists some of the differentials, however several opportunistic infections may be present secondarily and the best course of action is to review bird movements, husbandry, and signalment of the affected birds and submit several fresh cadavers to a pathologist for in depth assessment.

10.4.3 Trauma

Growing feathers have a vascular shaft and trauma may lead to significant haemorrhage. Owners can apply corn starch or tie cotton above the site of damage as a first aid measure to stop bleeding. On presentation, the affected feather can be removed by grasping with haemostats close to the base and applying firm traction along the direction of growth whilst supporting the surrounding soft tissues with the other hand.

Cat bites are true emergencies as not only can the physical trauma be great, but *Pasteurella multocida* is a common inhabitant of cat mouths and can cause rapid septicaemia and death in birds (de Matos and Morrisey 2005). Cleaning of wounds should be done under anaesthesia for all but the most minor injuries. Analgesia and antibiotic therapy should be administered in all cases of cat bites, and fluoroquinolones and sulphonamides are appropriate for *Pasteurella* cover (de Matos and Morrisey 2005).

Fractures are not uncommon as there is little soft tissue cover over the bones of the limbs. Supportive care, treatment of shock, and analgesia should be promptly instituted prior to immobilisation of the fracture site. Tibiotarsal fractures make up the majority of injuries and can be managed with Altman tape splints. The feathers are plucked over the lower leg and the leg is flexed in a perching position with the fracture reduced (Calvo Carrasco 2019). Horizontal overlapping strips of silk or similar adhesive tape are then placed medially and laterally in two or more layers. These layers are manually compressed to conform around the leg and immobilise the fracture. Tissue glue can be applied to increase rigidity if necessary (Calvo Carrasco 2019). The tibiotarsus, stifle and intertarsal joint are all included to provide fracture stability. The tape splint is removed after three weeks when healing is typically complete. Good success is reported with this technique in birds of less than 200 g body weight, with return of limb function in 92% (Wright et al. 2018). Failures were predominantly seen in cases where cat or dog bites were responsible, deep pain response was absent in the foot or the splint was removed before 14 days (Wright et al. 2018). For comminuted fractures, use of K-wires or hypodermic needles as intramedullary pins, combined with an external fixator or tape splint will provide superior fixation.

Renal neoplasia is common in budgerigars and is a major differential for birds presenting with unilateral lameness.

Table 10.3 Differential diagnoses for flock mortality events.

Viral diseases	Avian polyoma virus, paramyxovirus, reovirus, adenovirus, avian bornavirus (PDD), herpesvirus, circovirus (PBFD), avian influenza
Bacterial diseases	*Yersinia pseudotuberculosis, Salmonella* spp., *Mycobacteria (Mycobacteria avium-intracellulare* complex, *M. genavense), Chlamydia psittaci, Campylobacter, Mycoplasma, Pasteurella,* pathogenic *E. coli*
Protozoal diseases	*Toxoplasma gondii, Trichomonas* spp.*, Hexamita, Giardia, Eimeria* spp.*, Cryptosporidia, Leucocytozoon, Encephalitozoon hellem*
Parasitic diseases	Northern fowl mite, red mite, *Sternosoma* tracheal mites, *Capillaria*, Ascarids, Cestodes, trematodes
Fungal diseases	Intestinal candidiasis, systemic candidiasis (rare in adults), *Aspergillosis, Macrorhabdus ornithogaster*
Intoxication	Ingested metal intoxication, chemical/Teflon fume exposure, plant ingestion (e.g. avocado, ivy)
Environmental causes	Hypothermia, predation, starvation (lack of food, inaccessible food – either by position or dominance of other birds), traumatic injury, inappropriate nutrition (iodine deficiency, hyper/hypovitaminosis D), acute/chronic stress

10.4.4 Nutritional Deficiency

Nutritional deficiencies are reportedly common in cockatiels fed on an un-supplemented seed diet (Foreman et al. 2015).

Seeds contain negligible Vitamin A though they do contain small quantities of carotene precursors. It is not uncommon for budgies on an unsupplemented, poorly varied diet to develop deficiency. Budgies require 12 µg daily, and can tolerate up to 750 µg (Baker 1990). Cockatiels require 600 µg Vitamin A per kg of food and anecdotal reports of clinical deficiency are widespread. However, cockatiels fed on a Vitamin A free diet showed only minor evidence of immunosuppression over a two-year period of evaluation suggesting dietary requirements are lower than expected or hepatic storage of vitamin A is sufficient to maintain cockatiels for a prolonged period (Koutsos et al. 2001b). Common symptoms of deficiency include squamous metaplasia of epithelium, keratinisation of mucous membranes, immunosuppression, susceptibility to respiratory infections, salivary gland abscessation, poor quality plumage, and loss of condition (Lowenstine 1986).

Hypervitaminosis A resulting from long-term excessive supplementation can also be a concern and presents with similar clinical signs to deficiency. Cockatiels fed 3000 µg/ kg food, or greater, showed an increase in vocalisations, feather changes, pancreatitis, hyperexcitablity, and altered immune function (Koutsos et al. 2001b).

Intake of diets with greater than 1% calcium, in combination with high Vitamin D3 levels (>2000 IU/kg) have resulted in fatal renal mineralisation in small psittacines (Fudge 2004), but deficiency of calcium is more common. Progressive demineralisation of bone renders birds susceptible to pathological fractures. Seeds, particularly millet, canary seeds and corn, contain insufficient calcium to meet the needs of birds, but providing cuttlefish or oyster shell grit allows self-supplementation. Budgies and cockatiels appear able to tolerate lower calcium diets than other birds, successfully breeding on diets of 0.35 and 0.85% calcium respectively, whereas chickens require 3.3% calcium for the same functions (Earle and Clarke 1991; Roudybush 1996). Vitamin D levels in seeds may be insufficient, impeding calcium uptake in birds irrespective of dietary content and so exposure to natural sunlight or artificial UV-B lighting is advisable to allow endogenous Vitamin D formation.

Iodine deficiency and secondary goitre is well recognised in budgerigars on a seed diet. Thyroidal enlargement results in clinical signs of an audible respiratory click, dyspnoea, and occasionally crop stasis. Hypo-, or hyperthyroidism is not noted. Iodine supplementation, as short-term administration of iodine solution in water or orally, and long-term with provision of cuttlefish, is curative (Merryman and Buckles 1998).

10.4.5 Renal Disease

The avian kidneys are fused to the dorsal body wall, within the synsacrum, and are closely associated with nerves from both the sacral and lumbar plexi (Burgos-Rodríguez 2010). They are divided into cranial, middle, and caudal lobes but function as a single physiological unit. The ureter is fed by multiple ducts draining the renal parenchyma, and the semi-solid urates and liquid urine descend to the urodeum within the cloaca. Within the cloaca the urates may reflux into the terminal intestinal tract and urea, electrolytes, and water are reabsorbed.

A renal portal valve is located in the common iliac vein, which opens under influence of adrenaline to return blood from the hindquarters of the bird directly into the vena cava. This maintains central venous pressure at times of stress. When the bird is under no threat acetylcholine effects are dominant and the renal portal valve remains closed. This directs blood to the renal tubules, enabling maximal uric acid secretion, prior to blood returning to the heart. The presence of the renal portal system means that nephrotoxic drugs should not be administered in the hindquarters of the bird. Renally eliminated drugs hypothetically may not reach expected plasma levels if administered in the hindquarters though this has not been demonstrated convincingly.

Renal disease encompasses a wide variety of pathologies. Malnutrition is a common status in pet birds and can impact renal health. In budgerigars, a dietary calcium content of more than 0.7% results in renal calcification (Schmidt et al. 2003). Vitamin A deficiency results in squamous metaplasia of the lining of ureters and collecting ducts with a reduction in urate movement and increased potential for ureteral obstruction (Speer 1997). Atherosclerosis of glomerular vessels can result from an inappropriate diet and is frequently seen in cockatiels (Garner 2005).

Dehydration can lead to a reduction in urine production and urates may be retained in the tubules. If dehydration and obstruction persist then damage to the renal tissue can result.

Infectious disease can also result in renal disease. In cockatiels, chronic hepatitis (such as that seen with Chlamydiosis) has been associated with lipid accumulation in renal tissue (Schmidt et al. 2003). Adenovirus outbreaks in cockatiels have also been reported to cause renal enlargement, with large intranuclear inclusion bodies evident in tubule epithelial cells on histology (Fiskett and Reavill 2004). In budgerigars, the microsporidian parasite *Encephalitozoon hellem* has been associated with nephritis, and has zoonotic implications (Schmidt et al. 2003).

Renal neoplasia is a common pathology in budgerigars, with one study finding that 63.5% of neoplasms in this species were of renal origin (Neumann and Kummerfeld 1983).

Non-steroidal anti-inflammatory drugs induce renal change, with ketoprofen associated with renal necrosis in 75% of budgerigars treated for seven days. Meloxicam appeared to be better tolerated but minor histological lesions were still seen (Pereira and Werther 2007).

Heavy metal intoxication can be associated with renal compromise, particularly with lead ingestion.

Diagnostic urinalysis is not carried out routinely in birds as excreted urine and urates are modified in the urodeum and hindgut and are contaminated with faeces. Catheterisation of the ureters to obtain an unmodified sample is not practical in small birds. As a consequence blood parameters are used as indirect indicators of renal function. Serum uric acid levels increase when renal tubule function reduces below 30% and increases may be pre-renal, renal, or post-renal in origin (Burgos-Rodríguez 2010). Urea measurement can be used as an assessor of pre-renal compromise as dehydrated birds reabsorb urea for osmoregulation and circulating levels rise. Aspartate transaminase (AST) levels in renal tissue in budgerigars are very high so this enzyme may be useful in indicating severity of a suspected renal insult, however it is not specific (Burgos-Rodríguez 2010). Endoscopic renal biopsy is recommended for obtaining a diagnosis of the cause of renal damage, and the approach is through the left caudal thoracic air sac. Although this technique is relatively straightforward in larger psittacines, in smaller species access and visibility are reduced. In many cases empirical therapy is initiated without a firm diagnosis. Enteral and/or parenteral fluid therapy are the mainstay of support. Weight and urine output should be monitored closely to avoid fluid overload. Where suspicion of infection or intoxication is present, targeted therapy for these factors is also initiated.

10.4.6 Gout

In birds, gout is a consequence of renal compromise rather than the disruption to metabolic pathways that is seen in mammals. Uric acid is the primary nitrogen waste product produced by birds, comprising 60–80% of nitrogen excretion (Tung et al. 2006). The avian kidney tubules secrete uric acid and any factors that compromise renal function or reduce renal perfusion can result in decreased secretion and increased plasma concentrations of uric acid. Common causes are dehydration, Vitamin A deficiency, infectious agents, neoplasia, and a high protein diet. When plasma levels are elevated, acid crystals can precipitate in tissues, most commonly in viscera or around joints.

With articular gout, the feet are commonly affected as the extremities are cooler, reducing the solubility of circulating uric acid. Clinical signs include lameness, altered perching posture, swollen limbs or feet, and difficulty flying or climbing. Diagnosis is by aspiration of swellings under general anaes-thesia, to demonstrate the monosodium urate crystals microscopically (grossly evident as thick white paste), and by demonstration of an elevated serum uric acid level. Treatment involves management of the primary cause of renal compromise, alongside fluid administration for diuresis, analgesia using opioid agents and consideration of use of medications to moderate uric acid levels. Allopurinol blocks synthesis of uric acid from its precursors of xanthine and hypoxanthine, and so helps to lower serum uric acid levels, however it has been associated with nephrotoxicity and induction of gout in red tail hawks (Lumeij et al. 1998). Urate oxidase catalyses conversion of urate into water soluble products to hasten elimination and has shown promise in managing hyperuricaemia (Abuchowski et al. 1981). Currently it is only available from human pharmacies and costs may limit usage. Colchicine inhibits xanthine conversion to reduce uric acid synthesis but has been associated with adverse effects (Abuchowski et al. 1981). Reducing protein content and increasing Vitamin A and fluid content of the diet may be beneficial adjunctive measures.

Visceral gout is less common in small psittacines (Goodman 1996), and has no pathognomonic clinical signs. Birds may appear non-specifically unwell with signs of discomfort, anorexia, lethargy, and fluffed up feathers. Increased radiopacity of viscera, particularly the kidneys, may be seen on radiographs but diagnosis is presumptive in a bird with elevated serum uric acid levels and suggestive clinical presentation. Treatment is as for articular gout.

10.4.7 Trichomoniasis

This protozoal infection is common in budgerigars and occasionally noted in cockatiels. Vomiting, crop distension, halitosis, weight loss and, rarely, dyspnoea may be seen. Thickened white plaques may be noted over the mucosa. Motile trichomonads are evident on light microscopy of scrapes from lesions or samples of crop contents. Treatment is with metronidazole (Phalen 2005).

10.4.8 Spiral Bacteria

Spiral bacteria have been associated with oral and upper respiratory tract infections in cockatiels but remain poorly understood. Some birds appear to carry these bacteria asymptomatically. Clinical infection is more common in birds less than two years of age, displaying colour mutations, or on a poor diet suggesting that these bacteria are opportunistic pathogens (Wade et al. 2003). Clinical signs may include lethargy, anorexia, choanal inflammation, sneezing, nasal discharge, conjunctivitis, and sinusitis (often presenting as periocular swelling) (Evans et al. 2008). Diagnosis is by demonstration of bacteria on cytology. Swabs taken from affected areas stained with Romanowsky or Gram stains show a spirally curved, gram-negative rod of $0.5 \times 8–16\,\mu m$ in size (Evans et al. 2008). Wet preparations show a motile rod that demonstrates motion in a corkscrew movement without flexion. Culture has so far proved unsuccessful though PCR analysis has suggested that the bacterium may be associated with the *Helicobacter* genus (Wade 2005). Treatment is by doxycycline administration, directly or in water and all birds within a group should be treated to avoid persistence of subclinical carriers.

10.4.9 Sinusitis and Upper Respiratory Infection

Upper respiratory infections are common in cockatiels and may involve spiral bacteria, *Chlamydia*, and a variety of opportunistic pathogens. Symptoms often include sneezing, nasal discharge, ocular discharge, and fluctuant swelling around the eye as a consequence of fluid accumulation within the periocular sinus. Treatment involves antibiotic therapy based on cytology and culture and sensitivity, and *Chlamydia* testing is advisable. For chronic cases with intractable sinusitis, surgical debridement and flushing of the sinus is required. In a small number of cases in young cockatiels, infection has been noted to progress to the temporomandibular joint and result in an inability of animals to open their beak, in these cases euthanasia is advisable (Fitzgerald et al. 2001).

10.4.10 Respiratory Tract Obstruction

Fungal granulomas on the syrinx are uncommon in small psittacines but can cause rapid onset of progressive dyspnoea. Fungal respiratory infections with aspergillosis are described in detail in Chapter 11.

Peracute dyspnoea is more commonly associated with inhalation of small seeds, particularly millet. Open beak breathing, extending wings, and evident respiratory distress develop after feeding with a partial obstruction to the trachea. The seed can be visualised with transillumination of the neck using a bright, non-heating, light source (Figure 10.9). General anaesthesia is induced and suction used to clear the obstruction per os.

10.4.11 Mycobacteria

Experimental infections of budgerigars imply a higher susceptibility to *Mycobacteria bovis* than *Mycobacteria avium, Mycobacteria fortuitum, Mycobacteria tuberculosis,* and *Mycobacteria intracellulare* (Ledwoń et al. 2008). Intradermal tuberculin testing was unsuccessful at identifying infected birds in this study. Cockatiels are uncommonly affected by

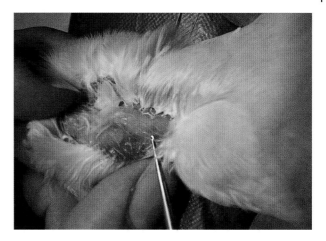

Figure 10.9 Tracheal foreign body in a cockatiel. A millet seed was identified and removed using a 10 ml syringe and cannula for suction.

Mycobacteria, but periocular granulomas appear the most frequent presentation (Fiskett and Reavill 2003).

10.4.12 Knemidokoptes

Knemidokoptes pilae infection is common in budgerigars. A proliferative white, honeycomb pattern develops on non-feathered skin, usually around the beak and occasionally on the legs (Figure 10.10) (Fiskett and Reavill 2004). In chronic infections beak deformities are common. Mites are transmitted readily and infestations may be asymptomatic until secondary factors cause immunosuppression. Diagnosis is confirmed by microscopy of scrapes from affected areas demonstrating mites (Figure 10.11). Treatment is with topical or systemic ivermectin.

10.4.13 Chlamydia/Psittacosis

Chlamydia psittaci is an obligate intracellular bacterium widespread in pet parrots and capable of infecting many bird families and also their human carers. Clinical and subclinical infection is commonly seen in cockatiels and budgerigars (Smith et al. 2010). Dorrestein and Wiegman (1989) demonstrated shedding in 10% of captive budgerigars using an ELISA antigen detection method. Cockatiels are reportedly more likely to be asymptomatic carriers (Phalen 2006)

Infected birds shed elementary bodies (resilient spore-like forms) in feather dust, faeces, and bodily fluids and these can survive for weeks to months in organic material (West 2011). Inhaled or ingested elementary bodies convert to reticulate bodies capable of intracellular replication. A bacteraemia develops and migration to organs, primarily the liver and respiratory system, leads to disseminated infection and clinical signs.

(a)

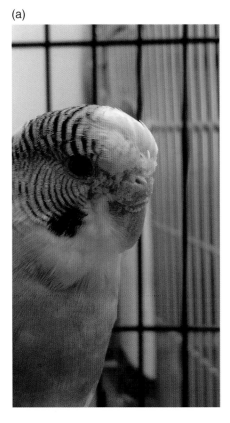

(b)

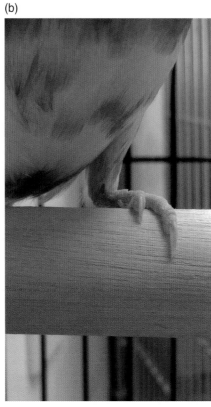

Figure 10.10 (a) *Knemidokoptes* infestation causing hyperkeratosis of the cere and rhinotheca (upper beak). (b) More subtle lesions on the tarsal skin in the same bird.

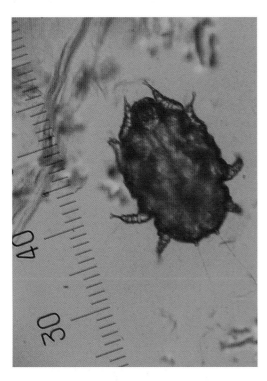

Figure 10.11 *Knemidokoptes* mite identified on microscopy of a superficial scraping from a hyperkeratotic beak.

Not all birds develop clinical disease and asymptomatic carriers can act as a reservoir of infection, or develop disease at a later stage if immune function is suppressed by disease or stressors. Where clinical disease is seen it can include conjunctivitis, nasal discharge, dyspnoea, lethargy, anorexia, diarrhoea, yellow/green urates, or, rarely, neurological symptoms. On imaging (or at post-mortem) hepatomegaly, splenomegaly, and air sacculitis are common findings. A leucocytosis with monocytosis may be present on haematology (Lierz 2005).

Diagnostic methods include PCR for *C. psittaci* and serology. PCR is most commonly performed on faecal matter collected over three to five days. This can result in false negatives especially in asymptomatic carriers due to intermittent shedding, but can be useful to screen for disease within groups/aviaries of birds on pooled samples. Individual birds are better tested on PCR using a swab rolled over the conjunctival, choanal, and cloacal mucous membranes, but serology is preferred for higher sensitivity. A small volume of blood is needed (0.05–0.1 ml) and antibody levels can be determined using in-house kits (Immunocomb; Biogal, Israel) or external laboratory testing. A positive serological result in a bird is considered of potential significance, unless the bird has been recently treated for psittacosis. Culture from organs or swabs, fluorescent antibody testing of cytology preparations or tissue samples are also possible.

Treatment of psittacosis involves supportive care such as assist feeding and oxygen therapy, and appropriate antibiotic therapy to attempt to eliminate the pathogen. Tetracycline antibiotics, most frequently doxycycline, are used for a continuous six week treatment and are effective in the majority of cases. In experimental trials, a 30 days doxycycline course was sufficient for treating budgerigars, and 21 days for cockatiels (Guzman et al. 2010; Smith et al. 2010) but the longer course is generally administered due to the lack of supporting information in natural infections and potential for poorer compliance outside of a controlled laboratory setting. Doxycycline is commercially produced as an oral liquid, a depot weekly injection as 'Vibravenos' in Europe (though availability is limited and importation documentation is required to obtain the product in the UK) and an in-water powder treatment as well as tablet forms. In-water-treatment is not recommended in budgerigars due to difficulties reaching therapeutic concentrations due to the low volumes of water consumed and reduced palatability of water at higher doxycycline concentrations. Coating seed in oil and doxycycline powder was accepted well by budgerigars in one study but may be impractical to replicate reliably in the home environment (Flammer et al. 2003). Doxycycline can be bound and inactivated by calcium salts so supplementation (including mineral blocks and cuttlefish) should be temporarily withdrawn during treatment. All birds sharing an air space should be treated even when asymptomatic. Azithromycin has shown promise as an alternative therapy in cockatiels (Guzman et al. 2010). It is recommended to repeat testing following treatment to confirm absence of bacteria on PCR or a decline in serum antibody levels to support successful treatment.

10.4.14 Megabacteria

'Megabacteria' (*Macrorhabdus ornithogaster*, or avian gastric yeast) are large rod-shaped, gram-positive yeast (Moore et al. 2001). Cockatiels are rarely infected but budgerigars commonly develop gastrointestinal disease. Infection tends to be localised to the mucosal glands of the isthmus – the junction between the proventriculus and ventriculus. Symptoms include weight loss, vomiting, diarrhoea, lethargy, and death, though some infected birds remain asymptomatic. In an endemic situation chick mortality can exceed 50% (Madani et al. 2014).

Macrorhabdus does not grow on conventional fungal media. Diagnosis is made by demonstration of the organism on cytology of faeces, vomit, crop contents, or post-mortem on scrapings or impression smears from the mucoid lining of the isthmus (Flammer 2007). Treatment

is difficult as no method has high success in eliminating the organism long-term. Oral amphotericin B has resulted in cessation of clinical signs and shedding of megabacteria but birds often return to shedding the organisms in future (Moore et al. 2001; Hoppes 2012). In-water Amphotericin B is poorly effective so birds should be individually medicated twice daily by gavage administration, which is impractical in larger flocks (Phalen et al. 2002).

Cider vinegar has been advocated anecdotally but has been shown to have no effect on infections (Lublin 1998). Nystatin was found to be effective in goldfinches but this has not been replicated in any other species (Filippich and Hendrikz 1998). Azoles have limited efficacy – only fluconazole showed promise in treatment but therapeutic levels were shown to be toxic to budgerigars and tolerated doses were inadequate for treatment (Phalen et al. 2002).

Sodium Benzoate has been postulated to be a new treatment for *Macrorhabdus* and reduces morbidity and mortality (Madani et al. 2014). 500–1000 mg/l of drinking water has been advocated but concerns have been raised with toxicity at this level, particularly in parent-fed nestlings or in species that have higher fluid requirements than xerophilic budgerigars (Hoppes 2012; Madani et al. 2014).

Long-term removal of infection from a population can be achieved by removing eggs from infected parents, cleaning the egg surface with a 5% povidone iodine solution and artificially incubating the eggs to give infection-free chicks (Moore et al. 2001). Environmental disinfection is difficult to do so infection free birds should be reared and kept in uncontaminated aviaries.

10.4.15 Candidiasis

Candidiasis occurs in cockatiels with immunosuppression or disruption to normal intestinal bacterial populations (Fiskett and Reavill 2004). Poor food hygiene, co-morbidities, stress, or prolonged antibiotic administration may be primary factors. Presence of budding or mycelial forms of yeast on cytology of faeces or crop contents is indicative. Administration of oral nystatin is typically effective.

10.4.16 Feather Dystrophy

The circovirus responsible for Psittacine beak and feather disease (PBFD) is recognised as a common pathogen in budgerigars. Acute disease is often seen in young parrots, with immunosuppression, feather abnormalities, and high mortality but this presentation appears rare in budgerigars (Fudge 2004). Chronic disease in adults, with progressive dystrophy of feathers at subsequent moults appears more common in this species. A subclinical state has also been noted in budgerigars and other parrots, where virus is shed asymptomatically, contaminating the environment and infecting other birds (Ritchie 1995; Rahaus and Wolff 2003). These birds typically show no clinical signs but may be predisposed to repeated mild secondary infections and can progress to the chronic disease status. Diagnosis is by submission of samples for PCR detection of the virus, and feather and cloacal swab samples are more sensitive for viral detection than blood samples in budgerigars (Hess et al. 2004).

Cockatiels are uncommonly affected by PBFD and an innate resistance to infection has been purported as the cause of unusually low infection rates (Shearer et al. 2008). Low numbers of confirmed infections have been reported (Khalesi et al. 2005; Shearer et al. 2008) and the virus identified by Shearer et al. (2008) appears antigenically distinct from other psittacine circoviruses.

Polyoma virus can cause lack of feather development and high mortality, predominantly in chicks of 10–28 days (Kingston 1992). Neonatal mortality in outbreaks varies from 30 to 100%, with acute death, or following a period of symptoms including anorexia, coelomic distension, subcutaneous haemorrhage, ataxia, and failure of feather development (Fiskett and Reavill 2004). Renomegaly, hepatomegaly, cardiomegaly, hydropericardium, and multifocal haemorrhages may be noted post-mortem and diagnosis can be confirmed by PCR detection of the virus. Survivors may become long-term carriers, shedding virus when stressed (Fiskett and Reavill 2004).

10.4.17 Diabetes Mellitus

Diabetes mellitus has been reported in a cockatiel secondary to herpesvirus related pancreatitis, and in a budgerigar with islet cell carcinoma (Ryan et al. 1982; Phalen et al. 2007). Zinc, mycotoxins, bacterial infection, and paramyxovirus-3 may also be inducing factors (Phalen et al. 2007). Polyuria, polydipsia, polyphagia, and weight loss are common clinical signs (Desmarchelier and Langlois 2008). Hyperglycaemia (reference range in budgerigars: 14–29.3 mmol/l) and elevated fructosamine (preliminary psittacine reference range: 113–238 μmol/l) and low insulin levels (psittacine reference range: 5.8–11.3 μU/ml) may be found on blood analysis (Bonda 1996; Scope et al. 2005; Gancz et al. 2007; Desmarchelier and Langlois 2008). Elevated urine specific gravity (reference range for cockatiels 1.005–1.020) and glucosuria (none present normally) are expected on urinalysis (Phalen et al. 2007). There is little available information on medical management of diabetes mellitus in small psittacines. Attempted therapy in a Nanday conure and a Chestnut fronted macaw with insulin, and use of glipizide in a cockatiel were unsuccessful

(Pilny and Luong 2005; Phalen et al. 2007; Desmarchelier and Langlois 2008).

10.4.18 Neoplasia

Budgies have a high incidence of neoplasia with historic published figures varying between 15.8 and 24.2%, (Blackmore 1966). Lipomas, renal and gonadal tumours have been consistently found to be amongst the most prevalent though a wide range of neoplasms have been reported infrequently.

Lipomas are benign adipose growths that are locally invasive. They are common in budgerigars and seen frequently in cockatiels. They are more common in obese birds and are typically found around the neck and over the sternum (Figure 10.12). They may alter balance when perching, or flight ability. Surgical removal is possible where they are disrupting normal activity, but these growths may be highly vascular and recurrence is common. Liposarcomas have been reported in cockatiels and budgerigars and these tend to be firmer and more vascular. They behave more aggressively and may be present at multiple sites (Reavill 2004).

Xanthomas are soft, yellow subcutaneous masses of cholesterol deposits. They are benign but tend to invade surrounding tissues. They are very common in cockatiels and are seen frequently in female budgerigars (Reavill 2004). Surgical resection is the treatment of choice and complete excision is typically curative, but due to the large size of growths may result in large skin deficits and failure of wound closure. Dietary changes, weight reduction and bandaging affected areas may be used for adjunctive therapy, or palliation where surgery is not an option (Fudge 2004).

Poorly differentiated mesenchymal neoplasms are an uncommon entity in cockatiels (Ellis 2001). Massive, discrete

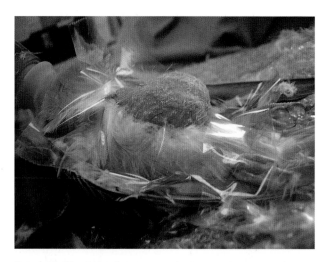

Figure 10.12 Large lipoma over the keel and ventrum of a budgerigar, resulting in inability to fly and pododermatitis due to altered perching.

masses are present in the lungs and cranial coelom arising from mediastinal tissues and invade surrounding tissues, including the vertebrae. Diagnosis is typically made post-mortem and there is suspicion of a viral aetiology (Reavill 2004).

Young to middle-aged budgerigars are commonly affected by renal tumours including nephroblastoma, adenocarcinoma, carcinoma, and adenoma (Neumann and Kummerfeld 1983). These rarely metastasise or affect renal function but the rapidly enlarging mass causes compression of other structures (Fiskett and Reavill 2004). Progression is rapid, over weeks to months and clinical signs tend to be unilateral lameness from nerve compression, or vomiting and weight loss associated with ventral displacement and compression of the ventriculus. Surgical treatment carries high mortality and no medical therapy is available.

Gonadal tumours are also common in budgerigars and cockatiels (Reavill 2004). Testicular neoplasms tend to be unilateral, large masses (Figure 10.13), though may occasionally be bilateral. Seminomas, sertoli cell tumours, and interstitial cell tumours have been reported and present in a similar way to renal neoplasms, though oestrogen secreting masses can cause hyperostosis and cere colour change to brown. Orchidectomy in small birds has high complication and mortality rates (Hadley 2010; Mans and Pilny 2014).

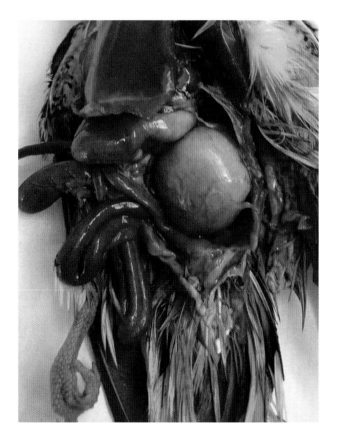

Figure 10.13   Testicular neoplasm in a young male budgerigar with unilateral leg paresis. Source: courtesy of Mikel Sabater.

Deslorelin GnRH agonist implants have been used to palliate Sertoli cell neoplasms in budgerigars and appeared to alleviate symptoms in functionally active neoplasms (Straub and Zenker 2013).

Ovarian neoplasia is common in cockatiels and budgerigars (Reavill and Schmidt 2003; Keller et al. 2013). Clinical signs may be absent, or include coelomic effusion, hind limb paresis, or dystocia (Reavill and Schmidt 2003). Prognosis is guarded as ovariectomy is a challenging procedure as access to the ovarian vessels is hampered by anatomy and the proximity of the cranial renal artery and common iliac vein create further risk of severe haemorrhage (Echols 2002). Partial ovariectomy may be possible for focal lesions (Bowles 2002) and ligation of the common iliac vein to enable ovariectomy has been described (Echols 2002).

Pituitary chromophobe tumours were historically reported to be common in young budgerigars but appear to be rare in current populations. Pituitary adenocarcinomas and adenomas have been described in cockatiels (Wheler 1992). Clinical signs include bilateral ocular proptosis, blindness, feather colouration changes, polydipsia, ataxia, seizures, and death (Schlumberger 1954; Reavill 2004). Diagnosis is by exclusion, or at post-mortem and prognosis is grave.

Budgies and cockatiels appear over-represented with some neoplasms, including haemangiomas, pancreatic adenocarcinomas, dermal and intestinal squamous cell carcinomas, proventricular adenocarcinomas, thyroid neoplasms, ovarian and oviductal carcinomas, and dermal fibrosarcomas (Helmer et al. 2000; Reavill and Schmidt 2003; Reavill 2004; Chen and Bartick 2006). Cockatiels have been reported to be affected by an unusual congenital neoplasm, malignant intraocular teratoid medulloepithelioma, presenting as buphthalmos (Schmidt et al. 1976; Bras et al. 2005). Preen gland carcinomas are reportedly common in older budgerigars and excision may be curative if carried out before local invasion or metastasis occurs (Fudge 2004).

Treatment of neoplasms has included radiotherapy, and systemic or topical chemotherapy including vincristine, chlorambucil, cyclophosphamide, prednisolone, doxorubicin, and L-asparaginase however positive outcomes are rare (Reavill 2004). Leuprolide acetate (a GnRH agonist) has been used to palliate ovarian neoplasia in cockatiels and appeared to improve survival in some cases (Nemetz 2010; Keller et al. 2013).

10.4.19   Intoxications

Teflon (PTFE) is well documented as a fatal toxin in psittacine birds and is reportedly more common in cockatiels, budgerigars, conures, and lovebirds (Fiskett and Reavill

2004). Overheated Teflon releases airborne toxins with inhalation resulting in acute pulmonary oedema and pulmonary haemorrhage. Treatments attempted include antibiotics, diuretics, corticosteroids, antibiotics, oxygen therapy but therapy is invariably unsuccessful.

Lead may be ingested by captive birds free-flying in a home. Some decorative ornaments, stained glass windows, fishing weights, solder, ammunition, and paints contain lead and may be investigated by curious birds. Ingestion results in primarily neurological symptoms including weakness, ataxia, blindness, and seizures, though haematochezia, haematuria, polyuria, and regurgitation may also be seen (Denver et al. 2000). Radiographs identify radiodense metal fragments in many cases, though ingestion of small particles, such as paint flakes, may be more challenging to confidently identify. Blood samples can be collected and submitted to a commercial laboratory for lead assay, to definitively confirm the metal present whilst presumptive treatment begins.

Treatment is chelation therapy and encouraging elimination of remaining fragments within the intestinal tract with minimal further absorption. Chelation involves administration of sodium calcium edetate (EDTA) by intramuscular (or intravenous) injection in most cases, but D-penicillamine or dimercaprol can be used to enhance chelation though these have greater potential for side effects. Meso-2,3-dimercaptosuccinic acid (DMSA) is an alternative chelation agent and can be given orally. DMSA has been used successfully in budgerigars, but in a study in cockatiels it caused regurgitation, death at high doses, and no convincing enhancement of chelation over EDTA, either when used alone or with EDTA (Denver et al. 2000; Lupu and Robins 2009). Surgical removal of fragments is not advisable and endoscopic retrieval is not practical in small birds, so using materials to hasten elimination helps reduce the length of treatment. Provision of grit appears the most effective way of hastening metal elimination from the intestinal tract though administering oily foods also has a minor beneficial effect (Lupu and Robins 2009).

A case of intoxication by the plant Crown vetch has been reported in a budgerigar, with vomiting, tachypnoea, and progressive weakness, tremors, and ataxia (Campbell 2006). Administration of activated charcoal, alongside assist feeding and fluid therapy lead to marked improvement over 24 hours and no long-term effects were seen. Crown vetch is widely used in North America for controlling soil erosion but is an uncommon plant in the UK. Avocado, black locust, clematis, lily-of-the-valley, oleander, philodendron, poinsettia, Virginia creeper, and yew are also reported as plants toxic to budgerigars (Hargis et al. 1989; Bauck and LaBonde 1997; Frazier 2000; Campbell 2006).

10.4.20 Reproductive Pathology

Reproductive problems are common in both cockatiels and budgerigars (Romagnano 2005), and, other than testicular neoplasia, primarily affect female birds.

Dystocia ('egg binding') is an acute onset condition in most cases as the egg passage from ovary to laying is only 48 hours in these species. Causes include hypocalcaemic suppression of oviductal motility, obesity, salpingitis, oversized or irregular egg shape, neoplasia, or weakness secondary to systemic illness (Clayton and Ritzman 2006). Oviductal torsion has also been reported, with cockatiels appearing disproportionately affectted (Harcourt-Brown 1996). Presenting signs of dystocia include unproductive nesting behaviour or straining, a distended coelom, wide-based stance, tachypnoea, and a weak or collapsed status. These birds are often in a critical condition and clinical examination should be brief and in the presence of supplemental oxygen therapy if respiratory changes are evident. An egg may be palpable in the caudal coelom (or occasionally visible in the cloaca), but soft-shelled or cranially located eggs may not be clearly identifiable (Bowles 2002). Stabilisation with analgesia, fluid therapy, oxygen and assist feeding of a simple sugar or critical care solution should be a priority. Once stabilised, anaesthesia and investigation should follow. Radiography and palpation are often sufficient for initial appraisal but ultrasound and cloacal/oviductal endoscopy can add further information. For eggs visible through the vent, perforation using a large gauge hypodermic needle, aspiration of contents and application of gentle pressure to implode the egg allows piecemeal retrieval of egg shell but carries a small risk of cloacal trauma from egg shell fragments. Transcutaneous drainage of eggs is not advisable due to risk of oviductal damage, egg shell retention and egg content leakage. For inaccessible eggs of normal appearance, medical therapy with calcium followed by prostaglandins or oxytocin may allow progression of laying but if a torsion or obstruction is present then an oviductal rupture may result. A surgical approach to these cases, or those where medical therapy is not appropriate, is challenging due to patient size but is often the optimal management. The egg can be removed via a salpingotomy, but salpingectomy is preferred for avoidance of recurrence. Only a left oviduct exists in parrots, hence a left-sided approach is usually taken with the incision parallel and caudal to the last rib with the left leg retracted backwards. The incision to access the coelomic cavity will result in air sac exposure, resulting in anaesthetic gas leakage into the environment and potentially unstable anaesthesia so constant close monitoring and adjustment of anaesthesia depth is required. Within the coelomic cavity the oviduct is identifiable as a plicated tubular structure running cranial to caudal, and presence of an egg allows easy identification. For salpingotomy an incision is made over the egg, all debris removed and an inverting pattern used for closure. Salpingectomy requires blunt dissection of the ventral ligament and careful haemostasis of the more vascular dorsal ligament. This is easiest achieved by ligation of the oviduct at its caudal boundary with the cloaca to allow dissection and greater manipulation, followed by progressive ligation of vessels of the dorsal ligament. Use of bipolar electrocautery forceps or haemoclip application is preferred where available as individual vessel ligation is time-consuming and intricate. The cranial extent of the oviduct has a large artery which requires ligation or clipping, before the oviduct can be removed completely. The ovary is left in place as lack of endocrine stimulation from the oviduct is believed to result in quiescence but there is a potential complication of ectopic ovulation and future coelomitis (Clayton and Ritzman 2006). Concurrent ovariectomy is inadvisable as an elective procedure due to the high mortality associated with this procedure (Echols 2002).

Chronic egg laying is common in both cockatiels and budgerigars. Long day length (including extended exposure to artificial light), increased temperature, presence of a mate, bonding to a human in hand-reared birds, and provision of nesting materials are key stimulating factors and can encourage chronic laying (Hadley 2010). Persistent laying of larger or more frequent clutches results in metabolic drain and predisposition to other reproductive changes such as dystocia or coelomitis. Initial management is by removing stimulating factors, including moderating owner handling and behaviour, and supplementing calcium but many cases continue to lay regardless. Endocrine manipulation using GnRH analogues is a useful tool in controlling egg laying. Leuprolide acetate injections have been used but have now largely been replaced by deslorelin implants. The implant is placed subcutaneously (most commonly between the scapulae), under anaesthesia, and constant high levels of GnRH result in cessation of reproductive cycling. Duration of action varies greatly and may be as short as three months in birds but this is often long enough for management changes to be fully implemented. Some birds may need no further implants, others require repeat management at certain times of the year (Hadley 2010). For refractory cases salpingectomy is indicated.

Egg yolk coelomitis is seen as a fluid distension of the coelomic cavity and may occur with or without observed reproductive behaviour. Aspiration of fluid should be carried out cautiously under anaesthesia with ultrasound guidance, as inadvertent perforation of viscera or incomplete drainage and movement of residual fluid into the air sacs can result in patient death. A clear or turbid yellow fluid is commonly grossly identifiable, and heterophils, macrophages, yolk, and fat globules are often evident on microscopy (Caruso et al. 2002). Most cases involve a sterile response to yolk material but culture of aspirates is prudent as sepsis can result from an undetected infection. Cystic ovarian disease, neoplasia, and oophoritis may be inciting factors and medical suppression of ovarian activity or salpingectomy is advisable to manage these cases long-term.

10.4.21 Viral Infection

Proventricular dilation disease (PDD) is a virally induced auto-immune neuropathy. Infection with avian bornavirus results in immune response against viral proteins that cross react with neurotransmitter proteins causing generalised neurological symptoms or, more commonly, focal changes within the gastrointestinal tract. Birds may be clinically normal, or demonstrate weight loss, passage of undigested food in faeces (Figure 10.14), regurgitation, ataxia, altered proprioception, seizures, or sudden death. Radiographs often demonstrate a dilation of the proventriculus. Cockatiels are susceptible but budgerigars are unusual amongst psittacines by demonstrating an apparent resistance to infection (Gancz et al. 2010).

Diagnosis is by demonstration of virus by PCR on choanal and cloacal swabs, and serology to identify an active immune response. It is important to be aware that presence of virus does not automatically confirm bornavirus as the cause of symptoms as birds can be asymptomatically infected. Radiographs show a dilated proventriculus in around 70% of cases and this is strong evidence of an

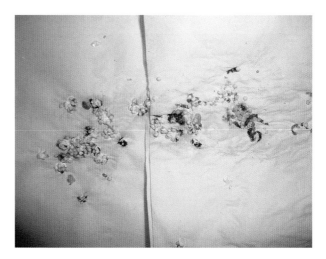

Figure 10.14 Undigested seed in the faeces of a cockatiel – this is a common consequence of bornaviral infection but candidiasis was responsible in this case.

active, relevant infection (Gancz et al. 2010). Biopsy of the intestinal tract, generally the crop as this is accessible and carries a less severe risk of complications with dehiscence, may confirm active neuritis with a lymphoplasmacytic infiltrate of nerves.

Treatment of clinical cases involves feeding of an easily assimilated diet and administration of anti-inflammatory therapy to reduce the immune-mediated inflammation of the nerves. Celecoxib has been advocated as the preferred NSAID due to its COX-2 specific activity for GI symptoms, and amantadine has been used to reduce symptoms and prolong life expectancy where CNS symptoms are present (Gancz et al. 2010). PDD is discussed in more detail in Chapter 11.

Psittacine herpes virus (PsHV-1 or Pacheco's disease) causes severe acute hepatic necrosis and high mortality in clinical cases. Subclinical cases are also possible and birds remain infected for life. Budgerigars and cockatiels are less susceptible to PsHV-1 than African and South American parrot species. Diagnosis is made by PCR detection of virus on oral and cloacal swab samples. Acyclovir can be used, alongside supportive therapy, to treat clinical cases and prognosis is guarded.

10.5 Preventative Health Measures

No preventative measures are carried out routinely though faecal screening for parasites (and *M. ornithogaster*) is prudent to carry out. Annual screening is sufficient for indoor birds but birds with a recent history of parasitism, or in outdoor aviaries, should be screened more frequently. It is advisable to test new birds for *C. psittaci* and for birds moving in to a multibird household screening for other pathogens such as circovirus, polyomavirus, and *Macrorhabdus* is recommended.

10.6 Radiographic Imaging

For survey radiographs a laterolateral and a ventrodorsal view are typical obtained with positioning as demonstrated in Figure 10.15. Clarity is limited in these species due to their small size. With familiarity, or a good reference manual, soft tissue changes such as masses, air sac lesions and increases in organ size may be noted. Splenomegaly is an indication of active, sustained immune response. Hepatomegaly is a common finding and may be nutritional or related to hepatitis, hepatic lipidosis, or neoplasia. Administering barium by crop tube helps delineate the intestinal tract, providing more detail on this and the surrounding viscera.

Radiography is particularly useful in identifying ingested metals and calcified eggs and these are often clinically relevant. Polyostotic hyperostisis is a physiological phenomenon seen in reproductively active female birds. Increased mineralisation of the medullary cavities of the radius, ulna, femur, tibiotarsus, or vertebrae is noted on radiographs (Hadley 2010). It may support suspicion of a reproductive pathology (or functional gonadal neoplasia in male birds) when pronounced, or be an incidental finding in a reproductively active female bird.

Radiographic anatomy in psittacines is detailed further in Chapter 11.

(a)

(b)

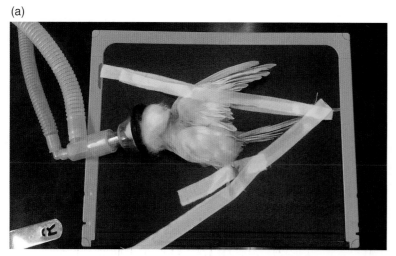
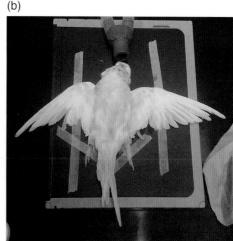

Figure 10.15 (a) Positioning of a budgerigar for a laterolateral radiograph. (b) Positioning of a budgerigar for a ventrodorsal radiograph.

Formulary

Anaesthesia

Isoflurane	3–5% for induction, 1–2% for maintenance		Primary method of anaesthesia, rapid induction, depth of anaesthesia able to be altered and fast recovery
Sevoflurane	5–8% for induction, 3–4% for maintenance		Primary method of anaesthesia, rapid induction, depth of anaesthesia able to be altered and fast recovery
Ketamine and xylazine	20 mg/kg (K) and 10 mg/kg (X) IM		30–40 minutes of anaesthesia (Gandomania et al. 2009)
Midazolam and butorphanol	3 mg/kg of each, intranasal		Sedation (Doss et al. 2018)

Analgesia

Meloxicam	0.1–1 mg/kg IM, SC, PO	q12h	Use lower dose in budgerigars (Pollock et al. 2005; Pereira and Werther 2007)
Butorphanol	1–4 mg/kg IM	q4h	Pollock et al. (2005)

Buprenorphine and hydromorphone: no apparent analgesic effect in cockatiels (Guzman et al. 2018; Houck et al. 2018)

Antimicrobials

Doxycycline	25–50 mg/kg PO	q24h for 45 days	Drug of choice for Chlamydiosis (de Matos and Morrisey 2005)
Doxycycline	25 mg/kg PO	q12h for 3 weeks	For spiral bacteria (Wade 2005)
Doxycycline	400 mg/l in drinking water		Suitable for cockatiels to treat Chlamydiosis or spiral bacteria, does not maintain plasma concentrations in budgerigars (Powers et al. 2000; Flammer et al. 2003; Evans et al. 2008)
Enrofloxacin	15 mg/kg PO, IM	q24h	Good gram-negative cover. May eliminate signs of Chlamydiosis but does not clear infection (de Matos and Morrisey 2005)
Amoxicillin	150–175 mg/kg PO, IM	q8h	(de Matos and Morrisey 2005)
Trimethoprim-sulphamethoxazole	120 mg/kg (combined dose) PO, IM, SC	q12h	(Flammer 2013)
Azithromycin	40 mg/kg PO	q48h for 21 days	Appeared to eliminate Chlamydiosis (Guzman et al. 2010)

Antifungals

Amphotericin B	10–100 mg/kg PO	q12h for 30 days	For *Macrorhabdus* treatment (de Matos and Morrisey 2005)
Nystatin	100 000–300 000 IU/kg PO	q12h for 7–14 days	(de Matos and Morrisey 2005) Used for intestinal candidiasis. Ineffective against *Macrorhabdus*
Sodium benzoate	1 g/l water		For *Macrorhabdus*. Initial dose of 500 mg/l water may avoid reduced intake (Madani et al. 2014)

Antiparasitics

Metronidazole	50 mg/kg/day PO	Can be divided into two doses of 25 mg/kg daily	For Trichomoniasis
Ivermectin	200 μg/kg PO, SC, topically		For *Knemidokoptes* mite infestations or nematodes (de Matos and Morrisey 2005)

Miscellaneous

Sodium calcium edetate (EDTA)	40 mg/kg IM	q12h	Preferred chelation, has been used for up to 21 days with no adverse effects (Denver et al. 2000)
DMSA	25–40 mg/kg PO	q12h	Chelation. Fatal to cockatiels at higher doses of 80 mg/kg (Denver et al. 2000)
Celecoxib	20 mg/kg PO	q24h	For bornaviral infection (PDD) (Gancz et al. 2010)
Amantadine	10–20 mg/kg PO	q24h	For bornaviral infection (PDD) (Gancz et al. 2010)

(Continued)

(Continued)

Calcium gluconate	50 mg/kg IM	q12h	For management of calcium deficiency or uterine inertia
Prostaglandin E2	0.02–0.1 mg/kg topically		For management of dystocia (Hadley 2010)
Oxytocin	5–10 IU/kg IM		For management of dystocia (Hadley 2010)
prostaglandin F2a	0.02–0.1 mg/kg IM		For management of dystocia (Hadley 2010)
Deslorelin implant	4.7 mg SC	q4–5m	For management of reproductive pathology in females (Straub and Zenker 2013)
Leuprolide acetate	1500 to 3500 mg/kg IM	q 2–3wks	For management of reproductive pathology in females (Mans and Pilny 2014)
Allopurinol	10–15 mg/kg PO	q4–12h	Used to treat gout (Rupiper 1993)
Urate oxidase	100–200 IU/kg IM	q24h	Used to treat gout (Poffers et al. 2002)
Colchicine	0.0 to 0.04 mg/kg PO	q12–24h	For gout (Pollock 2006)
Glipizide	1 mg/kg PO	q24h	For treatment of diabetes mellitus in a cockatiel- poor response (Phalen et al. 2007)

References

Abuchowski, A., Karp, D., and Davis, F.F. (1981). Reduction of plasma urate levels in the cockerel with polyethylene glycol-uricase. *The Journal of Pharmacology and Experimental Therapeutics* 219 (2): 352–354.

Ayala-Guerrero, F. (1989). Sleep patterns in the parakeet *Melopsittacus undulatus*. *Physiology & Behavior* 46 (5): 787–791.

Baker, J. (1990). Dangers in vitamin overdose. *Cage Aviary Birds* 31 (March): 5–6.

Bauck, L. and LaBonde, J. (1997). Toxic diseases. In: Avian Medicine and Surgery (eds. R.B. Altman, S.L. Clubb, G.M. Dorrestein, et al.), 612. Philadelphia, PA: WB Saunders Co.

Blackmore, D.K. (1966). The clinical approach to tumours in cage birds—I. *Journal of Small Animal Practice* 7 (3): 217–223.

Bonda, M. (1996). Plasma glucagon, serum insulin, and serum amylase levels in normal and a hyperglycemic macaw. Proceedings of the Annual Conferenve of the Association of Avian Veterinarians, 77, 88.

Bowles, H.L. (2002). Reproductive diseases of pet bird species. *The Veterinary Clinics of North America. Exotic Animal Practice* 5 (3): 489–506.

Bras, I.D., Gemensky-Metzler, A.J., Kusewitt, D.F. et al. (2005). Immunohistochemical characterization of a malignant intraocular teratoid medulloepithelioma in a cockatiel. *Veterinary Ophthalmology* 8 (1): 59–65.

Brzezinski, I.L. (2003). Handraising cockatiels. *AFA Watchbird* 30 (2): 38–41.

Burgos-Rodríguez, A.G. (2010). Avian renal system: clinical implications. *The Veterinary Clinics of North America. Exotic Animal Practice* 13 (3): 393–411.

Buttemer, W.A., Hayworth, A.M., Weathers, W.W. et al. (1986). Time-budget estimates of avian energy expenditure: physiological and meteorological considerations. *Physiological Zoology* 59 (2): 131–149.

Calvo Carrasco, D. (2019). Fracture management in avian species. *Veterinary Clinics: Exotic Animal Practice* 22 (2): 223–238.

Campbell, T.W. (2006). Crown vetch (*Coronilla varia*) poisoning in a budgerigar (*Melopsittacus undulatus*). *Journal of Avian Medicine and Surgery* 20 (2): 97–101.

Caruso, K., Cowell, R., Meinkoth, J. et al. (2002). Abdominal effusion in a bird. *Veterinary Clinical Pathology* 31: 127–128.

Chen, S. and Bartick, T. (2006). Resection and use of a cyclooxygenase-2 inhibitor for treatment of pancreatic adenocarcinoma in a cockatiel. *Journal of the American Veterinary Medical Association* 228 (1): 69–73.

Clayton, L.A. and Ritzman, T.K. (2006). Egg binding in a cockatiel (*Nymphicus hollandicus*). *Veterinary Clinics: Exotic Animal Practice* 9 (3): 511–518.

Denver, M.C., Tell, L.A., Galey, F.D. et al. (2000). Comparison of two heavy metal chelators for treatment of lead toxicosis in cockatiels. *American Journal of Veterinary Research* 61 (8): 935–940.

Desmarchelier, M. and Langlois, I. (2008). Diabetes mellitus in a nanday conure (*Nandayus nenday*). *Journal of Avian Medicine and Surgery* 22 (3): 246–255.

Dorrestein, G.M. and Wiegman, L.J. (1989). Inventory of the shedding of *Chlamydia psittaci* by parakeets in the Utrecht area using ELISA. *Tijdschrift voor Diergeneeskunde* 114: 1227–1236.

Doss, G.A., Fink, D.M., and Mans, C. (2018). Assessment of sedation after intranasal administration of midazolam and midazolam-butorphanol in cockatiels (*Nymphicus hollandicus*). *American Journal of Veterinary Research* 79 (12): 1246–1252.

Earle, K.E. and Clarke, N.R. (1991). The nutrition of the budgerigar (*Melopsittacus undulatus*). *The Journal of Nutrition* 121 (suppl_11): S186–S192.

Echols, M.S. (2002). Surgery of the avian reproductive tract. *Seminars in Avian and Exotic Pet Medicine* 11 (4): 177–195.

Ellis, C. (2001). What is your diagnosis? *Journal of Avian Medicine and Surgery* 15 (1): 60–63.

Evans, E.E., Wade, L.L., and Flammer, K. (2008). Administration of doxycycline in drinking water for treatment of spiral bacterial infection in cockatiels. *Journal of the American Veterinary Medical Association* 232 (3): 389–393.

Farabaugh, S.M. and Dooling, R.J. (1996). Acoustic communication in parrots: laboratory and field studies of budgerigars, Melopsittacus undulatus. In: Ecology and Evolution of Acoustic Communication in Birds (eds. D.E. Kroodsma and E.H. Miller), 97–117. Ithaca, NY; London: Comstock.

Ficken, R.W., van Tienhoven, A.V., Ficken, M.S. et al. (1960). Effect of visual and vocal stimuli on breeding in the budgerigar (*Melopsittacus undulatus*). *Animal Behaviour* 8 (1–2): 104–106.

Filippich, L.J. and Hendrikz, J.K. (1998). Prevalence of megabacteria in budgerigar colonies. *Australian Veterinary Journal* 76 (2): 92–95.

Fiskett, R. and Reavill, D. (2003). Mycobacteria Conjunctivitis in Cockatiels (Nymphicus hollandicus). In: Proceedings of the 7th EAAV Conference, Tenerife: 54–57.

Fiskett, R.A.M. and Reavill, D.R. (2004). Disease conditions and clinical signs of pet birds. In: *Proceedings of Annual Conference,* Association of Avian Veterinarians: 245–263.

Fitzgerald, S.D., Hanika, C., and Reed, W.M. (2001). Lockjaw syndrome in cockatiels associated with sinusitis. *Avian Pathology* 30 (1): 49–53.

Flammer, K. (2007). How I manage fungal diseases in companion birds. In: BSAVA Congress Proceedings, 12–15. Birmingham UK: BSAVA.

Flammer, K. (2013). Antimicrobial drug use in companion birds. In: Antimicrobial Therapy in Veterinary Medicine (eds. P.M. Dowling, S. Giguère and J.F. Prescott), 589. Ames, IA: Wiley-Blackwell.

Flammer, K., Trogdon, M.M., and Papich, M. (2003). Assessment of plasma concentrations of doxycycline in budgerigars fed medicated seed or water. *Journal of the American Veterinary Medical Association* 223 (7): 993–998.

Foreman, A.L., Fallon, J.A., and Moritz, J.S. (2015). Cockatiel transition from a seed-based to a complete diet. *Journal of Avian Medicine and Surgery* 29 (2): 114–119.

Frazier, D.L. (2000). Avian toxicology. In: Manual of Avian Medicine (eds. G.H. Olsen and S.E. Orosz), 228–263. St. Louis, MO: Mosby.

Fudge, A.M. (2004). The budgerigar, an important patient and family member. Proceedings of Annual Conference, Association of Avian Veterinarians: 245–263.

Gancz, A.Y., Wellehan, J.F., Boutette, J. et al. (2007). Diabetes mellitus concurrent with hepatic haemosiderosis in two macaws (*Ara severa, Ara militaris*). *Avian Pathology* 36 (4): 331–336.

Gancz, A.Y., Clubb, S., and Shivaprasad, H.L. (2010). Advanced diagnostic approaches and current management of proventricular dilatation disease. *Veterinary Clinics: Exotic Animal Practice* 13 (3): 471–494.

Gandomania, M.J., Tamadon, A., Mehdizadeh, A. et al. (2009). Comparison of different ketamine-Xylazine combinations for prolonged anaesthesia in budgerigars (*Melopsittacus undulatus*). *VetScan* 4 (1): 21.

Garner, M.M. (2005). Lipid deposition disorders in cockatiels (Nymphicus hollandicus). In: Proceedings of the of Association of Avian Veterinarians 26th Annual Conference, Monterey (CA), 249–252.

Goodman, G.J. (1996). Metabolic disorders. In: Diseases of Cage and Aviary Birds, 3e (eds. W. Rosskopf and R. Woerpel), 477–478. Philadelphia, PA: Williams & Wilkins.

Guzman, D.S.M., Diaz-Figueroa, O., Tully, T. Jr. et al. (2010). Evaluating 21-day doxycycline and azithromycin treatments for experimental Chlamydophila psittaci infection in cockatiels (*Nymphicus hollandicus*). *Journal of Avian Medicine and Surgery* 24 (1): 35–45.

Guzman, D.S.M., Houck, E.L., Knych, H.K.D. et al. (2018). Evaluation of the thermal antinociceptive effects and pharmacokinetics after intramuscular administration of buprenorphine hydrochloride to cockatiels (*Nymphicus hollandicus*). *American Journal of Veterinary Research* 79 (12): 1239–1245.

Hadley, T.L. (2010). Management of common psittacine reproductive disorders in clinical practice. *Veterinary Clinics: Exotic Animal Practice* 13 (3): 429–438.

Hänse, M., Schmidt, V., Schneider, S. et al. (2008). Comparative examination of testicular biopsy samples and influence on semen characteristics in budgerigars (*Melopsittacus undulatus*). *Journal of Avian Medicine and Surgery* 22 (4): 300–309.

Harcourt-Brown, N.H. (1996). Torsion and displacement of the oviduct as a cause of egg-binding in four psittacine birds. *Journal of Avian Medicine and Surgery* 10 (4): 262–267.

Hargis, A.M., Stauber, E., Casteel, S. et al. (1989). Avocado (*Persea americana*) intoxication in caged birds. *Journal of the American Veterinary Medical Association* 194: 64–66.

Hawkins, P. (2001). Laboratory birds: refinements in husbandry and procedures. *Laboratory Animals* 35: S1–S163.

Hawkins, P., Morton, D.B., Cameron, D. et al. (2001). Laboratory birds: refinements in husbandry and procedures. *Laboratory Animals* 35 (Suppl 1): 1–163.

Helmer, P.J., Carpenter, J.W., and Hoskinson, J.J. (2000). What is your diagnosis? *Journal of Avian Medicine and Surgery* 14 (3): 200–203.

Hess, M., Scope, A., and Heincz, U. (2004). Comparitive sensitivity of polymerase chain reaction diagnosis of psittacine beak and feather disease on feather samples, cloacal swabs and blood from budgerigars (Melopsittacus undulates, Shaw 18005). *Avian Pathology* 33 (5): 477–481.

Hoppes, S. (2012). Treatment of *Macrorhabdus ornithogastor* with sodium benzoate in budgerigars (*Melopsittacus undulates*). AAV Proceedings, 67.

Houck, E.L., Guzman, D.S.M., Beaufrère, H. et al. (2018). Evaluation of the thermal antinociceptive effects and pharmacokinetics of hydromorphone hydrochloride after intramuscular administration to cockatiels (*Nymphicus hollandicus*). *American Journal of Veterinary Research* 79 (8): 820–827.

del Hoyo, J., Elliot, A., and Sargatal, J. (1997). Handbook of the Birds of the World, vol. 4. Lynx Editions: Barcelona, Spain.

Jaensch, S.M., Cullen, L., and Raidal, S.R. (2001). The pathology of normobaric oxygen toxicity in budgerigars (*Melopsittacus undulatus*). *Avian Pathology* 30 (2): 135–142.

Jones, D. (1987). Feeding ecology of the cockatiel, *Nymphicus hollandicus*, in a grain-growing area. *Australian Wildlife Research* 14: 105–115.

Kalmar, I.D., Janssens, G.P., and Moons, C.P. (2010). Guidelines and ethical considerations for housing and management of psittacine birds used in research. *ILAR Journal* 51 (4): 409–423.

Keller, K.A., Beaufrere, H., Brandão, J. et al. (2013). Long-term management of ovarian neoplasia in two cockatiels (*Nymphicus hollandicus*). *Journal of Avian Medicine and Surgery* 27 (1): 44–52.

Khalesi, B., Bonne, N., Stewart, M. et al. (2005). A comparison of haemagglutination, haemagglutination inhibition and PCR for the detection of psittacine beak and feather disease virus infection and a comparison of isolates obtained from loriids. *Journal of General Virology* 86 (11): 3039–3046.

Kingston, R.S. (1992). Budgerigar fledgling disease (papovavirus) in pet birds. *Journal of Veterinary Diagnostic Investigation* 4 (4): 455–458.

Koutsos, E.A., Matson, K.D., and Klasing, K.C. (2001a). Nutrition of birds in the order Psittaciformes: a review. *Journal of Avian Medicine and Surgery* 15 (4): 257–275.

Koutsos, E.A., Pham, H.N., Millam, J.R. et al. (2001b). Vocalizations of cockatiels (Nymphicus hollandicus) are affected by dietary vitamin a concentration. Proceedings of the 35th International Congress of the ISAE, Davis, CA, 116.

Ledwoń, A., Szeleszczuk, P., Zwolska, Z. et al. (2008). Experimental infection of budgerigars (*Melopsittacus undulatus*) with five mycobacterium species. *Avian Pathology* 37 (1): 59–64.

Lierz, M. (2005). Systemic infectious disease. In: BSAVA Manual of Psittacine Birds, 2e (eds. N. Harcourt-Brown and J. Chitty), 155–169. Gloucester: BSAVA.

Lowenstine, L.J. (1986). Nutritional disorders of birds. In: Zoo and Wild Animal Medicine (ed. M.E. Fowler), 201–212. Philadelphia, PA: WB Saunders.

Lublin, A. (1998). A five-year survey of megabacteriosis in birds of Israel and a biological control. In: Proceedings of the Annual Conference of the Association of Avian Veterinarians, 241–245. St Paul, MN: Association of Avian Veterinarians.

Lumeij, J.T., Sprang, E.P.M., and Redig, P.T. (1998). Further studies on allopurinol-induced hyperuricaemia and visceral gout in red-tailed hawks (*Buteo jamaicensis*). *Avian Pathology* 27 (4): 390–393.

Lupu, C. and Robins, S. (2009). Comparison of treatment protocols for removing metallic foreign objects from the ventriculus of budgerigars (*Melopsittacus undulatus*). *Journal of Avian Medicine and Surgery* 23 (3): 186–193.

Madani, S.A., Ghorbani, A., and Arabkhazaeli, F. (2014). Successful treatment of macrorhabdosis in budgerigars (*Melopsittacus undulatus*) using sodium benzoate. *Journal of Mycology Research* 1 (1): 21–27.

Mans, C. and Pilny, A. (2014). Use of GnRH-agonists for medical management of reproductive disorders in birds. *Veterinary Clinics: Exotic Animal Practice* 17 (1): 23–33.

de Matos, R. and Morrisey, J.K. (2005). Emergency and critical care of small psittacines and passerines. *Seminars in Avian and Exotic Pet Medicine* 14 (2): 90–105.

Merryman, J.I. and Buckles, E.L. (1998). The avian thyroid gland. Part two: a review of function and pathophysiology. *Journal of Avian Medicine and Surgery* 12: 238–242.

Moore, R.P., Snowden, K.F., and Phalen, D.N. (2001). A method of preventing transmission of so-called "megabacteria" in budgerigars (*Melopsittacus undulatus*). *Journal of Avian Medicine and Surgery* 15 (4): 283–287.

Myers, S.A., Millam, J.R., Roudybush, T.E. et al. (1988). Reproductive success of hand-reared vs. parent-reared cockatiels (*Nymphicus hollandicus*). *The Auk* 105 (3): 536–542.

Nemetz, L. (2010). Leuprolide acetate control of ovarian carcinoma in a cockatiel (Nymphicus hollandicus). In: Proceedings of the Annual Conference of the Association of Avian Veterinarians: 333–338

Neumann, U. and Kummerfeld, N. (1983). Neoplasms in budgerigars (*Melopsittacus undulatus*): clinical, pathological and serological findings with special consideration of kidney tumours. *Avian Pathology* 12: 353–362.

Neumann, D., Kaleta, E.F., and Lierz, M. (2013). Semen collection and artificial insemination in cockatiels (*Nymphicus hollandicus*) – a potential model for Psittacines. *Tierärztliche Praxis. Ausgabe K, Kleintiere/Heimtiere* 41 (02): 101–105.

Nicol, C.J. and Pope, S.J. (1993). A comparison of the behaviour of solitary and group-housed budgerigars. *Animal Welfare* 2 (3): 269–277.

Pereira, M.E. and Werther, K. (2007). Evaluation of the renal effects of flunixin meglumine, ketoprofen and meloxicam in budgerigars (*Melopsittacus undulatus*). *The Veterinary Record* 160 (24): 844.

Phalen, D.N. (2005). Parasitic diseases. Proceedings of the North American Veterinary Conference, 8–12 January 2005, Orlando, FL: 1188–1190.

Phalen, D.N. (2006). Preventive medicine and screening. In: Clinical Avian Medicine (eds. G.J. Harrison and T.L. Lightfoot), 573–585. Florida: Spix Pub.

Phalen, D.N., Tomaszewski, E., and Davis, A. (2002). Investigation into the detection, treatment, and pathogenicty of avian gastric yeast. In: Proceedings of the 23rd Annual Conference of the Association of Avian Veterinarians, 49–51. Monterey, CA: Association of Avian Veterinarians.

Phalen, D.N., Falcon, M., and Tomaszewski, E.K. (2007). Endocrine pancreatic insufficiency secondary to chronic herpesvirus pancreatitis in a cockatiel (*Nymphicus hollandicus*). *Journal of Avian Medicine and Surgery* 21 (2): 140–146.

Pilny, A.A. and Luong, R. (2005). Diabetes mellitus in a chestnut-fronted macaw (*Ara severa*). *Journal of Avian Medicine and Surgery* 19 (4): 297–302.

Poffers, J., Lumeij, J.T., and Redig, P.T. (2002). Investigations into the uricolytic properties of urate oxidase in a granivorous (*Columba livia domestica*) and in a carnivorous (*Buteo jamaicensis*) avian species. *Avian Pathology* 31 (6): 573–579.

Pollock, C. (2006). Diagnosis and treatment of avian renal disease. *The Veterinary Clinics of North America. Exotic Animal Practice* 9 (1): 107–128.

Pollock, C., Carpenter, J.W., and Antinoff, N. (2005). Birds. In: Exotic Animal Formulary, 3e (ed. J.W. Carpenter), 135–264. Philadelphia: Elsevier Saunders.

Powers, L.V., Flammer, K., and Papich, M. (2000). Preliminary investigation of doxycycline plasma concentrations in cockatiels (*Nymphicus hollandicus*) after administration by injection or in water or feed. *Journal of Avian Medicine and Surgery* 14 (1): 23–31.

Rahaus, M. and Wolff, M.H. (2003). Psittacine beak and feather disease: a first survey of the distribution of beak and feather virus inside the population of captive psittacine birds in Germany. *Journal of Veterinary Medicine. B, Infectious Diseases and Veterinary Public Health* 50: 368–371.

Reavill, D.R. (2004). Tumors of pet birds. *Veterinary Clinics: Exotic Animal Practice* 7 (3): 537–560.

Reavill, D. and Schmidt, R. (2003). Tumors of the psittacine ovary and oviduct: 37 cases. In Proceedings of the Annual Conference of the Associaion of Avian Veterinarians: 67–69

Ritchie, B.W. (1995). Psittacine beak and feather disease. In: Avian Viruses (ed. B.W. Ritchie), 223–252. Lake Worth, FL: Wingers Publishing.

Romagnano, A. (2005). Reproduction and paediatrics. In: BSAVA Manual of Psittacine Birds, 2e (eds. N.H. Harcourt-Brown, J. Chitty and BSAVA), 222–233. Gloucester: BSAVA.

Roudybush, T. (1996). Nutrition. In: Diseases of Cage and Aviary Birds (eds. W. Rosskopf and R. Woerpel), 218–234. Baltimore, MD: Williams & Wilkins.

Rupiper, D.J. (1993). Allopurinol in simple syrup for gout. *Journal of the Association of Avian Veterinarians* 7 (4): 219–220.

Ryan, C.P., Walder, E.J., and Howard, E.B. (1982). Diabetes mellitus and islet cell carcinoma in a parakeet. *Journal of the American Animal Hospital Association* 18 (1): 139–142.

Samour, J.H. (2002). The reproductive biology of the budgerigar (*Melopsittacus undulatus*): semen preservation techniques and artificial insemination procedures. *Journal of Avian Medicine and Surgery* 16 (1): 39–49.

Schlumberger, H.G. (1954). Neoplasia in the parakeet: I. Spontaneous chromophobe pituitary tumors. *Cancer Research* 14 (3): 237–245.

Schmidt, R.E., Becker, L.L., and McElroy, J.M. (1976). Malignant teratoid medulloepithelioma in two cockatiels. *Journal of the American Veterinary Medical Association* 189: 1105–1106.

Schmidt, R.E., Reavill, D.R., and Phalen, D.N. (2003). Urinary system. In: Pathology of Pet and Aviary Birds (eds. R. Schmidt, D.R. Reavill and D.N. Phalen), 95–107. Ames, IA: Lowa State Press.

Scope, A., Schwendenwein, I., and Frommlet, F. (2005). Influence of outlying values and variations between sampling days on reference ranges for clinical chemistry in budgerigars (*Melopsittacus undulatus*). *Veterinary Record* 156 (10): 310–314.

Shearer, P.L., Bonne, N., Clark, P. et al. (2008). Beak and feather disease virus infection in cockatiels (*Nymphicus hollandicus*). *Avian Pathology* 37 (1): 75–81.

Shields, K.M., Yamamoto, J.T., and Millam, J.R. (1989). Reproductive behavior and LH levels of cockatiels (*Nymphicus hollandicus*) associated with photostimulation, nest-box presentation, and degree of mate access. *Hormones and Behavior* 23 (1): 68–82.

Smith, K.A., Campbell, C.T., Murphy, J. et al. (2010). Compendium of measures to control *Chlamydophila psittaci* infection among humans (psittacosis) and pet birds (avian chlamydiosis). http://nasphv.org/documents CompendiaPsittacosis.html (accessed 10 June 2018).

Speer, B.L. (1997). Diseases of the urogenital system. In: Avian Medicine and Surgery (eds. R.B. Altman, S.L. Clubb, G.M. Dorrestein, et al.), 625–644. Philadelphia: WB Saunders.

Stamps, J., Clark, A., Kus, B. et al. (1987). The effects of parent and offspring gender on food allocation in budgerigars. *Behaviour* 101 (1): 177–199.

Stamps, J., Kus, B., and Clark, A. (1990). Social relationships of fledgling budgerigars, Melopsitticus undulatus. *Animal Behaviour* 40 (4): 688–700.

Straub, J. and Zenker, I. (2013). First experience in hormonal treatment of sertoli cell tumors in budgerigars (*M. undulates*) with absorbable extended release GnRH chips (Suprelorin) First International Conference on Avian, Herpetological and Exotic Mammal Medicine.Wiesbaden, 20–26 April: 299–301.

Tung, J., Mullin, M., and Heatley, J.J. (2006). What is your diagnosis. *Journal of Avian Medicine and Surgery* 20 (1): 39–43.

Wade, L. (2005). Identification of spiral bacteria (*Helicobacter* sp.) in cockatiels. In: Proceedings of the Annual Conference of the Mid-Atlantic State Association of Avian Veterinarians: 229–238.

Wade, L., Simpson, K., McDonough, P. et al. (2003). Identification of oral spiral bacteria in cockatiels (Nymphicus hollandicus). In: Proceedings of the Annual Conference of the Association of Avian Veterinarians: 23–25.

West, A. (2011). A brief review of *Chlamydophila psittaci* in birds and humans. *Journal of Exotic Pet Medicine* 20: 18–20.

Wheler, C. (1992). Pituitary tumors in cockatiels. *Journal of the Association of Avian Veterinarians* 6 (2): 92–92.

Wolf, P. and Kamphues, J. (1997). Water intake of pet birds—basic data and influencing factors. First International Symposium on Pet Bird Nutrition: 74.

Wright, L., Mans, C., Olsen, G. et al. (2018). Retrospective evaluation of Tibiotarsal fractures treated with tape splints in birds: 86 cases (2006–2015). *Journal of Avian Medicine and Surgery* 32 (3): 205–210.

Wyndham, E. (1980a). Environment and food of the budgerigar *Melopsittacus undulatus*. *Austral Ecology* 5 (1): 47–61.

Wyndham, E. (1980b). Diurnal cycle, behaviour and social organization of the budgerigar Melopsittacus undulatus. *Emu* 86: 25–33.

Wyndham, E. (1981). Breeding and mortality of budgerigars *Melopsittacus undulatus*. *Emu-Austral Ornithology* 81 (4): 240–243.

11

Grey Parrots
Marie Kubiak

11.1   Introduction

Grey parrots include the Congo grey parrot (*Psittacus erithacus*) (Figure 11.1) and the less commonly kept Timneh grey parrot (*Psittacus timneh*) (Figure 11.2). These have historically been considered subspecies of *P. erithacus* but in 2012 were proposed to be distinct species though this change is not universally accepted (Taylor 2012). *P. erithacus* inhabits Central and Western Africa whereas *P. timneh* originates from Western Africa. Capture of these birds for the pet trade has had a devastating effect on wild populations and these birds are now included on CITES Appendix I, effectively prohibiting trade in wild caught animals. Captive bred animals (or those legally obtained before CITES changes came into action) can still be legally traded, or used for commercial display, in the UK with an Article 10 certificate obtained from DEFRA (APHA 2017). Biological parameters for these birds are given in Table 11.1.

11.1.1   Husbandry

Grey parrots form flocks of up to 10 000 birds, inhabiting lowland African forests, nesting at height in tree cavities (Parr and Juniper 2010). Juveniles remain as part of the flock and grow up supported and able to learn their complex behavioural repertoire and survival skills from adults around them. In captivity they are commonly kept as single pet animals in a cage within a household environment and behavioural problems are frequently reported.

Under laboratory conditions, a 6 m long pen is recommended for a pair of grey parrots, with less than 3 m being considered unacceptable (Hawkins et al. 2001). Similar standards should be provided by pet bird owners and traditional parrot cages should be regarded only as a sleeping area, with birds allowed access to a larger room (under supervision if necessary) or self-contained aviary on a daily basis to exhibit their range of natural behaviours, including flight (Figure 11.3). Cages should be made of a non-toxic metal and positioned away from doors and walls, allowing good visualisation of the room and encouraging interaction with humans in the house. A range of temperatures (16–25 °C) are tolerated by indoor birds. Birds housed in outdoor aviaries require protection from adverse weather conditions, with a fully enclosed indoor section and supplemental heating for temperate climes. Full spectrum lighting is recommended for grey parrots as hypocalcaemia due to Vitamin D deficiency is commonly seen in these species and can be prevented with as little as 4 hours exposure daily to ultraviolet-B lighting of wavelength 315–285 nm (Stanford 2005). Lamps should be secure with no access to bulb or wiring and of a flicker frequency undetectable to birds.

Free-living grey parrots feed on a wide variety of nuts, fruits, and seeds with small quantities of leaves, invertebrates, and flowers also taken (Parr and Juniper 2010). Timneh greys have been shown to select a nutritionally incomplete, high-fat diet given free choice (Ullrey et al. 1991). Offering a complete pelleted diet or variety of sprouted pulses, alongside fresh fruit and vegetables will meet the majority of nutritional needs for grey parrots and reduce detrimental effects of selective feeding. Commercially available seeds (especially sunflower seeds) are best avoided, other than as occasional rewards due to their poor nutritional content. It is still common for pet grey parrots to be fed on a predominantly seed-based diet with associated chronic nutritional deficiencies and malnutrition is a common factor in many disease processes and reproductive failures (Ullrey et al. 1991). Changing the diet abruptly is rarely successful. In the wild, inexperienced juveniles learn from adult flock members which foods are safe, but in captivity pet birds rarely have this social learning. Birds are therefore often reluctant to accept a perceived risk with unrecognised foods. Seeing humans eating the new food (or simulating this), being hand fed by an owner or having the new item mixed in with other established foods may reduce

Handbook of Exotic Pet Medicine, First Edition. Edited by Marie Kubiak.
© 2021 John Wiley & Sons Ltd. Published 2021 by John Wiley & Sons Ltd.
Companion website: www.wiley.com/go/kubiak/exotic_pet_medicine

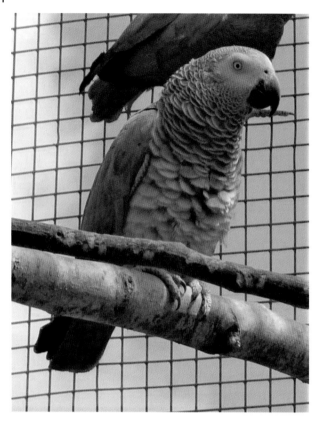

Figure 11.1 Congo grey parrot with black beak and red tail (*Source:* photo courtesy of Drayton Manor Park Zoo).

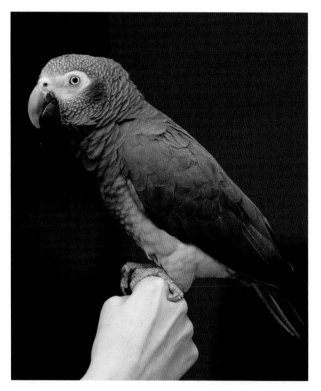

Figure 11.2 Timneh grey parrot, note the pale beak and maroon tail (*Source:* photo courtesy of Marcus Hurst).

Table 11.1 Biological parameters.

	Congo grey	Timneh grey
Body length	28–39 cm	22–28 cm
Weight	410–500 g	250–350
Plumage	Medium grey with red tail	Dark grey with burgundy tail
Beak colouration	Solid black	Pale centre to upper beak
Conservation status	Endangered	Vulnerable
Sexual maturity	3–5 years	3–5 years
Clutch size	2–5 eggs	3–5 eggs
Incubation period	21–30 days	28–30 days
Fledging age	12 weeks	12 weeks
Longevity	40–60 years	30–50 years
Heart rate	340–600	340–600
Respiratory rate	25–45/min	25–45/min

the apprehension and aid diet change. Additionally only providing the old food for 5–10 minute periods three times daily and having the new diet available at all times may help. Dietary change is best delayed in sick birds as a temporary reduction in intake at transition can be detrimental.

Enrichment is a crucial part of keeping a highly intelligent and active species and should be provided on a daily basis. Interaction with other birds and free flight have been found to be the most valued opportunities for grey parrots (van Zeeland et al. 2013a). Conversely, destructible items (such as branches and paper toys), indestructible toys, and auditory stimuli were not valued. This supports the strong need for social interaction ideally with other birds (though human contact may be sufficient in imprinted birds), together with exercise, access to a flight, and foraging opportunities. Providing toys within a cage and background noise from a radio or television is not sufficient stimulation for a single parrot, although this has historically been recommended. Foraging enrichment and flight can be combined easily by concealing valued food items in multiple, unpredictable locations around a bird-safe area and letting the bird investigate and find them. Once this activity is established, birds will continue to forage even when no food is stashed, reducing the time available for developing or demonstrating abnormal behaviours. Feeding times can also be increased for caged birds by increasing complexity of food access with puzzle toys, hanging food holders, scattered food, or wrapping or combining food with safe non-edible items. Flight ability should not be removed from captive birds (e.g. by wing clipping/confinement) as it is highly detrimental to their mental well-being and physical fitness.

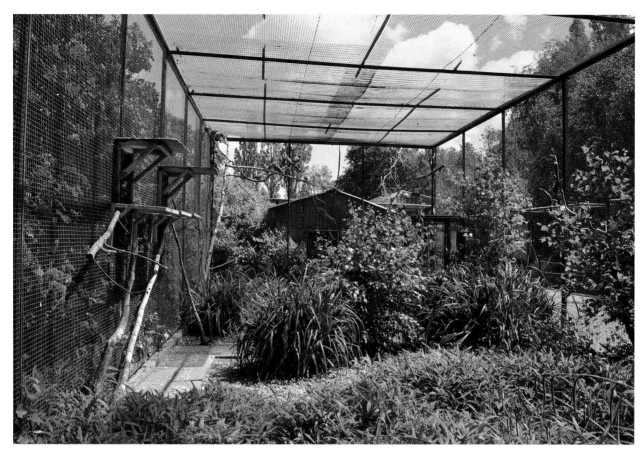

Figure 11.3 A large naturalistic enclosure for a flock of birds allows demonstration of the full repertoire of behaviours (*Source:* photo courtesy of Drayton Manor Park Zoo).

11.1.2 Breeding

Pairs form at sexual maturity and are monogamous. Nests in the wild are made in tree cavities, 10–30 m above the ground. Eggs are laid at 2–5 day intervals whilst the male guards the nest site and feeds the hen. Chicks are altricial and are fed and cared for by both parents for the first 12 weeks of their lives. Once fledged, chicks move away from the nest site, but remain as part of the family social group within the flock.

In captivity, birds tend to be paired in aviaries for breeding and use nest boxes in lieu of tree cavities. Failure to breed is common and may be due to pair incompatibility, lack of learned behavioural repertoire, pathology of the reproductive tract, or inappropriate conditions to support breeding. Chicks are typically hand-reared by owners to imprint them onto humans and provide birds to the pet trade that are tolerant of human contact. These birds then identify themselves as humans in the absence of parental contact and are more affectionate and docile for the first few years of their life. Hand-rearing may involve artificial incubation of eggs, tube/spoon feeding, and no contact with adult birds, or allowing parents to feed and rear

offspring for a reduced period prior to removal and then assist feeding chicks through to weaning. Grey parrots that are hand-reared have more problems bonding with other birds and less successful breeding, and are more likely to show sexual behaviours towards humans (Sistermann 2000). They also demonstrate poorer overall health, increased aggression, and develop attention-seeking behaviours or stereotypies more frequently than parent-reared birds (Schmid et al. 2006). Allowing parent-rearing is better for the mental well-being of both parents and offspring and regular human contact and handling of chicks can still result in a bird that is tolerant of human contact yet capable of behaving normally and interacting with other birds (Schmid et al. 2006).

11.2 Clinical Evaluation

Prey species will mask any overt evidence of ill health and so on initial presentation parrots may appear in good health. However, as they relax, subtle signs of illness may become evident. It is useful to observe the bird in its cage initially and take a detailed history from the owner before carrying out a clinical examination. During this time the bird's apparent status may change and the symptoms shown will influence the focus of questions or examination. See Table 10.2 in Chapter 10 for common abnormalities on evaluation.

11.2.1 History-Taking

A thorough evaluation of husbandry is essential as in many cases husbandry is a primary factor in disease development. Rearing method, previous health screens, diet (including any supplements, and actual intake of food offered), access to UV-B lighting or natural sunlight, time outside the cage, contact with any other bird, changes in behaviour or droppings, and reproductive history are all important.

11.2.2 Handling

Before handling any birds, ensure that the room is secure with no hazards such as open windows or fans running. Young imprinted birds may tolerate a complete examination under gentle restraint (Figure 11.4), but the majority of birds will resent this. It is easiest to catch birds in a small cage, under dim light conditions and by wrapping a towel around the back of the bird to restrain the neck as a priority (Figure 11.5). The ideal grip is to hold the neck securely between thumb and index finger with the towel wrapped gently around the body to minimise movement and prevent damage to wings and feathers. The keel should never be immobilised as this will limit respiratory function. These birds can give a firm bite so a secure head restraint is necessary for handler safety. Having an assistant restrain the bird allows for a two handed examination.

11.2.3 Sex Determination

These species are sexually monomorphic and sex determination is possible by reproductive history or DNA sexing on blood or plucked feather samples. Moulted feathers lack sufficient remaining genetic material for DNA sex determination. Laparoscopic examination of gonads has been used historically for sex determination but is an invasive procedure and is no longer recommended.

11.2.4 Clinical Examination

Handling should be limited to the minimum duration to avoid undue stress to the patient. Systematic appraisal is carried out with assessment including in particular the choanal papillae (mucosal spines lining the slit in the roof of the oral cavity), plumage, body condition, alignment and

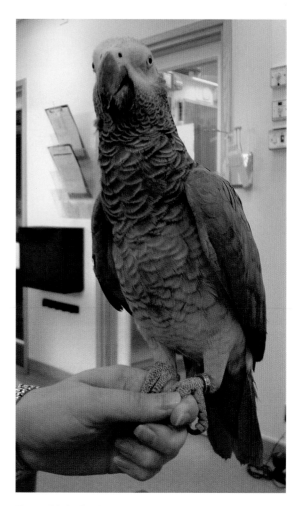

Figure 11.4 Docile birds will tolerate cursory examination under light restraint. Here the toes are being gently held to maintain the bird on the hand.

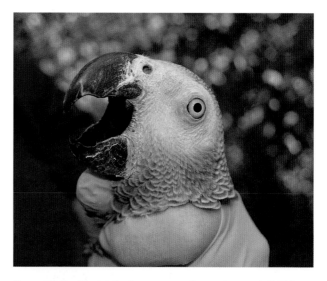

Figure 11.5 The beak of a grey parrot can give a painful bite so restraint of the neck is a priority (*Source:* photo courtesy of Drayton Manor Park Zoo).

symmetry of long bones, and coelomic palpation. In critically unwell birds examination should be deferred until the bird can be stabilised where possible.

11.3 Basic Techniques

11.3.1 Medication Administration

Oral medications can be administered on food, syringed directly into the mouth, or by instilling medication into the crop using a gavage or crop tube. For a right-handed administrator, the blunt tipped metal tube is passed into the mouth on the bird's left side, advanced over the tongue and across the mouth to the bird's right side to avoid the glottis and slid down the oesophagus into the crop. The end of the tube should be palpated at the base of the neck and the glottis confirmed visibly clear of the tube before administering medication or food.

Injectable medications can be given intramuscularly into the pectoral muscles, or subcutaneously into the loose skin in the inguinal region or between the scapulae.

11.3.2 Sample Collection

Blood sampling is easiest achieved under anaesthesia as the restraint required is resented and accidental venous lacerations can be catastrophic. Blood samples are commonly collected from the superficial ulnar vein, the right jugular or the smaller left jugular. A 1 ml syringe with 25G needle is used, and the needle can be bent at a 30° angle to facilitate venous access. The superficial ulnar vein is identified on the inner aspect of the elbow following extension of the wing (Figure 11.6). The scant feathers overlying it can be damped or plucked, and a sample collected with gentle negative pressure to avoid collapsing the vein. Afterwards, firm pressure using a finger or a cotton bud is necessary for 60 seconds as large haematomas may form, especially in hypocalcaemic birds. The right jugular vein is located in a featherless tract on the side of the neck and the feathers can be lightly damped with water or surgical spirit to allow better visualisation. The jugular is gently compressed with a thumb at the level of the thoracic inlet and the bird's neck is rotated until the vein overlies the vertebral column. The needle is inserted from caudal to cranial and the sample collected. Digital pressure is applied afterwards to the venepuncture site for 30 seconds – if the puncture site is not over the vertebrae then reliable compression is difficult to achieve. The site should be closely examined afterwards as significant haematomas can develop in the loose skin and blood loss can be significant.

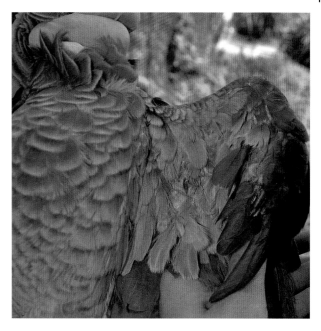

Figure 11.6 The superficial ulnar (or basilar) vein is identified within a sparsely feathered area of skin on the medial elbow.

The nails can be clipped short to yield small volumes of blood in a conscious or anaesthetised bird, followed by chemical cautery. These samples are likely to be contaminated with urates, debris from the nail and osteocytes that may affect results obtained. This procedure is also painful and is best avoided.

11.3.3 Nutritional Support

If not feeding and maintaining weight, grey parrots should be assist fed every 4–6 hours. Hand rearing and critical care liquid foods for parrots are commercially available. 10–15 ml/ kg body weight can be given in a single administration but individual energy requirements can be calculated. Baseline calorific requirements for hospitalised birds are:

$$155 \times BW^{0.73} \, (BW = \text{bodyweight in kg}) \, (\text{Koutsos et al. 2001}).$$

Sick birds will typically require 1.5–2× baseline requirements for maintenance of weight and metabolic processes. Birds should be weighed twice daily, ideally at similar times and prior to feeding/fluids and feeding frequency and volumes adjusted to weight alterations.

11.3.4 Fluid Therapy

Intravenous catheters are challenging to place and maintain in birds due to interference, although superficial ulnar vein placement may be tolerated as it is underneath the wing when it is in a normal flexed position. Under anaesthesia a 24/26G intravenous cannula is placed in the superficial ulnar vein (or, less commonly, the right jugular) and a lightweight bung secured in the hub. A tab of adhesive tape can be closed around the bung and hub, and the corners of this tab sutured to the skin or anchored around feather shafts.

For collapsed birds where venous access is not possible, an intraosseous catheter can be placed. Under anaesthesia and with analgesia, the carpus is flexed and a 23–25G hypodermic needle placed into the distal ulna using gentle pressure and rotation of the bevel to push through the bone. Once in the medullary cavity there should be no resistance to advancement. Flushing the needle confirms patency and position within the bone. If the needle is obstructed by a bone plug, withdrawal and placement of a fresh needle is necessary (de Matos and Morrisey 2005). The proximal tibiotarsus can also be used for intraosseous catheter placement.

Maintenance requirements are estimated to be 50 ml/kg/day (de Matos and Morrisey 2005), but ongoing losses, fluid deficits, and fluid provided in food should be considered when calculating daily requirements. Bolus administration of up to 10 ml/kg of warmed fluids repeatedly through the day is preferred over continuous infusion as drip lines restrict movement and are poorly tolerated. Normal saline or lactated Ringers solution are generally appropriate and may be supplemented by vitamin and amino acid solutions.

11.3.5 Anaesthesia

Fasting for one to two hours prior to anaesthesia is preferred to ensure there is no food in the crop which can result in regurgitation and aspiration. Premedication is rarely used in birds though it is useful to reduce stress and duration of induction (Kubiak et al. 2016). Butorphanol and midazolam can be administered by intramuscular injection, or intranasally to provide sedation and relaxation (Lennox 2011).

High concentration of isoflurane or sevoflurane via facemask results in anaesthesia in 30–60 seconds. Once unresponsive then birds can be intubated and maintained on a lower percentage of volatile agent. The tongue is gently extended forward to visualise the glottis and a 2–3 mm soft, uncuffed tube is placed and secured with a bandage tie placed around the tube, crossed under the lower beak and tied at the back of the neck.

Reflex monitoring is particularly useful in birds. The corneal reflex is elicited by touching the surface of the eye with a lubricated cotton bud, causing the third eyelid to move across the globe. This movement should be slow; if fast then the patient is at a light plane of anaesthesia, if absent then they are too deep or the reflex dulled by repeated use (the other eye should then be checked for comparison). Toe pinch responses are seen at lighter planes of anaesthesia.

Capnography is very useful in birds as hypoventilation is common with inhalant anaesthesia and progressive hypercapnoea can develop despite apparently normal respiratory movements (Figure 11.7). Measuring end tidal CO_2 ($ETCO_2$) using capnography has been shown to be effective at approximating arterial CO_2 levels in Congo grey parrots, although readings consistently overestimated arterial CO_2 by 5 mmHg (Edling 2006). When recorded $ETCO_2$ exceeds 60 mmHg then assisted ventilation is likely to be necessary, with the aim to maintain CO_2 levels at 35–45 mmHg (Hernandez-Divers 2007). Patient ventilation is best in lateral recumbency as keel and rib movements are least compromised in this position. Cardiac auscultation using traditional stethoscopes is simple

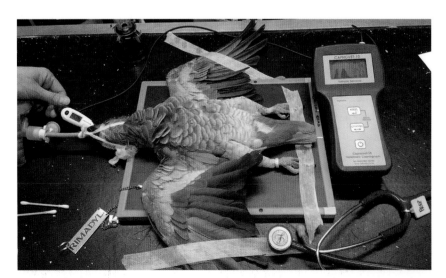

Figure 11.7 Anaesthetised Congo grey parrot positioned for radiography. Note the oesophageal thermometer, sidestream capnography and cotton buds for corneal reflex assessment.

with the bell placed over the keel or the back. Temperature monitoring is important as birds can lose (or gain) heat rapidly. Cloacal probes may not accurately reflect core temperature and oesophageal temperature measurements are preferred (Nevarez 2005). Pulse oximetry can be carried out on the leading edge of the wing to track changes in haemoglobin saturation trends, but absolute values and heart rates obtained are often inaccurate (Schmidt et al. 1998). Blood pressure can be monitored using the indirect method with the cuff placed between feathers on the mid humerus and inflated. A Doppler probe is placed over the ulnar artery and the cuff deflated until blood flow can be detected. Cuff position can affect the readings so the pressure should not be taken as an absolute figure, but blood pressure monitored repeatedly with the cuff remaining in the same position to detect changes in the individual patient (Zehnder et al. 2009).

On recovery, volatile agents are turned off and patients remain intubated on 100% oxygen until breathing well by themselves and conscious head movements are made. Extubation occurs when the patient no longer tolerates the tube in place. Birds should then be held in an upright posture to minimise risks of regurgitation until they are able to stand (Figure 11.8).

A pre-warmed recovery area should be available and critical care incubators work well for this, but must be secure and have an appropriate perch for the species. Once able to perch and climb steadily patients can be returned to their hospital cage and checked regularly to ensure they are stable and need no further intervention.

11.3.6 Euthanasia

Administration of a gaseous anaesthetic followed by intravenous injection of pentobarbitone is recommended (Leary et al. 2013). Conscious intravenous injection of pentobarbitone can be carried out where birds are collapsed, and intraperitoneal injection is an alternative only in anaesthetised birds. Physical methods of euthanasia are not appropriate.

11.3.7 Hospitalisation Requirements

Birds can be admitted in their own cage for hospitalisation if it is safe, allows uncomplicated capture for treatments, and there is sufficient space to place this within an appropriate ward. If birds are accepted as patients then it is sensible to have one or more basic short-term hospitalisation cages available (Figure 11.9). These should be a minimum of 90 cm × 60 cm × 60 cm with bars less than 2 cm apart,

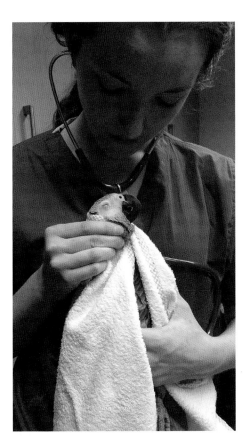

Figure 11.8 Monitoring of the recovering patient, maintained in an upright position with ongoing auscultation.

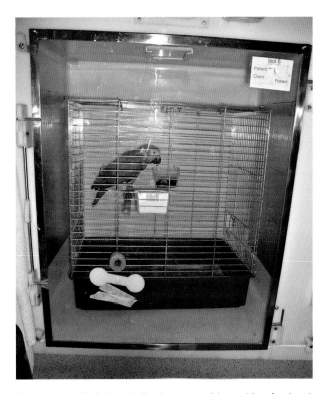

Figure 11.9 Basic hospitalisation cage with perching, food and water. Note the transparent secondary door with access point for oxygen supply or nebuliser inflow.

with perches, accessible food and water supplies and a ideally a retreat area with visual barriers. Where possible cages should be elevated as birds may feel vulnerable at floor level. Larger cages, or collapsible aviary structures, are necessary for birds hospitalised for longer periods.

Cages should be sited away from predators such as cats and dogs, in a quiet room.

11.4 Common Medical and Surgical Conditions

See Chapter 10 for the approach to dealing with a collapsed bird.

11.4.1 Non-infectious Conditions

11.4.1.1 Hypocalcaemia

Dietary deficiency of calcium or vitamin D3 (as seen with seed diets), absence of ultraviolet light, or excessive dietary phosphorus can result in hypocalcaemia and nutritional secondary hyperparathyroidism (NSHP) (de Matos 2008). With reduced serum calcium, parathyroid hormone secretion increases to raise serum calcium levels. Mineral is resorbed from bone with replacement by fibrous connective tissue and calcium and phosphorus are released into the circulation (de Matos 2008). Chronic lack of available calcium results in progressive depletion of bone mineral to maintain circulating levels. Grey parrots appear heavily predisposed to clinical hypocalcaemia and suggested causative factors include disruption to osteoclast function, inherited defects in vitamin D receptors, inappropriate diet, or greater reliance on ultraviolet lighting (Stanford 2005; de Matos 2008). Clinical signs include laying abnormal eggs, dystocia, infertility, pathological fractures, skeletal deformities, poor feather condition, weakness, tremors, ataxia, and seizures. Incidence is high, with 44% of Congo grey parrots presented for other concerns found to have skeletal deformities on radiography (Harcourt-Brown 2003).

Clinical history of seed diet and lack of ultraviolet light, alongside clinical signs are highly suggestive of NSHP. Radiographs may identify deformities, poor mineralisation, and pathological fractures as prognostic indicators. Serum calcium levels may be normal as parathyroid hormone maintains circulating levels until bone stores are depleted. Total calcium levels are of limited diagnostic value as a large proportion of total calcium is albumin-bound and physiologically inactive. Ionised calcium is more sensitive and can be used to support diagnosis and to monitor response to therapy. The reference cage for grey parrots has been demonstrated to be 0.96–1.22 mmol/l (Stanford 2003a). Alkaline phosphatase and phosphorus

are commonly elevated. Vitamin D (as 25-hydroxycholecalciferol) in hypocalcaemic grey parrots has been reported as 7.74–12.88 nmol/l, compared to birds with appropriate diet and UV-B lighting with levels of 104–137 nmol/l (Stanford 2003b, 2005).

Treatment of seizuring birds, involves Vitamin D and parenteral calcium administration concurrently (Hochleithner et al. 1997). Hypocalcaemic seizures typically respond rapidly to calcium administration. Refractory seizures may indicate a separate neuropathy such as clinical bornaviral or paramyxoviral infection, ischaemic compromise, intoxication, neoplasia, traumatic injury, or congenital hydrocephalus (Shivaprasad 1993; Beaufrère et al. 2011).

Chronic NSHP cases require short-term supplementation, long-term dietary changes, provision of ultraviolet light, and management of any secondary consequences such as dystocia. Birds with severe bone deformities that will result in permanent compromise to welfare or mobility require euthanasia.

Use of a compete pelleted diet has been shown to significantly increase ionised calcium and Vitamin D in grey parrots (Stanford 2007) and is recommended for maintenance of this species.

Renal secondary hyperparathyroidism has not been reported in birds (de Matos 2008).

11.4.1.2 Hypovitaminosis A

Seeds contain negligible Vitamin A and an unsupplemented seed diet will result in deficiency. Common symptoms include squamous metaplasia of epithelial surfaces (including the respiratory tract, oral cavity, and gastrointestinal tract) with associated increased susceptibility to infections, mucosal abscessation, keratin rhinolith formation (Figure 11.10), poor quality plumage, and loss of condition (Lowenstine 1986). Diagnosis is based upon clinical signs and nutritional evaluation. Treatment is by managing secondary complications and improving the diet. At least 50% formulated diet is needed to avoid deficiency in Vitamin A in pet parrots (Hess et al. 2002).

11.4.1.3 Cardiac Disease/Atherosclerosis

Congestive heart failure incidence has been reported as 9.7% in parrots, and one case series reported a predilection for cardiomyopathy in juvenile grey parrots (Oglesbee and Oglesbee 1998; Juan-Sallés et al. 2011). Cor pulmonale secondary to fungal pneumonia has been reported in two parrots, and overall right-sided failure predominates (Oglesbee and Oglesbee 1998). Cardiac cases typically present in congestive heart failure as subtle earlier signs are masked by patient instinct, lack of any specific symptoms, and a sedentary lifestyle.

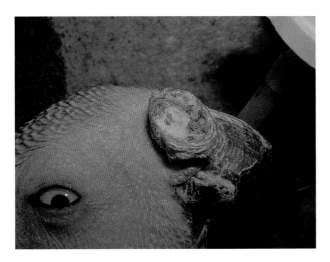

Figure 11.10 Rhinolith formation in the nare of a Congo grey. This is commonly associated with Vitamin A deficiency but localised infection, including aspergillosis may be involved.

Clinical signs include non-specific signs such as regurgitation, weakness, poor growth in juveniles, and intestinal hypomotility, as well as more recognisable changes such as coelomic distension and hyperpnoea (Juan-Sallés et al. 2011). On clinical examination, rales, ascites, or cyanosis of the periorbital skin may be evident. Arrhythmias may not be detectable on auscultation due to the rapid heart rate. Clinical investigation follows that for domestic species with radiography, echocardiography, and electrocardiogram (ECG) used to evaluate cardiac morphology and function. Echocardiography uses a midline window caudal to the sternum with the probe angled cranially, using the liver as a stand-off, avoiding the laterally placed air-filled lungs and air sacs. The resulting longitudinal view precludes M-mode assessment and instead B-mode evaluation is used exclusively. A 7.5 MHz (or higher frequency) probe with a small coupling area is needed (Pees and Krautwald-Junghanns 2005). For ECG a paper speed of at least 100 mm/s is needed to accommodate the high heart rate, but otherwise interpretation is similar to more familiar species (Nap et al. 1992). Asymptomatic arrhythmias, or those induced by anaesthesia, may be incidental findings and need to be interpreted cautiously in clinically well birds (de Wit and Schoemaker 2005). Occasional sinoatrial arrest may be a normal finding in birds, but sinoatrial arrest associated with syncope and third degree AV block has been reported in grey parrots (Lumeij and Ritchie 1994). Therapy for arrhythmia, cardiomyopathy, or congestive heart failure mimics that of domestic animals and specific dosing regimens for birds are poorly established or validated. Treatment typically comprises medication to improve cardiac function, drainage of fluid, management of underlying causes, and supportive measures. Diuresis is used where volume overload or effusion is present, but as the majority of avian nephrons lack a loop of Henle, furosemide is less effective than in mammals (Lierz 2003).

Atherosclerosis is common in grey parrots but reported incidence varies from 12.6 to 92.4%, with around a quarter of cases classified as severe (Kempeneers 1987; Bavelaar and Beynen 2003a). Cholesterol deposits progressively accumulate in arterial walls narrowing the lumen, increasing resistance to blood flow, reducing vessel elasticity, and creating turbulence. Thrombus formation appears a rare consequence (Bohorquez and Stout 1972). Severity and incidence of lesions increases with age and the brachiocephalic trunks and ascending aorta are most commonly affected. Atherosclerosis may be asymptomatic if mild to moderate, but as it progresses it can result in neuropathy, lethargy, secondary cardiac disease or sudden death. Sudden death is reported as the most common consequence in diagnosed cases, but many cases are diagnosed as an incidental finding or co-morbidity complicating interpretation of significance (Dorrestein et al. 1977; Bavelaar and Beynen 2004a). Failure to dissect vessels at post-mortem examination results in atherosclerosis being frequently overlooked (Dorrestein et al. 2006). Radiography may demonstrate increased opacity or even mineralisation of vessels, particularly the aorta, and concurrent cardiac enlargement (Mans and Brown 2007). Echocardiography can be used but images of high enough quality to appraise vessel walls are difficult to achieve. Indirect assessment by detection of chamber dilation may support diagnosis. Left ventricular dilation, secondary to increased aortic rigidity is typical, but right atrial and ventricular dilation have been reported in a grey parrot with pulmonary arterial atherosclerosis (Sedacca et al. 2009). Biochemistry may support clinical suspicion where high cholesterol levels are present. In other avian species plasma cholesterol levels correlate with severity of atherosclerosis (Bavelaar and Beynen 2004b). Captive grey parrots have higher circulating cholesterol levels than most other psittacine species (8.4 +/− 2.6 mmol/l) which may reflect poor diet in captivity, or a physiologically higher cholesterol level, either of which may contribute to the atherosclerosis predisposition seen in this species (Bavelaar and Beynen 2004a). Induction of hypercholesterolaemia in grey parrots fed a high fat diet would support dietary origin (Bavelaar and Beynen 2003b), but inactivity and social stress are hypothesised to increase incidence and are both common in captive birds (Ratcliffe and Cronin 1958). Presence of *Chlamydia psittaci* antigen within lesions in affected birds supports the potential role of Chlamydial infection as a risk factor for atherosclerosis development (Pilny et al. 2012). Alpha-linolenic acid levels are lower in birds with atherosclerosis but a protective effect of this fatty acid has not been convincingly demonstrated (Bavelaar and Beynen 2003a).

In poultry beta blockers have shown a protective effect but do not aid clearance of existing lesions whereas calcium channel blockers nifedipine and verapamil resulted in a decrease in severity and extent of atherosclerotic lesions (García-Pérez et al. 2005). Statins are reported as useful in avian patients to lower cholesterol but studies to determine appropriate dosing are lacking. Rosuvastatin, a long-acting human statin, has been trialled in Amazon parrots, but the oral preparation failed to reach therapeutic concentrations in the majority of subjects, even at greater than 40 times the human dose (Beaufrère et al. 2015). Isoxuprine, a peripheral vasodilator, has been used in an Amazon parrot to resolve clinical signs associated with atherosclerosis (Simone-Freilicher 2007). Avoiding high fat foods, such as sunflower seeds, is advisable for prevention or management of atherosclerosis.

11.4.1.4 Feather Damaging Behaviour (FDB/'Plucking')

FDB is a very common problem in pet grey parrots with 39.4% of those presenting to UK clinics affected (Jayson et al. 2014). Although a common presenting complaint, FDB is a frustrating syndrome associated with a vast range of causative factors that can involve significant clinical investigation, time, and management to attempt to control and may never resolve.

Affected parrots present with varying intensity of self-trauma, from mild over-preening to complete feather removal with self-inflicted soft tissue injuries (Figure 11.11). The duration of changes may be as short as a few days or over many years.

The first step in assessing a case involves taking a detailed history with particular evaluation of rearing details (i.e. hand-reared, wild-caught, or parent reared bird), source of bird, diet, housing, relationship and interactions with humans and other animals in the household, daily routine (including time alone and sleep patterns) and the owner's response to FBD when observed. The physical examination proceeds as normal, but also includes location of feather loss, whether feather shafts are removed or broken, appearance and quality of remaining feathers, assessment of skin over body and feet and evaluation of beak and nails.

Table 11.2 shows the more common factors associated with clinical FDB and it is important to be aware that more than one factor can be present in a bird so a thorough diagnostic assessment is advisable at the outset. The author uses whole body radiographs (ventrodorsal and laterolateral views) and collection of a blood sample (for haematology, biochemistry, and *C. psittaci* serology) under general anaesthesia as a broad health screen to assess for presence of pathological factors. Further tests for additional specific pathogens or diseases are indicated based on findings of history, clinical examination and the initial health screen, but will vary between cases.

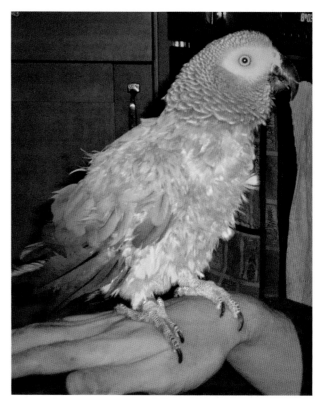

Figure 11.11 Moderate feather destructive behaviour, with shortening and removal of feathers over the ventrum and overpreening damage to wing and tail feathers.

If a medical cause is identified then specific therapy can be instigated, but it is important to make owners aware that even after resolution of a health problem established stereotypies can remain.

Managing behavioural causes is often more complex as a clear cause is rarely established.

Stressors may be identified on husbandry review, or by observing patterns associated with initiation of FDB episodes. These may include lack of sleep, perceived predation risk (from household pets or visible wildlife), or failure of expected social responses from human companions. Imprinted birds perceive themselves as human, resulting in inability to communicate and interact effectively with either humans or other birds and significant stress as a consequence. 'Breeder frustration', typically a consequence of imprinted birds showing unreciprocated courtship behaviours to human handlers, is commonly blamed for FDB, but this is poorly supported by scientific evidence (Jayson et al. 2014). Unfortunately the psychological changes inflicted by hand-rearing are irreversible.

Exercise, a predictable routine, regular bird or human contact and extensive enrichment are key factors in reducing stress and maintaining stimulation and reducing time for 'filler' behaviours. In captivity, birds have ready access

Table 11.2 Presenting signs, diagnostic approach and treatment of feather destructive behaviour presentations.

	Appearance	Diagnosis	Treatment
Psittacine beak and feather disease (PBFD/circovirus)	Loss of down feathers on flanks, contour, wing and tail feathers moult through as dystrophic or discoloured feathers. Beak appears dull and may be brittle.	PCR on feather pulp	None available.
Alloopreening	Companion preens bird exuberantly, typically over the head and neck.	Position of feather loss, presence of companion, observation of behaviour.	Separation from companion possible but likely to cause significant stress to both birds. Offer alternative activities in the form of enrichment.
Stereotypical behaviour	Typically seen in hand-reared pet birds with removal of contour feathers typically over ventrum and legs. Can develop secondary to any other trigger for FDB.	Elimination of other causes, thorough history evaluation and behavioural review	See text – environmental changes main focus.
Malnutrition	Feathers are fragile, discoloured and easily broken, often with horizontal 'stress bars'. Damaged feathers may be removed by the bird.	Assess diet, examine feathers and skin.	Implement gradual change onto balanced nutrition.
Exposure to strong scents	Overpreening and feather removal over all areas in response to adsorption of smells into feathers. Distinct smell often noted (e.g. smoke, air freshener, cooking fumes).	Examination, review of husbandry	Stop exposure to strong smells or airborne irritants.
Internal discomfort	FDB focused over the area of discomfort	Other changes associated with painful focus, e.g. swelling, lameness. Radiography, ultrasound to identify pathology, e.g. atherosclerosis, osteoarthritis, hepatitis, air sacculitis	Manage primary condition, analgesia
Dermatitis	Inflamed appearance to skin, open exudative lesions. Commonly in axillary region.	Cytology and culture of lesions.	Management of primary condition. Temporary placement of restraint collar to prevent self-trauma may need to be considered in severe or chronic cases. Neoplasia may present as ulcerative skin disease.
Neuropathy	Overpreening may be focal or generalised as a response to neuropathic pain, or a lack of negative feedback from normal preening.	Radiography and bloodwork to identify common causes (heavy metal intoxication, Chlamydiosis, proventricular dilation syndrome, sciatic nerve compression with renal or reproductive disease or spinal lesions)	Treatment of primary cause or targeted analgesia.
Presence of damaged feathers	Damaged feathers may be present on examination, or may have been removed by the bird	Known trauma commonly precedes the self-removal of damaged feathers. Common causes are flight injuries causing broken feathers, or wing clipping resulting in sharp ends to wing feathers impinging on skin when the wing is closed.	Imping (transplanting an old moulted feather into the shaft of the damaged feather) is recommended for functional replacement of wing and tail feathers. Removal of, or cutting short, damaged feathers may be of less value.
Ectoparasites	Very rarely seen in companion parrots. Hyperkeratosis of skin with dermal mites, opacity and fragility of feather quills with quill mites, lice or feather mites evident on feathers (particularly on the inside of the wing) may be seen.	Lice or eggs visible on feather shafts, mites evident on microscopy of feather pulp or skin scrapes.	Ivermectin injections or spray

to food, rarely have chick rearing responsibilities and have less social contact. Long periods of the day therefore have no necessary activity to occupy birds and lower priority behaviours, such as preening, increase to fill this time and may escalate to abnormal behaviour patterns seen in FDB. Enrichment (see husbandry section) helps to fill these time periods and provides mental stimulation, not only reducing FDB but also appears to prevent the development of FDB in parrots (Meehan et al. 2003; Lumeij and Hommers 2008).

Introducing another bird can help in some cases, however an imprinted parrot will lack species identity and behaviours and may not integrate with other birds. Optimising the husbandry is often the most important management of behavioural cases, but is poorly appreciated by owners so the value must be made clear and follow up discussions used to assess progress and maintain owner motivation.

Additional measures include physical restraint using collars and pharmacological intervention.

Normal preening triggers physiological endogenous endorphin release and temporary calmative effects, often elicited on exposure to stressors. Chronic stress however can result in excessive preening, reliance on induced endorphin release, and a suggested induction and self-perpetuation of FDB as a coping mechanism (Van Ree et al. 2000). Bird collars are used to prevent abnormal preening and break this cycle, but they also restrict normal behaviours. As such, collars should only be considered where there is significant self-trauma. Physical restraint should never be used as a long-term solution as it will not have any effect on the primary stressors. Less restrictive options such as blunting the beak tip or applying an acrylic beak tip prosthesis may be short-term alternatives in birds demonstrating self-mutilation.

Pharmacological suppression of behaviours is rarely used due to lack of information on pharmacokinetics and efficacy. No pharmacological therapy should be initiated without a thorough assessment of the patient's management and health and addressing other causes. Pharmacological options are included in the formulary table.

The tricyclic anti-depressant Clomipramine has shown some promise in reducing FDB in cockatoos but has also been associated with neurological side effects so should be used with caution and at low starting doses (Seibert et al. 2004; Seibert 2007).

Selective serotonin reuptake inhibitors appear to have limited application. Available Paroxetine oral preparations show poor absorption in parrots and although Fluoxetine reduces FDB initially many treated birds relapse (Mertens 1997; Van Zeeland et al. 2013b).

Haloperidol is a catecholamine and dopamine receptor antagonist used to treat human compulsive disorders.

Positive results have been reported in self-traumatising cockatoos, but grey parrots develop disorientation so it is not recommended (Lennox and Van der Hayden 1993).

Benzodiazepines provide limited benefit in FDB reduction, and improvements are commonly due to sedation rather than management of the underlying psychological or biochemical changes. They should only be used short-term, where mutilation or anxiety justify application (Seibert 2007).

As endogenous opioid endorphins may be a key part of compulsive FDB, opioid antagonists have been suggested for treatment to remove the positive feedback associated with preening. Naltrexone therapy has shown promise in combined treatments, but needs further investigation (Turner 1993).

11.4.1.5 Neoplasia

Neoplasia is sporadically described in grey parrots, with individual case reports predominating. The majority occur in parrots of 20 years or older, but neoplasia has also been reported in young birds. Round cell tumours include a bursal lymphoma and a bilateral periorbital lymphoma with poor response to radiation therapy in both cases (Paul-Murphy et al. 1985; Wyre and Quesenberry 2007). Further periorbital neoplasms include a bilateral periorbital liposarcoma and a successfully resected retrobulbar adenoma (Graham et al. 2003; Simova-Curd et al. 2009). Multifocal neoplasms include metastatic renal and bronchial carcinomas, multifocal malignant melanoma, and a disseminated fibrosarcoma (Riddell and Cribb 1983; Latimer et al. 1996; André and Delverdier 1999; Shrader et al. 2016). Additional case reports describe a discrete malignant melanoma, bilateral aural adenocarcinomas, dermal squamous cell carcinoma unresponsive to cisplatin and a uropygial gland carcinoma successfully managed with excision and radiotherapy (Andre et al. 1993; Klaphake et al. 2006; Pignon et al. 2011; Houck et al. 2016).

In Timneh grey parrots two case reports of a beak squamous cell carcinoma managed with radiation therapy, and a metastatic air sac cystadenocarcinoma are described (Azmanis et al. 2013; Swisher et al. 2016). Cutaneous papillomas have been reported in both Timneh and Congo grey parrots and are associated with a papillomavirus (O'Banion et al. 1992).

Zehnder et al. (2016) describe potential chemotherapy dosing regimens but consultation with an oncologist for individual cases is advisable.

11.4.2 Infectious Diseases

11.4.2.1 Axillary Dermatitis

Ulcerative dermatitis can occur with FDB self-trauma (see above), or as a primary infectious condition. For this latter presentation, *Staphylococcus aureus* is a common finding with methicillin resistant strains rarely identified (Briscoe et al. 2008).

A specific presentation seen in grey parrots (and less frequently in small psittacine birds and Harris Hawks), is that of axillary or patagial dermatitis. Affected birds present with ulcerative lesions under the wing, affecting the axilla and/or the ventral surface of the proximal wing and this may be advanced by the time of identification as lesions are shielded by the wing. Cause is poorly understood with excessive humidity, nutritional deficiency, hypersensitivity, and primary infectious dermatitis postulated as potential causes. Culture in established cases typically yields multiple pathogens including *Staphylococci, Strepococci*, and *Pseudomonas* spp., as well as *Malassezia* and *Candida* yeasts (Powers and Van Sant 2006).

Treatment is challenging as primary cause is unclear, ongoing self-trauma and skin mobility in this region hinders healing, and topical therapy is often poorly tolerated by patients. Reducing contamination and allowing wounds to heal by secondary intention is often the only course of action as thin, damaged and infected skin with large deficits is not able to be closed by primary intention. Systemic antibiotic therapy should be administered based on culture results, and topical antifungal agents may be required. Emollients and broad spectrum antimicrobial disinfectants such as dilute chlorhexidine or medical honey may aid local healing in the early stages of therapy. Bandaging the affected area should be avoided as contracture of the patagial tendons on the leading edge of the wing is a likely consequence of wing immobilisation. Reduced air flow and increased humidity within bandages may also favour microbial growth. Where self-trauma prevents healing, collars can be placed temporarily to restrict access.

A similar presentation is seen with squamous cell carcinomas and fibrosarcomas in this region and neoplasia may be a separate disease entity or a consequence of chronic tissue trauma. Biopsy collection for histopathology should be considered, though in cases with concurrent infection secondary changes predominate. Histopathology is therefore more sensitive after resolution of infection and is often reserved for cases that fail to respond positively to medical therapy.

11.4.2.2 Psittacine Beak and Feather Disease (PBFD)

PBFD is caused by a circovirus and infection can occur by inhalation, ingestion, or vertical transmission (Ritchie et al. 1991). The virus is very stable, resistant to disinfectants and able to remain infectious for years. Dividing cells are targeted so developing feathers and bone marrow are typically affected. Disease course is very variable and tends to be dependent on age of bird at infection:

Acute: Sudden death or rapidly fatal secondary infections are seen in neonates.

Subacute: Anorexia, regurgitation, lethargy, diarrhoea, secondary infections and death are seen in both young and adult grey parrots (Schoemaker et al. 2000). Rapid development of loss of powder down, feather malformation, and colour changes may also occur. Anaemia, hepatopathy and secondary infections (typically Aspergillosis) may be identified (Schoemaker et al. 2000). Birds occasionally survive this presentation and become chronically infected.

Chronic: Adult birds showing progressive feather abnormalities are the most common presentation seen in practice. Dystrophic feathers gradually begin to replace normal ones as they are moulted and growing feathers become distorted and fragile, feather sheaths retained and grey feathers replaced with orange ones. A lack of down feathers results in altered preening, dull plumage, and glossy beak, and immunosuppression results in opportunistic infections.

Some infected adult birds may clear infection. Others become asymptomatic carriers, shedding virus, and may progress to the chronic disease status.

Diagnosis is by PCR detection of the virus in feather pulp from plucked feathers, or tissue samples from the thymus, bursa, bone marrow, or liver at post-mortem examination (Dahlhausen and Radabaugh 1993). False negatives may occur from feather samples in early infection, or if an uncommon variant (notably PBFD2 from Lories) is responsible. Asymptomatic birds testing positive on routine screens should be retested after three months to differentiate carriers from challenged birds that clear infection. Blood samples can also be tested by PCR but profound leucopaenia decreases the circulating viral load and may reduce sensitivity. Bone marrow aspirate samples are preferable in severely leucopaenic birds.

Therapy for PBFD is typically unsuccessful and chronically infected birds usually die within four years from refractory secondary infections. Euthanasia may be necessary on welfare grounds or to prevent transmission of infection. Avian interferon has shown promise in treating juvenile leucopaenic infected grey parrots (Stanford 2004) but is not commercially available.

Prevention involves quarantine and repeat testing of new birds coming in to disease free collections. Quarantine alone is ineffective due to carrier status and slow development of clinical signs in adult birds. Experimental vaccines have appeared promising but extensive trials and commercial production have not followed (Raidal et al. 1993; Shearer 2009).

11.4.3 Chlamydia/Psittacosis

C. psittaci is an obligate intracellular bacterium commonly identified as a primary or opportunistic pathogen in many parrot species, causing asymptomatic carriage, respiratory symptoms, or non-specific illness. Importantly is it also zoonotic and can cause serious illness in immunocompromised humans. It is described in greater detail in Chapter 10. Diagnosis of individual birds focuses on identification of antibodies using serology or the organism using PCR techniques. Treatment is a six-week course of doxycycline for affected birds and any in-contacts.

11.4.4 Aspergillosis

Aspergillosis is a respiratory infection caused by fungi from the Aspergillus genus, predominantly *Aspergillosis fumigatus*. Aspergillosis is the most common respiratory disease of captive birds (Redig 1993) and grey parrots appear highly susceptible (Redig 2005).

Aspergillus spores are ubiquitous, but disease may develop if birds are exposed to overwhelming quantities through poor hygiene or a build-up of organic material, or if they are immunosuppressed.

Symptoms of disease may be non-specific, especially where infection is confined to the air sacs. Lethargy, inappetance, loss of weight, green faeces, and polyuria/polydipsia may result. Tracheal or syringeal lesions may cause a loss or change in voice, and should be considered a true emergency as obstruction may rapidly develop. Pulmonary aspergillosis results in dyspnoea or acute death. Aspergillus sinusitis may also be noted with periorbital swelling and nasal discharge and appears a unique phenomenon to this species (Redig 2005).

Diagnosis is confirmed by direct visualisation of the fungal granulomas on tracheal or air sac endoscopy or by identification of large air sac lesions on radiographs in advanced disease. Hyperinflation of the air sacs, hepatomegaly, and small opacities within the air sacs may support a diagnosis but are not pathognomonic. Haematological findings are inconsistent but may include leucocytosis, heterophilia, monocytosis, lymphopaenia, or a non-regenerative anaemia. Serum protein electrophoresis initially shows increased beta globulins and decreased albumin concentration, followed by beta and/or gamma globulin increases in chronic disease (Jones and Orosz 2000).

ELISA analysis to detect galactomannan (a soluble component of the aspergillus cell wall released during growth) has been proposed as a specific test. However, sensitivity and specificity were found to be 67% and 73% respectively (with a cut off of 0.5) in one study so this test should be used alongside other methodologies to support a diagnosis (Cray et al. 2009).

Serological techniques have low sensitivity, but may have a supportive role in diagnosing non-invasive cases of chronic aspergillosis or monitoring response to therapy (Martinez-Quesada et al. 1993; Redig 2005).

Prognosis is grave for pulmonary aspergillosis, and fair for syringeal and air sac lesions treated promptly. Debulking of accessible lesions will hasten recovery and is often essential in syringeal infections. Endoscopic resection is possible but requires placing an air sac cannula to maintain respiratory function during syringeal access. Tracheotomy allows better access in cases where the endoscopic approach is unsuccessful. Air sac lesions can be debrided piecemeal, endoscopically. Submission of samples for culture and sensitivity testing is advisable as resistance has been seen to some treatments.

Systemic antifungal therapy is needed for all cases and itraconazole has previously been considered the first line medication but anecdotal reports of toxicity in grey parrots mean that alternatives such as terbinafine are preferred in these species. Newer generation drugs such as voriconazole have been used with a significant improvement in treatment success. As these antifungal agents are predominantly fungistatic rather than fungicidal they must be continued for a minimum of eight weeks to achieve resolution. Nebulisation using antifungal agents, or broad spectrum bird-safe disinfectants is of benefit, particularly for upper respiratory infections. Effective concentration of nebulised particles reduces for lower respiratory tract sites and exposure times should be increased (Tell et al. 2012).

11.4.5 Proventricular Dilation Disease (PDD)

Infection with avian bornavirus causes neural inflammation with a highly variable incubation period of days to years (Gancz et al. 2010). Birds may be clinically normal, or demonstrate weight loss, passage of undigested food in faeces, regurgitation, ataxia, altered proprioception, paresis, torticollis, blindness, seizures, or sudden death (Berhane et al. 2001). Dilation of the proventricular wall may be seen at post-mortem (Figure 11.12).

Diagnosis typically uses both serology and PCR. Combined choanal and cloacal swabs are recommended for antemortem PCR testing though intermittent shedding can give false negative results. For post-mortem testing, brain, crop, proventriculus, ventriculus, and adrenal gland tissues are preferred (Rinder et al. 2009).

It is important to be aware that presence of virus or antibody response does not automatically confirm bornavirus as the cause of symptoms as birds can be asymptomatically infected. Exclusion of other causes of neuropathy, such as heavy metal intoxication and Chlamydiosis, is prudent. Biopsy of the intestinal tract demonstrating lymphoplasmacytic genglioneuritis alongside a positive PCR or serological result is strongly supportive of clinical bornaviral disease. The crop is typically chosen as the biopsy site as access and sample collection are far simpler than for the

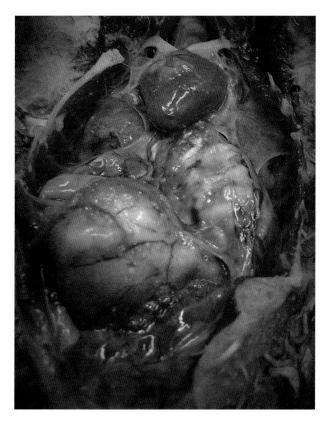

Figure 11.12 Marked dilation and thinning of the proventricular wall in a bird with PDD resulting in a translucent appearance and distention with retained food.

proventriculus and ventriculus, and post-operative dehiscence has less catastrophic consequences.

Imaging is widely used as a non-invasive alternative, but changes seen are not pathognomonic for bornaviral disease. Radiographs show food retention and a dilated proventriculus in around 70% of cases and this is strong evidence of an active, relevant infection (Gancz et al. 2010). Positive contrast studies can increase sensitivity over plain radiographs. Barium contrast fluoroscopy where available is valuable in identifying the reduced motility, increased transit time, focal hypomotility, or dilation of the proventriculus that may be seen.

Treatment of clinical cases involves reducing the inflammatory response to the virus that is predominantly responsible for symptoms. Corticosteroids are contraindicated in birds due to the profound leucopaenia induced with a high risk of secondary infections, particularly Aspergillosis. Non-steroidal anti-inflammatory drugs (NSAIDs) have shown promise in reducing symptoms, presumably by reduction in inflammatory response but there is some evidence that they may have antiviral properties (Lee et al. 2011). Celecoxib has been advocated as the preferred NSAID due to its COX-2 specific activity for GI symptoms though this is available as capsules and requires compounding to provide a usable form. Meloxicam is clinically inferior to celecoxib but is readily available in a stable liquid formulation (Gancz et al. 2010). NSAIDs are generally well tolerated but monitoring of biochemistry for renal changes is sensible and medication should be stopped if melaena or haematochezia is noted. The antiviral agent amantadine has been used alongside NSAIDs to reduce symptoms and prolong life expectancy where CNS symptoms are present (Gancz et al. 2010). Metoclopramide can be used where hypomotility or regurgitation are present but can cause excitation in some birds.

Feeding of an easily assimilated diet may aid in maintaining body condition and meeting nutritional requirements. Secondary infections of the intestinal tract are seen and microscopy or culture of faecal samples can allow targeted treatment with antibiotic or antifungal agents.

Monitoring of cases with gastrointestinal symptoms may be possible by following weight and body condition changes. Weight assessment alone may be inaccurate as intestinal food retention may artificially increase weight in deteriorating cases. Birds should be considered infected lifelong.

Positive birds in a single pet environment have little potential for viral transmission but if owners have contact with other parrots then they should take measures to prevent transfer, such as hand washing and changing clothes. Within a large collection or breeding facility, established infection is hard to eliminate and screening birds prior to introduction to attempt to maintain a PDD-free flock is preferable. If intending to produce a bornavirus free population in a flock with confirmed infection (or unknown status), birds should be tested by PCR and serological techniques and positive birds permanently isolated or euthanased. Negative birds should be subjected to repeat testing as the long incubation period and intermittent shedding can result in false negatives, especially early in the disease process. Often this approach is not practical or acceptable to owners and intermittent losses from clinical PDD are to be expected.

11.4.6 Reovirus

Reoviruses lead to immunosuppression and secondary infections. Young grey parrots are considered highly susceptible and infection results in pancytopaenia, petechiation, enteritis, pneumonia, hepatitis, and necrotic splenitis (Spenser 1991; Sanchez-Cordon et al. 2002). In one outbreak of reovirus in grey parrots, morbidity was 80% and mortality (associated with co-infections of herpesvirus and aspergillosis in some birds) was 30% (Sanchez-Cordon et al. 2002). Diagnosis is generally post-mortem but may be complicated by presence of other pathogens. Serology and PCR

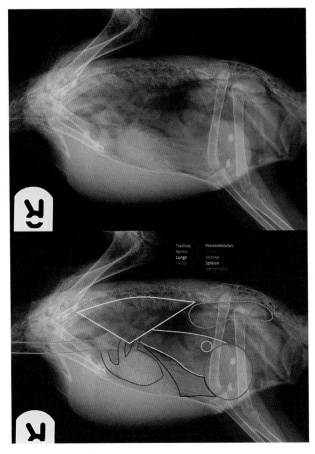

Figure 11.13 Right lateral radiographic view with visceral positions highlighted.

(of choanal and cloacal swabs) can be performed ante-mortem. Treatment is primarily supportive with additional management of secondary infections.

11.5 Preventative Health Measures

No preventative measures are carried out routinely though faecal screening for parasites is prudent to carry out for birds with a history of parasitism, or in outdoor aviaries. It is advisable to test new birds for *C. psittaci* and for birds moving in to a multibird household screening for other pathogens such as circovirus and avian bornavirus is recommended.

11.6 Radiographic Imaging

Survey radiographs are commonly used as a broad diagnostic screen for birds presenting with non-specific signs, or to investigate specific concerns. The ventrodorsal and right lateral views are most commonly used. Visceral anatomy is detailed in Figures 11.13 and 11.14.

On the ventrodorsal view, the heart and liver overlap to form an hourglass shape. Focal distortion of this silhouette can help pinpoint the location of the abnormality. Due to the overlap of liver and heart, it is rarely possible to accurately measure heart length. The width of the

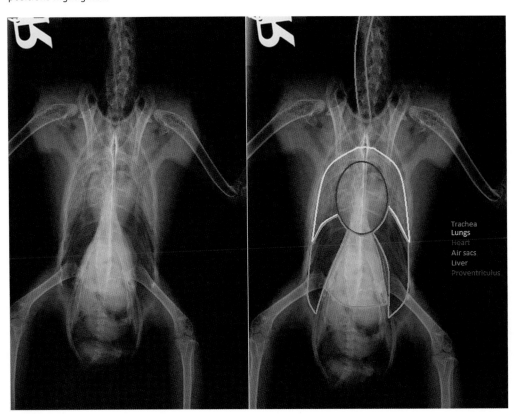

Figure 11.14 Ventrodorsal radiographic view with visceral positions highlighted.

cardiac silhouette is used instead and at its widest point this has been shown to be 54–57% of the width of the body cavity at the same level in grey parrots (Straub et al. 2002).

On the lateral view the great vessels are better defined and opacity or mineralisation suggestive of atherosclerosis can be identified. Ascites results in a loss of distinction between viscera and compression of the air sacs. The proventricular height at the level of the spinal-synsacral junction should be no greater than 48% of the maximum dorsoventral keel height and enlargement may indicate a foreign body, PDD, bacterial or fungal infection, or neoplasia (Dennison et al. 2008).

Fluoroscopy with barium contrast agents is useful for evaluating gastrointestinal motility and structure, and highlighting the proventricular lumen. Gastrointestinal transit time has been demonstrated to be four to six hours in grey parrots using this methodology (Kubiak and Forbes 2012). Prolonged transit time, retention of contrast in the proventriculus or distention of the proventriculus is often

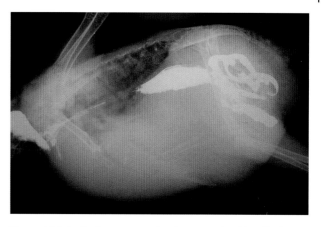

Figure 11.15 Barium contrast has been used to identify the source of diffusely increased coelomic soft tissue. A hepatic mass was indicated and a carcinoma diagnosed on biopsy.

seen in clinical bornaviral cases. Contrast can also be used to determine the anatomical source of soft tissue masses within the coelom (Figure 11.15).

Formulary

Medication	Dose	Dosing interval	Additional comments
Anaesthesia			
Butorphanol	1 mg/kg IM	–	Used as pre-medication in combination prior to volatile induction (Kubiak et al. 2016)
Midazolam	0.3 mg/kg IM	–	
Isoflurane	5% to induce, 2–3% for maintenance	–	Used alone, or following pre-medication (Kubiak et al. 2016)
Analgesia			
Butorphanol	2 mg/kg PO/IM/SC	q4hrs	(Paul-Murphy et al. 1999)
Buprenorphine	–		Ineffective (Paul-Murphy et al. 1999)
Carprofen	3 mg/kg IM	bid	Short-lived effects in Amazon parrots (Paul-Murphy et al. 2009)
Meloxicam	1 mg/kg IM/PO	bid	Based on dose in Amazon parrots (Cole et al. 2009)
Antibiotics			
Amoxicillin clavulanate	125 mg/kg PO/IM	tid	Based on Amazon parrot pharmacokinetics (Orosz et al. 2000)
Enrofloxacin	10 mg/kg PO	bid	In water therapy poorly effective (Flammer and Whitt-Smith 2002)
Doxycycline	800 mg/l water	continuous dosing for 6 weeks	For treatment of Chlamydiosis (Flammer et al. 2001)
	25 mg/kg PO	sid for 6 weeks	For treatment of Chlamydiosis (Rinaldi 2014)
Antifungals			
Voriconazole	12–18 mg/kg PO	bid	Timneh grey parrots (Flammer et al. 2008)
Itraconazole	5–10 mg/kg PO	sid	Anecdotally associated with hepatitis, not routinely used (Orosz 2003)

(Continued)

(Continued)

Medication	Dose	Dosing interval	Additional comments
Amphotericin B	1 mg/kg IV	bid/tid	Can be used topically on lesions. Precipitates with sodium salts so must be diluted in sterile water for administration
Terbinafine	10–15 mg/kg PO	bid	(Redig 2005)
Fluconazole	10–20 mg/kg PO	q24–48h	Timneh grey parrots (Flammer and Papich 2006)
F10 Disinfectant	1 : 250 solution in saline for nebulisation	2–4 times daily	30–60 mins sessions for upper respiratory tract and lung, 2–4hrs for air sac infections (Tell et al. 2012)

Treatment of cardiovascular disease

Enalapril	0.5–1.25 mg/kg PO	bid	Mainstay of therapy (Pees and Krautwald-Junghanns 2004; Pees et al. 2006)
Furosemide	0.1–0.2 mg/kg PO/IM	sid/bid	(Ritchie and Harrison 1994)
Benazepril	0.5 mg/kg PO	sid	(Sedacca et al. 2009)
Pimobendan	0.25 mg/kg PO	bid	(Sedacca et al. 2009)
Digoxin	0.02–0.1 mg/kg initially, 0.01 mg/kg for maintenance	sid	Used for stabilisation and rarely for long-term therapy of dilated cardiomyopathy, ventricular tachycardia, and in birds diagnosed with sinus or atrioventricular node disease (Pees and Krautwald-Junghanns 2004; Pees and Krautwald-Junghanns 2009)
Ephedrine	0.5 mg/kg PO	tid	Used for bradycardia and second-degree AV block (de Wit and Schoemaker 2005)
Isoxuprine	10 mg/kg PO	sid	Used for vasodilation in atherosclerosis (Simone-Freilicher 2007) or for peripheral vasodilation with soft tissue injury

Miscellaneous

Interferon gamma (avian origin)	1 000 000 iu IM	sid for 90d	Species specific interferon required but not readily available. Used for treating PBFD (Stanford 2004)
Diazepam	1–2 mg/kg IM	as needed	For seizure control (Beaufrère et al. 2011). Lower doses of 0.5–0.6 mg/kg q8–24hrs for management of feather destructive behaviours (van Zeeland and Schoemaker 2014b)
Celecoxib	20 mg/kg PO	sid	For management of PDD (Clubb 2006)
Amantidine	10–20 mg/kg PO	sid	For control of neurological symptoms associated with PDS (Gancz et al. 2010)
Metoclopramide	0.5 mg/kg PO/IM	bid	Prokinetic, used in hypomotility but can cause excitation (Clubb 2006)
Calcium borogluconate	10 mg/kg IM	sid	(Stanford 2003b)
35 mg/ml Calcium gluconate with 25 iu/ml cholecalciferol (ZolcalD)	1 ml/kg PO	sid for 10d	For management of chronic NSHP
Paroxetine HCl	2–4 mg/kg po	sid/bid	Relapse common and oral uptake poor with many preparations (Van Zeeland et al. 2013b)
Clomipramine	0.5–3.0 mg/kg PO	sid/bid	Dose started at low end but can be tapered up if no side effects are seen but FDB symptoms persist (Juarbe-Díaz 2000; Seibert 2007)
Naltrexone	1.5 mg/kg PO	bid/tid	Opioid receptor antagonist that may block the endorphin release that reinforces compulsive behaviour (van Zeeland and Schoemaker 2014b)
Ivermectin	0.2 mg/kg PO, IM	Every 2wks	A minimum of two treatments are required for ectoparasites, 3–4 treatments are often necessary (van Zeeland and Schoemaker 2014a)

References

André, J.P. and Delverdier, M. (1999). Primary bronchial carcinoma with osseous metastasis in an African grey parrot (*Psittacus erithacus*). *Journal of Avian Medicine and Surgery* 13 (3): 180–186.

Andre, J.P., Delverdier, M., Cabanie, P. et al. (1993). Malignant melanoma in an African grey parrot (*Psittacus erithacus erithacus*). *Journal of the Association of Avian Veterinarians* 7 (2): 83–85.

APHA (2017). African Grey Parrot traders: Information needed to support an application for an Article 10 Certificate http://ahvla.defra.gov.uk/documents/cites/cites-news030317.pdf (accessed 12 April 2018).

Azmanis, P., Stenkat, J., Hübel, J. et al. (2013). A complicated, metastatic, humeral air sac cystadenocarcinoma in a timneh African grey parrot (*Psittacus erithacus timneh*). *Journal of Avian Medicine and Surgery* 27 (1): 38–43.

Bavelaar, F.J. and Beynen, A.C. (2003a). Severity of atherosclerosis in parrots in relation to the intake of α-linolenic acid. *Avian Diseases* 47 (3): 566–577.

Bavelaar, F.J. and Beynen, A.C. (2003b). Influence of amount and type of dietary fat on plasma cholesterol concentrations in African grey parrots. *Journal of Applied Research in Veterinary Medicine* 1 (1): 1–8.

Bavelaar, F.J. and Beynen, A.C. (2004a). Atherosclerosis in parrots. A review. *Veterinary Quarterly* 26 (2): 50–60.

Bavelaar, F.J. and Beynen, A.C. (2004b). The relation between diet, plasma cholesterol and atherosclerosis in pigeons, quails and chickens. *International Journal of Poultry Science* 3 (11): 671–684.

Beaufrère, H., Nevarez, J., Gaschen, L. et al. (2011). Diagnosis of presumed acute ischemic stroke and associated seizure management in a Congo African grey parrot. *Journal of the American Veterinary Medical Association* 239 (1): 122–128.

Beaufrère, H., Papich, M.G., Brandão, J. et al. (2015). Plasma drug concentrations of orally administered rosuvastatin in Hispaniolan Amazon parrots (*Amazona ventralis*). *Journal of Avian Medicine and Surgery* 29 (1): 18–24.

Berhane, Y., Smith, D.A., Newman, S. et al. (2001). Peripheral neuritis in psittacine birds with proventricular dilatation disease. *Avian Pathology* 30 (5): 563–570.

Bohorquez, F. and Stout, C. (1972). Aortic atherosclerosis in exotic avians. *Experimental and Molecular Pathology* 17 (3): 261–273.

Briscoe, J.A., Morris, D.O., Rankin, S.C. et al. (2008). Methicillin-resistant Staphylococcus aureus–associated dermatitis in a Congo African grey parrot (*Psittacus erithacus erithacus*). *Journal of Avian Medicine and Surgery* 22 (4): 336–343.

Clubb, S.L. (2006). Clinical management of psittacine birds affected with proventricular dilation disease. Procedings of the Annual Conference of the Association of Avian Veterinarians: 85–90.

Cole, G.A., Paul-Murphy, J., Krugner-Higby, L. et al. (2009). Analgesic effects of intramuscular administration of meloxicam in Hispaniolan parrots (*Amazona ventralis*) with experimentally induced arthritis. *American Journal of Veterinary Research* 70 (12): 1471–1476.

Cray, C., Reavill, D., Romagnano, A. et al. (2009). Galactomannan assay and plasma protein electrophoresis findings in psittacine birds with aspergillosis. *Journal of Avian Medicine and Surgery* 23 (2): 125–135.

Dahlhausen, B. and Radabaugh, S. (1993). Update on psittacine beak and feather disease and avian polyomavirus testing. Procedings of the Annual Conference of the Association of Avian Veterinarians, Nashville: 5–7.

Dennison, S.E., Paul-Murphy, J.R., and Adams, W.M. (2008). Radiographic determination of proventricular diameter in psittacine birds. *Journal of the American Veterinary Medical Association* 232 (5): 709–714.

Dorrestein, G.M., Zwart, P., Borst, G.H.A. et al. (1977). Disease and causes of death in birds. *Tijdschrift voor Diergeneeskunde* 102 (7): 437–447.

Dorrestein, G.M., Fricke, C., and Krautwald-Junghanns, M.E. (2006). Atherosclerosis in African grey parrots (Psittacus erithacus) and Amazons (*Amazona* species). Procedings of the Annual Conference of the Association of Avian Veterinarians: 95–98.

Edling, T.M. (2006). Anesthesia and monitoring. In: *Clinical Avian Medicine*, vol. 1 (eds. G.J. Harrison and T.L. Lightfoot), 747–760. Palm Beach, Fl: Spix Publishing.

Flammer, K. and Papich, M. (2006). Pharmacokinetics of fluconazole after oral administration of single and multiple doses in African grey parrots. *American Journal of Veterinary Research* 67 (3): 417–422.

Flammer, K. and Whitt-Smith, D. (2002). Plasma concentrations of enrofloxacin in psittacine birds offered water medicated with 200 mg/L of the injectable formulation of enrofloxacin. *Journal of Avian Medicine and Surgery* 16 (4): 286–290.

Flammer, K., Whitt-Smith, D., and Papich, M. (2001). Plasma concentrations of doxycycline in selected psittacine birds when administered in water for potential treatment of *Chlamydophila psittaci* infection. *Journal of Avian Medicine and Surgery* 15 (4): 276–282.

Flammer, K., Nettifee Osborne, J.A., Webb, D.J. et al. (2008). Pharmacokinetics of voriconazole after oral administration of single and multiple doses in African grey parrots (*Psittacus erithacus* timneh). *American Journal of Veterinary Research* 69 (1): 114–121.

Gancz, A.Y., Clubb, S., and Shivaprasad, H.L. (2010). Advanced diagnostic approaches and current management of proventricular dilatation disease. *The Veterinary Clinics of North America. Exotic Animal Practice* 13 (3): 471–494.

García-Pérez, B., Ayala, I., Castells, M.T. et al. (2005). Effects of nifedipine, verapamil and diltiazem on serum biochemical parameters and aortic composition of atherosclerotic chickens. *Biomedicine & Pharmacotherapy* 59 (1–2): 1–7.

Graham, J.E., Werner, J.A., Lowenstine, L.J. et al. (2003). Periorbital liposarcoma in an African grey parrot (*Psittacus erithacus*). *Journal of Avian Medicine and Surgery* 17 (3): 147–153.

Harcourt-Brown, N. (2003). Incidence of juvenile osteodystrophy in hand-reared grey parrots (*Psittacus e erithacus*). *The Veterinary Record* 152 (14): 438.

Hawkins, P., Morton, D.B., Cameron, D. et al. (2001). Laboratory birds: refinements in husbandry and procedures. *Laboratory Animals* 35 (Suppl 1): 108.

Hernandez-Divers, S.J. (2007). Avian Anesthesia. Atlantic Coast Veterinary Conference, Atlantic City, NJ, 9–11 October.

Hess, L., Mauldin, G., and Rosenthal, K. (2002). Estimated nutrient content of diets commonly fed to pet birds. *Veterinary Record* 150 (13): 399–404.

Hochleithner, M., Hochleithner, C., and Harrison, G.J. (1997). Evidence of hypoparathyroidism in hypocalcemic African grey parrots. *The Avian Examiner* Special Suppl. HBD International Ltd (Spring).

Houck, E.L., Keller, K.A., Hawkins, M.G. et al. (2016). Bilateral aural adenocarcinoma in a Congo African grey parrot (*Psittacus erithacus erithacus*). *Journal of Avian Medicine and Surgery* 30 (3): 257–262.

Jayson, S.L., Williams, D.L., and Wood, J.L. (2014). Prevalence and risk factors of feather plucking in African grey parrots (*Psittacus erithacus erithacus* and *Psittacus erithacus timneh*) and cockatoos (*Cacatua* spp.). *Journal of Exotic Pet Medicine* 23 (3): 250–257.

Jones, M.P. and Orosz, S.E. (2000). The diagnosis of aspergillosis in birds. *Seminars in Avian and Exotic Pet Medicine* 9 (2): 52–58.

Juan-Sallés, C., Soto, S., Garner, M.M. et al. (2011). Congestive heart failure in 6 African grey parrots (*Psittacus e erithacus*). *Veterinary Pathology* 48 (3): 691–697.

Juarbe-Díaz, S.V. (2000). Animal behavior case of the month. *Journal of the American Veterinary Medical Association* 216 (10): 1562–1564.

Kempeneers, P. (1987). Atherosclerosis in parrots. Student Scription, Department of Pathology, Faculty of Veterinary Medicine, Utrecht University.

Klaphake, E., Beazley-Keane, S.L., Jones, M. et al. (2006). Multisite integumentary squamous cell carcinoma in an African grey parrot (*Psittacus erithacus erithacus*). *The Veterinary Record* 158 (17): 593.

Koutsos, E.A., Matson, K.D., and Klasing, K.C. (2001). Nutrition of birds in the order Psittaciformes: a review. *Journal of Avian Medicine and Surgery* 15 (4): 257–275.

Kubiak, M. and Forbes, N.A. (2012). Fluoroscopic evaluation of gastrointestinal transit time in African Grey parrots. *Veterinary Record* 171 (22): 563.

Kubiak, M., Roach, L., and Eatwell, K. (2016). The influence of a combined butorphanol and midazolam premedication on anesthesia in psittacid species. *Journal of Avian Medicine and Surgery* 30 (4): 317–324.

Latimer, K.S., Ritchie, B.W., Campagnoli, R.P. et al. (1996). Metastatic renal carcinoma in an African grey parrot (*Psittacus erithacus erithacus*). *Journal of Veterinary Diagnostic Investigation* 8 (2): 261–264.

Leary, S., Underwood, W., Anthony, R. et al. (2013). *AVMA Guidelines for the Euthanasia of Animals: 2013 Edition*. Schaumburg, IL: American Veterinary Medical Association.

Lee, S.M., Gai, W.W., Cheung, T.K. et al. (2011). Antiviral effect of a selective COX-2 inhibitor on H5N1 infection in vitro. *Antiviral Research* 91 (3): 330–334.

Lennox, A.M. (2011). Sedation as an alternative to general anesthesia in pet birds. Proceedings of the Conference of the Association of Avian Veterinarians.

Lennox, A. and Van der Hayden, N. (1993). Haloperidol for use in treatment of psittacine self-mutilation and feather plucking. Proceedings of the Conference of the Association of Avian Veterinarians, Nashville: 119–120.

Lierz, M. (2003). Avian renal disease: pathogenesis, diagnosis, and therapy. *The Veterinary Clinics of North America. Exotic Animal Practice* 6 (1): 29–55.

Lowenstine, L.J. (1986). Nutritional disorders of birds. In: *Zoo & Wild Animal Medicine*, 2e (ed. M.E. Fowler), 202–205. Philadelphia: W.B. Saunders.

Lumeij, J.T. and Hommers, C.J. (2008). Foraging 'enrichment' as treatment for pterotillomania. *Applied Animal Behaviour Science* 111: 85–94.

Lumeij, J.T. and Ritchie, B.W. (1994). Cardiology. In: *Avian Medicine: Principles and Application* (eds. B.W. Ritchie, G.J. Harrison and L.R. Harrison), 695–722. Lake Worth, FL: Wingers Publishing.

Mans, C. and Brown, C.J. (2007). Radiographic evidence of atherosclerosis of the descending aorta in a grey-cheeked parakeet (*Brotogeris pyrrhopterus*). *Journal of Avian Medicine and Surgery* 21 (1): 56–62.

Martinez-Quesada, J., Nieto-Cadenazzi, A., and Torres-Rodriguez, J.M. (1993). Humoral immunoresponse of pigeons to *Aspergillus fumigatus* antigens. *Mycopathologia* 124 (3): 131–137.

de Matos, R. (2008). Calcium metabolism in birds. *The Veterinary Clinics of North America. Exotic Animal Practice* 11 (1): 59–82.

de Matos, R. and Morrisey, J.K. (2005). Emergency and critical care of small psittacines and passerines. *Seminars in Avian and Exotic Pet Medicine* 14 (2): 90–105.

Meehan, C.L., Millam, J.R., and Mench, J.A. (2003). Foraging opportunity and increased complexity both prevent and reduce psychogenic feather picking by young Amazon parrots. *Applied Animal Behaviour Science* 80: 71–85.

Mertens, P.A. (1997). Pharmacological treatment of feather picking in pet birds. Proceedings 1st International Conference on Veterinary Behavioural Medicine, Birmingham, UK, International Veterinary Behaviour Meeting: 209–211.

Nap, A.M.P., Lumeij, J.T., and Stokhof, A.A. (1992). Electrocardiogram of the African grey (*Psittacus erithacus*) and Amazon (*Amazona* spp.) parrot. *Avian Pathology* 21 (1): 45–53.

Nevarez, J.G. (2005). Monitoring during avian and exotic pet anesthesia. *Seminars in Avian and Exotic Pet Medicine* 14 (4): 277–283.

O'Banion, K., Jacobson, E.R., and Sundberg, J.P. (1992). Molecular cloning and partial characterization of a parrot papillomavirus. *Intervirology* 33 (2): 91–96.

Oglesbee, B.L. and Oglesbee, M.J. (1998). Results of postmortem examination of psittacine birds with cardiac disease: 26 cases (1991-1995). *Journal of the American Veterinary Medical Association* 212 (11): 1737–1742.

Orosz, S.E. (2003). Antifungal therapy in avian species. *The Veterinary Clinics of North America. Exotic Animal Practice* 6: 337–350.

Orosz, S.E., Jones, M.P., Cox, S.K. et al. (2000). Pharmacokinetics of amoxicillin plus clavulanic acid in blue-fronted Amazon parrots (*Amazona aestiva aestiva*). *Journal of Avian Medicine and Surgery* 14 (2): 107–112.

Parr, M. and Juniper, T. (2010). *Parrots: A Guide to the Parrots of the World*. Robertsbridge, UK: Pica Press.

Paul-Murphy, J., Lowenstine, L., Turrel, J.M. et al. (1985). Malignant lymphoreticular neoplasm in an African gray parrot. *Journal of the American Veterinary Medical Association* 187 (11): 1216–1217.

Paul-Murphy, J.R., Brunson, D.B., and Miletic, V. (1999). Analgesic effects of butorphanol and buprenorphine in conscious African grey parrots (*Psittacus erithacus erithacus* and *Psittacus erithacus timneh*). *American Journal of Veterinary Research* 60 (10): 1218–1221.

Paul-Murphy, J.R., Sladky, K.K., Krugner-Higby, L.A. et al. (2009). Analgesic effects of carprofen and liposome-encapsulated butorphanol tartrate in Hispaniolan parrots (*Amazona ventralis*) with experimentally induced arthritis. *American Journal of Veterinary Research* 70 (10): 1201–1210.

Pees, M. and Krautwald-Junghanns, M.E. (2004). Therapy of cardiac diseases: possibilities and limitations. Proceedings of the Conference of the Association of Avian Veterinarians, New Orleans: 35–39.

Pees, M. and Krautwald-Junghanns, M.E. (2005). Avian echocardiography. *Seminars in Avian and Exotic Pet Medicine* 14 (1): 14–21.

Pees, M. and Krautwald-Junghanns, M.E. (2009). Cardiovascular physiology and diseases of pet birds. *The Veterinary Clinics of North America. Exotic Animal Practice* 12 (1): 81–97.

Pees, M., Kuhring, K., and Demiraij, F. (2006). Bioavailability and compatibility of enalapril in birds. Proceedings of the 27th Annual Association of Avian Veterinarians Conference. San Antonio, TX: 7–11.

Pignon, C., Azuma, C., and Mayer, J. (2011). Radiation therapy of uropygial gland carcinoma in psittacine species. Proceedings of the 32nd Annual Confrence of the Association of Avian Veterinarians, Seattle, WA: 263.

Pilny, A.A., Quesenberry, K.E., Bartick-Sedrish, T.E. et al. (2012). Evaluation of *Chlamydophila psittaci* infection and other risk factors for atherosclerosis in pet psittacine birds. *Journal of the American Veterinary Medical Association* 240 (12): 1474–1480.

Powers, L.V. and Van Sant, F. (2006). Axillary and patagial dermatitis in African Grey parrots (Psittacus erithacus). Proceedings of the 27th Annual Association of Avian Veterinarians Conference, San Antonio, TX: 101–105.

Raidal, S.R., Firth, G.A., and Cross, G.M. (1993). Vaccination and challenge studies with psittacine beak and feather disease virus. *Australian Veterinary Journal* 70 (12): 437–441.

Ratcliffe, H.L. and Cronin, M.T.I. (1958). Changing frequency of arteriosclerosis in mammals and birds at the Philadelphia zoological garden: review of autopsy records. *Circulation* 18 (1): 41–52.

Redig, P. (1993). Avian aspergillosis. In: *Zoo and Wild Animal Medicine: Current Therapy*, 3e (ed. M.E. Fowler), 178–181. Philadelphia: WB Saunders.

Redig, P. (2005). Mycotic infections in birds I: aspergillosis. In: *The North American Veterinary Conference Proceedings*, 1192–1194. Gainesville, FL: Eastern States Veterinary Association.

Riddell, C. and Cribb, P.H. (1983). Fibrosarcoma in an African grey parrot (*Psittacus erithacus*). *Avian Diseases* 27 (2): 549–555.

Rinaldi, M.L. (2014). Therapeutic review: doxycycline. *Journal of Exotic Pet Medicine* 23 (1): 107–112.

Rinder, M., Ackermann, A., Kempf, H. et al. (2009). Broad tissue and cell tropism of avian bornavirus in parrots with proventricular dilatation disease. *Journal of Virology* 83 (11): 5401–5407.

Ritchie, B.W. and Harrison, G.J. (1994). Formulary. In: *Avian Medicine: Principles and Application* (eds. B.W. Ritchie, G.J. Harrison and L.R. Harrison), 457–478. Lake Worth, FL: Wingers Publishing.

Ritchie, B., Niagro, F., Latimer, K. et al. (1991). Routes and prevalence of shedding of psittacine beak and feather disease virus. *American Journal of Veterinary Research* 52 (11): 1804–1809.

Sanchez-Cordon, P.J., Hervas, J., de Lara, F.C. et al. (2002). Reovirus infection in psittacine birds (*Psittacus erithacus*): morphologic and immunohistochemical study. *Avian Diseases* 46 (2): 485–492.

Schmid, R., Doherr, M.G., and Steiger, A. (2006). The influence of the breeding method on the behaviour of adult African grey parrots (*Psittacus erithacus*). *Applied Animal Behaviour Science* 98 (3): 293–307.

Schmidt, P.M., Gobel, T., and Trautvetter, E. (1998). Evaluation of pulse oximetry as a monitoring method in avian anesthesia. *Journal of Avian Medicine and Surgery* 12 (2): 91–98.

Schoemaker, N., Dorrenstein, G., Latimer, K. et al. (2000). Severe leukopaenia and liver necrosis in young African grey parrots (*Psittacus erithacus erithacus*) infected with psittacine circovirus. *Avian Diseases* 44 (2): 470–478.

Sedacca, C.D., Campbell, T.W., Bright, J.M. et al. (2009). Chronic cor pulmonale secondary to pulmonary atherosclerosis in an African Grey parrot. *Journal of the American Veterinary Medical Association* 234 (8): 1055–1059.

Seibert, L. (2007). Pharmacotherapy for behavioural disorders in pet birds. *Journal of Exotic Pet Medicine* 16 (1): 30–37.

Seibert, L.M., Crowell-Davis, S.L., Wilson, G.H. et al. (2004). Placebo-controlled clomipramine trial for the treatment of feather picking disorder in cockatoos. *Journal of the American Animal Hospital Association* 40: 261–269.

Shearer, P.L. (2009). Development of novel diagnostic and vaccine options for beak and feather disease virus (BFDV). Doctoral dissertation, Murdoch University. http://researchrepository.murdoch.edu.au/id/eprint/691 (accessed 21 May 2018).

Shivaprasad, H.L. (1993). Diseases of the nervous system in pet birds: a review and report of diseases rarely documented. Proceedings of the Annual Conference of the Association of Avian Veterinarians, Nashville, TN: 213–222.

Shrader, T.C., Carpenter, J.W., Cino-Ozuna, A.G. et al. (2016). Malignant melanoma of the syrinx and liver in an African grey parrot (*Psittacus erithacus erithacus*). *Journal of Avian Medicine and Surgery* 30 (2): 165–171.

Simone-Freilicher, E. (2007). Use of isoxsuprine for treatment of clinical signs associated with presumptive atherosclerosis in a yellow-naped Amazon parrot (*Amazona ochrocephala auropalliata*). *Journal of Avian Medicine and Surgery* 21 (3): 215–219.

Simova-Curd, S., Richter, M., Hauser, B. et al. (2009). Surgical removal of a retrobulbar adenoma in an African grey parrot (*Psittacus erithacus*). *Journal of Avian Medicine and Surgery* 23 (1): 24–28.

Sistermann, R. (2000). *Untersuchung zur Sexuellen Pra¨gung Handaufgezogener Grosspapageien.* Aachen: Institut fur Biologie II/Lehrstuhl fur Zoologie-Tierphysiologie.

Spenser, E.L. (1991). Common infectious diseases of psittacine birds seen in practice. *Veterinary Clinics of North America: Small Animal Practice* 21 (6): 1213–1230.

Stanford, M.D. (2003a). Measurement of ionised calcium in grey parrots (*Psittacus* e. *erithacus*): the effect of diet. Proceedings of the European Association of Avian Veterinarians 7th European meeting, Tenerife, Spain, 22–26 April: 269–275.

Stanford, M.D. (2003b). Measurement of 25-hydroxycholecalciferol in captive grey parrots (*Psittacus e erithacus*). *The Veterinary Record* 153: 58–59.

Stanford, M. (2004). Interferon treatment of circovirus infection in grey parrots (*Psittacus e erithacus*). *Veterinary Record* 154: 435–436.

Stanford, M. (2005). Calcium metabolism in grey parrots: the effects of husbandry. Diploma of Fellowship Thesis, Royal College of Veterinary Surgeons Library.

Stanford, M. (2007). Clinical pathology of hypocalcaemia in adult grey parrots (*Psittacus e erithacus*). *Veterinary Record* 161 (13): 456.

Straub, J., Pees, M., and Krautwald-Junghanns, M.E. (2002). Measurement of the cardiac silhouette in psittacines. *Journal of the American Veterinary Medical Association* 221 (1): 76–79.

Swisher, S.D., Phillips, K.L., Tobias, J.R. et al. (2016). External beam radiation therapy of squamous cell carcinoma in the beak of an African grey parrot (*Psittacus timneh*). *Journal of Avian Medicine and Surgery* 30 (3): 250–256.

Taylor, J. (2012). Grey parrot (Psittacus erithacus) has been split into grey parrot (P. erithacus) and Timneh grey parrot (*P. timneh*): are both eligible for uplisting? *Birdlife International*, Archived 2011–2012 topics. http://www.birdlife.org (accessed 4 June 2018).

Tell, L.A., Stephens, K., Teague, S.V. et al. (2012). Study of nebulization delivery of aerosolized fluorescent microspheres to the avian respiratory tract. *Avian Diseases* 56 (2): 381–386.

Turner, R. (1993). Trexan (naltrexone hydrochloride) use in feather picking in avian species. Proceedings of the Annual Conference of the Association of Avian Veterinarians, Nashville, TN: 116–118.

Ullrey, D.E., Allen, M.E., and Baer, D.J. (1991). Formulated diets versus seed mixtures for psittacines. *The Journal of Nutrition* 121 (suppl_11): S193–S205.

Van Ree, J.M., Niesink, R.J.M., van Wolfswinkel, R.L. et al. (2000). Endogenous opioids and reward. *European Journal of Pharmacology* 405: 89–101.

Van Zeeland, Y.R.A., Schoemaker, N.J., Vinke, C.M. et al. (2013a). Evaluating motivation for enrichment of Grey parrots (Psittacus erithacus erithacus): A preliminary report. In: Y.R.A. van Zeeland, The feather damaging Grey parrot: An analysis of its behaviour and needs, PhD thesis, Utrecht University.

Van Zeeland, Y.R.A., Schoemaker, N.J., Haritova, A. et al. (2013b). Pharmacokinetics of paroxetine, a selective serotonin reuptake inhibitor, in Grey parrots (*Psittacus erithacus erithacus*): influence of pharmaceutical formulation and length of dosing. *Journal of Veterinary Pharmacology and Therapeutics* 36 (1): 51–58.

van Zeeland, Y.R. and Schoemaker, N.J. (2014a). Plumage disorders in psittacine birds – part 1: feather abnormalities. *European Journal of Companion Animal Practice* 24 (1): 34–47.

van Zeeland, Y.R. and Schoemaker, N.J. (2014b). Plumage disorders in psittacine birds – part 2: feather damaging behaviour. *European Journal of Companion Animal Practice* 24 (2): 24–36.

de Wit, M. and Schoemaker, N.J. (2005). Clinical approach to avian cardiac disease. *Seminars in Avian and Exotic Pet Medicine* 14 (1): 6–13.

Wyre, N.R. and Quesenberry, K.E. (2007). Bursal Lymphosarcoma in a 4-year-old Congo African Grey Parrot (Psittacus erithacus), Proceedings of the 28th Annual Association of Avian Veterinarians Conference. Providence, RI.

Zehnder, A.M., Hawkins, M.G., Pascoe, P.J. et al. (2009). Evaluation of indirect blood pressure monitoring in awake and anesthetized red-tailed hawks (*Buteo jamaicensis*): effects of cuff size, cuff placement, and monitoring equipment. *Veterinary Anaesthesia and Analgesia* 36 (5): 464–479.

Zehnder, A., Graham, J., Reavill, D.R. et al. (2016). Neoplastic diseases in avian species. In: *Current Therapy in Avian Medicine and Surgery* (ed. B.L. Speer), 107–141. St Louis, MO: Elsevier.

12

Birds of Prey
Alberto Rodriguez Barbon and Marie Kubiak

Raptors is a general term to include birds of prey of the orders Accipitriformes, Falconiformes, and Strigiformes (hawks, falcons, eagles, vultures, and owls). These birds are carnivorous with beaks and feet adapted for catching and prehending animals. This chapter will focus on raptors that the practitioner is more likely to encounter; hawks, falcons, and owls. Biological parameters of common species are shown in Table 12.1.

Falcons are fast flying, streamlined birds adapted to hunt prey in flight. Their wings and tails are relatively long with a triangular shape, giving great agility and speed. The upper beak (rhinotheca) has a pronounced tomium on each side for gripping and shearing food (Ford 2010). Commonly kept species of falcon include the Peregrine falcon (*Falco peregrinus*, Figure 12.1), Saker falcon (*F. cherrug*) and Gyr falcon (*F. rusticolus*, Figure 12.2). It is common to find hybridisation of these species in birds used for falconry.

Hawks can be divided in two major groups: forest hawks and soaring hawks. Forest hawks, such as the Northern goshawk (*Accipiter gentilis*, Figure 12.3), are adapted for quick acceleration and sharp turns, aided by their short round wings and long tails. Soaring hawks, such as the Common buzzard (*Buteo buteo*), are a very diverse group adapted to different habitats, with a common feature of broad, fan-shaped wings.

Owls are predominantly crepuscular to nocturnal and are visibly different to the diurnal raptors. They have a large head and stocky body, large forward-facing eyes and asymmetrically placed ears (Figure 12.4). Their prey is predominantly small terrestrial mammals or birds and their plumage allows for close to silent flight for ambush predation. There is great variety in size, from the 30 g elf owl (*Micrathene whitneyi*) to the Eurasian Eagle owl (*Bubo bubo*) (Figure 12.5) which can weigh up to 4 kg.

12.1 Husbandry

Diurnal birds of prey are usually kept in free flying aviaries, or tethered to bow or block perches outside during the day and housed in covered areas overnight. Tethered birds are usually equipped with leather anklets (aylmeri), closed around the metatarsus by a metal rivet. Leather straps (jesses), go through the metal rivet and are joined to a rotating metal joint, the swivel, that connects to a leash of variable length, securing the bird to the perch (Figure 12.6). Owls are more commonly maintained in aviaries and are rarely tethered.

Aviaries should allow for flight and walls should be made of sufficient gauge steel mesh that animals cannot escape and rodents, mammalian predators (e.g. cats, mustelids, and foxes), and wild birds are kept out. There should be an area of the aviary with a solid roof and walls for protection from adverse weather conditions and species adapted to warmer climates may require additional heating in winter. For nervous species, screening or regularly spaced batons may be needed over the mesh walls to avoid collisions and damage to the face, feet, or feathers (Figure 12.7). A substrate of gravel is often preferred for hygiene and aesthetics, but a solid base of concrete or impermeable membrane underneath will help prevent wildlife incursion.

Raptors used for falconry are usually trained to hunt and during training and hunting falconers use weight management. Weight is reduced to encourage the bird to feed on the fist, and this is achieved progressively. Initially the bird is tethered and picked up whilst feeding. Once the bird is confident with this process, it is encouraged to jump to the fist to feed. Hawks are then usually trained by progressively increasing the distance to the fist. Falcons are trained using different types of lures, which consist of food attached to a

Handbook of Exotic Pet Medicine, First Edition. Edited by Marie Kubiak.
© 2021 John Wiley & Sons Ltd. Published 2021 by John Wiley & Sons Ltd.
Companion website: www.wiley.com/go/kubiak/exotic_pet_medicine

Table 12.1 Biological parameters of common species.

Common name	Scientific name	Male weight range (g)	Female weight range (g)	Clutch size	Incubation time (days)	Nestling period (days)
Northern goshawk	*Accipiter gentilis*	570–1110	820–2000	2–4	28–38	34–35
Harris' hawk	*Parabuteo unicinctus*	630–880	910–1200	1–5	31–36	44–48
Common buzzard	*Buteo buteo*	530–980	700–1200	2–4	33–35	50–55
Peregrine falcon	*Falco peregrinus*	550–660	740–1120	2–5	29–32	35–42
Gyr falcon	*Falco rusticolus*	960–1300	1400–2000	1–5	34–36	45–50
Lanner falcon	*Falco biarmicus*	500–600	700–900	3–5	32–34	35–47
Saker falcon	*Falco cherrug*	730–990	970–1300	2–6	32–36	45–50
Barn owl	*Tyto alba*	440–500	510–630	4–7	32–34	50–70
Eurasian Eagle owl	*Bubo bubo*	1400–2500	1700–3300	1–3	31–36	25–45

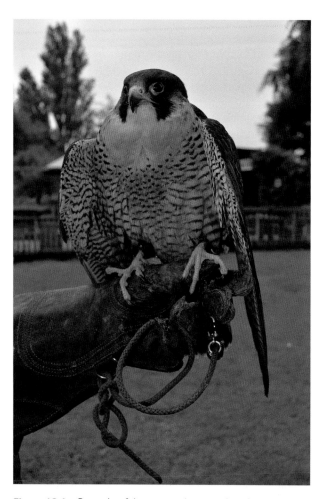

Figure 12.1 Peregrine falcon, note the restraint of the legs by the jesses being held short.

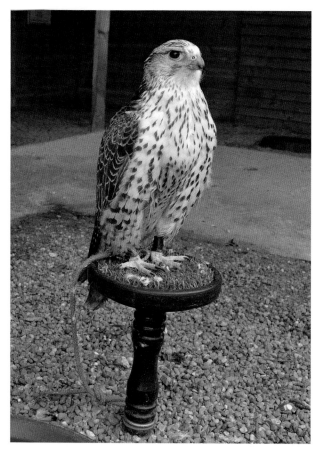

Figure 12.2 Gyr falcon.

pair of wings to mimic a prey item, that are swung around to encourage the bird to fly.

Raptors eat whole carcass diets with rodents, poultry, and rabbits commercially available. The indigestible portion, such as fur and feathers, is regurgitated or cast as a pellet, around 12 hours after being fed (Figure 12.8). Reducing the indigestible elements in the diet by actions such as skinning the prey is important when medicating animals orally to prevent casting and potential associated regurgitation of medication.

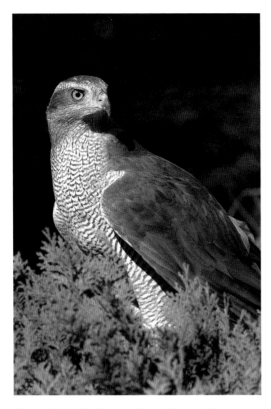

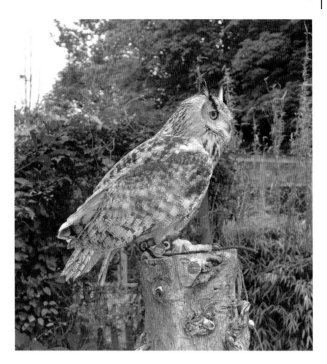

Figure 12.5 Turkmenian eagle owl, a subspecies of the Eurasian eagle owl.

Figure 12.3 Northern goshawk (*Source:* Photo courtesy of Gemma Atherton).

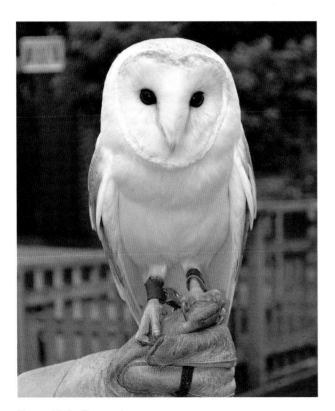

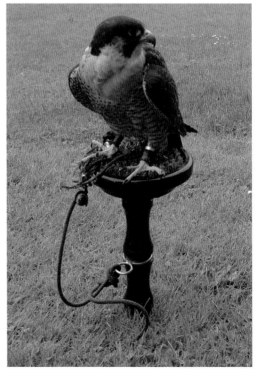

Figure 12.6 Peregrine falcon tethered on block perch.

Figure 12.4 Barn owl.

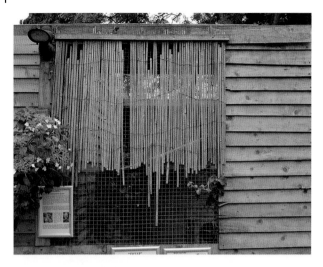

Figure 12.7 Batons placed over mesh to minimise stress from external stimuli and reduce damage associated with collisions.

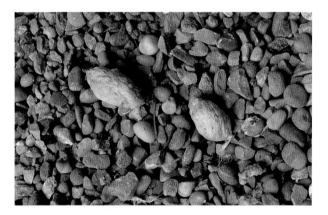

Figure 12.8 Cast pellets, consisting of indigestible components of the diet.

12.2 Clinical Evaluation

12.2.1 History Taking

It is important to allocate adequate time to take a thorough clinical history before attempting examination. Valuable information is gathered, and the time spent collecting a clinical history from the owner will allow the bird to settle in the new environment, and informative clinical signs are more likely to be evident in a relaxed bird.

General information includes age, sex, bird source (wild-caught/captive bred), rearing method (imprinted to humans/parent-reared), weight (current weight, flying, and moult weights), reproductive status, flight performance, frequency and duration of flying, and appearance of droppings (referred to as mutes by falconers).

Diet information required includes food items offered (frequency, quantity, variations over the year), food source,

storage and thawing conditions (if maintained frozen), mineral and vitamin supplements, casting appearance, frequency and time after feeding, and type of prey hunted recently.

The aviary size, layout and location, substrate material and replacement/cleaning frequency, perching material, number, location and type, presence of other birds in the aviary or nearby, overall hygiene and disinfectants used are also relevant. It is beneficial to review pictures of the husbandry conditions where available.

The use of relevant terminology (e.g. mutes, casting) and asking for certain information whilst obtaining a medical history from a raptor used in falconry is a good opportunity to demonstrate familiarity with the species presented.

12.2.2 Handling

Handling of birds of prey competently is important not just due to the potential injuries that may be inflicted on the handler with their feet and beak, but to build a good relation between client and veterinarian. A skilled and confident handling will instil the owner with confidence. Species and individuals vary greatly in temperament, with owls generally being more docile than hawks and falcons.

Falconry birds are usually carried to the practice in a closed box or tethered to a perch and hooded. The most common approach is to request the owner to have the bird on the fist holding the leash and jesses short to prevent foot movement (Figure 12.1). The bird is approached from behind with a towel extended over the hands and forearms of the handler. A common reaction by the birds if they notice the handler is to extend their wings and vocalise, hooding or dimming the lights may help avoid this. The towel is wrapped around the wings to prevent wing flapping, and once secure, one hand is moved to hold the distal portion of the legs. The metatarsi are approached from behind and the second or middle finger can be placed between both legs whilst the rest of the fingers grasp firmly both metatarsi (Figure 12.9). Once the feet are secured, the falconer can release the leash and jesses. The head is restrained with the other hand as some raptors may bite. The feet should always be directed away from the body to prevent being grabbed by talons, this action is referred as footing by falconers.

If the bird needs to be retrieved directly from the box it is important to assess the position of the bird first, with the preferred position as the bird facing away from the handler. The hands should be protected prior to attempting capture. Although protective gloves can be used this may damage the feathers and limit the handler dexterity. A thick folded towel over the hands can offer sufficient protection and allow restraint of the bird in the box. Some birds may lie on their backs and try to grab the handler with their talons, in these situations the bird can be allowed to grab the loose towel whilst the metatarsi are targeted by the handler.

If the handler gets caught by one of the feet, trying to unlock the foot grip can be challenging and result in

damage to the raptor, releasing the bird is the best option in this situation.

12.2.3 Sex Determination

Sexual dimorphism is pronounced in falcons and hawks, with females larger than males (Figure 12.10) (Wheeler and Greenwood 1983). Although the difference is obvious when male and female are observed together, it can be challenging when the veterinarian is not experienced with a particular species due to the absence of other obvious external differences. In owls the insectivorous species tend to exhibit less marked size dimorphism than carnivorous species (Mueller 1986).

Plumage colour is different between males and female in some species such as the European and American kestrels, or the sparrow hawk, but this form of sexual dimorphism is relatively uncommon or quite subtle. Animal weight can be used as a guide but with caution due to variations of weight depending on the medical condition or husbandry aspects including falconry training (weight management) and some overlap between the sexes for many species. Table 12.1 includes weights of males and females of common species.

12.2.4 Clinical Examination

Weight should be always obtained as part of the clinical examination, although falconers tend to keep accurate records that can be reviewed whilst obtaining a medical history.

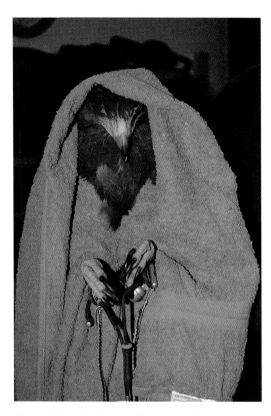

Figure 12.9   Casting of a Harris hawk for restraint.

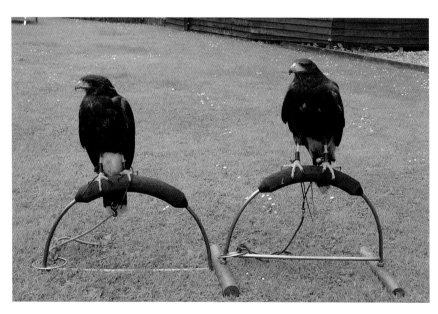

Figure 12.10   Harris hawks on bow perches. Note the smaller size of the male on the left.

A large portion of the clinical examination should be carried out prior to restraint by visual examination; physical restraint is likely to affect the behaviour of the animal making some aspects less rewarding. Clinical examination can be carried out in a restrained individual in most cases, but for large or aggressive birds, or inexperienced handlers, an assistant restraining the bird may facilitate examination.

12.2.4.1 Beak and Oral Cavity

The clinician should be familiar with the normal shape and length of each part of the beak, rhinotheca, covering the maxilla, and gnathotheca, covering the mandible, especially where trimming (also referred to as coping) is requested. Visual abnormalities such as cracks and chips may be linked to inadequate nutrition or abnormal metabolism. Examination of the oral cavity should include the tongue, glottis, and the choanal slit and papillae (in the roof of the mouth).

12.2.4.2 Ears

The external ear canal is covered with feathers and not directly visible without displacing feathers cranially. Symmetry, discharge, and presence of foreign material or parasites should be assessed.

12.2.4.3 Eyes

Sight is a key sense in raptors, visual examination should establish normal movement of the eyelids, with the lower eyelid more mobile, and the nictitating membrane. Symmetry, shape, presence of ocular discharge, or periorbital swellings (often associated with periocular sinus pathologies) can be evaluated. Pupillary light reflexes can be observed but interpretation can be complicated due to voluntary myosis and mydriasis. The pecten (a vascular structure responsible for providing nutrients to the retina) is visible in the posterior chamber on ophthalmic examination, haemorrhage may occur from this structure following head trauma.

12.2.4.4 Respiratory Tract

The area around the nostrils can be evaluated for presence of discharge or obstruction. An operculum is present in most species within the openings of the nares and should not be misinterpreted as a pathological finding (Figure 12.11) (Tully 1995). Changes in the vocalisation may be suggestive of tracheal or syringeal abnormalities. Open mouth breathing, acquiring orthopnoeic postures with the neck overextended and wings slightly open, or increased dorsoventral movement of the tail feathers are commonly associated with dyspnoea. Auscultation is

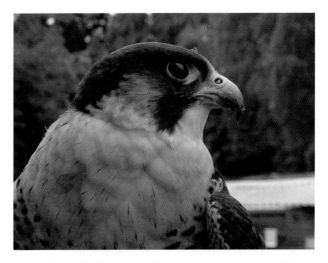

Figure 12.11 A fleshy operculum is present in each nostril and should not be interpreted as an abnormality on examination.

possible but is affected by the rigid nature of the lungs in avian species, preventing the detection of certain sounds noted in mammalian species. Abnormal noises such as clicking may indicate inflammation and adhesions in the air sacs.

A short endurance test can be carried out in falconry birds to evaluate the cardiorespiratory function. The initial heart and respiratory rate are established prior to making the bird flap vigorously for 30 seconds. The respiratory and heart rates should return to resting level after approximately two minutes in a healthy bird (Samour 2006). Exercise may also exacerbate any respiratory noise and repeating auscultation immediately afterwards may increase auscultation sensitivity (Tully 1995).

12.2.4.5 Gastrointestinal Tract

The proximal oesophagus and crop can be palpated to establish the presence of food, inflammation, or masses. In owls, the ventriculus and small intestine can be palpated within the caudal coelom. Feathers around the cloaca should be clean; soiling may be related to gastrointestinal and genitourinary pathologies, or unusual posture or perching. The cloaca can be examined by palpation externally and internally in larger species or visually by partially everting the cloaca mucosa.

12.2.4.6 Genitourinary System

Due to the anatomical location of kidneys and reproductive system in the dorsal coelom, a thorough examination is difficult. Eggs may be palpable in the caudal coelom when egg binding is present, or oviposition is imminent, but should be clearly differentiated from the ventriculus during palpation.

12.2.4.7 Droppings Evaluation

Material expelled through the cloaca is a combination of faeces, urates, and urine, the ratios between the three components may provide information regarding the hydration status or related to polyuria and food intake. Changes in colour, especially in urates and faeces can indicate specific pathologies.

12.2.4.8 Cardiovascular System

Cardiac rate and rhythm can be assessed by auscultation. Heart rate can be affected by environmental conditions, related to the physical examination and husbandry factors such as the levels of fitness associated with the falconry training.

12.2.4.9 Musculoskeletal

Posture should be assessed visually prior to palpation; asymmetries in the wing posture may indicate distortions, fractures, and dislocations whilst leg positioning and digit grip whilst perching aid evaluation of the hindlimbs. Palpation of wings and legs and evaluation of the joints' range of movement should be carried out symmetrically starting from proximal to distal as it is will increase the chances of detecting any abnormalities.

12.2.4.10 Feathers and Uropygial Gland

Feather status can be assessed visually and through feather manipulation; damage to tail feathers and tips of primary feathers may indicate abnormal perching, inappropriate housing, or suboptimal movements of inexperienced birds during hunting. Self-destructive feather damage can be observed in some species, notably Harris Hawks (Figure 12.10), due to abnormal behaviours. Fret marks (horizontal bars across the feather) may indicate nutritional or environmental abnormalities during the previous moult. The uropygial or preen gland is located in the lumbar area, cranial to the insertion of the tail feathers, its shape and size can be evaluated and its normal function and secretion appearance established by applying gentle pressure.

12.3 Basic Techniques

12.3.1 Blood Sampling

Common blood sampling sites in birds of prey are the right jugular vein, the ulnar/basilar vein, and the metatarsal vein. Blood sampling can cause significant stress in conscious birds of prey as firm physical restraint will be required, and this may be an important consideration in sick birds especially those suffering from cardiorespiratory conditions.

For right jugular vein sampling the bird should be securely restrained (by an assistant for larger species), sedated, or anaesthetised. The neck is extended and feathers on the right side separated to identify the featherless apterium overlying the vein (Owen 2011). If the vein is not visible, applying digital pressure to the left side of the neck will push the vein superficially to facilitate the direct observation of the blood vessel. The non-dominant hand applies pressure at the base of the neck to raise the vein whilst keeping the feathers away. The dominant hand collects the sample following needle insertion in a caudal-cranial direction. It is important to prevent any sudden movement from the patient that could cause a laceration in the vein and severe haemorrhage. Pressure is applied following blood sampling using the cervical vertebrae as support to prevent the formation of large haematomas.

For ulnar/basilar vein sampling the bird needs to be sedated or anaesthetised and placed in lateral recumbency with the wing extended (Owen 2011). The vein is located on the medial aspect of the wing, running parallel to the distal humerus and crossing over the proximal radius/ulna, 0.5–1 cm distal to the elbow joint. The vein is very superficial and can be easily observed after parting the feathers in the area. It is a very mobile vessel, which requires stretching the surrounding tissues gently in order to immobilise and raise the vein. Large haematomas are not uncommon, especially if excessive trauma (usually caused by bird movement) occurs, rendering the vessel useless for repeated phlebotomies (Owen 2011). Haemostasis can be challenging in conscious birds due to higher blood pressure, requiring application of digital pressure for several minutes on occasions.

For metatarsal vein access, the bird is firmly restrained, sedated, or anaesthetised and the leg extended. The vein is located in a palpable groove on the medial aspect of the metatarsus. Direct visualisation may be challenging in species with thick scales or feathers covering this area but is enhanced by applying pressure around the proximal metatarsus or distal tibiotarsus to raise the vein.

Heparin is preferred as an anticoagulant for both biochemistry and haematology as EDTA causes haemolysis of erythrocytes (Joseph 1999). Laboratory reference ranges exist for many of the commonly kept species, and consistency of haematology and biochemistry values across raptor species allows for extrapolation of values where a species-specific range is not available (Polo et al. 1992).

12.3.2 Fluid Therapy

Fluids can be administered through intravenous, intraosseous, subcutaneous, or oral routes. Maintenance fluid requirements are 50 ml/kg/day in adults and 75 ml/kg/day in juveniles (Heatley et al. 2001). Requirements are split in four to five slow bolus administrations through the day and isotonic crystalloids available for domestic species are suitable. Continuous fluid infusion can be challenging in avian species as entanglement with the giving set is likely to occur unless the patients can be closely monitored, though very sick subdued animals or hooded birds of prey may be suitable candidates.

Intravenous cannulae are well tolerated and can be placed in the metatarsal and ulnar/basilar veins. Securing the cannula in the medial metatarsal vein can be easily achieved with adhesive tape and the cannula remains accessible (especially in tethered birds), but additional contamination may occur due to proximity with the substrate. For the ulnar/basilar vein, a tab of tape around the cannula is sutured to the skin either side, and around the shaft of one of the secondary feathers to prevent the catheter from bending. An additional wing bandage can also be placed to secure the cannula. For this location usage of an accessible three-way stopcock connected to a Heidelberger extension is beneficial or the bird has to be restrained to access the cannula.

Intraosseous catheters are well tolerated and allow for rapid rehydration of debilitated patients (Dubé et al. 2011). The humerus and femur may be pneumatised, communicating with the respiratory system, and should never be used for fluid therapy. The proximal tibiotarsus or distal ulna are used in birds over 100 g, but placement in smaller individuals has a higher risk of causing iatrogenic fractures. 19–23 gauge hypodermic needles can be used, although specialised intraosseous needles use a stylet which will reduce the likelihood of blockage by osseous material during placement. Anaesthesia and aseptic conditions are required for placement, ongoing analgesia necessary, and catheters should be secured with a bandage (Dubé et al. 2011).

Subcutaneous fluid administration is sufficient for patients with less than 5% dehydration, where no external evidence of dehydration is evident, and boluses should not exceed 20 ml/kg. The skin is thin, relatively inelastic and closely associated to the subcutaneous tissues limiting the locations for the administration of large volumes of fluids. Subcutaneous fluids are best administered in the precrural fold, which is accessed by extending the leg to reveal medial skin folds on the cranial aspect of the femur, and small volumes can also be given superficially in the interscapular region. The interscapular location is used when air sac endoscopy or air sac tube placement has been carried out, or is likely to be required.

Oral fluids can be administered through crop tubing (see Section 12.3.3) but are not appropriate for debilitated animals, or those with greater than 5% dehydration.

12.3.3 Nutritional Support

The Basal metabolic rate (BMR) in kcal/day is calculated based on bodyweight:

$$BMR = 78 \times \left[\text{weight} \left(kg \right) \right]^{0.75}$$

The maintenance energy requirements (MER) in raptors are considered to be 1.25 times the BMR, and sick birds will require more energy, between 1.5 and 2 × MER (Quesenberry and Hillyer 1994).

Whole prey can be offered if the animal has good appetite, skinned day-old chicks can be used for short periods of time during hospitalisation.

For assisted feeding, the amount of food can then be calculated based on energy in the food and split into two to three feeds through the day. Birds should be weighed on a daily basis during hospitalisation and feed intake adapted based on changes.

Commercial carnivore liquid formulas can be administered through a crop tube with ease for non-feeding animals. Blunt metal or plastic tubes can be used for this purpose. An assistant restrains the patient to avoid footing injury or patient trauma. The non-dominant hand then holds the head with the thumb placed between the upper and lower beak at the oral commissure to maintain the mouth open. The other hand guides the tube along the oral cavity towards the oesophagus avoiding the midline glottis that can be clearly visualised at the base of the tongue. The tip of the tube can be palpated at the neck base to ensure that it is in the right location prior to food, fluid or medication administration.

12.3.4 Anaesthesia

Premedication is not common practice in these animals to reduce handling prior to anaesthesia, however sedation using midazolam can be beneficial in nervous individuals, 15–20 minutes prior to anaesthesia. Injectable agents can be used for induction but inhalational anaesthesia is preferred due to convenience and ability to alter depth of anaesthesia rapidly.

Initial induction is carried out under physical restraint by facemask. Endotracheal intubation is then easily carried out as the larynx can be clearly visualised caudal to the tongue base. Tracheal rings are complete and therefore the use of soft, uncuffed tubes is recommended to avoid iatrogenic tracheal damage. Gas flow should be approximately three times the respiratory volume of the patient, and 1–2 l/min is appropriate for mid-sized raptors on a non-rebreathing circuit (Redig et al. 2014).

Isoflurane, sevoflurane, and desflurane have been compared in red-tail hawks (*Buteo jamaicensis*), revealing lower respiratory rates with isoflurane and faster recovery of ocular tracking using sevoflurane and desflurane, though no differences were noted in cardiovascular parameters and temperature (Granone et al. 2012).

Pain recognition in raptors may be challenging and different behaviours may be displayed depending on the species and conditions. In wild red-tailed hawks suffering from skeletal injuries, head movement and beak clacks were reduced (Mazor-Thomas et al. 2014). Analgesia should be provided to any patient where pain could potentially be present, even where overt signs of pain are absent. Buprenorphine, butorphanol, fentanyl, gabapentine, hydromorphone, tramadol, and meloxicam have been evaluated in different bird of prey species.

12.3.5 Euthanasia

Sedation or anaesthesia, followed by intravenous administration of 150 mg/kg pentobarbitone is the recommended method of euthanasia. Intracoelomic or intrahepatic administration of barbiturates can be used when vascular access is not available but should be only carried out in anaesthetised animals based on welfare grounds (Leary et al. 2013).

12.3.6 Hospitalisation

Birds of prey should be hospitalised away from sight and sounds of potential predators like dogs and cats, and also prey animals, such as other avian species, rabbits and rodents. Designing the hospitalisation area with the cages fully enclosed, or covering the access to the cage with screens, will reduce stress for patients.

An appropriate perch should always be available for the hospitalised bird to prevent avoidable damage to tail feathers and the feet. A variety of sizes and types may be required, from falcon block perches, to bow perches resembling a branch, preferred by other species. Small sections of Astroturf can be used to cover the perch, increasing cushioning and allowing thorough cleaning and disinfection of the perching surface between patients (Figure 12.12).

The tail feathers should be protected during hospitalisation as damage and soiling of the feathers may limit the flying capabilities of the raptor until the next feather moult. Flexible plastic or card sheets can be folded around the tail to form a guard, which is taped to the proximal section of the tail feathers to hold it in place. Particularly in larger raptors, e.g. sea eagles or vultures, protection of the carpal region using padding may be advisable to prevent damage to the skin, feathers, and the joint in this region when confined.

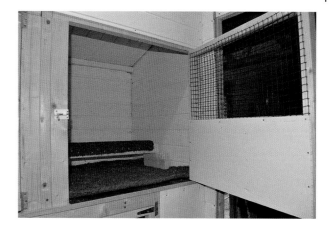

Figure 12.12 Basic hospital cage for small raptor species, note the AstroTurf cover, perch and partially screened door.

12.4 Common Conditions

12.4.1 Viral Diseases

12.4.1.1 Avian Influenza

Raptors may be infected from avian influenza by hunting or scavenging infected birds. Highly pathogenic avian influenza virus, H5N1, has been reported in wild European peregrine falcons, white-tailed sea eagles, and common buzzards associated with non-suppurative encephalitis (Van den Brand et al. 2015). Recently various raptors have succumbed to H5N8 infections (FLI 2017). Positive seroconversion has been observed in raptors in North America (Redig and Goyal 2012) and Middle East (Obon et al. 2009). Current recommendations are to maintain raptors away from wild birds and poultry when an influenza outbreak is imminent or ongoing. In this regard, hunting of avian prey should be suspended. However, there are likely to be welfare implications of maintaining birds in enclosed conditions for a prolonged period and a compromise may need to be reached. Vaccination of hybrid falcons using an inactivated H5N2-specific vaccine has been shown to prevent clinical disease after experimental infection with H5N1 (Lierz et al. 2007).

12.4.1.2 Newcastle Disease

Infection of raptors with this paramyxovirus (APMV-1) may follow contact with, or ingestion of infected prey (especially pigeons) and feeding of pigeons should be discouraged to prevent disease. This virus has shown two different presentations in birds of prey. The generalised form presents with varied symptoms including periorbital swelling and haemorrhagic diarrhoea, and the symptoms of the neurological form include tongue paresis, increased salivation, blindness, unilateral or bilateral paralysis of the nictitans membrane, clonic muscle contractions, ataxia, head tremors, seizures, and death (Samour 2014). Vaccination has been trialled in hybrid falcons, although a small percentage of the vaccinated birds failed to seroconvert. Vertical transmission of antibodies was demonstrated in eggs laid by vaccinated female falcons (Lloyd and Wernery 2008).

12.4.1.3 West Nile Disease

This flavivirus (WNV) is transmitted by mosquitoes and is established in North America, Europe, Africa, the Middle East, Western Asia, and Australasia (WHO 2017). Infection has not yet occurred within the UK and WNV remains a notifiable disease. The primary European vector, *Culex modestus*, has recently been identified within the South-East UK suggesting that incursion of WNV is possible (Golding et al. 2012).

Raptors are highly susceptible to infection and symptoms vary from inapparent to peracute fatal myocarditis and encephalitis (Ziegler et al. 2013). Pathogenicity appears to differ between raptor genera and species (Lopes et al. 2007). Young hawks appear more susceptible than adults, but deaths have been reported also in adults with goshawks appearing predisposed to clinical disease (Wunschmann et al. 2018; Sos-Koroknai 2019). Reports in falcons are more scarce (Wodak et al. 2011). Clinical disease with significant mortality is recognised in natural infection in owls, though experimental infection resulted in a mortality rate of only 14% in Eastern screech owls (Fitzgerald et al. 2003). Recently a dramatically increasing number of lethal infections have been reported in great grey owls and snowy owls (Michel et al. 2019). Clinical signs may be non-specific such as anorexia and weight loss, or associated with encephalitis including ataxia, head tremors, blindness, generalised seizures, and death. Once established in a bird, virus may be transmitted to other birds via the faecal oral route or by direct contact, leading to an epidemic situation (Komar et al. 2003). However, the main transmission involves arthropod vectors. Horizontal transfer did not occur with experimental infection in Screech owls despite confirmed viral shedding (Fitzgerald et al. 2003). Diagnosis is typically made post-mortem using PCR or immunohistochemistry on tissues, particularly the heart and nervous system. Ante-mortem diagnosis of active infection uses serology to demonstrate a rising titre, or viral isolation from blood, oral, and cloacal swabs and feather pulp (Nemeth et al. 2006; Lopes et al. 2007). Treatment of suspected cases is supportive only and presence of a significant antibody titre may be a positive prognostic factor, associated with a protective immune response (Nemeth et al. 2006). Commercially available equine vaccines and experimental DNA vaccines have been shown to reduce mortality,

viraemia, and levels of oral viral shedding in falcons (Angenvoort et al. 2014; Fischer et al. 2015)

12.4.1.4 Herpesvirus

Columbid herpesvirus-1 (CoHV-1) is the most common cause of clinical herpesvirus infections in raptors and disease has been described in many species (Gailbreath and Oaks 2008; Wunschmann et al. 2018). Infection in falcons and owls results from ingestion of asymptomatically infected pigeons with onset of clinical signs 7–10 days later. Feeding of pigeons should be discouraged to prevent the disease in raptors. The seroprevalence in the UK is low to moderate in falcons and owls and very low in hawks, with a greater proportion of seropositive wild birds compared to captive individuals (Zsivanovits et al. 2004). Clinical signs are non-specific, manifesting as weakness, anorexia, green faeces, and sudden death and different serovars demonstrate variable pathogenicity (Zsivanovits et al. 2004). Lesions in the liver, spleen, kidney, pharynx, and bone marrow, in the form of localised foci of necrosis, can be observed during the post-mortem examination (Graham et al. 1975; Ramis et al. 1994; Phalen et al. 2011).

Oral acyclovir has shown efficacy in experimentally infected avian species (Norton et al. 1991) and has also been used in raptors successfully (Joseph 1993). An attenuated vaccine has been trialled in common kestrels with seroconversion and protection demonstrated against experimental infection (Wernery et al. 1999). No vaccine is commercially available currently.

12.4.1.5 Poxvirus

Infection was initially reported in diurnal raptors in the Middle East, transmitted by biting insects or direct exposure in the presence of damaged skin (Samour and Cooper 1993), but infection occurs in many captive and wild raptor species, including owls, in other regions (Deem et al. 1997; Saito et al. 2009). Most exposed birds can mount an effective immune response preventing the development of clinical signs (Wrobel et al. 2016). In clinical cases, exudative proliferative lesions are observed on exposed skin of the head, especially eyelids and cere, and feet. Severe lesions may secondarily impair vision and tendon function in feet. Lesions may become colonised with bacterial and fungal organisms (Wunschmann et al. 2018). Surgical debridement of lesions and supplementation of vitamin A in early stages may mitigate the severity of lesions but most will self-resolve (Deem et al. 1997).

12.4.1.6 Adenovirus

Fatal adenovirus infections are commonly reported in falcons, although other raptors may be affected. Falconid adenovirus-1 has been characterised and established as cause of mortality across various falcon species (Oaks et al. 2005; Kovacs and Benko 2009; Wunschmann et al. 2018). Clinical adenoviral infection associated with Fowl adenovirus-4 has also been reported in wild black kites (*Milvus migrans*) scavenging poultry offal (Kumar et al. 2010). Clinical signs of adenoviral infections include lethargy, anorexia, haemorrhagic enteritis, and neurological changes but death can occur without any clinical signs (Kumar et al. 2010). Hepatomegaly and splenomegaly, with discrete white spots and haemorrhage in gastrointestinal tract, lungs, and reproductive tract can be observed at post-mortem (Zsivanovits et al. 2006; Wunschmann et al. 2018).

12.4.2 Parasitic Disease

12.4.2.1 Ticks

Ixodes frontalis has been associated with mortality in raptors (Monks et al. 2006). The ticks are usually attached around the head where self-removal is limited (Figure 12.13) and are accompanied by bruising and subcutaneous haemorrhages of variable severity. Pathophysiology that leads to the death of some animals is not clearly understood although it has been suggested that unknown bacteria may be involved leading to treatment with oxytetracyclines after removing the tick by some authors (Forbes 2008).

12.4.2.2 Nematodes

Capillaria nematodes are common in raptors, causing white caseous lesions on the tongue, oral mucosa, oesophagus, and occasionally the crop, small intestine, and caecum (Deem 1999). Its life cycle can be direct or indirect, utilising earthworms as intermediate hosts. Diagnosis is based on identification of the characteristic operculated eggs in faecal parasitology or identification of adults and eggs from scrapes collected from oropharyngeal lesions (Globokar et al. 2017). Treatment with fenbendazole or ivermectin has been used successfully.

Syngamus trachea, commonly known as gape worm, can affect birds of prey. Adult worms complete their reproductive cycle in the trachea of the host causing localised irritation and clinical signs such as changes in vocalisations, head shaking, 'cough', or open mouth breathing. Worms can be visualised on tracheoscopy, or eggs identified in faecal samples. Treatment with ivermectin is recommended.

Serratospiculum seurati, *S. amaculata* and *S. tendo* are spirurid nematodes that infect air sacs in falcon and hawks. *Serratospiculum amaculata* has been described in prairie falcons (Ward and Fairchild 1972) whilst *S. seurati* has been described in a variety of species in the Middle East (Tarello 2006). In Europe, *S. tendo* has been reported in peregrine falcons and Northern goshawks (Santoro et al. 2016). Raptors are infected by ingesting beetles that have taken up embryonated eggs. L3 larvae penetrate the proventriculus and ventriculus colonising the air sacs, laid eggs travel to the lungs and are coughed up and swallowed being passed in faeces (Wunschmann et al. 2018). Adult parasites are found in the air sacs and females are relatively large, up to 20 cm long. Falcons affected show poor stamina and laboured breathing. Ivermectin and melarsomine (Tarello 2006) or moxidectin and surgical removal are used for treatment.

12.4.2.3 Trichomonas

Trichomonas gallinae infection occurs following feeding of infected prey, particularly pigeons (Deem 1999). The protozoa cause pale yellow necrotic lesions in the oral cavity and crop, and lesions are visually similar to those caused by *Capillaria*, Salmonellosis, candidiasis, pox, and herpesvirus (Wunschmann et al. 2018). Clinical signs include dysphagia and weight loss (Deem 1999). Fatalities have been observed, especially in young individuals with 14 deaths from 252 cases in one review (Naldo and Samour 2004). Diagnosis is made by direct visualisation of the motile parasites in wet mounts prepared from material scraped from lesions or via PCR. Metronidazole, ronidazole, and carnidazole are used as treatment.

12.4.2.4 Coccidia

Caryospora infections are common in falcons, causing diarrhoea, and less commonly haemorrhagic enteritis, weight loss, and exercise intolerance (Heidenreich 1997). Death may follow due to dehydration. A few reports exist of *Caryospora* infection in owls, including fatalities in Snowy owls (Papazahariadou et al. 2001). *Caryospora*

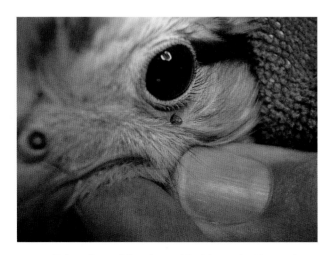

Figure 12.13 Crested Kara kara with tick attached below the lower eyelid.

species are host-specific and tend to be infective to a single genus (Upton and Sundermann 1990). Oocysts may be identified on faecal microscopy, with a subspherical appearance and sporulated oocysts demonstrating a single sporocyst containing eight sporozoites (Papazahariadou et al. 2001). Toltrazuril can be used for treatment, although the in-water poultry formulation may cause regurgitation and oesophagitis if administered neat due to its alkaline pH (Forbes 2008). Toltazuril resistance has been suspected, and clindamycin was a successful alternative therapy in one case (Jones 2010).

12.4.2.5 Cryptosporidium

Cryptosporidium infections appear rare in raptors, with infections described in falcons and Otus owls (*Otus scops*) (Rodríguez-Barbón and Forbes 2007; Van Zeeland et al. 2008; Molina-Lopez et al. 2010). Infections affect the respiratory system and cause associated clinical signs such as tachypnoea, increased respiratory effort and conjunctivitis (Molina-Lopez et al. 2010). Diagnosis is based on cytology or histopathology from affected tissues combined with PCR confirmation. Paromomycin, ponazuril, and azithromycin have been used for therapy with variable success (Rodríguez-Barbón and Forbes 2007).

12.4.2.6 Toxoplasma Gondii

Toxoplasma gondii has been detected in many raptor species without clinical signs of infection (Dubey 2002). Clinical toxoplasmosis has been identified in a single barred owl (*Strix varia*) that was hospitalised following a collision with a car (Mikaelian et al. 1997). The owl was demonstrating anorexia and lethargy and hepatitis associated with *Toxoplasma* tachyzoites was identified post-mortem. However, serological surveys and experimental infections suggest that raptors (including barred owls) are inherently resistant to developing clinical toxoplasmosis (Miller et al. 1972; Lindsay et al. 1991; Dubey et al. 1992; Mikaelian et al. 1997).

12.4.2.7 Haemoparasites

Haemoproteus, Leucocytozoon, Plasmodium, and *Babesia* spp. have been described in raptors (Forbes 2008). Overall prevalence of haemoparasitism in owls appears high but clinical disease is rare (Tavernier et al. 2005; Leppert et al. 2008). The pathogenicity of these parasites is usually low, but severe clinical disease and death have been described in isolated cases, especially in Northern owl species such as snowy owls (Evans and Otter 1998). Treatment with chloroquine or primaquine has been used.

Plasmodium subpraecox has been reported to cause clinical disease in a free-living Eastern Screech Owl (*Megascops*

asio), presenting with weakness, inability to fly, green diarrhoea, and dehydration (Tavernier et al. 2005). Traumatic injury to both eyes, anaemia, hepatomegaly and concurrent *Haemoproteus, Capillaria*, and trematode infestations were found on investigation. On analysis of blood smears, 90% of erythrocytes demonstrated *Plasmodium* infection. Treatment comprised blood transfusion and mefloquine and a rapid clinical improvement was seen.

12.4.3 Fungal Disease

12.4.3.1 Aspergillosis

Aspergillosis is one of the most common infectious respiratory pathologies birds of prey, with the most frequently isolated fungal species *Aspergillus flavus, A. fumigatus*, and *A. niger*. In one retrospective study, aspergillosis accounted for 2.2% of presented falcon cases, and 8% of mortalities (Naldo and Samour 2004).

Disease tends to occur when there is an increased spore load in the environment (decaying or damp organic material) or immunosuppressed birds. Some species appear predisposed, such as gyr falcons, snowy owls, and northern goshawks (Di Somma et al. 2007). Clinical signs include changes or loss of vocalisations, weight loss, increased respiratory effort following exercise (or constantly in advanced cases), open mouth breathing, and orthopnoeic postures. Diagnosis is reached though endoscopy of the trachea, syrinx, and/or air sacs, which allows direct visualisation and biopsy of caseous lesions (Fischer and Lierz 2015). Radiography and haematology are useful adjunctive tests but lack sensitivity and specificity until disease is advanced (Figure 12.14) (Redig 1993). Approach is similar to that in other species and is described in more detail in Chapter 11.

Treatment may combine medical options including antifungal drugs orally or parenterally (e.g. itraconazole or voriconazole) in combination with antifungal inhalation (e.g. enilconazole or F10) for several weeks. Additionally, surgical options such as debridement of lesions and application of topical antifungal treatment in the trachea and air sacs may be necessary. Placement of an air sac cannula is indicated in cases of significant reduction of the tracheal lumen, or during tracheal surgery, to maintain respiratory function.

12.4.3.2 Candidiasis

Candida albicans can cause mucosal ulceration and necrosis of the gastrointestinal tract. Lesions are most commonly identified in the oral cavity, but can develop in the crop and lower gastrointestinal tract complicating diagnosis. Clinical signs include anorexia, dysphagia, regurgitation, weight loss, and lethargy (Deem 1999). Diagnosis is made on microscopy of scrapes from lesions, preferably enhanced by quick staining using Romanovsky or methylene blue stains, and can be treated with nystatin or fluconazole. It is important to be aware that candidiasis is unusual as a pri-

mary pathogen and a primary factor such as prior antibiotic administration, or underlying immunosuppression is often present (Deem 1999).

12.4.3.3 Miscellaneous Infectious Disease

Suspected tetanus has been reported in a gyrfalcon presenting with hyperpnoea, hyperthermia, muscle spasticity, and ventral recumbency (Beaufrère et al. 2016). Concurrent pododermatitis was associated with presence of toxigenic *Clostridium tetani*, but no tetanus toxin could be detected in plasma.

12.4.4 Non-infectious Disease

12.4.4.1 Bumblefoot (Pododermatitis)

Bumblefoot has been recognised for decades as a common condition in captive birds of prey (Halliwell 1975; Riddle 1980). It is more frequently observed in falcons and appears rare in owls. Aetiology is multifactorial with described causes including obesity, poor nutrition, increased weight bearing in a single leg due to medical problems in the contralateral limb, immunosuppression or debilitation, wounds to the plantar aspect of the foot (often caused by excessively long talons or bites from prey), repeat landing trauma, poor perching design, or inadequate hygiene (Remple and Al-Ashbal 1993; Deem 1999). Clinical presentations and associated prognosis are detailed in Table 12.2 and shown in Figure 12.15. Once present this syndrome is progressive and highly unlikely to self-resolve (Remple 1993). Treatment failures are common due to persistence of infection in avascular tissue, ongoing trauma to weight-bearing surface, and an ineffective immune response to

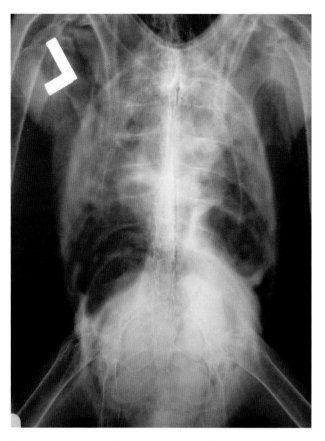

Figure 12.14 Ventrodorsal radiograph of Gyr falcon with air sac aspergillosis. Note the asymmetry and patchy opacity of the air sacs which should appear radiolucent.

Table 12.2 Grading system for bumblefoot in raptors.

Grade	Clinical signs	Prognosis	Treatment
1	Plantar epithelium flattening, hyperemia, localised keratosis	Very good	Address underlying causes, strict hygiene, topical disinfectants, application of creams to soften the skin, bandage application to reduce pressure over affected areas, increase activity to maintain perfusion
2	Subcutaneous tissue infections, scab formation, no signs of localised swelling	Good	As grade 1, plus careful removal of protruding material and addition of antibiotics based on culture and sensitivity.
3	Active inflammation with reddening, increased temperature and swelling of the foot, serous exudate in acute cases, tissue fibrosis in chronic scenarios, caseous material presence, tissue necrosis	Guarded	As grade 2, but surgical debridement is likely to be required
4	Deep infection affecting bone and tendons, arthritis and osteomyelitis	Poor	As grade 3, partial amputations may be required although this may affect weight distribution and aggravate the problem in the opposite limb. Euthanasia should be considered

(a)　　　　　　　　　　(b)　　　　　　　　　　(c)

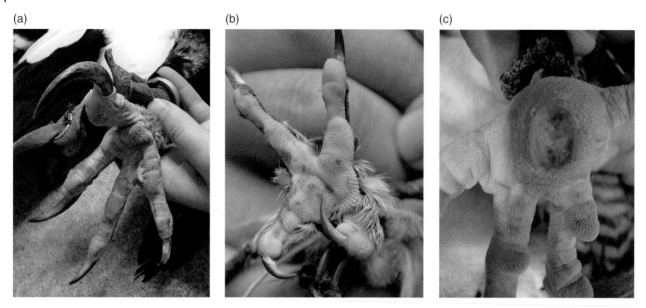

Figure 12.15　(a) Normal appearance of foot in an eagle. (b) Grade 2 bumblefoot in a long-eared owl. (c) Grade 4 bumblefoot with osteomyelitis confirmed radiographically.

lesions (Remple 1993). An aggressive approach may be advisable to achieve optimal results.

Management of any birds presented with bumblefoot should always involve a thorough husbandry review. Some management changes should be advised, including reducing weight of the bird down to its flying weight, providing artificial turf over perches to cushion the feet and allow thorough disinfection, and to continue exercising the bird.

The aims of treatment are to reduce inflammation, remove necrotic and avascular material, eliminate pathogens and facilitate healing.

Application of antiseptic and anti-inflammatory topical treatment on lesions in combination with bandage application may be enough in cases where localised inflammation is present but there is no damage of the epithelium. The aim of the bandage is to redistribute weight from the affected areas whilst reducing environmental contamination. Foam materials can be cut to shape to fit the size and position of the digits and, by cutting out the relevant section of foam, to reduce direct pressure on lesions. The toes can be kept extended, by creating a foam surface that it is cut to fit the extended foot position and held by tape to the toes. Alternatively, toes can be partially flexed by creating a ball of cotton wool reinforced with adhesive bandage, and taping the toes to the ball. Both methods can be alternated if the bandage is required for prolonged periods of time. Maintaining maximal perfusion of the feet is crucial and may be best achieved by flight training or jumping exercises. Additionally topical vasodilatory creams, laser therapy, and leeches have been used to increase vascularisation of the foot pad (Fischer 2011).

Systemic antibiotics may be required in some cases if bacterial involvement is suspected, ideally based on culture and sensitivity results. *Staphlycoccus aureus* is a common finding in these lesions and is not identified in wild birds which rarely suffer with bumblefoot (Remple and Al-Ashbal 1993). It appears that *S. aureus* is a reverse zoonosis in captive raptors that is associated with opportunistic colonisation of compromised tissues, fibrin deposition, and an incomplete immune response in raptors. If infection appears present, radiography is advisable at an early stage to detect extension of pathology into bone as this will have a negative effect on prognosis.

Rupture of the epithelial barrier is very likely to require surgical debridement of necrotic and fibrosed lesions within the soft tissues, as well as application and regular changes of bandages, topical antiseptic ointment application, and increased environment hygiene. Hydrocolloid bandages and ointments can also be used to encourage granulation of open lesions, but primary closure is preferred where possible. Culture and sensitivity from lesions is advised to inform medical management, although due to the encapsulated and poorly vascularised nature of some lesions, the use of intralesional antibiotic impregnated polymethylmethacrylate beads may be preferred to provide a high local concentration of antibiotic (Remple and Forbes 2002).

12.4.4.2　Lead Intoxication

Lead toxicity due to ingestion of prey that has been shot with lead-based ammunition is common in raptors (Cruz-Martinez et al. 2012). Clinical signs vary depending on the species' tolerance and if the exposure is acute or chronic (Redig and Arent 2008; Helander et al. 2009). They include neurological signs such as severe apathy, plantigrade stance, head tilt, ocular twitching, blindness, and seizures, as well as green discolouration of faeces, diarrhoea, haematuria, and gastrointestinal stasis (Fallon et al. 2017; Wunschmann et al. 2018). Diagnosis is made using serum lead levels. Levels should be <10 μg/dl, with 20–60 μg/dl suggestive of subclinical intoxication and levels >60 μg/dl strongly indicative of clinically significant intoxication (Kramer and Redig 1997; Fallon et al. 2017). Supportive haematological changes include a regenerative hypochromic anaemia with cytoplasmatic vacuolization of erythrocytes and heterophilia, whilst clinical chemistry may show hypoproteinemia and elevations in uric acid, lactate dehydrogenase, aspartate transaminase, and creatine kinase (Mautino 1997). Radiographs may demonstrate opaque metal fragments (Figure 12.16), but in some cases these will have been cast

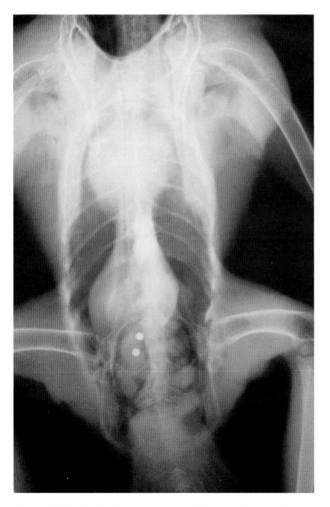

Figure 12.16 Radiodense fragments in the ventriculus of a hawk presenting with neurological symptoms. This is highly suggestive of lead intoxication.

with indigestible food parts or passed in faeces prior to development of clinical signs (Fallon et al. 2017).

Treatment involves supportive care and administration of chelation therapy such Calcium disodium ethylenediaminetetracetate [CaEDTA] (Fallon et al. 2017). Removal of metal particles from the gastrointestinal tract can be considered to prevent ongoing absorption and methods include endoscopic retrieval, proventricular and ventricular flushing under anaesthesia, and administration of laxatives (Heatley et al. 2001).

12.4.4.3 Sour Crop

In the majority of raptors (owls and ospreys excepted), the oesophagus has a well-developed dilation, termed the crop, used for food storage prior to movement into the proventriculus (Duke 1997). If there is a delay in crop emptying, meat is held at body temperature (41 °C) and will putrefy resulting in toxaemia and death (Stanford 2009). In one review of falcons, sour crop made up 0.02% of clinical presentations yet accounted for 2.3% of mortality (Naldo and Samour 2004).

The most common factors associated with sour crop development are overfeeding resulting in crop distension, a sudden diet change, ingluvitis (inflammation of the crop) dehydration, and debilitation. Birds may present with a distended crop and foul smell from the oral cavity and oral fluids, antibiotics and prokinetics can be administered if there is no suspicion of obstruction and the bird is clinically well. If presented collapsed once toxaemia has become established then prognosis is guarded. The patient must be promptly stabilised with fluid therapy, thermal support, and antibiotic administration, to allow the crop to be cleared of putrid meat under anaesthesia as soon as possible. The bird is intubated, the head is maintained elevated above the level of the crop and the food manually massaged back into the mouth and retrieved. Alternatively, the crop is surgically incised, emptied and flushed prior to closure in two layers. In very debilitated patients or if there is significant crop necrosis, an ingluviostomy tube may be placed for ongoing assisted feeding (Kubiak and Forbes 2011a).

12.4.4.4 Wing Tip Oedema

Wing tip oedema (WTO) is a seasonal condition affecting the metacarpus of raptors. Species from warm climates (e.g. Lanner falcons [*Falco biarmicus*] and Harris hawks) are most commonly affected, but any raptor exposed to extreme conditions can develop disease (Kubiak and Forbes 2011b). WTO is precipitated by a period of cold weather and young age, low body condition, and being tethered close to the ground appear predisposing individual factors. Birds present with one or both wings dropped or abducted, a loss of flight performance or swollen, wet, and cold wing tips (Kubiak and Forbes 2011b). Pitting oedema and blisters are often present over the distal wing (Figure 12.17). If untreated, the disruption to blood supply can progress to dry gangrene with the distal wing sloughing, permanently compromising flight.

Initial therapy on presentation involves attempting to re-establish circulation to the wing tip. This includes gentle focal warming, maintaining birds at 15–20 °C, and stimulating wing movement – including flight where possible. Large vesicles can be drained aseptically. Vasodilators such as isoxuprine and propentofylline may be of benefit, with isoxuprine reported to result in a significant increase in recovery rates from 21% to 90% (Forbes 1992; Lewis et al. 1993).

The condition can be avoided by maintaining birds free-flying in aviaries and providing supplemental heat to vulnerable individuals when temperatures are below 5 °C. Providing perching at least 50 cm from the ground is preferred to avoid prolonged proximity to frozen ground. Wet birds should be dried (e.g. by using a hair drier) upon return from hunting prior to placing the bird in its aviary during cold weather.

12.4.5 Ophthalmic Disease

Ocular lesions are common in free-living raptors, comprising 14.5% of all raptors presented for rehabilitation in one study (Murphy et al. 1982; Murphy 1987). Prevalence appears higher in owls, with 75% of free-living Tawny owls (*Strix aluco*) presented to a wildlife centre demonstrating ophthalmic lesions, and abnormalities found on ophthalmic evaluation in 83% of apparently healthy captive screech owls (*M. asio*) (Cousquer 2005; Harris et al. 2008). Trauma is responsible for 90% of the lesions and collisions with vehicles are the predominating cause (Murphy et al. 1982; Cousquer 2005).

Hyphaema is most common but ulceration, blepharitis, uveitis, retinal detachment, cataracts, and pecten trauma may also be seen and a full ocular exam is advisable in all trauma cases (Murphy 1987; Cousquer 2005). It should be noted that a menace response is inconsistently present in birds, the consensual pupillary light response is lacking and the iris contains striated muscle and a degree of voluntary control can be exerted over pupillary size (Murphy 1987). The pecten oculi is an anatomical structure unique to birds which projects from the optic disc into the posterior chamber (Mitkus et al. 2018). Its function is to provide

(a)

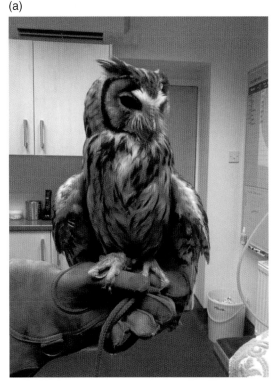

(b)

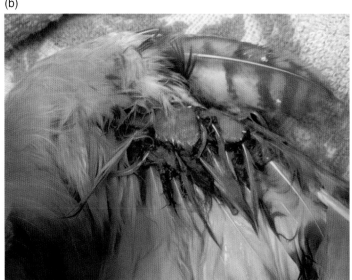

Figure 12.17 (a) Dropped wings on presentation of a striped owl. (b) On examination both wings demonstrated changes consistent with wing tip oedema.

oxygen and nutrients to the avascular retina and hence is highly vascular and mobile. Concussive trauma to the head or eye can result in pecten injury or detachment, with significant haemorrhage and consequential disruption to the visual axis and retinal health. Vitreous haemorrhages can take several months to resolve (Korbel 2000).

The majority of reported cases of corneal ulceration involve owls, reflecting anatomical predisposition with their large eye, prominent corneal surface, rostral eye placement and lack of a lacrimal gland resulting in a comparatively low level of tear production (Murphy 1987). Healing of superficial corneal ulcers is rapid, with resolution in three to five days (Murphy 1987). However deep ulceration is often accompanied by corneal thinning, ulceration, and bullous keratopathy, which can be difficult to manage. Successful treatment of advanced corneal ulceration with bullous keratopathy has been reported in two free-living Great horned owls (*Bubo virginianus*) using keratoplasty and a conjunctival pedicle graft (Gionfriddo and Powell 2006). Both cases required repeat surgeries and prolonged captivity but were eventually deemed suitable for release. A similar approach in the same species was associated in graft dehiscence and globe rupture in another case report (Andrew et al. 2002).

Cataracts may be seen as a degenerative change in geriatric raptors, or due to trauma, developmental abnormality, or inflammatory disease (Brooks 1997). Approaches include conservative management by adapting enclosures to support visual compromise, or invasive corrective procedures including needle aspiration, extracapsular extraction, and phacoemulsification (Kern 1997). A long-term follow up of diurnal raptors following phacoemulsification showed that 78% of treated eyes were visual and concluded that phacoemulsification was a viable technique for raptors (Sigmund et al. 2019). Phacoemulsification with implantation of an artificial lens has been reported in a great horned owl which was subsequently released and monitored for a further six months (Carter et al. 2007).

Glaucoma has been reported in two great horned owls. In one case, the glaucoma was suspected to be secondary to dysplasia of the iridocorneal angle and the owl was euthanised (Rayment and Williams 1997). In the second case, the glaucoma was considered secondary to a mature cataract and uveitis (Sandmeyer et al. 2007). Dorzolamide and timolol topical treatments were unsuccessful in reducing intraocular pressure and unilateral enucleation was necessary. Evisceration of globe contents was carried out and the preserved globe was filled with a silicon prosthesis for cosmetic reasons. Long-term outcome was not determined as the owl died from pneumonia five days later.

12.4.6 Cardiac Disease

Atherosclerosis has is reported to be the most common cardiovascular pathology in raptors and appears a disease of captivity (Jones 2013). Contributing factors include overfeeding, inadequate omega-3 fatty acid intake, reproductive pathology in females, lack of physical activity, and individual species' predisposition (Facon et al. 2014). Reported prevalence in falconiformes varies widely from 4 to 53%, with this variation suspected to be dependent on assessment criteria (Finlayson et al. 1962; Garner and Raymond 2003). Owls have less data available, but prevalence appears lower at 1.1–2.9% (Griner 1983; Garner and Raymond 2003). Birds may be asymptomatic, or develop non-specific symptoms such as lethargy, neurological changes, or respiratory compromise. In severe cases, secondary aortic rupture, myocardial infarction, or cardiomyopathy result in death (Garner and Raymond 2003; Shrubsole-Cockwill et al. 2008; Facon et al. 2014). Conclusive ante-mortem diagnosis remains difficult and comprises imaging techniques and serum biochemistry. Vascular opacity or mineralisation, and cardiomegaly, may be seen radiographically in advanced cases. Ultrasonography or CT can also be used to assess the aorta, brachiocephalic, and pulmonary arteries for lesions (Beaufrère 2013). Increased serum cholesterol and low-density lipoprotein levels may be noted on biochemistry. Electrocardiography may identify myocardial conduction disruption where ischaemia or cardiomyopathy is a secondary consequence of altered blood flow (Beaufrère 2013). Improving diet and gradually increasing activity are the mainstay of management. Statins have been used in parrots, but there is no pharmacokinetic data to support dosing schedules in raptors.

Little published information is available on myocardial diseases in captive raptors. In the authors' experience cardiomegaly is a common finding at post-mortem in geriatric owls and ante-mortem clinical signs include reduced flight ability and regurgitation of large meals. In one study in red tailed hawks, transoesophageal echocardiography was considered superior to the transcoelomic approach for assessing cardiac morphology. However, even with this approach there was significant variation between individual clinicians when assessing cardiac measurements and this was considered a relatively unreliable technique for objective assessment (Beaufrère et al. 2012). Ultrasonography remains valuable in subjective assessment of suspected cardiac pathology with altered contractility, chamber size, and effusions able to be identified.

12.4.7 Fractures

A full review of fracture repairs is outside the scope of this chapter, but the most frequent presentations are discussed.

Tibiotarsal fractures are the most common type of orthopaedic injury seen in captive raptors (Harcourt-Brown 1996). These are predominantly an injury of newly tethered birds, as birds unaccustomed to tethering may bate (fly away from) their perch before being stopped mid-flight by the tethering leash. This is associated with shearing forces applied to the legs and fracture of the tibiotarsus at the level of the distal fibular crest due to an inherent weakness at this point (Harcourt-Brown 1996). Birds typically present as unilaterally non-weight bearing, with bilateral injury rare. Palpable instability is common though extensive soft tissue swelling and bruising may hinder this. Radiography is necessary to confirm diagnosis and plan surgery.

A tie-in hybrid fixator (Figure 12.18) combines an intramedullary (IM) and external skeletal fixator (ESF)

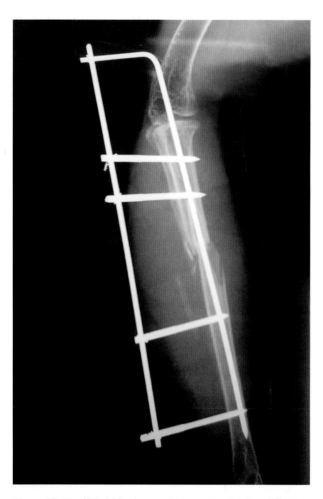

Figure 12.18 Hybrid fixator used to repair a tibiotarsal fracture in a Harris hawk.

to provide rotational and longitudinal stability, without the restriction of a splint (Redig 2000). This type of fixation has a reported success rate of 84% for tibiotarsal fractures in raptors (Bueno et al. 2015). For the open technique, an incision is made on the medial aspect of the leg and the muscle layers bluntly reflected to access the fracture site. An IM pin is passed retrograde into the proximal fragment and out of the cranial aspect of the flexed stifle, then advanced normograde into the distal fragment. For the closed approach, the IM pin is inserted through the lateral condyle of the proximal tibiotarsus and advanced whilst the fragments are manually held in alignment (Muller and Mohammed 2015). Following either approach two threaded ESF pins (or Kirshner wires for small species) are then placed lateral to medial in both the proximal and distal fragments through both cortices, but not through the soft tissue and skin on the medial aspect, resulting in a type I ESF. The proximal end of the IM pin is bent at around 90°, 5 mm from the exit point, and directed laterally, to allow the ESF and IM pins to be joined with a straight bar. This is secured with a FESSA system, or cerclage wires overlain with methylmethacrylate at the junctions (Muller and Mohammed 2015). The IM pin is removed 10 days following initial surgery if radiographs and palpation confirm callus formation and absence of complications, and the ESF pins two weeks later.

As tibiotarsal fractures are primarily due to poor management, husbandry changes can reduce occurrence. Birds should not be tethered prior to skeletal maturity, especially Harris hawks, with a minimum age of four months advisable prior to tethering (Maier and Fischer 2018). Short leashes limit flight distance and, hence, speed and force achieved. Bow perches increase incidence as potential flight length is greater compared with block perches, which are preferable for initial tethering (Kubiak and Forbes 2011b). Confinement at first tethering reduces the stimulus (and limits the distance) for flight and, hence, trauma at impact; this can later be increased as the bird adapts to tethering.

Coracoid fractures are occasionally seen as a consequence of in-flight collisions (Scheelings 2014). Birds typically present with an inability to fly and a dropped wing may be evident on examination (Holz 2003). Radiography of the pectoral girdle using orthogonal views allows assessment of this short bone that runs from the cranial sternum to the head of the humerus (Redig and Ponder 2016). Concurrent injuries to the surrounding bones and soft tissues are common complicating factors. Much has been reported on comparative success of surgical fixation and conservative management. Surgical fixation using normograde placement of an IM pin has been associated with variable success rates (34–75%) and one study reported an intraoperative mortality rate of 52%, relating to concurrent non-surgical soft tissue injuries (Holz 2003; Scheelings 2014). A recent review reported 97% success rate with conservative management of coracoid fractures in wild raptors (Cracknell et al. 2018). Conservative management in this review typically comprised two to three weeks confinement in a cage that did not permit full wing extension, plus analgesia, followed by movement to an aviary to allow flight resumption and release 24–27 days after presentation. No external coaptation was used and muscle mass support alone is considered adequate for this type of fracture (Scheelings 2014). Although individual studies show some variation in success rates for both approaches, the general consensus is that conservative management is appropriate for the majority of coracoid fractures (Redig and Ponder 2016).

Repair of humeral and femoral fractures is more challenging and is described in detail by Redig and Ponder (2016). Conventional treatment using body wrap bandages is usually not sufficient and surgery is necessary to restore full ability. In most cases an IM and ESF similar to the descriptions above for tibiotarsal fractures is applicable.

12.5 Preventative Health Measures

Submission of faecal samples on a regular basis, at least twice annually, for parasitological examination in raptors is advisable especially if birds are used for falconry as they are likely to have an increased exposure to wild specimens with higher burdens of parasites. The presence of parasites may not be an indication for treatment, especially if clinical signs are not present but may need to be considered in periods of higher stress for the bird such as the moult or falconry training, and in juvenile individuals.

12.6 Radiographic Imaging

Anaesthesia is often necessary in order to obtain adequate positioning for diagnostic radiography.

Whole body radiographs are obtained in ventrodorsal and lateral positions. For the ventrodorsal view the bird is placed in dorsal recumbency, with wings and legs partially extended. In order to obtain good symmetry, the keel and the vertebral column should be superimposed. Positioning for the lateral view is obtained by placing the bird in lateral recumbency extending the wings dorsally and legs caudally in an asymmetrical position to prevent overlapping; adequate positioning requires superposition of both coxofemoral joints.

There are few pharmacokinetic and pharmacodynamic studies that have been carried out in raptors and it is important that there may be significant variations between species despite the taxonomic proximity. The formulary offers a list of different drugs that have been evaluated in raptors or have been used regularly in practice.

Formulary

Drug	Dose mg/kg (unless indicated otherwise)	Route of administration	Frequency	Species	Comments	References
Anaesthesia						
Isoflurane	3.8% for induction, 1.2–1.5% for maintenance	Inhalation		Red tailed hawk	Mean induction time 226 s, rapid, smooth induction and recovery	Granone et al. (2012)
Sevoflurane	5.75% for induction, 2.2–2.4% for maintenance	Inhalation		Red tailed hawk	Mean induction time 218 s, faster normalisation of response to visual stimuli than with isoflurane	Granone et al. (2012)
Medetomidine/ketamine	0.1 (M), 10 (K)	IM		Common buzzard	Significant decreases in heart and respiratory rates, medetomidine reversed with 0.5 mg/kg atipamezole and recovery satisfactory/poor in all cases	Kilic and Paşa (2009)
Dexmedetomidine	25 µg/kg	IM		Common buzzard	Sedation for intubation, maintained on 1% isoflurane. Reversed with atipamezole for rapid recovery	Santangelo et al. (2009)
Dexmedetomidine	75 µg/kg	IM		Common kestrel	Sedation for intubation, maintained on 1% isoflurane. Reversed with atipamezole for rapid recovery	Santangelo et al. (2009)
Propofol	3.39–5.57 as 1 mg/kg/min infusion	IV		Red tailed hawk	Induction dose. 0.48 mg/kg/min used for maintenance by constant rate infusion. Respiratory suppression and prolonged recovery noted	Hawkins et al. (2003)
Propofol	10	IV		Common buzzard	Given over 1 minute to induce, repeated boluses of 2–4 mg/kg used for maintenance. Apnoea seen at induction	Kilic and Paşa (2009)
Propofol	2.65–4.07	IV		Great horned owl	Induction dose. 0.56 mg/kg/min used for maintenance by constant rate infusion. Respiratory suppression and prolonged recovery noted	Hawkins et al. (2003)
Tiletamine/zolazepam	10	IM		Great horned owl, Eastern screech owl	Rapid induction, prolonged recovery. Doses up to 40 mg/kg IM ineffective in red tailed hawks	Kreeger et al. (1993)
Tiletamine/zolazepam	40 mg/kg of 1 : 1 solution	PO		Common buzzard	Sedation protocol for free-living birds, using medicated bait	Janovsky et al. (2002)
Analgesia						
Buprenorphine hydrochloride	0.1–0.6	IM, IV	0.5–6 hours	American kestrel	Single dose pharmacokinetic study, no information on nociception	Ceulemans et al. (2014), Gustavsen et al. (2014)
Buprenorphine sustained release	1.8	IM, SC	24 hours	American kestrel	Single dose pharmacokinetic study, no information on nociception	Guzman et al. (2017)
Butorphanol	1–6	IM	NA	American kestrel	Single dose study, no effect increasing thermal withdrawal threshold, hyperaesthesia and agitation at high dose	Guzman et al. (2014a)
Butorphanol	0.5	IM, IV	1 hour	Red tailed hawk	Very short half life	Riggs et al. (2008)

Drug	Dose (mg/kg)	Route	Frequency	Species	Notes	Reference
Fentanyl	10–30 μg/kg/min	IV	NA	Red tailed-hawk	Reduced isoflurane MAC	Pavez et al. (2011)
Gabapentin	11	PO	12 hours	Prairie falcons	Self-mutilation therapy	Shaver et al. (2009)
Hydromorphone	0.1–0.6	IM. IV	3–6 hours	American kestrel	Single dose study, sedation at high doses	Guzman et al. (2013)
Tramadol	5	PO	1.5 hours	American kestrel	Single dose resulted in an increase in thermal withdrawal threshold	Guzman et al. (2014b)
Tramadol	11	PO	4 hours	Red tailed-hawk	Maintained human therapeutic plasma concentrations, no information regarding nociception	Souza et al. (2011)
Tramadol	11	PO	12 hours	American bald eagle	Sedation observed with multiple doses	Souza et al. (2009)
Meloxicam	0.5	IV, PO	NA	Red tailed-hawk	Very fast half life elimination 30 minutes average	Lacasse et al. (2013)
Antimicrobials						
Amoxicillin-clavulanate	150	PO, IM	12hrs	Raptors		Chitty (2002)
Acyclovir	80	PO	TID	Peregrine falcon	Juvenile birds, no significant improvement in herpesvirus related morbidity and mortality	Forbes and Simpson (1997)
Amikacin	15–20 per day	IM	divide daily dose every 8–12 hours	Red tailed-hawk	Single dose study,	Bloomfield et al. (1997)
Ceftiofur extended release	10–20	IM	36–96 hours	Red tailed-hawk	Plasma levels maintained for 36–45 hours at 10mg/kg, for 96 hours at 20mg/kg	Sadar et al. (2014)
Enrofloxacin	15	IM, PO	24 hours	Red-tailed hawk, great horned owl	Intravenous route resulted in adverse effects in great horned owls and is not recommended	Harrenstien et al. (2000)
Gentamicin	2.5	IM	8 hours	Red tailed-hawk, golden eagle	Single dose study	Bird et al. (1983)
Marbofloxacin	10	PO	24 hours	Eurassian buzzard	Using 0.25 μg/ml as MIC	Garcia-Montijano et al. (2003)
Piperacillin	100	IM	4–6 hours	Red tailed hawk	Using 8 μg/ml as MIC	Robbins et al. (2000)
Itraconazole	10	PO	24 hours	Red tailed hawk	Steady plasma concentrations after 2 weeks	Jones et al. (2000)
Ketoconazole	60	PO	12 hours	Eurasian buzzard	Aspergillosis treatment	Wagner et al. (1991)

(Continued)

(Continued)

Drug	Dose mg/kg (unless indicated otherwise)	Route of administration	Frequency	Species	Comments	References
Nystatin	100000IU	PO	8 hours	Raptors	Candidiasis	Deem (1999)
Terbinafine	22	PO	24 hours	Red tailed hawk	Single dose study, 0.8–1.6 8µg/ml as MIC	Bechert et al. (2010)
Voriconazole	10	PO	8 hours	Red tailed hawk	Multiple dose study, 1µg/ml as MIC	Gentry et al. (2014)
Voriconazole	12.5	PO	12 hours	Falcons	Based on successful treatment of clinical cases. Trough values may be below 1µg/ml	Di Somma et al. (2007), Schmidt et al. (2007)
Antiparasitics						
Carnidazole	50	PO	once	Unspecified	For Trichomoniasis. Alternate dose of 20mg/kg PO daily for two doses	Huckabee (2000)
Clindamycin	50	PO	12hrs for 5 days	Peregrine falcon	Alternative treatment for *Caryospora* infection resistant to toltrazuril	Jones (2010)
Fenbendazole	15–25	PO	24 hours	Falcons	5–8 days, elimination of *Serratospiculum* eggs and larvae from faeces. Toxic effects include severe immunosuppression. Use with caution in vultures.	Al-Timimi et al. (2009)
Imidocarb dipropionate	5–7	IM	Once repeat in 7 days	Peregrine falcon	*Babesia* treatment	Samour et al. (2005)
Ivermectin	0.4	IM	7days, 4 treatments	Golden eagle	*Micnemidocoptes* spp. treatment	Sadar et al. (2015)
Ivermectin	1	IM	Once	Falcons	Serratospiculum treatment, combined with melarsomine	Tarello (2006)
Ivermectin	2	IM	Once	Peregrine falcon	*Serratospiculum* treatment	Veiga et al. (2017)
Ivermectin	2	IM	Once	Falcons	*Capillaria* treatment	Tarello (2008)
Selamectin	23	TO	8days, 4 treatments	Golden eagle	*Micnemidocoptes* spp. treatment	Sadar et al. (2015)
Mefloquine	30	PO	At 0, 12, 24, and 48hrs	Eastern Screech Owl	For treatment of *Plasmodium* infection	Tavernier et al. (2005)
Melarsomine	0.25	IM	24 hours for 2 days	Falcons	*Serratospiculum* treatment, combined with ivermectin	Tarello (2006)
Metronidazole	100	PO	24 hours for 3 days	Falcons	*Trichomonas* treatment	Samour and Naldo (2003)
Paromomycin	100	PO	12 hours	Falcons	*Cryptosporidium* treatment	Rodríguez-Barbón and Forbes (2007)

Drug	Dose	Route	Frequency	Species	Indication	Reference
Ponazuril	20	PO	24 hours for 7 days	Falcons	*Cryptosporidium* treatment	Van Sant and Stewart (2009)
Primaquine	0.75	PO	24 hours for 5 days	Falcons	*Haemoproteus tinnunculi* treatment	Tarello (2007)
Toltrazuril	25	PO	Once	Falcons	Treatment for *Caryospora*. For endemic infections, targeted therapy of adults prior to laying and in juveniles at 21 and 35 days of age is recommended	Forbes and Fox (2000)
Miscellaneous						
Calcium disodium ethylenediaminetetracetate	50	IM	12 hours for 2–23 days	Falcons	Lead intoxication	Samour and Naldo (2002)
Pralidoxime (2-PAM)	100	IM	Once	Raptors	Monocrotophos toxicosis	Shlosberg (1976)
Vitamin K1	2.5	SC	12 hours	Red tailed hawk	Anticoagulant intoxication	Murray and Tseng (2008)
Allopurinol	25	PO	24 hours	Red tailed hawk	Failed to decrease plasma uric acid levels	Poffers et al. (2002a)
Urate oxidase	100–200 U/kg	IM	24 hours	Red tailed hawk	Lowered plasma uric acid	Poffers et al. (2002b)
Pimobendan	0.25	PO	12 hours	Harris hawk	Congestive heart failure management	Brandão et al. (2016)

References

Al-Timimi, F., Nolosco, P., and Al-Timimi, B. (2009). Incidence and treatment of serratospiculosis in falcons from Saudi Arabia. *Veterinary Record* 165 (14): 408–410.

Andrew, S.E., Clippinger, T.L., Brooks, D.E. et al. (2002). Penetrating keratoplasty for treatment of corneal protrusion in a great horned owl (*Bubo virginianus*). *Veterinary Ophthalmology* 5 (3): 201–205.

Angenvoort, J., Fischer, D., Fast, C. et al. (2014). Limited efficacy of West Nile virus vaccines in large falcons (*Falco* spp.). *Veterinary Research* 45 (1): 41.

Beaufrère, H. (2013). Avian atherosclerosis: parrots and beyond. *Journal of Exotic Pet Medicine* 22 (4): 336–347.

Beaufrère, H., Pariaut, R., Rodriguez, D. et al. (2012). Comparison of transcoelomic, contrast transcoelomic, and transesophageal echocardiography in anesthetized red-tailed hawks (*Buteo jamaicensis*). *American Journal of Veterinary Research* 73 (10): 1560–1568.

Beaufrère, H., Laniesse, D., Stickings, P. et al. (2016). Generalized tetanus in a gyrfalcon (*Falco rusticolus*) with pododermatitis. *Avian Diseases* 60 (4): 850–855.

Bechert, U., Christensen, J.M., Poppenga, R. et al. (2010). Pharmacokinetics of terbinafine after single oral dose administration in red-tailed hawks (*Buteo jamaicensis*). *Journal of Avian Medicine and Surgery* 24 (2): 122–130.

Bird, J.E., Miller, K.W., Larson, A.A. et al. (1983). Pharmacokinetics of gentamicin in birds of prey. *American Journal of Veterinary Research* 44 (7): 1245–1247.

Bloomfield, R.B., Brooks, D., and Vulliet, R. (1997). The pharmacokinetics of a single intramuscular dose of amikacin in red-tailed hawks (*Buteo jamaicensis*). *Journal of Zoo and Wildlife Medicine* 28 (1): 55–61.

Brandão, J., Reynolds, C.A., Beaufrère, H. et al. (2016). Cardiomyopathy in a Harris hawk (*Parabuteo unicinctus*). *Journal of the American Veterinary Medical Association* 249 (2): 221–227.

Brooks, D.E. (1997). Avian cataracts. *Seminars in Avian and Exotic Pet Medicine* 6: 131.

Bueno, I., Redig, P.T., and Rendahl, A.K. (2015). External skeletal fixator intramedullary pin tie-in for the repair of tibiotarsal fractures in raptors: 37 cases (1995–2011). *Journal of the American Veterinary Medical Association* 247 (10): 1154–1160.

Carter, R.T., Murphy, C.J., Stuhr, C.M. et al. (2007). Bilateral phacoemulsification and intraocular lens implantation in a great horned owl. *Journal of the American Veterinary Medical Association* 230 (4): 559–561.

Ceulemans, S.M., Guzman, D.S., Olsen, G.H. et al. (2014). Evaluation of thermal antinociceptive effects after intramuscular administration of buprenorphine hydrochloride to American kestrels (*Falco sparverius*). *American Journal of Veterinary Research* 75: 705–710.

Chitty, J.C. (2002). Birds of prey. In: *BSAVA Manual of Exotic Pets*, 4e (eds. A. Meredith and S. Redrobe), 179–192. British Small Animal Veterinary Association.

Cousquer, G. (2005). Ophthalmological findings in free-living tawny owls (*Strix aluco*) examined at a wildlife veterinary hospital. *Veterinary Record* 156 (23): 734–739.

Cracknell, J.M., Lawrie, A.M., Yon, L. et al. (2018). Outcomes of conservatively managed coracoid fractures in wild birds in the United Kingdom. *Journal of Avian Medicine and Surgery* 32 (1): 19–25.

Cruz-Martinez, L., Redig, P.T., and Deen, J. (2012). Lead from spent ammunition: a source of exposure and poisoning in bald eagles. *Human-Wildlife Interactions* 6: 94–100.

Deem, S.L. (1999). Infectious and parasitic diseases of raptors. *Compendium on Continuing Education for the Practicing Veterinarian* 21 (4): 329–338.

Deem, S.L., Heard, D.J., and Fox, J.H. (1997). Avian pox in eastern screech owls and barred owls from Florida. *Journal of Wildlife Diseases* 33 (2): 323–327.

Di Somma, A., Bailey, T., Silvanose, C. et al. (2007). The use of voriconazole for the treatment of aspergillosis in falcons (*Falco* species). *Journal of Avian Medicine and Surgery* 21 (4): 307–317.

Dubé, C., Dubois, I., and Struthers, J. (2011). Intravenous and intraosseous fluid therapy in critically ill birds of prey. *Journal of Exotic Pet Medicine* 20 (1): 21–26.

Dubey, J.P. (2002). A review of toxoplasmosis in wild birds. *Veterinary Parasitology* 106 (2): 121–153.

Dubey, J.P., Porter, S.L., Tseng, F. et al. (1992). Induced toxoplasmosis in owls. *Journal of Zoo and Wildlife Medicine* 23 (1): 98–102.

Duke, G.E. (1997). Gastrointestinal physiology and nutrition in wild birds. *Proceedings of the Nutrition Society* 56 (3): 1049–1056.

Evans, M. and Otter, A. (1998). Fatal combined infection with *Haemoproteus noctuae* and *Leucocytozoon ziemanni* in juvenile snowy owls (*Nyctea scandiaca*). *Veterinary Record* 143 (3): 72–76.

Facon, C., Beaufrere, H., Gaborit, C. et al. (2014). Cluster of atherosclerosis in a captive population of black kites (*Milvus migrans* subsp.) in France and effect of nutrition on the plasma lipid profile. *Avian Diseases* 58 (1): 176–182.

Fallon, J.A., Redig, P., Miller, T.A. et al. (2017). Guidelines for evaluation and treatment of lead poisoning of wild raptors. *Wildlife Society Bulletin* 41 (2): 205–211.

Finlayson, R., Symons, C., and TW-Fiennes, R.N. (1962). Atherosclerosis: a comparative study. *British Medical Journal* 1 (5277): 501.

Fischer, D. (2011). Sohlenballengeschwüre bei Vögeln – Ein häufiges Problem in menschlicher Haltung. *Wildtierzeit* 1: 24–28.

Fischer, D. and Lierz, M. (2015). Diagnostic procedures and available techniques for the diagnosis of aspergillosis in birds. *Journal of Exotic Pet Medicine* 24 (3): 283–295.

Fischer, D., Angenvoort, J., Ziegler, U. et al. (2015). DNA vaccines encoding the envelope protein of West Nile virus lineages 1 or 2 administered intramuscularly, via electroporation and with recombinant virus protein induce partial protection in large falcons (*Falco* spp.). *Veterinary Research* 46 (August 17): 87.

Fitzgerald, S.D., Patterson, J.S., Kiupel, M. et al. (2003). Clinical and pathologic features of West Nile virus infection in native North American owls (family Strigidae). *Avian Diseases* 47 (3): 602–610.

FLI (2017). Avian Influenza (AI)/Fowl Plague, May 02 2017 update, https://www.fli.de/en/news/animal-disease-situation/avian-influenza-ai-fowl-plague (accessed 2 August 2019).

Forbes, N.A. (1992). Wing tip oedema and dry gangrene in birds of prey. Proceedings of the Raptor Research Foundation Conference. Bellevue, WA, USA, 11–12 November.

Forbes, N. (2008). Raptors: parasitic disease. In: *BSAVA Manual of Raptors, Pigeons and Passerine Birds* (eds. J. Chitty and M. Lierz), 202–211. Gloucester, UK: British Small Animal Veterinary Association.

Forbes, N.A. and Fox, M.T. (2000). Control of endemic *Caryospora* species infestation of captive raptors. Proceedings of the Annual Conference of the Association of Avian Veterinarians: 173–179.

Forbes, N.A. and Simpson, G.N. (1997). A review of viruses affecting raptors. *The Veterinary Record* 141 (5): 123–126.

Ford, S. (2010). Raptor gastroenterology. *Journal of Exotic Pet Medicine* 19 (2): 140–150.

Gailbreath, K.L. and Oaks, J.L. (2008). Herpesviral inclusion body disease in owls and falcons is caused by the pigeon herpesvirus (Columbid herpesvirus 1). *Journal of Wildlife Diseases* 44 (2): 427–433.

García-Montijano, M., González, F., Waxman, S. et al. (2003). Pharmacokinetics of marbofloxacin after oral administration to Eurasian buzzards (*Buteo buteo*). *Journal of Avian Medicine and Surgery* 17 (4): 185–191.

Garner, M.M. and Raymond, J.T. (2003). A retrospective study of atherosclerosis in birds. Proceedings of the Annual Conference of the Association of Avian Veterinarians: 59–66.

Gentry, J., Montgerard, C., Crandall, E. et al. (2014). Voriconazole disposition after single and multiple oral doses in healthy, adult red-tailed hawks (*Buteo jamaicensis*). *Journal of Avian Medicine and Surgery* 28 (3): 201–209.

Gionfriddo, J.R. and Powell, C.C. (2006). Primary closure of the corneas of two great horned owls after resection of nonhealing ulcers. *Veterinary Ophthalmology* 9 (4): 251–254.

Globokar, M., Fischer, D., and Pantchev, N. (2017). Occurrence of endoparasites in captive birds between 2005 to 2011 as determined by faecal flotation and review of literature. *Berliner und Münchener Tierärztliche Wochenschrift* 130: 11–12.

Golding, N., Nunn, M.A., Medlock, J.M. et al. (2012). West Nile virus vector *Culex modestus* established in southern England. *Parasites & Vectors* 5 (1): 32.

Graham, D.L., Mare, C.J., Ward, F.P. et al. (1975). Inclusion body disease (herpesvirus infection) of falcons (IBDF). *Journal of Wildlife Diseases* 11: 83–91.

Granone, T.D., de Francisco, O.N., Killos, M.B. et al. (2012). Comparison of three different inhalant anesthetic agents (isoflurane, sevoflurane, desflurane) in red-tailed hawks (*Buteo jamaicensis*). *Veterinary Anaesthesia and Analgesia* 39 (1): 29–37.

Griner, L.A. (1983). Birds. In: *Pathology of Zoo Animals* (ed. L.A. Griner), 94–267. San Diego, CA: Zoological Society of San Diego.

Gustavsen, K.A., Guzman, D.S., Knych, H.K. et al. (2014). Pharmacokinetics of buprenorphine hydrochloride following intramuscular and intravenous administration to American kestrels (*Falco sparverius*). *American Journal of Veterinary Research* 75: 711–715.

Guzman, D.S., Drazenovich, T.L., Olsen, G.H. et al. (2013). Evaluation of thermal antinociceptive effects after intramuscular administration of hydromorphone hydrochloride to American kestrels (*Falco sparverius*). *American Journal of Veterinary Research* 74 (6): 817–822.

Guzman, D.S., Drazenovich, T., KuKanich, B. et al. (2014a). Evaluation of thermal antinociceptive effects and pharmacokinetics after intramuscular administration of butorphanol tartrate to American kestrel (*Falco sparverius*). *American Journal of Veterinary Research* 75 (1): 11–18.

Guzman, D.S., Drazenovich, T., KuKanich, B. et al. (2014b). Evaluation of thermal antinociceptive effects after oral administration of tramadol hydrochloride to American kestrels (*Falco sparverius*). *American Journal of Veterinary Research* 75 (2): 117–123.

Guzman, D.S., Knych, H.K., Olsen, G.H. et al. (2017). Pharmacokinetics of a sustained release formulation of buprenorphine after intramuscular subcutaneous administration to American kestrels (*Falco sparverius*). *Journal of Avian Medicine and Surgery* 31 (2): 102–107.

Halliwell, W.H. (1975). Bumblefoot infections in birds of prey. *The Journal of Zoo Animal Medicine* 6 (4): 8–10.

Harcourt-Brown, N.H. (1996). Foot and leg problems. In: *Manual of Raptors, Pigeons and Waterfowl* (eds. P.H. Beynon, N.A. Forbes and N.H. Harcourt-Brown), 147–168. Ames, IA: Iowa State University Press.

Harrenstien, L.A., Tell, L.A., Vulliet, R. et al. (2000). Disposition of enrofloxacin in red-tailed hawks (*Buteo jamaicensis*) and great horned owls (*Bubo virginianus*) after a single oral, intramuscular, or intravenous dose. *Journal of Avian Medicine and Surgery* 14 (4): 228–237.

Harris, M.C., Schorling, J.J., Herring, I.P. et al. (2008). Ophthalmic examination findings in a colony of screech owls (*Megascops asio*). *Veterinary Ophthalmology* 11 (3): 186–192.

Hawkins, M.G., Wright, B.D., Pascoe, P.J. et al. (2003). Pharmacokinetics and anesthetic and cardiopulmonary effects of propofol in red-tailed hawks (*Buteo jamaicensis*) and great horned owls (*Bubo virginianus*). *American Journal of Veterinary Research* 64 (6): 677–683.

Heatley, J.J., Marks, S., Mitchell, M. et al. (2001). Raptor emergency and critical care: therapy and techniques. *Compendium on Continuing Education for the Practising Veterinarian – North American Edition* 23 (6): 561–572.

Heidenreich, M. (1997). Parasitic diseases. In: *Birds of Prey, Medicine and Management* (eds. M. Heidenreich and Y. Oppenheim), 131–152. Oxford: Blackwell Science.

Helander, B., Axelsson, J., Borg, H. et al. (2009). Ingestion of lead from ammunition and lead concentrations in white-tailed sea eagles (*Haliaeetus albicilla*) in Sweden. *Science of the Total Environment* 407 (21): 5555–5563.

Holz, P.H. (2003). Coracoid fractures in wild birds: repair and outcomes. *Australian Veterinary Journal* 81 (8): 469–471.

Huckabee, J.R. (2000). Raptor therapeutics. *The Veterinary Clinics of North America. Exotic Animal Practice* 3 (1): 91–116.

Janovsky, M.A., Ruf, T.H., and Zenker, W.O. (2002). Oral administration of tiletamine/zolazepam for the immobilization of the common buzzard (*Buteo buteo*). *Journal of Raptor Research* 36 (3): 188–193.

Jones, R. (2010). Vet's personal perspective on debilitating disease in falcons. *Veterinary Times* 40 (33): 14–17.

Jones, M.P. (2013). Vascular diseases in birds of prey. *Journal of Exotic Pet Medicine* 22 (4): 348–357.

Jones, M.P., Orosz, S.E., Cox, S.K. et al. (2000). Pharmacokinetic disposition of itraconazole in red-tailed hawks (*Buteo jamaicensis*). *Journal of Avian Medicine and Surgery* 14 (1): 15–23.

Joseph, V. (1993). Raptor pediatrics. *Seminars in Avian and Exotic Pet Medicine* 2: 142–151.

Joseph, V. (1999). Raptor hematology and chemistry evaluation. *The Veterinary Clinics of North America. Exotic Animal Practice* 2 (3): 689–699.

Kern, T.J. (1997). Disorders of the special senses. In: *Avian Medicine and Surgery* (eds. R.B. Altman, S.L. Clubb and G.M. Dorrestein), 563–589. Philadelphia: WB Saunders Co.

Kilic, N. and Paşa, S. (2009). Cardiopulmonary effects of propofol compared with those of a medetomidine-ketamine combination in the common buzzards (*Buteo buteo*). *Revista de Medicina Veterinaria* 160 (3): 154–159.

Komar, N., Langevin, S., Hinten, S. et al. (2003). Experimental infection of North American birds with the New York 1999 strain of West Nile virus. *Emerging Infectious Diseases* 9 (3): 311.

Korbel, R.T. (2000). Disorders of the posterior eye segment in raptors – examination procedures and findings. In: *Raptor Biomedicine III*, 179–193. Lake Worth, FL: Zoological Education Network.

Kovacs, E.R. and Benko, M. (2009). Confirmation of a novel siadenovirus species detected in raptors: partial sequence and phylogenetic analysis. *Virus Research* 140 (1–2): 64–70.

Kramer, J.L. and Redig, P.T. (1997). Sixteen years of lead poisoning in eagles, 1980–95: an epizootiologic view. *Journal of Raptor Research* 31 (4): 327–332.

Kreeger, T.J., Degernes, L.A., Kreeger, J.S. et al. (1993). Immobilization of raptors with tiletamine and zolazepam (Telazol). In: *Raptor Biomedicine* (ed. P.T. Redig), 141–144. Minneapolis: University of Minnesota Press.

Kubiak, M. and Forbes, N. (2011a). Veterinary care of raptors: 1. Common conditions. *In Practice* 33 (1): 28–32.

Kubiak, M. and Forbes, N. (2011b). Veterinary care of raptors: 2. Musculoskeletal problems. *In Practice* 33 (2): 50–57.

Kumar, R., Kumar, V., Asthana, M. et al. (2010). Isolation and identification of a fowl adenovirus from wild black kites (*Milvus migrans*). *Journal of Wildlife Diseases* 46 (1): 272–276.

Lacasse, C., Gamble, K.C., and Boothe, D.M. (2013). Pharmacokinetics of a single dose of intravenous and oral meloxicam in red-tailed hawks (*Buteo jamaicensis*) and great horned owls (*Bubo virginianus*). *Journal of Avian Medicine and Surgery* 27 (3): 204–211.

Leary, S., Underwood, W., Anthony, R. et al. (2013). *AVMA Guidelines for the Euthanasia of Animals: 2013 Edition*. Schaumburg, IL: American Veterinary Medical Association.

Leppert, L.L., Dufty, A.M. Jr., Stock, S. et al. (2008). Survey of blood parasites in two forest owls, Northern Saw-whet Owls and Flammulated Owls, of western North America. *Journal of Wildlife Diseases* 44 (2): 475–479.

Lewis, J.C., Storm, J., and Greenwood, A.G. (1993). Treatment of wing tip oedema in raptors. *The Veterinary Record* 133 (13): 328.

Lierz, M., Hafez, H.M., Klopfleisch, R. et al. (2007). Protection and virus shedding of falcons vaccinated against highly pathogenic avian influenza A virus (H5N1). *Emerging Infectious Diseases* 13 (11): 1667.

Lindsay, D.S., Dubey, J.P., and Blagburn, B.L. (1991). *Toxoplasma gondii* infections in red-tailed hawks inoculated orally with tissue cysts. *The Journal of Parasitology* 77 (2): 322–325.

Lloyd, C. and Wernery, U. (2008). Humoral response of hybrid falcons inoculated with inactivated paramyxovirus-1 vaccine. *Journal of Avian Medicine and Surgery* 22 (3): 213–218.

Lopes, H., Redig, P., Glaser, A. et al. (2007). Clinical findings, lesions, and viral antigen distribution in great gray owls (*Strix nebulosa*) and barred owls (*Strix varia*) with spontaneous West Nile virus infection. *Avian Diseases* 51 (1): 140–145.

Maier, K. and Fischer, D. (2018). Krankheiten der Wüstenbussarde. Kapitel 15 [Diseases in Harris Hawks. Chapter 15]. In: *Harris Hawk - Faszination Wüstenbussard* (ed. C. Niehues), 209–220. Meldungen: Verlag J. Neumann Neudamm AG.

Mautino, M. (1997). Lead and zinc intoxication in zoological medicine: a review. *Journal of Zoo and Wildlife Medicine* 28 (1): 28–35.

Mazor-Thomas, J.E., Mann, P.E., Karas, A.Z. et al. (2014). Pain-suppressed behaviors in the red-tailed hawk (*Buteo jamaicensis*). *Applied Animal Behaviour Science* 152: 83–91.

Michel, F., Sieg, M., Fischer, D. et al. (2019). Evidence for West Nile virus and Usutu virus infections in wild and resident birds in Germany, 2017 and 2018. *Viruses* 11 (7): 674.

Mikaelian, I., Dubey, J.P., and Martineau, D. (1997). Severe hepatitis resulting from toxoplasmosis in a barred owl (*Strix varia*) from Québec, Canada. *Avian Diseases* 41 (3): 738–740.

Miller, N.L., Frenkel, J.K., and Dubey, J.P. (1972). Oral infections with Toxoplasma cysts and oocysts in felines, other mammals, and in birds. *The Journal of Parasitology* 58 (5): 928–937.

Mitkus, M., Potier, S., Martin, G.R. et al. (2018). Raptor vision. Oxford Research Encyclopedia of Neuroscience. https://doi.org/10.1093/acrefore/9780190264086.013.232 (accessed 2 January 2020).

Molina-Lopez, R.A., Ramis, A., Martin-Vazquez, S. et al. (2010). *Cryptosporidium baileyi* infection associated with an outbreak of ocular and respiratory disease in otus owls (*Otus scops*) in a rehabilitation centre. *Avian Pathology* 39 (3): 171–176.

Monks, D., Fisher, M., and Forbes, N.A. (2006). *Ixodes frontalis* and avian tick-related syndrome in the United Kingdom. *Journal of Small Animal Practice* 47 (8): 451–455.

Mueller, H.C. (1986). The evolution of reversed sexual dimorphism in owls: an empirical analysis of possible selective factors. *The Wilson Bulletin* 98 (3): 387–406.

Muller, M.G. and Mohammed, J. (2015). A new approach for tibiotarsal fractures in falcons with the FixEx tubulaire type FESSA system. Abu Dhabi Falcon Hospital. http://www.falconhospital.com/media/1461/fractures-tibiotarsus-in-falcons-fessa.pdf (accessed 6 April 2019).

Murphy, C.J. (1987). Raptor ophthalmology. *Compendium on Continuing Education for the Practicing Veterinarian* 9: 241–260.

Murphy, C.J., Kern, T., McKeever, K. et al. (1982). Ocular lesions in free-living raptors. *Journal of the American Veterinary Medical Association* 181 (11): 1302–1304.

Murray, M. and Tseng, F. (2008). Diagnosis and treatment of secondary anticoagulant rodenticide toxicosis in a red-tailed hawk (*Buteo jamaicensis*). *Journal of Avian Medicine and Surgery* 22 (1): 41–47.

Naldo, J.L. and Samour, J.H. (2004). Causes of morbidity and mortality in falcons in Saudi Arabia. *Journal of Avian Medicine and Surgery* 18 (4): 229–242.

Nemeth, N.M., Hahn, D.C., Gould, D.H. et al. (2006). Experimental West Nile virus infection in eastern screech owls (*Megascops asio*). *Avian Diseases* 50 (2): 252–258.

Norton, T.M., Gaskin, J., Kollias, G.V. et al. (1991). Efficacy of acyclovir against herpesvirus infection in Quaker parakeets. *American Journal of Veterinary Research* 52 (12): 2007–2009.

Oaks, J.L., Schrenzel, M., Rideout, B. et al. (2005). Isolation and epidemiology of falcon adenovirus. *Journal of Clinical Microbiology* 43 (7): 3414–3420.

Obon, E., Bailey, T.A., Di Somma, A. et al. (2009). Seroprevalence of H5 avian influenza virus in birds in the United Arab Emirates. *The Veterinary Record* 165 (25): 752.

Owen, J.C. (2011). Collecting, processing, and storing avian blood: a review. *Journal of Field Ornithology* 82 (4): 339–354.

Papazahariadou, M.G., Georgiades, G.K., Komnenou, A.T. et al. (2001). *Caryospora* species in a snowy owl (*Nyctea scandiaca*). *The Veterinary Record* 148 (2): 54–55.

Pavez, J.C., Hawkins, M.G., Pascoe, P.J. et al. (2011). Effect of fentanyl target-controlled infusions on isoflurane minimum anaesthetic concentration and cardiovascular function in red-tailed hawks (*Buteo jamaicensis*). *Veterinary Anaesthesia and Analgesia* 38 (4): 344–351.

Phalen, D.N., Holz, P., Rasmussen, L. et al. (2011). Fatal columbid herpesvirus-1 infections in three species of Australian birds of prey. *Australian Veterinary Journal* 89 (5): 193–196.

Poffers, J., Lumeij, J.T., Timmermans-Sprang, E.P.M. et al. (2002a). Further studies on the use of allopurinol to reduce plasma uric acid concentrations in the red-tailed hawk (*Buteo jamaicensis*) hyperuricaemic model. *Avian Pathology* 31 (6): 567–572.

Poffers, J., Lumeij, J.T., and Redig, P.T. (2002b). Investigations into the uricolytic properties of urate oxidase in a granivorous (*Columba livia domestica*) and in a carnivorous (*Buteo jamaicensis*) avian species. *Avian Pathology* 31 (6): 573–579.

Polo, F.J., Celdran, J.F., Peinado, V.I. et al. (1992). Hematological values for four species of birds of prey. *The Condor* 94 (4): 1007–1013.

Quesenberry, K.E. and Hillyer, E.V. (1994). Supportive care and emergency therapy. In: *Avian Medicine: Principles and Application* (eds. B.W. Ritchie, G.J. Harrison and L.R. Harrison), 382–416. Lake Worth, FL: Wingers.

Ramis, A., Major, N., Fumarole, M. et al. (1994). Herpesvirus hepatitis in two eagles in Spain. *Avian Diseases* 38: 197–200.

Rayment, L.J. and Williams, D. (1997). Glaucoma in a captive-bred great horned owl (*Bubo virginianus virginianus*). *Veterinary Record* 140 (18): 481–483.

Redig, P.T. (1993). General infectious diseases - avian aspergillosis. In: *Zoo & Wild Animal Medicine - Current Therapy*, 3e (ed. M.E. Fowler), 178–181. Denver, CO: Saunders.

Redig, P.T. (2000). The use of an external skeletal fixator-intramedullary pin tie-in (ESF-IM fixator) for treatment of long bone fractures in raptors. In: *Raptor Biomedicine III* (eds. J.T. Lumeij, J.D. Remple, P.T. Redig, et al.), 239–254. Lake Worth, FL: Zoological Education Network.

Redig, P.T. and Arent, L.R. (2008). Raptor toxicology. *The Veterinary Clinics of North America. Exotic Animal Practice* 11 (2): 261–282.

Redig, P.T. and Goyal, S.M. (2012). Serologic evidence of exposure of raptors to influenza a virus. *Avian Diseases* 56 (2): 411–413.

Redig, P.T. and Ponder, J. (2016). *Orthopedic Surgery. Avian Medicine*, 3e, 333–340. Missouri: Elsevier.

Redig, P.T., Willette, M., and Ponder, J. (2014). Raptors. In: *Zoo Animal and Wildlife Immobilization and Anesthesia* (eds. G. West, D. Heard and N. Caulkett), 459–472. Iowa, United States: Wiley Blackwell.

Remple, J.D. (1993). Raptor bumblefoot: a new treatment technique. *Raptor Biomedicine* 27: 154–155.

Remple, J.D. and Al-Ashbal, A.A. (1993). Raptor bumblefoot: another look at histopathology and pathogenesis. *Raptor Biomedicine* 17: 92–93.

Remple, J.D. and Forbes, N.A. (2002). Antibiotic-impregnated polymethyl methacrylate beads in the treatment of bumblefoot in raptors. In: *Raptor Biomedicine III* (eds. J.T. Lumeij, J.D. Remple, P.T. Redig, et al.), 255–263. Lake Worth, FL: Zoological Education Network.

Riddle, K.E. (1980). Surgical treatment of bumblefoot in raptors. In: *Recent Advances in the Study of Raptor Disease* (eds. J.E. Cooper and A.G. Greenwood), 67–73. West Yorkshire, UK: Chiron Publications.

Riggs, S.M., Hawkins, M.G., Craigmill, A.L. et al. (2008). Pharmacokinetics of butorphanol tartrate in red-tailed hawks (*Buteo jamaicensis*) and great horned owls (*Bubo virginianus*). *American Journal of Veterinary Research* 69 (5): 596–603.

Robbins, P.K., Tell, L.A., Needham, M.L. et al. (2000). Pharmacokinetics of piperacillin after intramuscular injection in red-tailed hawks (*Buteo jamaicensis*) and great horned owls (*Bubo virginianus*). *Journal of Zoo and Wildlife Medicine* 31 (1): 47–52.

Rodríguez-Barbón, A. and Forbes, N. (2007). Use of paromomycin in the treatment of a *Cryptosporidium* infection in a gyr falcon (Falco rusticolus) and a hybrid gyr/saker falcon (Falco rusticolus X Falco cherrug). Proceedings of the Annual Conference of the European Association of Avian Veterinarians: 191–197.

Sadar, M.J., Hawkins, M.G., and Drazenovich, T. (2014). Pharmacokinetic-pharmacodynamic integration of an extended-release ceftiofur formulation administered to red-tailed hawks (Buteo jamaicensis) Proceedings of the Annual Conference of the Association of Avian Veterinarians: 11.

Sadar, M.J., Sanchez-Migallon Guzman, D., Mete, A. et al. (2015). Mange caused by a novel *Micnemidocoptes* mite in a golden eagle (*Aquila chrysaetos*). *Journal of Avian Medicine and Surgery* 29 (3): 231–238.

Saito, K., Kodama, A., Yamaguchi, T. et al. (2009). Avian poxvirus infection in a white-tailed sea eagle (*Haliaeetus albicilla*) in Japan. *Avian Pathology* 38 (6): 485–489.

Samour, J. (2006). Management of raptors. In: *Clinical Avian Medicine* (eds. G.J. Harrison and T. Lightfoot), 915–956. Florida, USA: Spix Publishing.

Samour, J. (2014). Newcastle disease in captive falcons in the Middle East: a review of clinical and pathologic findings. *Journal of Avian Medicine and Surgery* 28 (1): 1–6.

Samour, J.H. and Cooper, J.E. (1993). Avian pox in birds of prey (order Falconiformes) in Bahrain. *The Veterinary Record* 132 (14): 343–345.

Samour, J.H. and Naldo, J. (2002). Diagnosis and therapeutic management of lead toxicosis in falcons in Saudi Arabia. *Journal of Avian Medicine and Surgery* 16 (1): 16–21.

Samour, J.H. and Naldo, J.L. (2003). Diagnosis and therapeutic management of trichomoniasis in falcons in Saudi Arabia. *Journal of Avian Medicine and Surgery* 17 (3): 136–144.

Samour, J.H., Naldo, J.L., and John, S.K. (2005). Therapeutic management of *Babesia shortii* infection in a peregrine falcon (*Falco peregrinus*). *Journal of Avian Medicine and Surgery* 19 (4): 294–296.

Sandmeyer, L.S., Breaux, C.B., McRuer, D.L. et al. (2007). Case report: a new technique for intraocular prosthesis implantation in a great horned owl (*Bubo virginianus*). *Journal of Exotic Pet Medicine* 16 (2): 95–100.

Santangelo, B., Ferrari, D., Di Martino, I. et al. (2009). Dexmedetomidine chemical restraint of two raptor species undergoing inhalation anaesthesia. *Veterinary Research Communications* 33 (1): 209–211.

Santoro, M., D'Alessio, N., Di Prisco, F. et al. (2016). The occurrence and pathogenicity of *Serratospiculum tendo* (Nematoda: Diplotriaenoidea) in birds of prey from southern Italy. *Journal of Helminthology* 90 (3): 294–297.

Scheelings, T.F. (2014). Coracoid fractures in wild birds: a comparison of surgical repair versus conservative treatment. *Journal of Avian Medicine and Surgery* 28 (4): 304–309.

Schmidt, V., Demiraj, F., Di Somma, A. et al. (2007). Plasma concentrations of voriconazole in falcons. *Veterinary Record* 161 (8): 265–268.

Shaver, S.L., Robinson, N.G., Wright, B.D. et al. (2009). A multimodal approach to management of suspected neuropathic pain in a prairie falcon (*Falco mexicanus*). *Journal of Avian Medicine and Surgery* 23 (3): 209–214.

Shlosberg, A. (1976). Treatment of monocrotophos-poisoned birds of prey with pralidoxime iodide. *Journal of the American Veterinary Medical Association* 169 (9): 989–990.

Shrubsole-Cockwill, A., Wojnarowicz, C., and Parker, D. (2008). Atherosclerosis and ischemic cardiomyopathy in a captive, adult red-tailed hawk (*Buteo jamaicensis*). *Avian Diseases* 52: 537–539.

Sigmund, A.B., Jones, M.P., Ward, D.A. et al. (2019). Long-term outcome of phacoemulsification in raptors—a retrospective study (1999-2014). *Veterinary Ophthalmology* 22 (3): 360–367.

Sos-Koroknai, V. (2019). Trends and incidence of West Nile Virus infection in goshawks (Accipiter gentilis) in a Hungarian wildlife rescue centre over the past 10 years, Proceedings of the EAZWV/IZW Joint conference, Kolmarden, Sweden, 14 June.

Souza, M.J., Martin-Jimenez, T., Jones, M.P. et al. (2009). Pharmacokinetics of intravenous and oral tramadol in the bald eagle (*Haliaeetus leucocephalus*). *Journal of Avian Medicine and Surgery* 23 (4): 247–253.

Souza, M.J., Martin-Jimenez, T., Jones, M.P. et al. (2011). Pharmacokinetics of oral tramadol in red-tailed hawks (*Buteo jamaicensis*). *Journal of Veterinary Pharmacology and Therapeutics* 34 (1): 86–88.

Stanford, M. (2009). Introduction to raptor management and husbandry. *In Practice* 31 (6): 267–275.

Tarello, W. (2006). Serratospiculosis in falcons from Kuwait: incidence, pathogenicity and treatment with melarsomine and ivermectin. *Parasite* 13 (1): 59–63.

Tarello, W. (2007). Clinical signs and response to primaquine in falcons with *Haemoproteus tinnuculi* infection. *The Veterinary Record* 161 (6): 204–206.

Tarello, W. (2008). Efficacy of ivermectin (Ivomec®) against intestinal capillariosis in falcons. *Parasite* 15 (2): 171–174.

Tavernier, P., Sagesse, M., Van Wettere, A. et al. (2005). Malaria in an eastern screech owl (*Otus asio*). *Avian Diseases* 49 (3): 433–435.

Tully, T.N. (1995). Avian respiratory diseases: clinical overview. *Journal of Avian Medicine and Surgery* 9 (3): 162–174.

Upton, S.J. and Sundermann, C.A. (1990). *Caryospora*: biology. In: *Coccidiosis of Man and Domestic Animals* (ed. P.L.L. Long), 187–204. Boca Raton: CRC Press.

Van den Brand, J.M., Krone, O., Wolf, P.U. et al. (2015). Host-specific exposure and fatal neurologic disease in wild raptors from highly pathogenic avian influenza virus H5N1 during the 2006 outbreak in Germany. *Veterinary Research* 5 (46): 24.

Van Sant, F. and Stewart, G.R. (2009). Ponazuril used as treatment for suspected *Cryptosporidium* infection in 2 hybrid falcons. Proceedings of the Annual Conference of the Association of Avian Veterinarians: 368–371.

Van Zeeland, Y.R.A., Schoemaker, N.J., Kik, M.J.L. et al. (2008). Upper respiratory tract infection caused by *Cryptosporidium baileyi* in three mixed-bred falcons (*Falco rusticolus* × *Falco cherrug*). *Avian Diseases* 52 (2): 357–363.

Veiga, I.B., Schediwy, M., Hentrich, B. et al. (2017). Serratospiculosis in captive peregrine falcons (*Falco peregrinus*) in Switzerland. *Journal of Avian Medicine and Surgery* 31 (3): 250–256.

Wagner, C.H., Hochleitner, M., and Rausch, W.D. (1991). Ketoconazole plasma levels in buzzards. In: *Proceedings of the Conference of the European Committee of the Association of Avian Veterinarians* (eds. A. Rubel and R. Baumgartner), 333–340. Utrecht: European Chapter of the Association of Avian Veterinarians.

Ward, F.P. and Fairchild, D.G. (1972). Air sac parasites of the genus *Serratospiculum* in falcons. *Journal of Wildlife Diseases* 8 (2): 165–168.

Wernery, U., Wernery, R., and Kinne, J. (1999). Production of a falcon herpesvirus vaccine. *Berliner und Münchener Tierärztliche Wochenschrift* 112 (9): 339–344.

Wheeler, P. and Greenwood, P.J. (1983). The evolution of reversed sexual dimorphism in birds of prey. *Oikos* 40 (1): 145–149.

WHO (2017). World Health Organisation West Nile Virus fact sheet. https://www.who.int/news-room/fact-sheets/detail/west-nile-virus (accessed 17 June 2019).

Wodak, E., Richter, S., Bagó, Z. et al. (2011). Detection and molecular analysis of West Nile virus infections in birds of prey in the eastern part of Austria in 2008 and 2009. *Veterinary Microbiology* 149 (3–4): 358–366.

Wrobel, E.R., Wilcoxen, T.E., Nuzzo, J.T. et al. (2016). Seroprevalence of avian pox and *Mycoplasma gallisepticum* in raptors in Central Illinois. *Journal of Raptor Research* 50 (3): 289–295.

Wunschmann, A., Armien, A.G., and Hofle, U. (2018). Birds of prey. In: *Pathology of Wildlife and Zoo Animals* (eds. K.A. Terio, D. McAloose and J.S. Leger), 717–740. London, UK: Academic Press.

Ziegler, U., Angenvoort, J., Fischer, D. et al. (2013). Pathogenesis of West Nile virus lineage 1 and 2 in experimentally infected large falcons. *Veterinary Microbiology* 161 (3–4): 263–273.

Zsivanovits, P., Forbes, N.A., Zvonar, L.T. et al. (2004). Investigation into the seroprevalence of falcon herpesvirus antibodies in raptors in the UK using virus neutralization tests and different herpesvirus isolates. *Avian Pathology* 33 (6): 599–604.

Zsivanovits, P., Monks, D.J., Forbes, N.A. et al. (2006). Presumptive identification of a novel adenovirus in a Harris hawk (*Parabuteo unicinctus*), a Bengal eagle owl (*Bubo bengalensis*), and a Verreaux's eagle owl (*Bubo lacteus*). *Journal of Avian Medicine and Surgery* 20 (2): 105–113.

13

Bearded Dragons
Marie Kubiak

There are six recognised species of bearded dragon within the *Pogona* genus, of which only one, the inland bearded dragon (*P. vitticeps)* is frequently kept as a companion animal and this chapter will focus on this species (Raiti 2012). The smaller Rankins dragon (*P. henrylawsonii*), the Eastern bearded dragon (*P. barbata*), and the hybridised Vittikins dragon are infrequently kept as captive pets but husbandry and veterinary care of these is similar. The biological parameters of commonly kept species are given in Table 13.1.

13.1 Husbandry

Bearded dragons are predominantly terrestrial lizards that occupy large home ranges, with areas of up to 44 600 m^2 reported for *P. barbata* (Wotherspoon 2007). *Pogona* species are also highly active foragers and will readily move outside their home range, regularly travelling distances of over 100 m daily (Thompson and Thompson 2003; Wotherspoon 2007). In contrast, published recommendations for a single or pair of captive adult bearded dragons are a minimum of 72 × 18 inches with a height of 24 inches (Grenard 2008) and a minimum floorspace of 72 × 24 inches for a group of three to four dragons. Juveniles are often kept in smaller enclosures of 36–48 inches length. These enclosure sizes will severely restrict natural behaviours and activity, and enclosures should be as large as is feasible, allowing sizeable areas for exercise and foraging.

Glass tanks are not suitable enclosures as heat retention and ventilation are poor, wooden tanks with multiple ventilation ports are more commonly used. Retreat areas with visual barriers within the enclosure are needed, with plants, tiered rock structures and commercially available wooden or ceramic hides amongst the suitable options. Bearded dragons are often observed basking on vertical structures in both the wild situation and in captivity, and a combination of vertical and horizontal structures placed under the basking spot is often well utilised (Figure 13.1) (Cannon 2003).

Males should not be housed together, to prevent conflict. Females can often be maintained in small groups, and a single male may be kept with one or more females, however repeated breeding and aggressive mating behaviour can lead to injury or debilitation in the females, and aggression may occur. Black colouration of the beard and head bobbing are often seen as a display of dominance and can precede aggression or mating, whereas arm-waving indicates submission (Boyer 2015). Bearded dragons do not appear to be social as adults so keeping a single individual is acceptable, however group rearing of hatchlings has been shown to be beneficial in learning behaviours in asocial reptile species and may be beneficial for bearded dragons (Ballen et al. 2014).

Adults can be kept on a substrate of fine sand with food provided in a bowl or on a stone surface to avoid inadvertent ingestion of substrate. Small quantities of sand ingested by a healthy lizard are passed uneventfully in the faeces. Large particulate substrates such as corn cob or gravel, or clumping calcium sands should be avoided due to the potential for intestinal obstruction with ingestion of small quantities (Klaphake 2010). Juveniles or debilitated animals are typically kept on paper or similar non-particulate substrate. Females housed with a male often readily breed, and females without access to a male may still produce infertile eggs, so an area with a 6–12 inch deep sand layer for egg laying should be provided. A wide, shallow water bowl should be provided for bathing and drinking opportunities but is rarely used. A humid hide with damp moss or vermiculite can be provided when shedding occurs.

As a diurnal basking species, an overhead heat source should be used to provide a basking spot of 35–40 °C at one

Handbook of Exotic Pet Medicine, First Edition. Edited by Marie Kubiak.
© 2021 John Wiley & Sons Ltd. Published 2021 by John Wiley & Sons Ltd.
Companion website: www.wiley.com/go/kubiak/exotic_pet_medicine

Table 13.1 Biological parameters of commonly kept species.

	Inland bearded dragon (*P. vitticeps*)	Rankins dragon (*P. henrylawsoni*)
Lifespan	7–12 years	6–8 years
Adult length (including tail)	45–60 cm	30 cm
Adult weight	230–520 g	60–120 g
Respiratory rate	14–28/min	–
Heart rate	40–90 bpm (98–148 bpm when restrained)	–
Basking spot temperature	35–40C	35–40C
Ambient daytime temperature	27C	25C
Ambient nighttime temperature	21C	21C
Humidity	30–40%	30–40%
Average clutch size	15–25	10–25
Gestation period	14–21d	28–42d
Incubation period	55–96d	50–85d

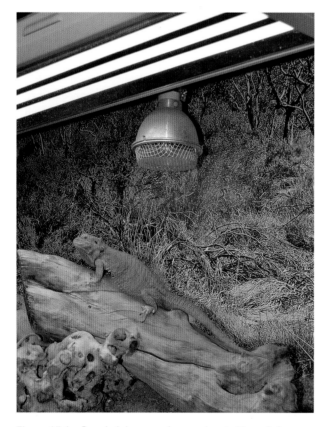

Figure 13.1 Bearded dragon using an elevated branch for basking note the close proximity of heat lamp and ultraviolet lights (*Source:* Photo courtesy of Drayton Manor Park Zoo).

end, creating a thermal gradient of 27–40 °C along the tank. This allows the bearded dragon to select an area of the enclosure based on the temperature required for its physiological status at that time. Small enclosure size will prevent achievement of a sufficient temperature gradient.

A thermostat is essential for any heat source to prevent overheating but will limit the durability of light bulb heat sources and can cause an irritating flicker effect as the bulb is turned on and off repeatedly. This is avoided by using ceramic heat sources as these have no light output. Any heat bulb must be protected by a guard or at sufficient height to prevent any possible contact. Night time temperatures should reduce to 21 °C to mimic natural circadian variations (Stahl 1999) and a heat mat placed on the side of the tank, a ceramic heat source, or an infrared bulb can provide thermal support without visible light. When asked about temperatures provided, owners will often state the temperature set on the thermostat but this may not reflect the temperatures within the enclosure. Temperatures should be manually checked regularly at both the basking spot and coolest area as thermostat malfunction or inadequate heater output may vary temperatures from the expected conditions.

An ultraviolet (UV) light is essential in bearded dragons as UV radiation of wavelength 290–320 nm is necessary for calcium homeostasis and immunocompetence, and is important in colour vision of reptiles (Raiti 2012; Baines 2018). The UV light output should be monitored at the basking level using a meter that measures UV-B wavelength light (Raiti 2012). Lights should be replaced for bearded dragons when they no longer maintain a UV-index of 2.9–7.4 (Baines et al. 2016). Where UV-B output is not being monitored, replacement of lights every six months is advisable but output will vary between light models and with age of light and appropriate levels may not be maintained. A light : dark cycle of 12 : 12 is suitable in summer, reducing to 10 : 14 in winter.

Bearded dragons are opportunistic omnivores, with seasonal availability of invertebrate prey and vegetation determining intake. Macmillen et al. (1989) found that adults' intake was predominantly plant material whereas young dragons had an equal intake of vegetable matter and insects. However, Oonincx et al. (2015) found a higher proportion of insect matter in adult *P. vitticeps* suggesting that intake is geographically and seasonally variable. Hatchlings are typically fed two to three times daily to maintain slow growth, and adults fed every one to two days to maintain body condition (De Vosjoli and Mailloux 1996). A wide variety of vegetables (including home-grown grasses and weeds) can be offered. Readily available feeder insects are limited and include crickets, locusts, cockroaches, and mealworms. These insects have a poor calcium: phosphorus ratio and low Vitamin D content, predisposing to disorders of calcium metabolism (Barker et al. 1998; Finke 2015). Dusting prey insects with calcium powder (substituted once weekly for a multi-vitamin powder), and pre-feeding insect prey on calcium-enriched insect diets may aid in improving nutritional value (Allen and Oftedal 1989). Providing a wide variety of insect prey, including earthworms, black soldier fly larvae, and wild-caught insects will also improve the relative calcium levels of the diet.

13.1.1 Breeding

Reproduction follows the rainy season in the wild, in September to March. In captivity, bearded dragons will breed year-round though a cooling period and increased environmental humidity encourage initiation of courtship. Receptive females will lay 6–40 eggs (average 15–25), two to three weeks after copulation and can lay further fertile clutches at four to six week intervals from retained sperm (Stahl 1999; Boyer 2015). Eggs incubated at 29 °C in moist substrate hatch after 55–75 days (Stahl 1999). Sex of offspring is primarily genetically determined with male homogamety (ZZ) and female heterogamety (ZW) identified in this species (Ezaz et al. 2005). However, if incubation temperatures exceed 32 °C, both ZZ and ZW embryos develop phenotypically as females (Deveson et al. 2017).

Hatchlings are left within the incubator for 24–48 hours to resorb the yolk sac prior to transfer (Stahl 1999). They can then be crèche-reared in small groups initially but if there is a size differential larger animals may attempt to cannibalise smaller individuals (Raiti 2012).

13.1.2 History Taking

Husbandry deficiencies remain a common factor in development of disease in this species and a full assessment of management and potential deficiencies are a crucial part of clinical assessment. A thorough review of husbandry takes time and consultation length should take this into account. Records of temperatures and UV-B readings (or providing the UV-B light for testing in the clinic), alongside photographs of the enclosure can aid in assessing husbandry more fully. Further relevant details include addition of new animals to the collection within the previous 12 months, onset of presenting complaint, and number of animals affected.

13.1.3 Handling

Bearded dragons are docile and very rarely will attempt to bite though sharp spines or nails can cause discomfort on handling. They can be held under the coelom with a hand or forearm to allow basic examination. With minimal restraint they will tend to remain still for a physical examination but will struggle if held tightly. The vagal response can be used as a temporary aid to handling or procedures such as radiography which require immobility. Pressure on the ocular globes result in an increase in parasympathetic drive and a temporary immobility. This can be achieved with manual pressure (Figure 13.2), or by compressing cotton wool balls over the eyes and securing them with a self-adhesive bandage.

13.1.4 Sex Determination

Adult males will typically be of longer body length with broader heads and develop male behaviours including head bobbing, darkening, and puffing out of the beard (Stahl 1999). Visible development of femoral pores along the medial aspect of the hindlimbs, and hemipene swellings at the tail base are highly suggestive of a mature male animal (Figure 13.3) but these characteristics can

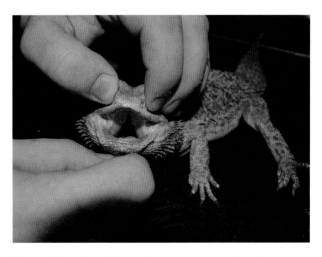

Figure 13.2 Use of the vagal response to permit oral examination – pressure is exerted on both ocular globes and results in reduced response to stimuli.

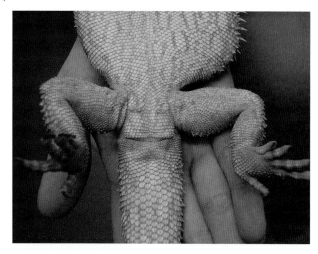

Figure 13.3   Male bearded dragon, note the developed femoral pores as well as hemipene swellings at the tail base.

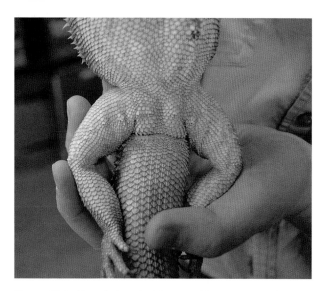

Figure 13.4   Female bearded dragon with lack of femoral pore development.

be subtle in inactive males. Females will have poorly developed femoral pores, a smaller cloacal opening, a flat tail base and may be smaller in size (Figure 13.4). The most reliable method of determining sex (without ultrasonographic or endoscopic gonad visualisation) is to evert the vent and check for the bilateral hemipenes found caudal to the vent opening in males. This usually requires an assistant to restrain the dragon in dorsal recumbency, and familiarity with the anatomy. Even this is not reliable in juveniles (particularly those <3 months) as hemipenes may be too small to easily identify. A probe can be inserted in the region of the hemipene, and in males it will pass more than 1 cm, but only 2–3 mm in females (Cannon 2003).

13.1.5   Clinical Examination

Observation within the carrier prior to handling is useful to assess activity, resting respiratory rate and response to a novel environment. A healthy bearded dragon should be alert, ambulatory, and capable of lifting the body and proximal tail clear of the ground (Raiti 2012). Basic evaluation consisting of visual assessment of the external structures, palpation of the limbs and coelom and examination of the skin can be carried out with minimal restraint. Placing the first and second finger either side of the head and the other fingers around the thorax will give firm restraint allowing oral and ophthalmic assessment. Oral examination is important as periodontal disease is not uncommon. The mouth can be opened by holding the upper jaw with one hand and gently pulling on the beard with the other. Placing the bearded dragon upright on the handler's chest where it will tend to remain static will facilitate this procedure. Autotomy, or tail dropping, does not occur in this species but they should never be restrained by the tail due to potential for traumatic injury.

13.2   Basic Techniques

13.2.1   Sample Collection

Faecal samples are often passed during transport or examination, but it is sensible to request owners bring a recent sample from the individual. A warm water bath or enema will also encourage defaecation. Faeces is brown and formed, and is accompanied by clear urine and soft white urates as renal excretory products.

Blood samples are straightforward to collect from the ventral coccygeal sinus and 0.8% of bodyweight can be taken (Cannon 2003). The bearded dragon can be held in ventral recumbency on a table with the tail lifted dorsally, or held upright with its back against an assistant to allow access to the ventral tail. The sinus is midline, just ventral to the coccygeal vertebrae and the sample can be collected at any point of the tail (though the proximal 5 cm is best avoided in males to avoid inadvertent trauma to the more lateral hemipenes). A needle is inserted at a 45° angle to the tail, angled forward to slide between scales, and advanced until the vertebrae are contacted. The needle is then incrementally withdrawn until blood flows into the hub. There is no need apply pressure to attempt to increase filling of the sinus. Once sufficient sample is obtained, the needle is withdrawn and manual pressure applied for 60 seconds. Both heparin and EDTA can be used as anticoagulants for samples.

13.2.2 Nutritional Support

Short periods of anorexia may be normal, relating to reproductive status or changes in environmental temperature, and rarely require nutritional support. Intervention should be considered for anorexia in excess of 10 days duration where the animal is clinically unwell, losing body condition or weight, or in an obese animal at high risk of hepatic lipidosis. In a dehydrated animal, rehydration should be carried out prior to feeding to avoid the potential of refeeding syndrome and associated electrolyte aberrations (Donoghue 2006).

Offering favoured food items such as locusts, edible yellow flowers and vegetables, and small pieces of fruit can stimulate a feeding response. Where this is absent, a mixture of carnivore and herbivore liquid diet, or omnivorous reptile formulas are suitable options for assist feeding. Nutritional requirements should be determined to ensure animals are receiving adequate nutrition, using manufacturer guidelines for convalescent liquid diets, or calculating approximate calorific requirements based on body weight:

$$\text{Standard Metabolic Rate (SMR) [Kcal/day]} = 28 \times \text{Mass (kg)}^{0.83} \text{ (Andrews and Pough 1985)}$$

Recuperating animals may have higher energy requirements than the baseline SMR dependent on the pathology present.

Small volumes can be fed by oral administration with the dragon restrained and mouth held open. Large volumes can be administered by gavage tube with the animal firmly restrained and a rigid plastic or metal tube passed down the oesophagus into the distal oesophagus or stomach. This method is stressful for the animal and risks trauma to the teeth and soft tissues so if prolonged support is expected to be needed, placement of an oesophageal feeding tube is advisable. For animals requiring large volumes, feeds should be divided into meals of a maximum of 10 ml/kg spread evenly through the day.

13.2.3 Fluid Therapy

Tacky saliva, pronounced skin folds, and sunken eyes are seen with >10% dehydration in this species. Azotaemia, hyperuricaemia, and an elevated PCV may be seen on bloodwork. Maintenance fluid requirements are 10–20 ml/kg/day (Nevarez 2009), and fluid deficits should be replaced alongside daily requirements over 3–4 days. Fluid administered within assist feeding should be taken into account to avoid over-administration (Music and Strunk 2016).

If the gastrointestinal tract is not compromised, oral fluids can be administered by the same methods as nutritional support or supplemented by wetting vegetable matter offered to self-feeding patients. Warm water baths (27–30 °C) can encourage drinking (Gibbons and Tell 2009).

Parenteral rehydration with warmed normal saline is often tolerated better than repeat force feeding of electrolyte solutions. Subcutaneous injections of fluid boluses are easily given over the flanks where loose skin is clearly visible and can be useful in gradual rehydration of noncritical patients. The intracoelomic route is not advisable as fluids are poorly absorbed and intravisceral administration, or traumatic injury are common (Gibbons and Tell 2009).

Intravenous fluid therapy is difficult to achieve repeatedly though off the needle boluses of fluids can be given into the ventral coccygeal sinus. A cut down technique can be used to place a cannula in the cephalic vein or ventral coccygeal sinus but these can be difficult to maintain in place in all but the most debilitated patients. Intraosseous fluid administration is often easier to manage, with placement of a hypodermic or spinal needle into the femur or tibia in patients with radiographically normal bone density. A needle is inserted via the greater trochanter (or tibial tuberosity) under sterile conditions and secured in place with tissue glue and adhesive bandage to allow repeated small boluses of fluids to be administered. Analgesia is mandatory for patients with intraosseous catheters in place.

13.2.4 Analgesia

Analgesia is often overlooked in reptilian patients as they may not demonstrate recognisable signs of pain and pharmacodynamic data on analgesic agents is lacking. As nociceptive pathways are present and mimic those in other taxa it should be assumed that stimuli considered nociceptive in mammals would induce pain in reptiles too and analgesia should be used routinely on this basis. Morphine has been shown to be effective in bearded dragons but butorphanol did not result in analgesia in this species (Sladky et al. 2008). Female bearded dragons appear to metabolise morphine faster requiring more frequent dosing (Greenacre et al. 2011). Oral tramadol reaches levels considered therapeutic in humans for only 45 minutes, but an analgesic metabolite persisted for over 36 hours (Greenacre et al. 2011). Oral administration gave faster absorption and higher serum levels than gavage administration. Meloxicam appears to have a short half-life and a single intramuscular injection resulted in negligible levels 18 hours post administration (Greenacre et al. 2011).

13.2.5 Anaesthesia

Fasting for 12–24 hours prior to anaesthesia will reduce the risk of regurgitation but this is an unusual complication in lizards and fasting is not recommended for animals that would be further debilitated by deprivation of food or oral fluids. Rehydration and acclimatising reptiles to a temperature within their physiological temperature range is sensible to enable optimal metabolism of any anaesthetic drugs.

Isoflurane or sevoflurane can be administered as a sole anaesthetic agent but chamber or mask induction results in unpredictable or slow induction (Bertelsen 2014). Propofol administered intravenously into the ventral coccygeal sinus gives rapid induction and 15–30 minutes of anaesthesia (Perrin and Bertelsen 2017), which can be extended with administration of isoflurane in oxygen. Alfaxalone is a more recently available injectable anaesthetic that is able to be given intravenously and by intramuscular injection. A single dose intravenously results in anaesthesia after 12–45 seconds (Knotek 2017) and at 12 mg/kg gives 20–75 minutes anaesthesia (Perrin and Bertelsen 2017). Incremental additional doses can be used to maintain anaesthesia for longer procedures. However, intubation and maintenance with isoflurane in oxygen is preferred to concurrently maintain oxygenation.

Volatile agents are useful for maintenance but reptiles have the ability to shunt blood from the right ventricle back into the systemic circulation, bypassing the lungs. This can mean that perfusion of the lungs, and associated volatile agent uptake, is variable and injectable agents may be required to augment anaesthetic maintenance in some cases. Atropine administered prior to anaesthesia has been shown to reduce shunting and lower the minimum anaesthetic concentration of isoflurane required in tortoises and this may be of benefit in other reptiles (Greunz et al. 2018).

It is typical for reptiles at a surgical plane of anaesthesia to be apnoeic and require ventilation and so intubation should be carried out for all procedures. The glottis is visible in the oral cavity on extending the tongue and can be accessed using a semi-rigid tube of 2–3 mm diameter. The glottis is mobile and soft endotracheal tubes may not pass into the trachea easily. Use of a stylet, or adapting a shortened dog urinary catheter or large gauge intravenous cannula improves tube rigidity for placement. Gentle ventilation should be used and visible movement of the body wall observed to confirm correct placement of the tube. If unilateral movement is observed then it is likely the tube has passed too far and into a single bronchus. The tube should be withdrawn slightly and ventilation re-evaluated to confirm symmetrical ventilation.

On completion of the procedure, the patient should remain intubated but ventilation source changed from oxygen to room air. Reptiles rely on a decrease in circulating oxygen to stimulate breathing so administering 100% oxygen prolongs recovery, though the extension of recovery has been shown not to be statistically significant (Odette et al. 2015). Ventilating with room air can be achieved with an Ambu-bag. Once breathing without assistance the reptile can be extubated and transferred to the recovery area.

A pre-warmed recovery area should be available and critical care incubators work well for this. Reptiles should remain monitored at an appropriate ambient temperature until mobile. Once able to move in a co-ordinated fashion patients can be returned to their vivarium.

13.2.6 Euthanasia

Intravenous injection of 400 mg/kg of pentobarbitone in the conscious animal, or via the intracardiac route in an anaesthetised animal, results in quick loss of consciousness and cessation of cardiac activity.

The reptile brain is able to withstand oxygen deprivation for prolonged periods and so once unconscious, destruction of the brainstem is advisable to prevent recovery. This has typically been achieved by pithing animals – passing a metal rod or large needle into the brain through the roof of the mouth and physically destroying the tissue. However this is not always accepted by pet owners and so the author now prefers to inject pentobarbitone into the brain. After administering the intravenous pentobarbitone and confirmation of lack of cardiac activity, a further injection of 100 mg/kg pentobarbitone is injected through the foramen magnum at the back of the cranium into the brainstem to achieve the same result as physical pithing.

13.2.7 Hospitalisation Requirements

Bearded dragons should be housed in a vivarium of a minimum of 36 × 24 inches for short-term management. Plastic vivaria are preferable as they are easier to clean thoroughly between patients. Newspaper or paper towel substrate helps maintain hygiene and should be changed daily. Heating and lighting should be similar to that provided in the home situation. An easily disinfected or disposable hide should be provided at each end of the viviarium. Small cardboard boxes with an entrance cut out of one side work well and can be replaced readily but should be sturdy enough to allow patients to climb. Inpatients should be examined and weighed daily and feeding and fluid administration adjusted daily based on clinical status.

13.3 Common Conditions

13.3.1 Anorexia

Anorexia is a non-specific finding in most pathological states in reptiles. A thorough evaluation of husbandry should be carried out, with particular emphasis on temperatures provided. Clinical examination will help determine if a pathological or physiological cause is likely but in many cases separation of the two is difficult. Broad further testing (bloodwork, imaging, faecal analysis) may be carried out to narrow the differential diagnoses as a wide range of underlying diseases may be causative.

Physiological anorexia accompanies winter brumation where a reduction in metabolic rate occurs in response to changes in temperature, light, UVB intensity, humidity, and air pressure. Anorexia or reduced appetite in the winter months in an otherwise healthy bearded dragon that is maintaining weight is not necessarily abnormal. If there are concerns that other factors are involved then increasing the temperature 2 °C above recommended standard levels and providing high intensity full spectrum lighting for 12 hours a day should reverse these changes and encourage feeding if no medical issues are present. Prolonged exposure to low environmental temperatures can induce an initial compensatory brumation-like phase, which if maintained long-term can result in debilitation, immunosuppression, and clinical decline. Anorexia is also seen as a physiological phenomenon in males in breeding season and in ovulating or heavily gravid females.

Prolonged anorexia of any cause can lead to mobilisation of internal fat to meet energy demands, with the secondary consequence of hepatic lipidosis. Obesity is a further risk factor. Once established, hepatic lipidosis results in a persisting anorexia and progressive debilitation even after resolution of the primary causative factor (Raiti 2012). Clinical presentation is non-specific (and may be obscured by the primary disease) with weight loss and weakness predominating, though coelomic distension due to hepatomegaly or ascites may be present (Divers and Cooper 2000). Liver enzyme values are often normal on biochemistry, but a lipaemia may be noted. A significant increase in bile acids in cases of hepatic lipidosis has been reported in green iguanas (Knotek et al. 2009), but has not been confirmed in this species. The liver is enlarged and hyperechoic on ultrasound examination and of pale colouration when visualised. Liver biopsy is needed to confirm diagnosis, with a left sided approach favoured to avoid the hepatic vein and gall bladder (Silvestre and Avepa 2013). Management consists of assist feeding, identification and management of the primary cause and hepatic support in severe cases (see formulary). Recovery can take several months (Boyer 2015).

13.3.2 Female Reproductive Pathology

Reproductive disorders are common, with 12% of female bearded dragons presented diagnosed with dystocia, follicular, or egg pathologies in one study (Schmidt-Ukaj et al. 2017). Prolapse of cloacal, oviductal or even intestinal tissue can be a consequence of reproductive pathology (Knotek et al. 2017).

13.3.2.1 Pre-Ovulatory Stasis/Follicular Stasis

This is believed to be primarily due to a lack of environmental or social cues to stimulate normal ovarian cycles (Stahl 2003; Knotek et al. 2017) though the author has seen two cases in this species associated with oviductal adenocarcinomas. With follicular stasis, one or more cycles of ovarian follicles are produced, enlarge, and fail to be ovulated. Large numbers of distended follicles accumulate bilaterally leading to compression of surrounding structures, metabolic drain, and risk of sepsis. Follicle rupture can result in severe oophoritis and coelomitis (Knotek et al. 2017).

There may be a history of increased digging or non-specific signs of lethargy and anorexia. On clinical examination a normal or enlarged coelom is often noted despite otherwise reduced body condition (Figure 13.5). Palpation and radiography identify poorly defined soft tissue structures in the mid-dorsal coelom. Ultrasonography demonstrates clusters of many round, fluid-filled structures

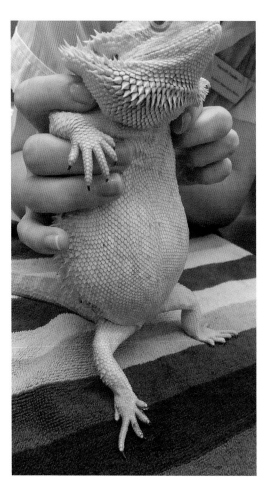

Figure 13.5 Distended coelom in a bearded dragon with follicular stasis.

within the coelom. Elevated total calcium, alkaline phosphatase, albumin, and protein may be noted on biochemistry, with anaemia and leukopenia often seen on haematology (McArthur 2001).

On the rare occasions that animals are presented early on in the disease progression, still feeding and with no loss in condition, conservative management can be attempted. This involves provision of correct conditions to induce normal progression of reproductive activity. A nesting substrate of sand or soil should be provided in several secluded areas of the vivarium, appropriate UVB lighting and calcium supplementation supplied and re-evaluation with follow up ultrasound examination every 10–14 days to assess whether follicular accumulations are decreasing in size and number.

In dragons that are in advanced disease, with anorexia and poor body condition then prompt surgical intervention is necessary. Poor prognosis has been reported in a study of elective ovariectomies in this species with death of four of seven bearded dragons (Christiansen et al. 2013). However this study involved animals in a student teaching laboratory with inexperienced surgeons and protracted surgical duration, the same procedure has been carried out in over 200 bearded dragons by the author with complications rarely seen.

The author favours a left paramedian approach to access both ovaries whilst avoiding the midline ventral abdominal vein, with the incision starting approximately 15 mm to the left of the midline at the level of the most caudal extent of the last rib (Figure 13.6). The skin is sharply incised with a scalpel blade, then the incision is extended 20–30 mm caudally using fine scissors to incise between scales. The thin underlying muscle layer is sharply dissected. The ventral abdominal vein should be identified and gently retracted if necessary before opening the thin, pigmented coelomic membrane. The ovaries are easily visualised due to their enlarged state and should be carefully exteriorised by grasping the connective tissue between follicles with atraumatic forceps, or by elevation using sterile cotton tip applicators. Direct pressure on follicles tends to result in leakage of inflammatory yolk proteins. The vascular supply within the ovarian ligament should then be ligated prior to sharp dissection to remove the ovary. Several ligatures are often necessary to encompass the three to eight vessels that branch from the aorta and renal veins (Alworth et al. 2011). Haemoclips can be used as a faster and more precise alternative to ligatures. It is important to avoid the vena cava, which is closely associated with the right ovary, and the renal vein and adrenal gland adjacent to the left ovary (Mader et al. 2006). The contralateral ovary can be exteriorised through the same incision and the procedure repeated. All ovarian tissue must be removed otherwise

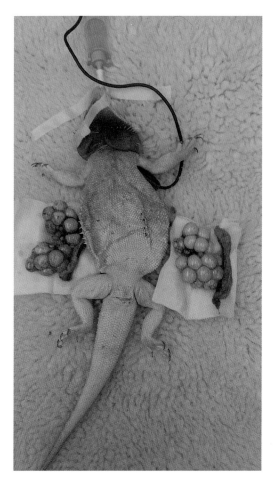

Figure 13.6 Bilateral ovariosalpingectomy carried out via a paramedian incision.

ovarian regeneration is possible from fragments left behind (Knotek et al. 2017). Unless the oviduct is abnormal then this is left in place (Alworth et al. 2011).

The coelomic membrane and muscle are closed together with a simple continuous pattern, taking care to avoid the vasculature (Alworth et al. 2011). Everting sutures, such as horizontal mattress sutures, should be used on the skin (Knotek 2017). Polydioxanone is typically used for reptile surgery due to its longer holding time. Sutures can be removed 6 wks post-surgery if healing is complete (Mader and Bennett 2006).

13.3.2.2 Egg Binding

Post-ovulatory stasis or egg binding is less common in this species. Retention of formed eggs can occur due to failure of an appropriate nesting site, hypocalcaemic oviductal inertia, large or abnormally shaped eggs, obesity, or oviductal pathology (Knotek et al. 2017). Animals may present with a distended coelom, indiscriminate digging, straining, hyperactivity, or lethargy. Administration of calcium followed by oxytocin may be effective for oviductal inertia, however where eggs are abnormally sized or shaped, chronically retained and potentially adherent to the oviduct, or oviductal pathology is present, oxytocin is contra-indicated. Additionally, if the animal is debilitated then oxytocin is unlikely to be effective. As a consequence conservative therapy is rarely successful (DeNardo 2006). Stabilisation and surgical intervention to remove retained eggs is advisable in most cases.

The surgical access is similar to that advised for ovariectomy, with exteriorisation of one oviduct at a time. Multiple incisions to the oviduct can be made to retrieve the eggs and salvage the oviducts for future breeding but it is faster to perform a salpingectomy and remove eggs and oviducts en bloc. The vessels in the mesosalpinx are individually ligated and the attachment of the oviduct to cloaca closed with a transfixing ligature prior to sharp dissection to remove the oviduct (Knotek et al. 2017). This is repeated for the other side, and a concurrent bilateral ovariectomy is recommended to prevent future ectopic ovulation (Alworth et al. 2011). Alternatively a second surgery to remove the ovaries can be scheduled weeks-months later when ovarian activity resumes and increased size enhances identification of all tissue (Knotek et al. 2017).

13.3.3 Intestinal Impaction

This is typically associated with inappropriate, particulate or calcium-based substrates but may also be predisposed to by hypocalcaemia and a secondary intestinal hypomotility (Klaphake 2010).

Clinical signs include coelomic distension, straining, anorexia, regurgitation, or failure to pass faeces. Owners may also have observed the animal eating substrate. Palpation of a firm mid-coelomic mass is highly suspicious and radiographs confirm accumulation of abnormal material. Small sand accumulations can often be passed with liquid paraffin administered orally, isotonic fluid enemas, hydration and correction of any calcium deficiency. Large gravel or bark pieces should be surgically removed, as they cannot be easily broken down and rough edges risk intestinal trauma and rupture.

The coeliotomy incision is made over the area of the impaction as the short mesentery often prevents extensive movement and full exteriorisation of the stomach or intestines. Enterotomy technique mimics that of mammalian patients though the smaller, more fragile tissues require gentle handling (Alworth et al. 2011). The enterotomy incision should be closed with an inverting pattern if this will not excessively narrow the lumen of the affected intestine, or appositional if necessary. Avoid rapidly absorbed suture materials as these risk dehiscence. Thorough flushing with warmed isotonic fluid should be carried out before

coelomic closure (Alworth et al. 2011). Antibiotics are commonly administered post-operatively.

13.3.4 Neoplasia

Various neoplasms have been reported in this species, with lymphoid and myelogenous leukaemia, and squamous cell carcinomas (SCC) most frequently identified (Suedmeyer and Turk 1996; Tocidlowski et al. 2001; Hannon et al. 2011; Jankowski et al. 2011).

Leukaemia can originate from any of the leucocyte cell lines and may present with non-specific signs, identification of a mass, or sudden death (Suedmeyer and Turk 1996; Tocidlowski et al. 2001; Gregory et al. 2004; Jankowski et al. 2011). Diagnosis of leukocyte neoplasms is based on identification of circulating neoplastic cells on a blood smear, or on cytology of mass aspirates or biopsies. Prognosis is grave. Cytosine arabinoside at $100 \, mg/m^2$ was trialled in one case of lymphoid leukaemia but patient death within 48 hours of initiating chemotherapy prevented assessment of therapeutic response (Jankowski et al. 2011).

SCC have a predilection for mucocutaneous junctions, particularly those around the eye with 75% affecting this region (Hannon et al. 2011). Excision, often with concurrent enucleation, remains the main therapeutic option. One report exists of successful treatment of a periocular SCC using cryotherapy (Boyer 2015). Topical therapy using imiquimod for a periocular SCC was initially positive, resulting in a reduction of mass size and clinical improvement, but acute deterioration refractory to further therapy occurred after a 75 day period (Pellett and Pinborough 2014).

Hepatic malignancies appear common in this species (Kubiak et al. 2020) and presenting signs are often vague (Figure 13.7). Anaplastic soft tissue sarcomas of mesenchymal origin (including fibrosarcomas, spindle cell sarcomas, nerve sheath tumours [neurofibrosarcoma], myxosarcoma, leiyomyosarcoma, and rhabdomyosarcoma) are common in agamids and can be difficult to differentiate (Garner et al. 2004; Kubiak et al. 2020). Chromatophoromas, haemangiomas, haemangiosarcomas, melanomas, and papillomas are also reported as externally identifiable neoplasms in this species (Kubiak et al. 2020). Biopsy of any evident mass should be encouraged with submission to a laboratory familiar with reptilian histopathology.

Gastric neuroendocrine carcinoma is an unusual endocrine neoplasm not reported in reptiles other than bearded dragons. Discrete neoplastic proliferations within the gastric mucosa secrete somatostatin (Lyons et al. 2010). Clinical signs present in young animals, typically of one to three years, and are often vague with malaise, anorexia, and vomition. The somatostatin release causes a persistent

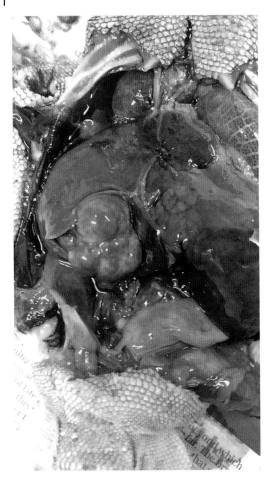

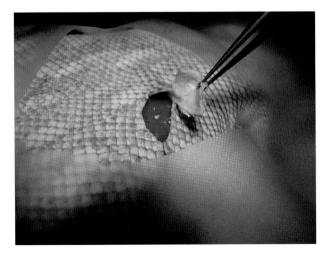

Figure 13.8 Elliptical biopsy collected for assessment of dermatitis. Note the lack of subcutaneous soft tissues.

Figure 13.7 Hepatocellular carcinoma in a bearded dragon with chronic anorexia, hepatic parameters were within normal limits on biochemistry and no mass was externally palpable.

hyperglycaemia, and this neoplasm should be considered for any clinically unwell bearded dragon with significant blood glucose elevation (>25mmol/l). Diagnosis is by endoscopic or surgical identification and biopsy of the small pale masses within the gastric mucosa. Prognosis is guarded due to the aggressive malignancy exhibited. Neuroendocrine carcinomas comprised 1.5% of bearded dragon neoplasms in one report with metastasis to the liver seen in all 10 cases evaluated (Ritter et al. 2009).

13.3.5 Dermatological Disease

Skin disorders are a common problem in clinical practice, often secondary to inappropriate husbandry conditions, hypovitaminosis A, trauma, thermal burns and excessive UV-B intensity, or UV of inappropriate wavelength (Gardiner et al. 2009; Hellebuyck et al. 2012). A moist, exudative dermatitis is most common but blisters, crusts, ulceration of the skin, granulomas, and firm abscess formation may also be noted. Opportunistic infections of

compromised skin are often indistinguishable from primary pathogens and a thorough approach, including culture and sensitivity and biopsy are advisable, particularly for severe or refractory cases (Figure 13.8).

Dermatological neoplasms, particularly SCC, can present as ulcerated thickened lesions with significant secondary infection.

Devriesea agamarum is an emerging primary skin pathogen of agamid lizards. It is associated with a crusting dermatitis in susceptible lizards but is recognised as an oral commensal in healthy bearded dragons (Hellebuyck et al. 2009a). As potential carriers, bearded dragons should not have direct or indirect contact with more susceptible species, particularly agamids of the *Uromastyx* genus (Devloo et al. 2011). Successful experimental infection following skin trauma has been demonstrated in bearded dragons, resulting in crusting, swelling, and plaque formation suggesting that spontaneous clinical disease is a possibility (Hellebuyck et al. 2009a). Diagnosis is by histological identification of the filamentous bacteria in crusts or biopsy samples and therapy with ceftazidime appears effective (Hellebuyck et al. 2009b; Lukac et al. 2013).

Fungal dermatitis presents similarly to bacterial causes and both may occur in tandem. In this species fungal infections may be predisposed to by excessive humidity, poor hygiene, or immunosuppression. The Chrysosporium anamorph of *Nannizziopsis vriesii* (CANV) has been identified as a pathogen in outbreaks of skin pathology in bearded dragons (Bowman et al. 2007; Hedley et al. 2010). It presents with yellow discolouration, vesicles, crusting and thickening of the skin, giving it its alternative name of 'Yellow fungus disease', and may spread systemically (Sigler et al. 2013). Biopsy for histopathology and fungal culture is needed to confirm diagnosis. Laboratories used should be familiar with this pathogen as misidentification, particularly as *Trichophyton* spp., has been reported (Bowman et al. 2007; Hedley et al. 2010). Treatment comprises topical and systemic antifungal therapy though mortality can be high. Related pathogens, *Nannizziopsis chlamydospora*, *Nannizziopsis draconii* and *Chrysosporium guarroi*, have also been reported to cause dermatitis in bearded dragons (Abarca et al. 2009; Stchigel et al. 2013; Schmidt-Ukaj et al. 2014) and approach is considered identical.

Dysecdysis is rarely a significant problem but lack of appropriate humidity, absence of abrasive enclosure décor, skin trauma, and dehydration can lead to retention of sloughed skin, which can result in constrictive bands of desiccated skin if the digits or tail are affected. Bathing to loosen retained shed, correction of husbandry, and rehydration is often sufficient, but persisting dysecdysis suggests a problem with skin integrity or debilitation from an underlying disease process and merits further investigation.

13.3.6 Atadenovirus Infection

Agamid Adenovirus-1 is well recognised as a cause of tremors, ataxia, immunosuppression, reduced growth and death in bearded dragons (Figure 13.9). As with many reptile viral infections, primary pathogenicity is unclear with environmental factors and co-infections suspected to play a significant role in individual response (Kim et al. 2002). PCR testing is available on choanal and cloacal swabs and detection alongside compatible clinical signs can support a diagnosis. However one small study showed that 5 of 27 bearded dragons in the UK had positive PCR results in the absence of any clinical signs (Kubiak 2013). It is recommended to screen breeding animals and remove positive individuals from breeding populations to decrease

prevalence. No treatment options are available and animals with compromised welfare due to advanced neurological symptoms should be euthanased.

13.3.7 Metabolic Bone Disease/Nutritional Secondary Hyperparathyroidism (NSHP)

Metabolic Bone Disease (MBD) is a group of conditions that can affect birds, reptiles, and mammals. NSHP appears the most common presentation in bearded dragons (Wright 2008), and is most common in growing animals (Klaphake 2010). Absence of UV lighting, vitamin and calcium supplementation, or appropriate heating, or competition for these resources, result in disruption to vitamin D synthesis and calcium absorption (Klaphake 2010). Insufficient available calcium induces endogenous release of parathyroid hormone, stimulating osteoclast activity and liberation of calcium salts from bone stabilises circulating ionised calcium levels. If the husbandry failings persist then chronic demineralisation results in pathological fractures and deformities of spine, limbs, or facial bones (Figure 13.10). Anorexia, intestinal hypomotility, tremors, limb paralysis, seizures, or chronic wasting are also commonly identified. The less common syndrome of renal secondary hyperparathyroidism can result in similar presentation with renal failure, due to inability of the kidneys to retain calcium and disruption of renal synthesis of calcitriol for vitamin D formation (Klaphake 2010).

Palpation of long bones and mandibles will demonstrate pathognomonic abnormal flexibility in advanced cases. Radiographs only detect changes when >30% reduction in bone density is present so are insensitive for early changes but remain useful in determining severity of demineralisation for prognosis (Klaphake 2010). Dual energy x-ray absorptiometry scans are superior at quantifying bone density but are not readily available and normal values are established for only a few species (Zotti et al. 2004). Serum total calcium

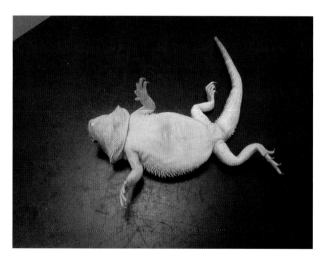

Figure 13.9 Lack of righting response in a juvenile bearded dragon with clinical adenoviral infection.

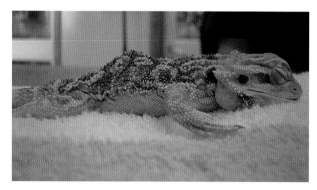

Figure 13.10 Pronounced kyphosis in a juvenile bearded dragon with NSHP.

levels may be normal, even in advanced cases but hyperphosphataemia (resulting in a serum calcium : phosphorus ratio <1 : 1) and elevated alkaline phosphatase are commonly identified.

Advanced cases should be euthanased due to permanent damage to bones and compromised feeding and mobility. Less marked changes can be treated with oral calcium and vitamin D, analgesia, UV lighting, appropriate temperatures, and removal of vivarium furniture to prevent injury. Radiographs should be taken every six weeks to monitor bone density and allow gradual withdrawal of medical treatment accordingly (Wright 2008). Medical management and husbandry changes appear sufficient to reverse mild–moderate changes in bearded dragons (Raiti 2012). Salmon calcitonin has been used in cases in other species where bone mineralisation does not progress after initial stabilisation. Calcitonin works by inhibition of osteoclast activity, resulting in net uptake of calcium into bone and should only be considered when circulating calcium levels have normalised yet persisting demineralisation of bone has been documented.

13.3.8 Constipation

Constipation, or obstipation, is a common reason for presentation in this species (Wright 2008). Clinical signs typically include failure to defaecate for over one week, straining, abdominal discomfort, and anorexia. A firm linear mass may be palpable in the caudal coelom on examination.

Urates are produced by the kidneys, are stored in the cloaca and retroflux into the colon for fluid and electrolyte reabsorption as an adaptation to arid climes. If they are not regularly egested with faeces then they can accumulate and progressively dehydrate to form a solid urolith, obstructing the colon. Common factors in urolith formation are dehydration or infrequent defaecation due to hypocalcaemia, obesity, endoparasitism, insufficient exercise, or a low fibre diet (Wright 2008). Gentle palpation during the clinical examination may elicit straining and passage of a firm cylinder of urates, followed by normal faeces. Warm water baths and repeated enemas of 10 ml/kg of warmed fluids may be necessary for more chronic cases.

Constipation may also result from other causes such as deformity of the spine or pelvic bones, intestinal stasis with hypocalcaemia, active folliculogenesis or ovarian pathology in females and intestinal obstructions such as substrate impaction, intussusception, abscessation, or neoplasia (Boyer 2015; Łojszczyk-Szczepaniak et al. 2018). In one review, endoparasites were present in over half of bearded dragons presenting with constipation and

evidence of NSHP was present in over one-third (Schmidt-Ukaj et al. 2017). As such, a thorough husbandry review and faecal parasitology is necessary in all cases and further diagnostics such as biochemistry, radiography, and coelomic ultrasound may also be indicated if no clear cause is evident.

13.3.9 Limb Swelling

A swollen joint or foot is a common presentation for bearded dragons. Differentials include osteomyelitis, articular gout, pseudogout, traumatic injury, neoplasia, and septic arthritis. Radiography can help achieve diagnosis but cytology and culture of biopsy or aspirate samples are often needed to determine cause of osteolytic changes.

Gout is typically a consequence of chronic renal compromise, often associated with excessive dietary protein, hypothermia, or chronic dehydration (Mader 2006). Uric acid is the main excretory product and with renal compromise, hyperuricaemia develops. Precipitates of uric acid crystals can occur in the organs with non-specific symptoms, or around joints resulting in visible areas of swelling. Aspirates from joint swellings show birefringent needle-shaped crystals which appear blue when using a polarising filter (Raiti 2012). Serum biochemistry often demonstrates a pronounced hyperuricaemia, and a concurrent hyperphosphataemia. Husbandry improvements, fluid therapy, analgesia, and medication to reduce serum uric acid levels are indicated and prognosis depends on the severity of the renal damage which may only be determined by renal biopsy.

Pseudogout involves deposition of crystalline material other than uric acid, most commonly calcium salts (Jones and Fitzgerald 2009). Although grossly identical in presentation to gout, polarised light microscopy and calcium stains differentiate crystals from uric acid. Pseudogout may be a consequence of excessive supplementation of calcium or Vitamin D, or renal compromise and can present concurrently with true gout (Jones and Fitzgerald 2009).

Septic arthritis of the digits is common, and is often suspected to be secondary to bacterial emboli disseminating from infections of the skin or gingiva (Raiti 2012). Osteolysis is often readily identifiable on radiographs. Culture and cytology of aspirates and long-term antibiotic therapy based on results is recommended, though amputation of individual digits may facilitate faster and more complete resolution. Mycobacterial osteomyelitis has been reported in this species, suspected to be caused by *Mycobacterium chelonae* and acid-fast staining of samples collected is advisable (Kramer 2006).

13.3.10 Periodontitis

Periodontal disease is recognised as a common syndrome in bearded dragons (McCracken and Birch 1994; Mott 2018). This genus of lizards has acrodont dentition, where teeth are fused to the mandibular or maxillary bone (Hedley 2016). The gingiva attach onto the bone and not the teeth, with only thin epithelium overlying the bone around the teeth rendering it vulnerable to injury or bacterial infection (Mans 2013). Prevalence of periodontal disease in UK bearded dragons has been demonstrated to be 48.89%, with older age, high or low body condition, and inclusion of fruit in the diet identified as correlations (Mott 2018). This same study found that type of insect fed or presence of vegetables in the diet had no discernible impact, suggesting that the pH or sugar content of fruit could be more significant than food softness.

Clinical signs include staining of the teeth, tartar and calculus accumulation, gingivitis, gingival regression, and osteomyelitis (Figure 13.11) (Raiti 2012; Boyer 2015). Owners may not identify changes until disease is severe when anorexia or abscessation become evident.

General anaesthesia is necessary for debridement of lesions, dental scaling and radiography to identify presence or extent of osteomyelitis (Hedley 2016). Samples should be collected for microbial culture to guide antibiotic therapy as a wide range of bacteria may be present. Analgesia should also be provided as this is likely a painful condition. Dietary improvement may slow progression of disease, and regular cleaning of any sulci resulting from gingival damage is needed to prevent ongoing infection from trapped food.

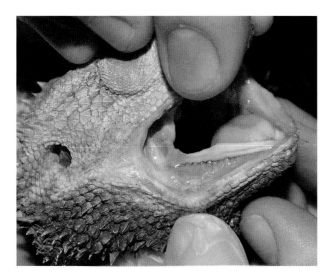

Figure 13.11 Mild-moderate periodontal disease with gingival regression, early tartar accumulation and focal cheilitis.

13.3.11 Cardiovascular Disease

Cardiac disease has been described as frequent in bearded dragons in one retrospective study (Reavill and Schmidt 2009) though case reports are scant. Schilliger et al. (2010) detail pericardial effusion and atherosclerosis in one bearded dragon and two further case reports detail arterial aneurysms in three dragons (Barten et al. 2006; Sweet et al. 2009). Many anecdotal reports of aneurysms also exist and the aorta or internal carotid artery appear most frequently involved (Boyer 2015). Animals typically present with a cervical or oral fluctuant swelling which has a pulsatile motion readily identified on Doppler auscultation. Animals may be asymptomatic, demonstrate lethargy and anorexia, or peracute death associated with rupture of the aneurysm. The source of the aneurysm is often deep to the swelling and difficult to identify and advanced imaging is advisable before contemplating intervention. Successful surgical correction has been described in one case (Barten et al. 2006) but was challenging with significant intraoperative haemorrhage requiring a blood transfusion.

Listeriosis has been reported to cause fatal cardiac infection in four bearded dragons (Vancraeynest et al. 2006; Denk and Stidworthy 2018). Clinical signs may include lethargy, dyspnoea, oedema, or sudden death (Denk and Stidworthy 2018). It is not known whether this syndrome is a consequence of opportunistic infection from commensal strains or food-borne infection.

Fireflies can contain toxic lucibufagin compounds and ingestion of a single *Photinus spp.* has been associated with fatal cardiotoxicity in bearded dragons (Knight et al. 1999). No therapeutic options have been identified.

13.3.12 Endoparasites

Oxyurids (pinworms) are frequently found on faecal examination of many reptile species and are rarely pathogenic (Figure 13.12). Low numbers in a clinically healthy animal may be left untreated. Diarrhoea, weight loss, anorexia, and reduced growth are consistent with excessive oxyurid loads and justify therapy if high numbers of ova are present in faeces. It should be noted that oxyurid number increases can be an indication of reduced immune function with husbandry deficiencies and concurrent health problems as potential primary concerns. Treatment is oral fenbendazole with a repeat faecal analysis recommended two weeks after the last treatment.

Isospora amphiboluri is the most common species of coccidia in bearded dragons (Singleton et al. 2006). It is pathogenic at moderate levels, with disease more common in juveniles, and detected infections should be

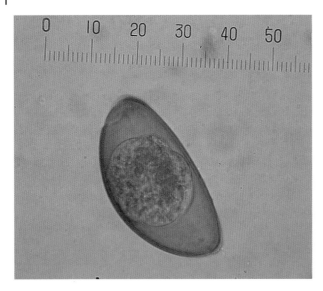

Figure 13.12 Oxyurid identified on faecal flotation in Zinc sulphate solution.

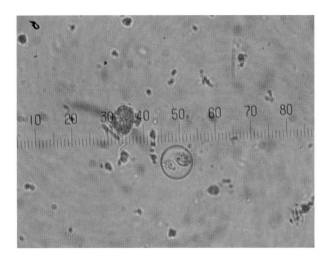

Figure 13.13 *Isospora* oocyst identified on faecal flotation.

treated. Inflammation within the small intestine causes diarrhoea, reduced growth, weight loss, haematochezia and, occasionally, neurological signs (due to thiamine deficiency following uptake by coccidia) (Scullion and Scullion 2009). Oocysts are consistently shed by infected animals and can be readily detected on faecal flotation analysis (Figure 13.13).

Reduction of infection using oral potentiated sulphonamides or toltrazuril eliminates clinical signs, but clearance may not be achieved (Scullion and Scullion 2009). Daily removal of faeces before oocysts have a chance to undergo sporogony to produce the infective form will help reduce future flare-ups.

Microsporidial intracellular protozoal parasites, morphologically similar to *Encephalitozoon* species, have been reported to cause anorexia, lethargy, neurological signs,

and acute death in bearded dragons (Richter et al. 2013). Infection can be direct via ingestion of infective spores from faeces of infected dragons, indirectly by contamination of feeder insects or fomites, or by vertical transmission (Mitchell and Garner 2011). Diagnosis is by histopathology demonstrating the multifocal granulomas and presence of gram-positive, acid-fast staining organisms with a dark polar cap (Jacobson et al. 1998). Although treatment can be attempted using fenbendazole no published protocols are available and the prognosis is guarded (Reavill and Schmidt 2009).

Protozoa of the genus *Cryptosporidium* have been identified in the faeces of bearded dragons but surprisingly are not known to cause pathology in this species. Paromomycin has been demonstrated to terminate shedding of oocysts in experimentally infected bearded dragons, and treatment is recommended in multi-species households to avoid transmission to more susceptible species (Grosset et al. 2011).

Entamoeba infection appears highly pathogenic in bearded dragons with development of disseminated visceral granulomas following parasite migration (Klingenberg 2004). Detection of motile *Entamoeba* trophozoites on a direct faecal examination aids diagnosis. Prognosis is guarded but metronidazole can be used to attempt treatment.

13.3.13 Ectoparasites

Ophionyssus natricis ('snake mite') and Pterygosomid mites are occasionally seen on bearded dragons. The dark *Ophionyssus* mites prefer skin folds, particularly around the eyes and mouth whereas Pterygosomids are orange-red and found on the dorsal surface of the head and body. Topical therapy with fipronil or ivermectin is generally effective. Fipronil is commercially available with an alcohol solvent and must only be used in a well ventilated area to prevent intoxication. Enclosures must be thoroughly cleaned and treated with insecticides.

13.4 Preventative Health Measures

Routine faecal testing is advisable with direct examination and flotation techniques on a faecal sample carried out on a six monthly basis for clinically well animals, and three monthly for those with recent history of endoparasitism.

It is prudent to test breeding animals for Agamid Adenovirus-1 to aim to breed offspring free from the virus. Repeat testing is sensible in clinically well animals as shedding appears inconsistent.

Although testing for *Salmonella* appears a reasonable precaution, especially in households with small children, asymptomatic *Salmonella* carriage is widespread in reptiles, shedding is infrequent resulting in false negative cultures, and antibiotic treatment is not advisable. It is often more practical to advise owners to assume their pet reptile carries *Salmonella* and is intermittently shedding bacteria in faeces and to be vigilant with hygiene rather than screen on a routine basis (PHE 2014). For households with particularly vulnerable children, such as those under five years of age or with immunosuppression, or for businesses incorporating reptile handling, it can be prudent to screen for *Salmonella* with the aim of typing the strain identified in order to evaluate zoonotic risk more accurately.

13.5 Imaging

The single body cavity and lack of intervisceral fat deposits in reptiles result in lower radiographic image clarity compared to mammals and birds (Figure 13.14) (Silverman 2006), with lack of objective values further complicating interpretation (Łojszczyk-Szczepaniak et al. 2018). However, a recent study confirmed the clinical value of imaging techniques with a diagnosis made in over 70% of cases where radiography and ultrasound evaluations were performed (Łojszczyk-Szczepaniak et al. 2018). Radiography is most useful for evaluating the skeletal, respiratory and gastrointestinal systems, and identifying mineralised eggs. A dorsoventral view is preferred for survey radiographs. Lateral views with forelimbs extended cranially require restraint of patients and a horizontal beam, but are superior in evaluating the heart and lungs. Common radiographic findings are bony deformities associated with NSHP, osteomyelitis, fractures, pneumonia, and foreign body ingestion (Figures 13.15 and 13.16) (Raiti 2012).

Ultrasound is superior for evaluating liver and reproductive tract pathology (Łojszczyk-Szczepaniak et al. 2018). In anorexic animals with hepatic lipidosis, the normal heterogeneous appearance of the liver becomes homogeneous and similar in appearance to the fat bodies located in the lateral coelom, allowing presumptive diagnosis on ultrasound examination. Cholelithiasis has also been diagnosed ultrasonographically in a lethargic, anorexic bearded dragon (Ritzman and Garner 2009).

Echocardiography approach has been assessed in bearded dragons, with the left axillary window preferred for assessing cardiac anatomy and contractility, the right axillary window for pulmonary arterial flow assessment and both windows suitable for identification of valvular lesions or pericardial effusion (Silverman et al. 2016). Small quantities of pericardial fluid were identified in the majority of clinically normal animals and are assumed to be a normal finding.

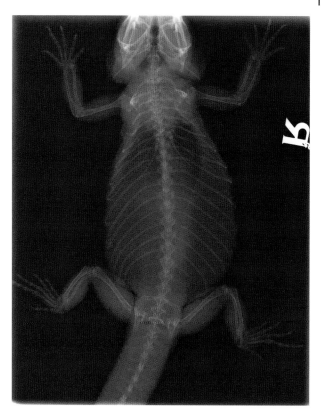

Figure 13.14 Dorsoventral view of normal bearded dragon, note the lack of coelomic contrast.

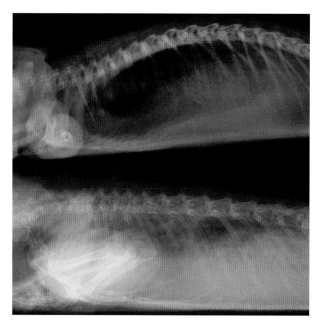

Figure 13.15 Laterolateral views of two bearded dragons; normal lung appearance (upper), diffuse bacterial pneumonia with mixed populations found on lung wash culture (lower).

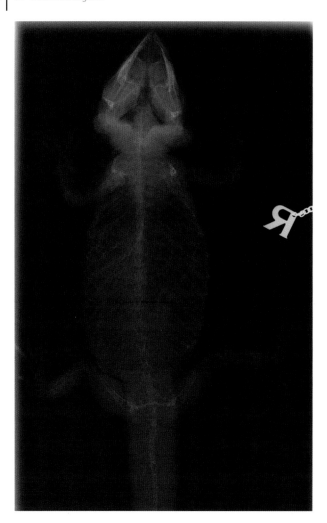

Figure 13.16 NSHP with marked demineralisation of the skeleton, long bone deformities and pathological fracture of left femur.

Formulary

Medication	Dose	Dosing interval	Additional comments
Anaesthesia			
Isoflurane	Inhalation of 3% in 100% oxygen		5–10 mins induction time reported though can be significantly longer (Odette et al. 2015)
Alfaxalone	5–12 mg/kg IV		Lower doses preferred for induction followed by maintenance with isoflurane. Anaesthesia duration of 22–75 mins at higher doses (Knotek 2017; Perrin and Bertelsen 2017)
Propofol	10 mg/kg IV		15–26 mins anaesthesia, invasive procedures typically require additional anaesthesia e.g. isoflurane (Perrin and Bertelsen 2017)
Dexmedetomidine and midazolam	0.1 mg/kg and 1 mg/kg respectively, SC or IM		Moderate sedation, rapid recovery after full reversal. 3 mg/kg ketamine can be added to deepen sedation (Mans 2015)
Atropine	1 mg/kg IM		Administered to reduce right–left shunting and improve efficacy of inhalation anaesthesia, based on tortoise dose (Greunz et al. 2018)

(Continued)

Medication	Dose	Dosing interval	Additional comments
Analgesia			
Morphine	5–10 mg/kg SC, IM	q24h in males, q8h in females	(Sladky et al. 2008; Greenacre et al. 2011)
Meloxicam	0.3 mg/kg PO, SC, IM	q12–18h	Presumed anti-inflammatory effects (Greenacre et al. 2011; Sladky and Mans 2012; Knotek et al. 2017)
Tramadol	5–10 mg/kg PO, IM, SC	q48h	(Greenacre et al. 2011)
Buprenorphine and butorphanol		No analgesic effects (Sladky et al. 2008; Sladky and Mans 2012)	
Antibiotics			
Trimethoprim-sulfa	30 mg/kg PO	q24 h for 7 d	(Jenkins 1991)
Ceftazidime	5 m/kg IM	q24h for minimum 18 days	Successful for eliminating *Devriesea agamarum* in Uromastyx (Hellebuyck et al. 2009b)
	10 mg/kg IM	q72hd for 5 doses	Successful for eliminating *Devriesea agamarum* in Uromastyx (Lukac et al. 2013)
	20 mg/kg IM	q72h	Used for gram-negative bacterial infections. Third generation cephalosporin, should not be first line antibiotic choice
Enrofloxacin	5–10 mg/kg PO, IM, SC	q24h	Injectable preparations can cause tissue necrosis (Gibbons et al. 2013). Fluoroquinolones should not be first line antitbiotics.
Oxytetracycline	6–10 mg/kg PO, IM	q24h	Injectable preparations can result in localised inflammation (Gibbons et al. 2013)
Metronidazole	20 mg/kg PO	q24–48h	Based on green iguana pharmacokinetics (Kolmstetter et al. 1998)
Amoxicillin	22 mg/kg PO	q24h	Often used in combination with an aminoglycoside (Frye 1991)
Amikacin	5 mg/kg initial dose then 2.5 mg/kg IM	q72h	Potentially nephrotoxic, ensure good hydration (Gibbons et al. 2013)
Antifungals			
Voriconazole	10 mg/kg PO	q24h for 7–10 weeks	(Van Waeyenberghe et al. 2010)
Itraconazole	5 mg/kg PO	q24h for 4–6 weeks	Higher mortality seen than with voriconazole (Van Waeyenberghe et al. 2010)
Antiparasitic agents			
Trimethoprim-sulfa	30 mg/kg PO	q24h for two doses, then q48h for 21 days	For coccidial treatment (Willette-Frahm et al. 1995)
Fenbendazole	33 mg/kg PO	q24h for 3d	For oxyurid treatment (Klingenberg 2004)
Metronidazole	20 mg/kg PO	q48h	For Entamoebiasis (Kolmstetter et al. 1998)
Toltrazuril	5–15 mg/kg PO	q24h for three doses	For coccidial treatment (Doneley 2006)
Praziquantel	5–8 mg/kg PO or IM		For cestodes (Klingenberg 2004)
Fipronil (0.29% spray)	2 ml/kg topically	q7d for 4 treatments	For ectoparasites, use in well ventilated environment and remove water bowl for 24 hrs after treatment

(Continued)

(Continued)

Medication	Dose	Dosing interval	Additional comments
Ivermectin	Dilute to 5 mg/l in water, spray animal and environment	q72–96h, up to 28 days	For ectoparasites (Klingenberg 2012)
	0.2 mg/kg PO, SC, IM	q14d	For ectoparasites (Gibbons et al. 2013)
Paromomycin	100 mg/kg/d PO for 7d then 360 mg/kg q48h for 10 days		For Cryptosporidia (Grosset et al. 2011)
Hepatic lipidosis therapy			
L-carnitine	250 mg/kg PO	q24h	(Boyer 2015) Used alongside assist feeding and management of co-morbidiities
Methionine	50 mg/kg PO	q24h	
S-adenosylmethionine	30 mg/kg PO	q24h	
Lactulose	0.5 ml/kg PO	q24h	
Silybun marianum (milk thistle extract)	4–15 mg/kg PO	q 8–12h	
Nandrolone	0.5 to 5 mg/kg IM		(Silvestre and Avepa 2013)
Miscellaneous			
Imiquimod 5%	topical application	q72h	Caused temporary regression of squamous cell carcinoma (Pellett and Pinborough 2014)
Allopurinol	50 mg/kg PO	q24h	Used to reduce serum uric acid levels in gout. Based on chelonian dose (Kolle 2001)
Probenecid	250 mg/kg PO	q12h	(Plumb 2008) Increases uric acid excretion to aid management of gout
Calcium gluconate	100 mg/kg SC, IM	q6–24h	(Gibbons et al. 2013) Oral supplementation with combined calcium and Vitamin D products preferred in non-critical patients
Oxytocin	1–5 U/kg IM	repeat after 1 hr if unsuccessful	(Divers 1996) Used for uterine inertia in the absence of egg adherence, egg deformity or oviductal pathology
Calcitonin	1.5 U/kg SC	q8h for 14–21 days	(Frye 1994). Used to induce bone mineralisation after resolution of hypocalcaemia in NSHP, rarely indicated and can induce hypocalcaemia.
Ranitidine	5 mg/kg SC, PO	q12–24h	Used to manage gastrointestinal atony occasionally seen after resolution of chronic obstipation

References

Abarca, M.L., Martorell, J., Castellá, G. et al. (2009). Dermatomycosis in a pet inland bearded dragon (*Pogona vitticeps*) caused by a *Chrysosporium* species related to *Nannizziopsis vriesii*. *Veterinary Dermatology* 20 (4): 295–299.

Allen, M.E. and Oftedal, O.T. (1989). Dietary manipulation of the calcium content of feed crickets. *Journal of Zoo and Wildlife Medicine* 20 (1): 26–33.

Alworth, L.C., Hernandez, S.M., and Divers, S.J. (2011). Laboratory reptile surgery: principles and techniques. *Journal of the American Association for Laboratory Animal Science* 50 (1): 11–26.

Andrews, R.M. and Pough, F.H. (1985). Metabolism of squamate reptiles: allometric and ecological relationships. *Physiological Zoology* 58 (2): 214–231.

Baines F. (2018). True full spectrum lighting for zoo animals. Proceedings of the British Veterinary Zoological Society, 9–11 November, Birmingham, UK: 20.

Baines, F., Chattell, J., Dale, J. et al. (2016). How much UV-B does my reptile need? The UV-Tool, a guide to the selection of UV lighting for reptiles and amphibians in captivity. *Journal of Zoo and Aquarium Research* 4 (1): 42.

Ballen, C., Shine, R., and Olsson, M. (2014). Effects of early social isolation on the behaviour and performance of juvenile lizards, *Chamaeleo calyptratus*. *Animal Behaviour* 88: 1–6.

Barker, D., Fitzpatrick, M.P., and Dierenfeld, E.S. (1998). Nutrient composition of selected whole invertebrates. *Zoo Biology*: Published in affiliation with the American Zoo and Aquarium Association 17 (2): 123–134.

Barten, S., Wyneken, J., Mader, D. et al. (2006). Aneurysm in the dorsolateral neck of two bearded dragons (*Pogona vitticeps*). Proceedings of the Association of Reptilian and Amphibian Veterinarians: 43–44.

Bertelsen, M.F. (2014). Squamates (snakes and lizards). In: *Zoo Animal and Wildlife Immobilization and Anesthesia* (eds. G. West, D. Heard and N. Caulkett), 233–244. Ames, IA: Blackwell Publishing.

Bowman, M.R., Paré, J.A., Sigler, L. et al. (2007). Deep fungal dermatitis in three inland bearded dragons (*Pogona vitticeps*) caused by the *Chrysosporium* anamorph of *Nannizziopsis vriesii*. *Medical Mycology* 45 (4): 371–376.

Boyer, T.H. (2015). Diseases of bearded dragons, In: Proceedings of the Pacific Veterinary Conference. Long Beach, CA, 18–21 June: 1–6.

Cannon, M.J. (2003). Husbandry and veterinary aspects of the bearded dragon (*Pogona* spp.) in Australia. *Seminars In Avian and Exotic Pet Medicine* 12 (4): 205–214.

Christiansen, E.F., Stoskopf, M.K., and Harms, C.A. (2013). Pre-and post-surgical evaluation of bearded dragons undergoing sterilization. *Journal of Herpetological Medicine and Surgery* 23 (3): 83–90.

De Vosjoli, P. and Mailloux, R. (1996). A simple system for raising juvenile bearded dragons indoors. *Vivarium* 7 (6): 42–55.

DeNardo, D. (2006). Reproductive biology. In: *Reptile Medicine and Surgery*, 2e (ed. D.R. Mader), 376–390. St Louis, MO: Elsevier Saunders.

Denk, D. and Stidworthy, M. (2018). Fatal Cardiac Listeriosis in Three Bearded Dragons (*Pogona vitticeps*), Proceedings of BVZS Conference, Birmingham, UK, 9–11 November: 90.

Deveson, I.W., Holleley, C.E., Blackburn, J. et al. (2017). Differential intron retention in Jumonji chromatin modifier genes is implicated in reptile temperature-dependent sex determination. *Science Advances* 3 (6): e1700731.

Devloo, R., Martel, A., Hellebuyck, T. et al. (2011). Bearded dragons (*Pogona vitticeps*) asymptomatically infected with *Devriesea agamarum* are a source of persistent clinical infection in captive colonies of dab lizards (*Uromastyx* sp.). *Veterinary Microbiology* 150 (3–4): 297–301.

Divers, S.J. (1996). Medical and surgical treatment of preovulatory ova stasis and postovulatory egg stasis in oviparous lizards. In: *Proceedings of the Association of Reptile and Amphibian Veterinarians (ARAV)*, 119–123. ARAV.

Divers, S.J. and Cooper, J.E. (2000). Reptile hepatic lipidosis. *Seminars in Avian and Exotic Pet Medicine* 9 (3): 153–164.

Doneley, B. (2006). Caring for the bearded dragon. In: Proceedings of the North American Veterinary Conference, Vol. 20: 1607–1611.

Donoghue, S. (2006). Nutrition. In: *Reptile Medicine and Surgery*, 2e (ed. D.R. Mader), 251–298. St. Louis, MO: Saunders Elsevier.

Ezaz, T., Quinn, A.E., Miura, I. et al. (2005). The dragon lizard *Pogona vitticeps* has ZZ/ZW micro-sex chromosomes. *Chromosome Research* 13 (8): 763–776.

Finke, M.D. (2015). Complete nutrient content of four species of commercially available feeder insects fed enhanced diets during growth. *Zoo Biology* 34 (6): 554–564.

Frye, F.L. (1991). *Reptile Care: An Atlas of Diseases and Treatments*. Neptune City: TFH Publications.

Frye, F.L. (1994). *Reptile Clinician's Handbook: A Compact Clinical and Surgical Reference*. Malabar, FL: Krieger Publishing Company.

Gardiner, D.W., Baines, F.M., and Pandher, K. (2009). Photodermatitis and photokeratoconjunctivitis in a ball python (*Python regius*) and a blue-tongue skink (*Tiliqua* spp.). *Journal of Zoo and Wildlife Medicine* 40 (4): 757–766.

Garner, M.M., Hernandez-Divers, S.M., and Raymond, J.T. (2004). Reptile neoplasia: a retrospective study of case submissions to a specialty diagnostic service. *The Veterinary Clinics of North America. Exotic Animal Practice* 7: 653–671.

Gibbons, P.M. and Tell, L.A. (2009). Problem solving in reptile practice. *Journal of Exotic Pet Medicine* 18 (3): 202–212.

Gibbons, P., Klaphake, E., and Carpenter, J.W. (2013). Reptiles. In: *Exotic Animal Formulary*, 4e (eds. J.W. Carpenter and C.J. Marion), 83–182. St Louis, MO: Saunders.

Greenacre, C.B., Cox, S., Yarborough, J. et al. (2011). Pharmacokinetics of morphine, Tramadol, meloxicam and Butorphanol in bearded dragons. Proceedings of the Association of Reptilian and Amphibian Veterinarians' 18th Annual Conference, Seattle, WA, 6–12 August: 172.

Gregory, C.R., Latimer, K.S., Fontenot, D.K. et al. (2004). Chronic monocytic leukemia in an inland bearded dragon, *Pogona vitticeps*. *Journal of Herpetological Medicine and Surgery* 14 (2): 12–16.

Grenard, S. (2008). *Bearded Dragon: Your Happy Healthy Pet*. Hoboken, NJ: Wiley Publishing Inc.

Greunz, E.M., Williams, C.J.A., Ringgaard, S. et al. (2018). Intracardiac shunting affects minimal alveolar concentration of isoflurane in the red-footed tortoise

(*Chelonoidis carbonaria*), Proceedings of the Joint EAZWV/AAZV/Leibniz-IZW Conference, Prague, 6–12 October: 123–124.

Grosset, C., Villeneuve, A., Brieger, A. et al. (2011). Cryptosporidiosis in juvenile bearded dragons (*Pogona vitticeps*): effects of treatment with paromomycin. *Journal of Herpetological Medicine and Surgery* 21 (1): 10–15.

Hannon, D.E., Garner, M.M., and Reavill, D.R. (2011). Squamous cell carcinomas in inland bearded dragons (*Pogona vitticeps*). *Journal of Herpetological Medicine and Surgery* 21 (4): 101–106.

Hedley, J. (2016). Anatomy and disorders of the oral cavity of reptiles and amphibians. *The Veterinary Clinics of North America. Exotic Animal Practice* 19 (3): 689–706.

Hedley, J., Eatwell, K., and Hume, L. (2010). Necrotising fungal dermatitis in a group of bearded dragons (*Pogona vitticeps*). *The Veterinary Record* 166: 464–465.

Hellebuyck, T., Martel, A., Chiers, K. et al. (2009a). *Devriesea agamarum* causes dermatitis in bearded dragons (*Pogona vitticeps*). *Veterinary Microbiology* 134 (3–4): 267–271.

Hellebuyck, T., Pasmans, F., Haesebrouck, F. et al. (2009b). Designing a successful antimicrobial treatment against Devriesea agamarum infections in lizards. *Veterinary Microbiology* 139 (1–2): 189–192.

Hellebuyck, T., Pasmans, F., Haesebrouck, F. et al. (2012). Dermatological diseases in lizards. *The Veterinary Journal* 193 (1): 38–45.

Jacobson, E.R., Green, D.E., Undeen, A.H. et al. (1998). Systemic microsporidiosis in inland bearded dragons (*Pogona vitticeps*). *Journal of Zoo and Wildlife Medicine* 29: 315–323.

Jankowski, G., Sirninger, J., Borne, J. et al. (2011). Chemotherapeutic treatment for leukemia in a bearded dragon (*Pogona vitticeps*). *Journal of Zoo and Wildlife Medicine* 42 (2): 322–325.

Jenkins, J.R. (1991). Medical management of reptile patients. *The Compendium on Continuing Education for the Practicing Veterinarian* 13: 980–988.

Jones, Y.L. and Fitzgerald, S.D. (2009). Articular gout and suspected pseudogout in a basilisk lizard (*Basilicus plumifrons*). *Journal of Zoo and Wildlife Medicine* 40 (3): 576–578.

Kim, D.Y., Mitchell, M.A., Bauer, R.W. et al. (2002). An outbreak of adenoviral infection in inland bearded dragons (*Pogona vitticeps*) coinfected with dependovirus and coccidial protozoa (*Isospora* sp.). *Journal of Veterinary Diagnostic Investigation* 14 (4): 332–334.

Klaphake, E. (2010). A fresh look at metabolic bone diseases in reptiles and amphibians. *The Veterinary Clinics of North America. Exotic Animal Practice* 13 (3): 375–392.

Klingenberg, R. (2004). Parasitology. In: *BSAVA Manual of Reptiles* (eds. S.J. Girling and P. Raiti), 319–329. Ames, IA: Wiley Blackwell.

Klingenberg, R. (2012). *Understanding Reptile Parasites*. Los Angeles, CA: i5 Publishing.

Knight, M., Glor, R., Smedley, S. et al. (1999). Firefly toxicosis in lizards. *Journal of Chemical Ecology* 25 (9): 1981–1986.

Knotek, Z. (2017). Induction to inhalation anaesthesia in agamid lizards with alfaxalone. *Veterinarni Medicina* 62 (01): 41–43.

Knotek, Z., Knotkova, Z., Hrda, A. et al. (2009). Plasma Bile Acids in Reptiles. Proceedings of the Association of Reptilian and Amphibian Veterinarians, Milwaukee: 124–127.

Knotek, Z., Cermakova, E., and Oliveri, M. (2017). Reproductive medicine in lizards. *The Veterinary Clinics of North America. Exotic Animal Practice* 20 (2): 411–438.

Kolle, P. (2001). Efficacy of allopurinol in European tortoises with hyperuricemia. Proceedings of the Association of Reptilian and Amphibian Veterinarians, 19–23 September, Orlando FL: 185–186.

Kolmstetter, C.M., Frazier, D., Cox, S. et al. (1998). Pharmacokinetics of metronidazole in the green iguana, *Iguana iguana*. *Bulletin of the Association of Reptilian and Amphibian Veterinarians* 8 (3): 4–7.

Kramer, M.H. (2006). Granulomatous osteomyelitis associated with atypical mycobacteriosis in a bearded dragon (*Pogona vitticeps*). *The Veterinary Clinics of North America. Exotic Animal Practice* 9 (3): 563–568.

Kubiak, M. (2013). Detection of agamid Adenovirus-1 in clinically healthy bearded dragons (*Pogona vitticeps*) in the UK. *Veterinary Record* 172 (18): 475–475.

Kubiak, M., Denk, D., and Stidworthy, M.F. (2020). Retrospective review of neoplasms of captive lizards in the United Kingdom. *Veterinary Record* 186 (1): 28–28.

Łojszczyk-Szczepaniak, A., Szczepaniak, K.O., Grzybek, M. et al. (2018). Causes of consultations and results of radiological and ultrasound methods in lizard diseases (2006–2014). *Medycyna Weterynaryjna* 74 (1): 65–69.

Lukac, M., Horvatek-Tomic, D., and Prukner-Radovcic, E. (2013). Findings of *Devriesea agamarum* associated infections in spiny-tailed lizards (*Uromastyx* sp.) in Croatia. *Journal of Zoo and Wildlife Medicine* 44 (2): 430–434.

Lyons, J.A., Newman, S.J., Greenacre, C.B. et al. (2010). A gastric neuroendocrine carcinoma expressing somatostatin in a bearded dragon (*Pogona vitticeps*). *Journal of Veterinary Diagnostic Investigation* 22 (2): 316–320.

Macmillen, R., Augee, M., and Ellis, B. (1989). Thermal ecology and diet of some xerophilous lizards from western New South Wales. *Journal of Arid Environments* 16 (2): 193–201.

Mader, D. (2006). Gout. In: *Reptile Medicine and Surgery*, 2e (ed. D. Mader), 793–800. St. Louis, MO: Saunders Elsevier Co.

Mader, D.R. and Bennett, R.A. (2006). Surgery: soft tissue, orthopedics and fracture repair. In: *Reptile Medicine and Surgery*, 2e (ed. D.R. Mader), 581–612. St Louis, MO: Saunders Elsevier.

Mans, C. (2013). Clinical update on diagnosis and management of disorders of the digestive system of reptiles. *Journal of Exotic Pet Medicine* 22 (2): 141–162.

Mans, C. (2015). Herpetology masterclass: Reptile sedation, anaesthesia and analgesia. Proceedings of ICARE, 18–23 April, Paris: 69–72.

McArthur, S. (2001). Follicular stasis in captive chelonians, *Testudo* spp. Proceedings of the Association of Reptilian and Amphibian Veterinarians, 19–23 September, Orlando FL: 75–86.

McCracken, H. and Birch, C. (1994). Periodontal disease in lizards: a review of numerous cases. Proceedings of the Association of Reptilian and Amphibian Veterinarians: 108–114.

Mitchell, M.A. and Garner, M. (2011). Microsporidiosis in bearded dragons: a case for vertical transmission. Proceedings of the Association of Reptilian and Amphibian Veterinarians: 123.

Mott, R. (2018). Prevalence and risk factors for periodontal disease in captive central bearded dragons (*Pogona vitticeps*) in the UK. Thesis for Bachelor of Veterinary Medicine, Royal Veterinary College.

Music, M.K. and Strunk, A. (2016). Reptile critical care and common emergencies. *The Veterinary Clinics of North America. Exotic Animal Practice* 19 (2): 591–612.

Nevarez, J. (2009). Lizards. In: *Manual of Exotic Pet Practice* (eds. M.A. Mitchell and T.N. Tully), 193. St. Louis, MO: Saunders Elsevier.

Odette, O., Churgin, S.M., Sladky, K.K. et al. (2015). Anesthetic induction and recovery parameters in bearded dragons (*Pogona vitticeps*): comparison of isoflurane delivered in 100% oxygen versus 21% oxygen. *Journal of Zoo and Wildlife Medicine* 46 (3): 534–540.

Oonincx, D.G.A.B., van Leeuwen, J.P., Hendriks, W.H. et al. (2015). The diet of free-roaming Australian central bearded dragons (*Pogona vitticeps*). *Zoo Biology* 34 (3): 271–277.

Pellett, S. and Pinborough, M. (2014). Squamous cell carcinoma in a central bearded dragon. *Companion Animal* 19 (7): 379–384.

Perrin, K.L. and Bertelsen, M.F. (2017). Intravenous Alfaxalone and Propofol anesthesia in the bearded dragon (*Pogona vitticeps*). *Journal of Herpetological Medicine and Surgery* 27 (3): 123–126

PHE (Public Health England) (2014). Reducing the risks of Salmonella infection from reptiles. PHE publications gateway number: 2014061, https://www.gov.uk/government/uploads/system/uploads/attachment_data/file/377731/Salmonella_in_reptiles_factsheet__2_.pdf (accessed 24 June 2019).

Plumb, D.C. (2008). Probenecid. In: *Plumb's Veterinary Drug Handbook*, 6e. Stockholm: Pharma Vet Inc.

Raiti, P. (2012). Husbandry, diseases, and veterinary care of the bearded dragon (*Pogona vitticeps*). *Journal of Herpetological Medicine and Surgery* 22 (3): 117–131.

Reavill, D. and Schmidt, R. (2009). A retrospective review of the diseases in family agamidae (agamas, bearded dragons, frilled dragon, water dragons). Proceedings of the Association of Reptilian and Amphibian Veterinarians: 111–116.

Richter, B., Csokai, J., Graner, I. et al. (2013). Encephalitozoonosis in two inland bearded dragons (*Pogona vitticeps*). *Journal of Comparative Pathology* 148 (2–3): 278–282.

Ritter, J.M., Garner, M.M., Chilton, J.A. et al. (2009). Gastric neuroendocrine carcinomas in bearded dragons (*Pogona vitticeps*). *Veterinary Pathology* 46 (6): 1109–1116.

Ritzman, T. and Garner, M. (2009). Cholelithiasis and surgical cholelith removal in a bearded dragon (*Pogona vitticeps*). Proceedings of the Association of Reptilian and Amphibian Veterinarians: 117.

Schilliger, L., Lemberger, K., Chai, N. et al. (2010). Atherosclerosis associated with pericardial effusion in a central bearded dragon (*Pogona vitticeps*). *Journal of Veterinary Diagnostic Investigation* 22 (5): 789–792.

Schmidt-Ukaj, S., Loncaric, I., Klang, A. et al. (2014). Infection with Devriesea agamarum and Chrysosporium guarroi in an inland bearded dragon (*Pogona vitticeps*). *Veterinary Dermatology* 25 (6): 555.

Schmidt-Ukaj, S., Hochleithner, M., Richter, B. et al. (2017). A survey of diseases in captive bearded dragons: a retrospective study of 529 patients. *Veterinární Medicína* 62 (9): 508–515.

Scullion, F.T. and Scullion, M.G. (2009). Gastrointestinal protozoal diseases in reptiles. *Journal of Exotic Pet Medicine* 18 (4): 266–278.

Sigler, L., Hambleton, S., and Paré, J.A. (2013). Molecular characterization of reptile pathogens currently known as members of the *Chrysosporium* anamorph of *Nannizziopsis vriesii* (CANV) complex and relationship with some human-associated isolates. *Journal of Clinical Microbiology* 51 (10): 3338–3357.

Silverman, S. (2006). Diagnostic imaging. In: *Reptile Medicine and Surgery* (ed. D.). Mader), 471–489. St. Louis, MO: Elsevier.

Silverman, S., Guzman, D.S.M., Stern, J. et al. (2016). Standardization of the two-dimensional transcoelomic echocardiographic examination in the central bearded dragon (*Pogona vitticeps*). *Journal of Veterinary Cardiology* 18 (2): 168–178.

Silvestre, A.M. and Avepa, A. (2013). Hepatic lipidosis in reptiles. Proceedings of the Southern European Veterinary Conference (SEVC), Barcelona, 17–19 October.

Singleton, C.B., Mitchell, M., Riggs, S. et al. (2006). Evaluating Quikon® Med as a Coccidiocide for inland bearded dragons (*Pogona vitticeps*). *Journal of Exotic Pet Medicine* 15 (4): 269–273.

Sladky, K.K. and Mans, C. (2012). Clinical analgesia in reptiles. *Journal of Exotic Pet Medicine* 21 (2): 158–167.

Sladky, K.K., Kinney, M.E., and Johnson, S.M. (2008). Analgesic efficacy of butorphanol and morphine in bearded dragons and corn snakes. *Journal of the American Veterinary Medical Association* 233 (2): 267–273.

Stahl, S.J. (1999). General husbandry and captive propagation of bearded dragons, *Pogona vitticeps*. *Bulletin of the Association of Reptilian and Amphibian Veterinarians* 9 (4): 12–17.

Stahl, S.J. (2003). Pet lizard conditions and syndromes. *Seminars in Avian and Exotic Pet Medicine* 12: 162–182.

Stchigel, A.M., Sutton, D.A., Cano-Lira, J.F. et al. (2013). Phylogeny of *chrysosporia* infecting reptiles: proposal of the new family Nannizziopsiaceae and five new species. *Persoonia: Molecular Phylogeny and Evolution of Fungi* 31: 86.

Suedmeyer, W.K. and Turk, J.R. (1996). Lymphoblastic leukemia in an inland bearded dragon, *Pogona vitticeps*. *Bulletin of the Association of Reptilian and Amphibian Veterinarians* 6 (4): 10–12.

Sweet, C., Linnetz, E., Golden, E. et al. (2009). What's your diagnosis? *Journal of the American Veterinary Medical Association* 234 (10): 1259–1260.

Thompson, S.A. and Thompson, G.G. (2003). The western bearded dragon, *Pogona minor* (Squamata: Agamidae): an early lizard coloniser of rehabilitated areas. *Journal of the Royal Society of Western Australia* 86: 1.

Tocidlowski, M.E., McNamara, P.L., and Wojcieszyn, J.W. (2001). Myelogenous leukemia in a bearded dragon (*Acanthodraco vitticeps*). *Journal of Zoo and Wildlife Medicine* 32 (1): 90–95.

Van Waeyenberghe, L., Baert, K., Pasmans, F. et al. (2010). Voriconazole, a safe alternative for treating infections caused by the *Chrysosporium* anamorph of *Nannizziopsis vriesii* in bearded dragons (*Pogona vitticeps*). *Sabouraudia* 48 (6): 880–885.

Vancraeynest, D., Pasmans, F., De Graef, E. et al. (2006). *Listeria monocytogenes* associated myocardial perforation in a bearded dragon (*Pogona vitticeps*). *Vlaams Diergeneeskundig Tijdschrift* 75 (3): 232–234.

Willette-Frahm, M., Wright, K.M., and Thode, B.C. (1995). Select protozoal diseases in amphibians and reptiles: a report for the infectious diseases committee, American Association of Zoo Veterinarians. *Bulletin of the Association of Reptilian and Amphibian Veterinarians* 5 (1): 19–29.

Wotherspoon, A.D. (2007). Ecology and management of eastern bearded dragon *Pogona barbata*. PhD thesis, University of Western Sydney, Richmond, Australia.

Wright, K. (2008). Two common disorders of captive bearded dragons (*Pogona vitticeps*): nutritional secondary hyperparathyroidism and constipation. *Journal of Exotic Pet Medicine* 17 (4 (October): 267–272.

Zotti, A., Selleri, P., Carnier, P. et al. (2004). Relationship between metabolic bone disease and bone mineral density measured by dual-energy X-ray absorptiometry in the green iguana (Iguana iguana). *Veterinary Radiology & Ultrasound* 45 (1): 10–16.

14

Geckos
Marie Kubiak

Geckos are a large infraorder of small lizards that comprise over 1300 species, making up 13–14% of all reptiles (Uetz 2009). Geckos tend to originate from warm tropical and desert regions of the world and have a morphologically consistent appearance, though colouration and ornamentation vary widely. Some species have shown remarkable ability to adapt and thrive to developing urbanisation of their natural habitats.

The leopard gecko (*Eublepharis macularius*) is by far the most popular species of captive gecko and is popular with both beginner and experienced herpetoculturists, with an ever increasing variety of colour morphs being selectively bred (Figure 14.1). This species is tolerant of captive conditions, docile, and readily breeds in captivity making it one of the better species to be kept as a companion animal. Other geckos are less commonly kept as pets but may include Tokay geckos (*Gekko gekko*), Day geckos (*Phelsuma* spp.), mourning geckos (*Lepidodactylus lugubris*), African fat-tail geckos (*Hemitheconyx caudicinctus*), and crested geckos (*Correlophus ciliatus*).

14.1 Husbandry

14.1.1 Housing

Male geckos housed together will often fight, leading to significant injuries. Most gecko species can be kept singly, in female groups, or as one male with multiple females but some species, e.g. Giant day geckos (*Phelsuma grandis*), are best kept singly to avoid aggression.

Terrestrial species such as leopard and fat-tailed geckos can be housed in traditional wooden or plastic vivaria with vent inserts to allow for air movement. Fish tank type, open-topped sealed glass enclosures are not suitable due to the lack of effective ventilation and typically small ground area.

Arboreal and semi-arboreal species, like tokay, crested, and day geckos, require greater height and secure branching to provide climbing opportunities (Figure 14.2).

Species from tropical climes require higher humidity. This can be achieved by a combination of regular hand-misting, automated sprayers/foggers, waterfalls, and drippers. Organic substrates and natural planting can help maintain stable humidity. Compromising ventilation to achieve suitable humidity should be avoided and maintaining good airflow through enclosures is essential. Wooden vivaria may warp or decay when humidity is maintained at high levels. More modern mesh enclosures can be useful but temperatures and humidity can be hard to maintain and inappropriate mesh size may result in injury to toes or allow animal escape. Large glass vivaria work well for many species if sufficient cover is provided and ventilation is maximised. Mesh roofing and front-opening non-sealed doors will achieve adequate ventilation in most cases but development of condensation, algal or mould growth should be considered as a potential indicator of poor airflow.

A moist hide should also be provided for terrestrial species to aid skin removal during shedding and this should be enclosed with a single entry/exit hole and contain moist substrate such as moss or soil. Arboreal species benefit from regular spraying of vegetation to provide humid pockets for similar shedding assistance. Environmental conditions for selected gecko species are given in Table 14.1.

14.1.2 Substrate

For terrestrial desert species such as the leopard gecko, sand and large rocks are close approximations to the natural environment. Sand is biologically inert, allows easy removal of faecal matter and is suitable for low humidity but risks intestinal impaction if ingested with food. To minimise risk of ingestion, livefood may be fed in a separate tank or

Handbook of Exotic Pet Medicine, First Edition. Edited by Marie Kubiak.
© 2021 John Wiley & Sons Ltd. Published 2021 by John Wiley & Sons Ltd.
Companion website: www.wiley.com/go/kubiak/exotic_pet_medicine

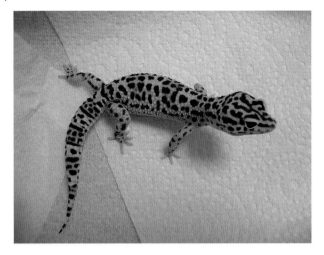

Figure 14.1 Wild colour morph leopard gecko.

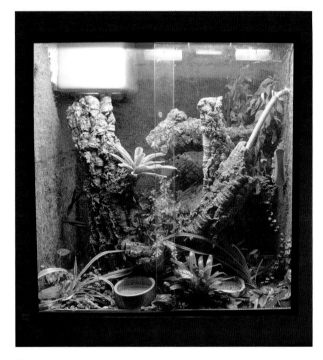

Figure 14.2 Vivarium for Tokay gecko providing climbing opportunities, visual barriers, basking spot, and ultraviolet lighting.

placed in a deep bowl. Fine reptile or children's play sand is superior to coarse grains and although calcium based sands are often advertised as digestible, impactions are still frequently seen so these should be used with caution. Particulate substrates such as bark, wood chips, corn cob, and gravel should be avoided in terrestrial species due to risk of accidental ingestion whilst feeding. Multiple hides or well-secured rocks should be available as leopard geckos tend to retreat into burrows or crevices during daylight hours (Thorogood and Whimster 1979).

Arboreal species are at lower risk of impaction as they tend to feed at higher levels in the tank and so bark can be a suitable substrate, as well as soil, coconut fibre, or moss substrates. A deep-littered soil substrate will enable growth of live plants which provide a more natural appearance to an enclosure and offer screening as well as climbing and drinking opportunities.

There is a growing trend towards replacing minimalist environments with a developed ecological niche. A spacious bioactive tank is sculpted and houses not just reptiles, but also invertebrates and plants. As such, natural soil substrates are growing in popularity due to ability to sustain plant life and house invertebrates. These invertebrates (typically earthworms, millipedes, woodlice, and springtails) live alongside the reptiles and are key in degrading organic matter, including reptile faeces, and maintaining hygiene with reduced need for human disturbance.

14.1.3 Heating

Leopard and fat-tail geckos are unusual lizards in their behaviour as they are crepuscular (active predominantly at dawn and dusk) and thigmotherms (absorbing heat through contact, from rocks that have been warmed by the sun) (Garrick 2008). A heat mat covering one-third to a half of the floor area is appropriate, and should be placed outside the tank to avoid direct contact. Alternatively an overhead heat lamp can be used, with rocks or slate tiles placed underneath to retain heat. Temperature must be controlled with a thermostat, with the thermostat probe placed on the heated substrate to prevent excessively high temperatures at the level of the animal.

Crested geckos are from cooler regions with temperatures required close to room temperature. It is advisable to provide a low output protected heat source to allow for provision of basking opportunity and thermal gradient during daytime hours. Mourning geckos can be kept in a similar way with a relatively low ambient temperature but a warmer daytime basking spot is needed and can be provided with a low output infra-red or visible light heat bulb. Geckos from warmer tropical climes such as day and tokay geckos require higher ambient temperatures, and use of higher output bulbs can achieve this and provide a basking spot. Overnight thermostatically controlled infra-red or ceramic bulbs, or a heat mat will be needed to maintain an appropriate ambient temperature.

14.1.4 Lighting

It is commonly assumed that crepuscular or nocturnal species do not require ultraviolet-B (UV-B) lighting. However, though leopard and fat-tail geckos will survive on dietary

Table 14.1 Environmental conditions for selected gecko species.

Common name	Scientific name	Temperature range required (°C)	Humidity (%)	Diet	Habitat	Suggested minimum enclosure size (L × W × H [cm])
Leopard gecko	*Eublepharis macularis*	20–32	30–40	Insects	Terrestrial desert	1 animal: 60 × 60 × 30, 1 pair: 90 × 60 × 30
Fat tail gecko	*Hemitheconyx caudicinctus*	20–30	30–40	Insects	Terrestrial desert	1 animal: 60 × 60 × 30, 1 pair: 90 × 60 × 30
Crested gecko	*Correlophus ciliatus*	18–25	60–90	Commercial diet supplemented with small numbers of insects and some fruit	Coastal subtropical forest, arboreal	1 animal: 60 × 30 × 60, 2 animals: 60 × 30 × 90
Tokay gecko	*Gekko gecko*	24–35 (22–26 at night)	60–80	Insects	Tropical, arboreal	1 animal: 80 × 30 × 100, 2 animals: 80 × 60 × 100
Mourning gecko	*Lepidodactylus lugubris*	18–28	60–70	Small insects, nectar, soft fruit and commercial liquid food	Coastal tropics, arboreal	1 animal: 30 × 30 × 30, colony of up to 6: 60 × 30 × 90
Giant day gecko	*Phelsuma grandis*	20–32	70–80	Commercial diet supplemented with small numbers of insects and some fruit	Tropical and subtropical forest, arboreal	1 animal: 60 × 30 × 90

calcium and vitamin D supplementation alone, circulating Vitamin D levels are significantly higher with UV-B exposure (Gould et al. 2018). Additionally a nocturnal house gecko species (*Hemidactylus garnoti*) was found to deplete calcium stores even on a high calcium diet without provision of UV-B lighting (Allen et al. 1993). Crepuscular and nocturnal species are still exposed to low levels of ultraviolet light at dawn and dusk in the wild and it is preferable to provide low intensity UV-B for the 10–12 hour photoperiod, with plenty of shaded areas to mimic their natural conditions. An alternative is to provide higher intensity UV-B lighting only for a 1 hour period at dusk and dawn, alongside visible light for the full photoperiod (Gould et al. 2018). These species are more efficient at endogenous Vitamin D formation than diurnal species, and extended exposure to high intensity UV-B lights is unnecessary and associated with apparent photodermatitis and increased shedding frequency (Carman et al. 2000; Wangen et al. 2013; Gould et al. 2018).

UV-B lighting is considered necessary for diurnal gecko species for calcium regulation. It is also recognised that some species have visual perception of ultraviolet light (Loew 1994) and this may be important in feeding and social cues. Tube or coil lamps are commonly used; mercury vapour lamps are an alternative but their high heat output can cause drying of substrate, low humidity and excessively high temperatures in small tanks.

14.1.5 Diet

Leopard, fat-tail, and tokay geckos are primarily insectivorous. Hatchlings will begin feeding on pinhead crickets within four to five days, after they have completed their first shed, and are voracious feeders (Boyer et al. 2013). A variety of appropriately sized insect prey should be offered to adults, with small locusts, crickets, mealworms, cockroaches, silkworms, and occasional waxworms suitable and readily available from reptile pet shops. Feeder insects should be 'gut-loaded' – this means offering fresh fruit and vegetables to insects prior to feeding to ensure optimal nutritional value.

Calcium supplementation should be applied to prey insects immediately before feeding (Boyer et al. 2013). A small container of calcium carbonate powder can be left in the vivarium and geckos have been observed to voluntarily ingest the powder (de Vosjoli et al. 1998). Multivitamin supplements should be used twice a month (Boyer et al. 2013).

Commercial powdered diets for frugivorous species are widely available, with day, mourning, and crested geckos commonly fed a moistened fruit powder mix alongside fresh fruit and supplemented insects.

Table 14.2 Biological parameters for selected geckos.

Common name	Scientific name	Gestation period (days)	Incubation period (days)	Lifespan (years)	Adult length, including tail (cm)	Adult weight (g)
Leopard gecko	*Eublepharis macularis*	21–28	45–60	6–15	20–25	75–110
Fat tail gecko	*Hemitheconyx caudicinctus*	21–28	43–70	10–20	18–25	50–110
Crested gecko	*Correlophus ciliatus*	30	65–120	15–20	15–22	35–70
Tokay gecko	*Gekko gecko*	30–60	65–200	8–15	25–40	120–250
Mourning gecko	*Lepidodactylus lugubris*	N/A	55–65	10–15	5–8	0.3–3
Giant day gecko	*Phelsuma grandis*	30	47–82	6–8	20–30	50–100

A shallow water dish should be provided in the cool end of the tank but geckos will rarely make use of this, instead obtaining all their fluid from food or, in the case of arboreal species, as droplets from vegetation or from direct spraying. Water should be refreshed daily to prevent algal and bacterial growth.

14.1.6 Breeding

Most common species will breed in captivity and even single females may lay eggs so a laying site should always be provided to avoid egg retention problems. Leopard, fat-tail, and crested geckos will dig into moist substrate to bury eggs so an enclosed chamber partly filled with moist soil, vermiculite, or moss can be used. Tokay, mourning, and day geckos need vertical surfaces such as cork pieces to adhere their eggs to, and may still choose to adhere eggs onto tank walls. Information on reproductive parameters in common species are included in Table 14.2. Crested geckos, leopard geckos, fat-tailed geckos, and day geckos demonstrate temperature dependent sex-determination with egg incubation temperature influencing gender development (Gamble 2010). Tokay geckos appear to utilise genetic sex determination with sex chromosomes identified (Trifonov et al. 2011), however anecdotal reports suggest that incubation temperature still appears to influence sex of offspring. Mourning geckos are parthenogenic with unmated females producing fertile eggs that result in female offspring (Radtkey et al. 1995).

Most information available relates to leopard geckos. Females can breed from 30 to 35 g, are spontaneous ovulators, will mate repeatedly and with more than one male before laying eggs (de Vosjoli 2004). These multiple matings increase fecundity and fertility, and one clutch of two eggs can have two different sires (Kratochvíl and Frynta 2007; LaDage et al. 2008; Stevens 2008). Females are able to store sperm for up to a year to enable fertilisation of subsequent clutches (LaDage et al. 2008). Up to eight clutches of two eggs may be produced in a year (LaDage et al. 2008). Once eggs

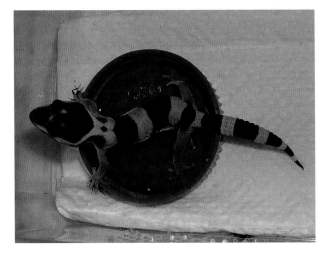

Figure 14.3 Neonate wild morph leopard gecko. Juveniles are independent of parents and will feed after their first moult at a few days of age.

have been laid there is no parental involvement in incubation or rearing hatchlings (Figure 14.3). Egg incubation at 24–28 °C results in female offspring, 32–32.5 °C results in males and intermediate temperatures produce both sexes (Viets et al. 1993). Above 34 °C, females are again produced but fertility of females incubated at warmer temperatures may be reduced (Gutzke and Crews 1988). Incubation duration depends on temperature, with one study demonstrating hatching at 72 days when incubating eggs at 26 °C, and 36 days when incubating at 32.5 °C (Viets et al. 1993).

Parthenogenic mourning geckos lay eggs that hatch genetically identical daughters (Cuellar and Kluge 1972). Fecundity is higher in social groups compared to animals housed individually though dominant animals may suppress maturation of subordinate animals. Keeping two adults together is most successful for breeding (Brown and Sakai 1988; Brown and O'Brien 1993). Females are sexually mature at 9.5 months (Brown and O'Brien 1993). No defined season is seen and two eggs (rarely a single egg) are laid on vertical surfaces in the enclosure (Sabath 1981; Griffing et al. 2018). Removing eggs to incubate them artificially is possible if the surface they are adhered to can be moved. The author leaves the eggs in place in the enclosure to hatch however in smaller enclosures cannibalism of juveniles may occur by adults. Eggs at 25.5 °C take 65 days to hatch, whereas those at 22 °C take 103 days (Brown and Duffy 1992). Hatchlings are 15–20 mm in length and can be kept in identical conditions to adults.

14.2 History Taking

Critical evaluation of husbandry is crucial as inappropriate management is a common factor in many disease processes. Temperatures provided, type of heat source, lighting, diet, supplementation, humidity, and enclosure dimensions should all be established and compared to requirements.

Low temperatures can result in anorexia, immunosuppression, and secondary infections whereas high temperatures can result in thermal burns, dehydration, and reclusive behaviour. Diet should be evaluated for suitability with particular focus on levels of Vitamins A and D, and calcium provided.

As with all species, clinical signs, duration of signs, and any co-morbidity or mortality in other reptiles in the house remain important.

14.2.1 Handling

Leopard geckos, fat tailed geckos, and crested geckos are generally docile but if threatened may bite and will grip firmly though injuries are minor. They should be restrained from above with a finger firmly placed either side of the head and their body held with the rest of the fingers (Figure 14.4). Gentle handling is necessary as the skin of many gecko species is thin and can tear with forceful restraint. Tokay geckos are typically highly aggressive and should be handled with caution, using leather gloves or a small towel to avoid injury to handler, and the teeth or fragile skin of the animal (Figure 14.5).

Day geckos and smaller species can be visually examined in a clear plastic box to avoid handling trauma to delicate skin or escape.

Never grasp the tail of geckos as in many species this can be dropped as a defensive response (see Autotomy).

14.2.2 Sexing

Sex determination of adults varies between species.

Mature male leopard geckos are larger than females and have visible development of pre-anal pores in a V-shape cranial to the vent, and hemipene swellings caudal to the vent (Figure 14.6) (Stevens 2008). Females and juveniles have poorly developed pores, a flat tail base and are slightly

(b)

(a)

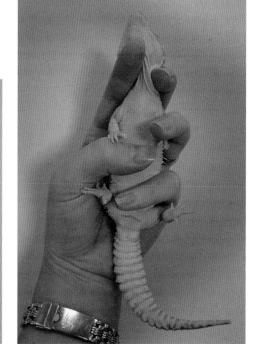

Figure 14.4   (a, b) Restraint of an albino leopard gecko for examination.

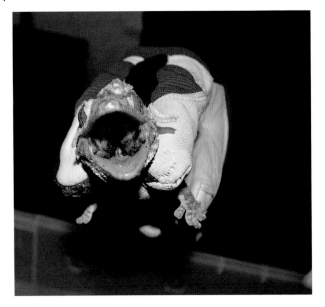

Figure 14.5 Tokay geckos tend to be more aggressive and initial capture often requires a towel or glove to avoid bite injuries to the hand.

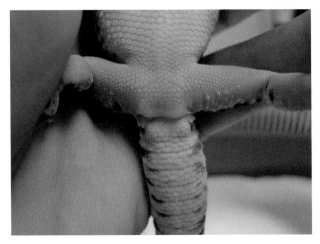

Figure 14.7 Female leopard gecko with absence of developed pores.

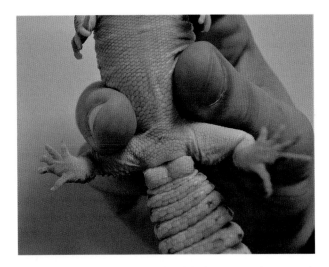

Figure 14.6 Male leopard gecko with clear pre-anal pores and hemipene swellings at tail base. Also note the loss of toe tips on the right hind foot.

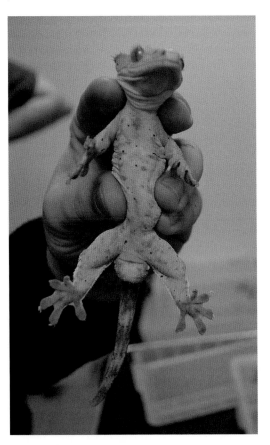

Figure 14.8 Male crested gecko with pronounced hemipene swellings caudal to vent.

smaller in size (Figure 14.7). African fat-tailed geckos and Tokay geckos have similar characteristics, and in crested geckos the pores are less prominent but hemipene swellings are more pronounced and are evident from around six months of age (Figure 14.8). Giant day gecko males have well-defined femoral pores on the ventral surface of the hind legs, often with profuse waxy secretions and hemipene swellings are subtle, whereas females have only small pore depressions along the hindlimbs and lack of hemipene swellings. In day and mourning geckos, endolymphatic sacs may also be visible as lateral cervical swellings in mature females.

14.2.3 Clinical Examination

An initial visual examination in the carrier is advisable to determine any major concerns (e.g. marked dyspnoea, lack of response, significant orthopaedic conditions) that may necessitate immediate intervention and delay a full clinical examination.

In docile species, such as leopard geckos, where handling is appropriate, an initial evaluation can be carried out with minimal restraint by allowing the gecko to walk across hands or an examination table to assess mobility and co-ordination. A full restrained examination then follows. Sex determination, body weight, and body condition assessment should be carried out on any patient presenting even if apparently clinically well. A routine examination comprises visual evaluation and palpation from head to vent.

Coelomic palpation can identify masses such as substrate impaction or mature eggs but is often unrewarding for other conditions. Visualisation of viscera through the ventral skin in species with little pigmentation may identify hepatomegaly, gall bladder distension, or reproductive activity. This assessment can be enhanced using transillumination, where a bright, non-heating, light source is focused on the lateral aspect of the gecko whilst the viscera are evaluated from the ventral aspect. Oral examination is aided by the natural defensive gape posture assumed by geckos and this is often elicited by gentle restraint around the neck (Figure 14.5). Inserting a small card between the rostral lips can encourage mouth opening in more stoic animals.

Common areas of pathology are the mouth, eyes, vent, and intestinal tract and these should always be evaluated in detail where possible.

14.3 Basic Techniques

14.3.1 Blood Sample Collection

Blood volume varies from 4 to 8% of body weight in reptiles and size of individual may preclude blood sample collection (Martinez-Jimenez and Hernandez-Divers 2007). A maximum sample of 0.5 ml per 100 g body weight (including any haematoma volume) is considered appropriate (McBride and Hernandez-Divers 2004). The most commonly used site for venepuncture in lizards is the ventral coccygeal vein. However, in conscious geckos autotomy compromises tail handling and general anaesthesia is needed for sampling. Additional sites include the jugular vein, cranial vena cava, and ventral abdominal vein but due to fragility, blind access to deep veins and patient size, anaesthesia remains advisable for these sites. Haemostasis can be difficult to achieve following sample collection from these sites.

14.3.2 Nutritional Support

Short periods of anorexia require no intervention in most cases as reptile metabolic rate is slow and physiological anorexia is frequently noted in animals during breeding season. Prolonged anorexia (missing more than seven scheduled feeds) with associated weight loss, or anorexia in an unwell animal necessitates intervention. Force feeding should not be instigated without full consideration of all patient factors as this procedure is often highly stressful to the patient. Rehydration should be carried out prior to feeding to avoid refeeding syndrome and associated electrolyte aberrations (Donoghue 2006).

Liquid commercial diets are readily available for many frugivorous or omnivorous species, intended for everyday home use and these can also be used for assist feeding. Fruit purees and juices are high in sugar and low in fibre so are not suitable long-term but in the absence of alternatives can be beneficial in initial stabilisation of frugivorous species. Insectivores can be fed a blended insect mix prepared in the clinic, but no commercial insectivore liquid diet is currently available. A mixture of carnivore and herbivore/omnivore critical care diets can approximate nutritional requirements of insectivorous geckos and are a convenient option.

In many gecko species liquid will be licked from the lips and a drop of a liquid diet can be placed onto the lip margin. This is a slow method of providing food but is less stressful and is well accepted in individuals that will tolerate human proximity. Where large volumes are necessary or the patient will not accept the drip method, restraint for oral or gavage tube administration can be used. If repeated administrations of food or oral medication are expected to be necessary then surgical placement of an oesophageal feeding tube is considered preferable in animals of suitable size.

Nutritional requirements should be calculated to ensure animals are receiving appropriate nutrition from manufacturer guidelines for commercial preparations or based on calorific requirements:

Standard Metabolic Rate (SMR) [KJ/day] $= 21.69 \times$ Mass $(kg)^{0.8}$ (Andrews and Pough 1985)

Sick animals able to digest food generally require $1-3 \times$ SMR depending on the type of pathology present. However, in chronically anorexic animals feeding only 20% of the SMR is advisable for several days until normal GI function resumes (Martinez-Jimenez and Hernandez-Divers 2007).

14.3.3 Fluid Therapy

Geckos produce uric acid as the renal end-product and dehydration can lead to elevation of serum uric acid levels, predisposing to visceral and articular gout (Figure 14.9). Sick animals should be assumed to be dehydrated with estimated losses replaced over three to four days alongside administration of maintenance requirements. Maintenance requirements for geckos are 15 ml/kg/day and fluid administered within assist feeding should be taken into account (Music and Strunk 2016).

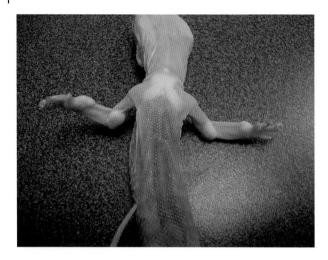

Figure 14.9 Articular gout in a leopard gecko, with precipitation of uric acid following chronic dehydration due to excessively high environmental temperatures.

If the gastrointestinal tract is not compromised, oral fluids can be administered by the same methods as nutritional support. Patients should be kept within their preferred optimum temperature zone to allow normal intestinal absorption.

Normal saline is suitable for parenteral rehydration and any fluids should be warmed before administration. Subcutaneous fluids can be given in most gecko species but extreme care should be taken in species with fragile skin (e.g. day geckos) as the skin can easily tear on handling or injection. The lateral body tends to have the most available free skin so is the site of choice for fluid boluses.

Intracoelomic fluids are best avoided due to the risk of inadvertent visceral trauma on injection but in very small species this route may be the only available option. The lizard is held in dorsal recumbency with the head lower than the body and the needle enters the coleomic cavity in the right lower quadrant, just cranial to the pelvis (Divers 1999).

Intravenous routes are difficult to access in geckos due to patient size and the need for surgical techniques to place catheters for repeated administration.

Intraosseous catheters are easier to place in medium-large geckos but this route should be avoided where metabolic bone disease (MBD) is present due to the high risk of pathological fractures. The femur can be used with a needle inserted via the greater trochanter under sterile conditions, or the tibial tuberosity used for access to the tibial medullary cavity. Hypodermic needles are typically used due to small patient size. Continuous infusion is not possible with small patients and repeated small bolus injection of fluids is recommended, with concurrent analgesia.

14.3.4 Anaesthesia

Gaseous anaesthesia using volatile agents such as isoflurane or sevoflurane can be a slow method of induction. Reptiles' respiratory drive is stimulated by a decrease in circulating oxygen and so provision of a volatile agent in 100% oxygen reduces respiratory rate, resulting in a prolonged or unsuccessful induction (Redrobe 2004). Using a small, airtight chamber for induction so that oxygen levels progressively deplete can speed the process.

Agents designed for intravenous use alone, such as propofol, are not easily administered in a conscious patient so use is restricted to geckos with an intravenous or intraosseous catheter already placed.

Intramuscular or subcutaneous administration of sedative or anaesthetic agents is most commonly utilised. Ketamine has been widely used historically (Bertelsen 2007) but tends to result in prolonged sedation and recovery periods when used as a sole agent, though used at low doses in combination with other agents such as benzodiazepines or alpha-2 agonists it can be useful for sedation. Alfaxalone appears a reliable anaesthetic in reptiles and although typically administered intravenously it can also be administered by intramuscular or subcutaneous routes facilitating use in small gecko species with poorly accessible veins. In leopard geckos, the addition of midazolam reduced the alfaxalone dose required and allowed partial reversibility of sedation (Doss et al. 2017). Injection into the forelimb improves sedation compared to hindlimb injections, due to avoidance of rapid hepatic and renal clearance (Fink et al. 2018). Further details are given in the formulary.

Reptiles typically become apnoeic at a surgical plane of anaesthesia so it is recommended to place an endotracheal tube to allow manual or mechanical ventilation of patients. This provides oxygen and allows maintenance of anaesthesia using volatile agents. Due to patient size standard small animal tubes are not suitable, but intravenous cannulae can be utilised instead for small patients. Ventilation frequency should reflect the natural respiratory rate for the species so observation of individuals prior to anaesthesia can help plan ventilation rates for unfamiliar species.

Small patients can lose heat rapidly and a hypothermic reptile will exhibit a reduction in metabolic rate and prolonged recovery from anaesthesia. A warm ambient temperature and use of monitored active heating from a thermostatically controlled heat mat is recommended during surgery to prevent hypo- or hyperthermia.

Monitoring during anaesthesia is limited but at a surgical plane of anaesthesia, the toe pinch withdrawal should be absent and a slow blink present in response to corneal contact (in gecko species with eyelids). Monitoring of changes in heart rate will also give an indication of a lightening or excessively deep plane of anaesthesia. A Doppler flow monitor placed in the left axilla, or under the manubrium will allow continuous assessment of heart rate.

During recovery, cardiac monitoring and thermal support should continue until the patient is responsive and able to ambulate and regulate temperature independently. Ventilation with room air may result in faster recovery from inhalational anaesthesia than ongoing ventilation with oxygen.

14.3.5 Euthanasia

Anaesthesia followed by intracardiac or intracoelomic injection of 60–100 mg/kg pentobarbitone is considered acceptable, though response following administration via the intracoleomic route can be slow (Leary et al. 2013). Use of intracoelomic injection of buffered tricaine methanesulfonate (MS222) has also been described in geckos as an alternative to pentobarbitone (Conroy et al. 2009).

Lack of cardiac function does not confirm death as reptiles can tolerate cardiac arrest and hypoxia with ongoing brain function. As a consequence it is prudent to carry out 'pithing', or brainstem destruction following chemical euthanasia to prevent recovery. This is carried out by inserting a needle or rod into the brainstem, usually through the roof of the mouth, and mechanically disrupting the tissues. The author has found injection of pentobarbitone into the brainstem through the foramen magmum equally effective, technically simpler, and less cosmetically destructive for pet animals but this should only be carried out in an unconscious animal with no cardiac activity.

Decapitation alone is not considered a suitable method of euthanasia. In small species accurate, rapid concussive force to the cranium to forcefully destroy the brain, or instantaneous freezing in liquid nitrogen (only for animals weighing less than 4 g) is acceptable where no chemical option is available (Leary et al. 2013).

14.3.6 Hospitalisation Requirements

Basic vivaria are necessary for hospitalisation of gecko patients following similar requirements as for standard husbandry but some minor amendments are advisable to maintain clinical standards of hygiene. Vivaria made from moulded plastic with no crevices and ridges are ideal as they are easily cleaned and disinfected and prevent animals from retreating into inaccessible positions. Normal substrate is often replaced by kitchen roll or newspaper which can be changed daily. Branching for arboreal species can be simulated using plastic or wooden rods which can be disposed of or disinfected between patients.

14.4 Common Conditions

14.4.1 Non-Infectious Conditions

14.4.1.1 Anorexia

This is a common but non-specific presenting sign and may be a physiological response to reproductive activity or seasonal changes, or an indication of a disease process. Anorexia in an animal that is maintaining weight and not showing any other symptoms merits husbandry review, clinical examination, and ongoing monitoring. Where a husbandry deficit is identified, correction of management often results in gradual resumption of feeding. In an animal losing weight then additional measures include a screen for parasites, raising environmental temperatures to the higher end of the range for the species, and prompt investigation of any abnormalities detected on clinical evaluation.

Hepatic lipidosis is a consequence of chronic anorexia that results in persisting anorexia even if the inciting cause has resolved. A pale appearance to the liver on transillumination, or a hyperechoic appearance on ultrasound examination is highly suggestive of hepatic lipidosis. Assist feeding can help prevent or manage established hepatic lipidosis in animals presenting with chronic anorexia. Confimation of diagnosis and identification of additional hepatic pathology is made by endoscopic or surgical liver biopsy (Divers and Cooper 2000). Surgical biopsy collection has been associated with complications of wound breakdown, coelomic haemorrhage, and peri-operative mortality in apparently healthy animals (Cojean et al. 2018a) and as a consequence this technique may not be appropriate to carry out in a debilitated animal.

14.4.1.2 Nutritional Secondary Hyperparathyroidism (NSHP)

NSHP is a common pathology, particularly in leopard geckos (Gould et al. 2018). Insect prey available in captivity are relatively deficient in Vitamin D and calcium, with a disproportionately high phosphorus content. Failure to supplement these with Vitamin D and calcium results in dietary imbalance (Barker et al. 1998). This is compounded by a lack of UV-B lighting or adequate temperatures, disrupting endogenous Vitamin D formation. Vitamin D is necessary for effective calcium absorption and homeostasis (Webb and Holick 1988). Without adequate vitamin D or calcium available, serum calcium levels reduce and bones are progressively demineralised (under the effects of parathyroid hormone) to liberate calcium into the circulation. Animals present with pathological fractures, twisted or bent long bones, spinal deformities, a flaccid tail, inability to feed due mandibular softening and pain, neurological

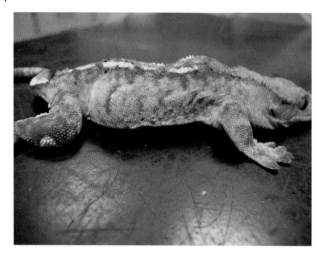

Figure 14.10 Kyphosis in a crested gecko with NSHP due to lack of UVB lighting.

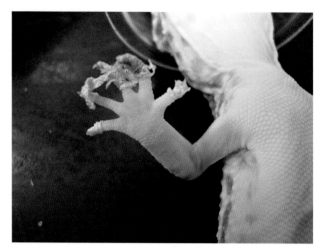

Figure 14.11 Retention of skin on toes is a common consequence of dysecdysis, and loss of toe tips often results due to avascular necrosis (see Figure 14.6).

symptoms, or chronic wasting (Figure 14.10). Palpation of long bones and mandibles will demonstrate the deformities and abnormal flexibility typical for MBD. Radiographs are useful in determining severity of demineralisation but are only diagnostic in moderate–severe disease, with lower sensitivity in small species (Klaphake 2010). Blood calcium levels may be normal, even in advanced cases but phosphorus levels are often elevated (Klaphake 2010).

Advanced cases should be euthanased due to permanent deformities to bones and compromised feeding and mobility. Less marked changes can be treated with oral calcium and vitamin D liquid supplementation, provision of UV-B lighting, appropriate temperatures, and removal of vivarium furniture to avoid injury. Even if other cagemates appear normal they are likely to be subclinically affected and husbandry changes must be implemented for all.

14.4.1.3 Vitamin A Deficiency Associated Diseases

Insects are low in Vitamin A (Barker et al. 1998), and lack of supplementation and gut-loading of prey can result in hypovitaminosis A which may take months to manifest (Kroenlein et al. 2008). The resulting squamous metaplasia of epithelium can render animals susceptible to respiratory infections, renal degeneration, and affect skin health. Overdose with Vitamin A can lead to iatrogenic skin pathology so gradual replenishment of Vitamin A stores using correct nutrition and long-term low dose oral supplementation is the safest treatment. Leopard geckos are able to assimilate oral B-carotene, a Vitamin A precursor, to Vitamin A (Cojean et al. 2018a) and hence feeding prey on carotene rich foods alongside supplementation of Vitamin A at manufacturer recommended levels is advisable.

14.4.1.3.1 Dysecdysis The failure to shed normally is a common problem particularly in leopard geckos. Juveniles shed frequently, up to every ten days during rapid growth phases, and adults typically shed every three to four weeks (Thorogood and Whimster 1979). Fluid is secreted between the old and new skin to enable separation of the old skin. The shed skin is removed in large pieces over one to two hours and eaten by the gecko.

When dysecdysis occurs, shed skin tends to be retained on smaller areas such as the toes and eyelids. Contraction of desiccated retained skin can result in avascular necrosis and loss of toes, or keratitis if the eyelids are affected (Figures 14.6, 14.11 and 14.12). Treatment is removal of retained skin by soaking the affected area in warm water and gently teasing loose fragments away with damp cotton buds and atraumatic forceps.

Prevention of complications from shedding in a clinically normal animal is by provision of an appropriate diet with Vitamin A supplementation and ensuring adequate hydration and humidity to facilitate separation of the old and new skin. A humid hide should be provided during shedding and recluse areas should be available at all times.

14.4.1.3.2 Stomatitis Stomatitis is common in leopard geckos (Reavill and Griffin 2014), typically as a secondary condition, predisposed to by hypovitaminosis A or injury to the gingiva. Affected animals may present for anorexia, facial swelling, or concurrent changes affecting the eyes. Hypovitaminosis A in leopard geckos causes accumulation of metaplastic epithelium in the oral glands located at the oral commissures, resulting in distension of the glands and ducts. At an early stage removal of plugs of debris and dietary improvements can resolve the problem. At a later

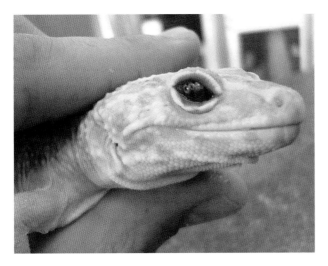

Figure 14.12 Keratitis secondary to retention of skin of the eyelids with dysecdysis. This is a particularly common problem in leopard geckos.

stage extensive damage with secondary abscessation develops and requires surgical debridement, analgesia, and antibiotic administration.

14.4.1.4 Ophthalmic Disease

The Eublepharidae family of geckos are unusual in that they have mobile eyelids, whereas other gecko families have a clear spectacle covering the eye. This anatomical difference results in a higher incidence of ophthalmic disease in Eublepharid geckos, such as leopard and fat-tail geckos. In one study, ophthalmic cases accounted for 46% of leopard geckos presented to an exotic animal clinic, with the majority affected by keratitis or conjunctivitis (Wiggans et al. 2018). Animals often present with discharge, blepharospasm, retained skin pieces within the palpebral aperture, and corneal neovascularisation, oedema, or ulceration (Figure 14.12). Older animals, males, animals without a heat source, and those with no dietary vitamin A supplementation are significantly more likely to be affected (Wiggans et al. 2018). Conjunctival squamous metaplasia has been identified on histology of affected animals, and was linked to a lack of Vitamin A provision (Wiggans et al. 2018). Vitamin A deficiency also results in orbital gland metaplasia and dysfunction (Millichamp et al. 1983). The combination of changes seen predisposes to retention of shed eyelid skin in the conjunctival fornix with secondary inflammation and potential for bacterial or fungal colonisation. For ocular surface disease, eyes should be gently bathed with a sterile aqueous solution and any caseous debris removed from underneath the eyelids. Cytology of material is necessary to identify infections and guide treatment choice. Topical antibacterial or antifungal preparations are often sufficient for localised

infections. Recovery can be prolonged with recurrences occurring at subsequent sheds unless the underlying causative factors are addressed.

Anterior uveitis, phthisis bulbi, an abnormally shallow anterior chamber, third eyelid deformity and lower eyelid defect have also been reported as uncommon cases in leopard geckos (Wiggans et al. 2018).

Species such as crested or tokay geckos that have a transparent spectacle covering the cornea instead of eyelids tend to develop a different spectrum of diseases. Retained spectacles with a dull, irregular appearance over the surface of the eye can occur as part of dysecdysis and these should be bathed and gently removed or left until the next shed. In Tokay geckos, hypopyon associated with *Klebsiella pneumoniae* (Bonney et al. 1978) and subspectacular bacterial infections with *Proteus vulgaris* and *Klebsiella oxytoca* have been described (Brannian and Greve 1987). Surgical wedge resection of the ventral aspect of the spectacle allows drainage and application of topical therapy for subspectacular bacterial infections. Unilateral retinal degeneration has also been reported in a tokay gecko (Schmidt and Toft 1981).

14.4.1.5 Vitamin E/Selenium Deficiency

Weakness, lethargy, and decreased appetite has been reported in satanic leaf tailed geckos (*Uroplatus phantasticus*) associated with a suspected nutritional deficiency of vitamin E and/or Selenium, resulting in myopathy in the absence of bone demineralisation (Gabor 2005).

14.4.1.6 Neurological Disease

Leopard geckos with the colour pattern 'Enigma' frequently exhibit neurological symptoms, including seizures (Cojean et al. 2018b). This appears to be a dominant trait associated with selective breeding. No treatment is possible.

Cerebral xanthomatosis has been reported in a northern green gecko (*Naultinus grayi*) and four leaf-tailed geckos (*Uroplatus henkeli*, *U. sikorae*, *U. fimbriatus*) (Garner et al. 1999). Neurological symptoms were seen in two animals including torticollis, stargazing, dorsal recumbency, and seizures, two animals showed non-specific signs including anorexia and weight loss, and sudden death was the only sign in one animal. Xanthomas were found around viscera in most cases and the lateral or third ventricles of the brain in all animals, and were associated with hydrocephalus in three animals. All affected animals were female and it was hypothesised that yolk coelomitis, folliculogenesis, follicular degeneration, or diet may be a factor in the ectopic accumulations of cholesterol seen in these cases (Garner et al. 1999). Leopard geckos have also been diagnosed with xanthomas in the brain, lungs, liver, and coelom (Boyer et al. 2013).

14.4.1.7 Male Reproductive Disease

Retained plugs of debris within the hemipene can be expressed under sedation (Boyer et al. 2013). Material is removed via the normal hemipene orifice located on the caudal aspect of the vent. If untreated these can develop to abscesses with a swollen erythematous tail base, lethargy, anorexia, and straining commonly noted (Figure 14.13). Analgesia and antibiotic therapy should be initiated, with expression of inspissated purulent material carried out under anaesthesia. Extreme cases may require a surgical approach, with incisions made over the abscess pocket to remove impacted material. The incisions are flushed and left open to heal by secondary intention. Vitamin A provision should be assessed in these cases.

Where the hemipene has been traumatised (often during mating) and tissue is no longer vital or appears to have significant infection then amputation is justified (Boyer et al. 2013; Knotek et al. 2017). Fertility may be reduced by unilateral amputation and certainly would be heavily compromised with bilateral amputation but urination is unaffected. The hemipene is fully everted through the natural opening with gentle traction, under general anaesthesia or sedation with local anaesthesia. A transfixing ligature of monofilament absorbable material is placed at the hemipene base and the remainder sharply dissected free. Post-operative analgesia and antibiotic cover is recommended.

14.4.1.8 Female Reproductive Disorders

Pre-ovulatory stasis with accumulation of distended follicles on the ovaries is unusual in this group. Lipogranulomatous oophoritis has been reported in a New Caledonian

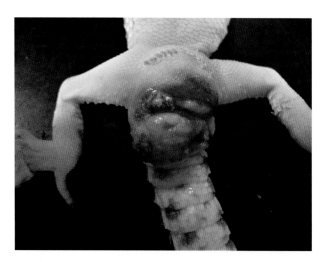

Figure 14.13 Hemipene abscessation in a leopard gecko, note the inspissated material extruding both from the natural orifice just caudal to the vent and through a fistula on the tail.

gecko (*Rhacodactylus leachianus*), and Salmonella-associated oophoritis in a viviparous Duvaucel's gecko (*Hoplodactylus duvaucelii*) (Le Souëf et al. 2015; Kophamel et al. 2018). For infectious, inflammatory, or neoplastic ovarian disease, ovariectomy remains the treatment of choice (Kophamel et al. 2018). The gecko is anaesthetised and placed in dorsal recumbency. A paramedian incision is made in the skin of the ventrum to avoid the midline abdominal vein (Di Giuseppe et al. 2017), at the level of the caudalmost rib and extended 1–2 cm caudally. The underlying thin muscles and coelomic membrane are bluntly dissected to access the coelom (Knotek et al. 2017). The ovaries can be identified on the dorsal aspect of the coelom, and are elevated with ligatures placed on the blood vessels prior to removal. Use of haemoclips makes surgery easier and faster (Di Giuseppe et al. 2017). Care should be taken to remove all ovarian tissue completely as even very small ovarian remnants can result in resumption of egg production in future. All yolk and inspissated debris should be removed, and the coelom flushed with warmed fluids to avoid post-operative coelomitis. The coelomic membrane and muscles are closed in a single layer, and the skin closed with everting sutures. Long-lasting suture materials such as polydioxanone are preferred as skin healing can take six weeks.

Failure to lay formed eggs due to a lack of an appropriate nesting site, inability of the oviduct to contract due to debilitation or calcium deficiency, or oversized eggs is common in geckos (Hochleithner and Holland 2014). Geckos often present with anorexia, a distended coelom, indiscriminate digging, straining, or lethargy (Di Giuseppe et al. 2017). The large eggs may be clearly visible through the ventral body wall (Hall and Lewbart 2006). Administration of oral calcium syrup or intramuscular calcium gluconate followed an hour later by oxytocin is often successful in lizards with oviductal inertia alone. In cases of oviductal torsion, oversized eggs or adhesion of eggs to the oviduct wall, medical therapy can exacerbate problems so should be carried out with caution and with ongoing observation of the patient, ideally in the hospital. Surgical intervention is necessary if clinical deterioration or a failure of medical treatment to elicit oviposition occurs, or if the gecko is collapsed and weak at presentation as medical treatment is then unlikely to be effective.

In these critical cases fluid therapy, analgesia, and calcium is administered, followed by surgical management. Surgery entails a coeliotomy and salpingotomy (or salpingectomy) to remove eggs and this can be challenging in very small species (Di Giuseppe et al. 2017). A paramedian longitudinal incision is made on the ventrum. Eggs within the oviduct can be removed via a salpingotomy, with an incision made longitudinally on the antimesosalpingeal aspect where blood vessels are sparse. Gentle traction using atraumatic forceps can aid removal of the eggs but should be done cautiously to avoid rupture and release of inflammatory yolk material into the coelom. Using moist sterile cotton buds to push and guide eggs is preferable. Once the egg is removed, the salpinx can be closed with a fine (4-0 or smaller) monofilament suture material in a continuous pattern. Polydiaxanone is typically used due to strength retention and persistence over a six week period as reptile healing is slow. If two eggs are present then this technique is repeated for the contralateral salpinx. Both salpinges should be inspected before closure to ensure there is no persisting torsion or other abnormality and salpingectomy carried out if pathology is present. For this, the vessels on the mesosalpinx are ligated or clipped and a transfixing ligature placed at the junction with the cloaca prior to sharp dissection to remove the oviduct. Elective ovariectomy at the time of intervention should always be offered to prevent recurrence and must be carried out following salpingectomy otherwise yolk coelomitis from subsequent ovulations will result.

Where surgery is not possible, transcutaneous ovocentesis of eggs to reduce their size and facilitate oviposition has been described in leopard geckos. Under anaesthesia, a 23G butterfly catheter is inserted into the centre of the egg using a ventrolateral approach, and negative pressure applied by a 6 ml syringe (Hall and Lewbart 2006). This approach is likely to be unsuccessful for oviductal adhesion, torsion, or advanced inertia and risks iatrogenic damage to viscera or coelomitis from leakage of inflammatory yolk proteins (Di Giuseppe et al. 2017). The author has used this approach successfully in a small number of select cases of uterine inertia, alongside calcium provision. Collapsed eggs were passed within 48 hours, but surgical intervention remains preferable due to limitations, risks, and lack of prevention of recurrence of this approach.

Tamoxifen and indomethacin have both been trialled in female leopard geckos to inhibit reproductive activity (DeNardo and Helminski 2001). Tamoxifen resulted in at least 81 days of inhibition of ovarian activity, with no oviposition for a full breeding season even after vitellogenesis resumed. Indomethacin inhibited ovarian activity for a full year but resulted in generalised oedema in half the treated animals. Although the intracoelomic implantation of these medications is less invasive than ovariectomy, the need for repeat procedures and potential for side effects of indomethacin mean that ovariectomy is still the preferred preventative approach for reproductive disease in geckos. The GnRH agonist, deslorelin, has not proven effective in suppressing reproductive activity in female leopard geckos (Knotek et al. 2017).

14.4.1.9 Neoplasia

Leopard geckos have a decreased disposition towards development of neoplasia compared to other lizard species (Kubiak et al. 2020) but little data exists on prevalence in other gecko species. Case reports include disseminated mast cell neoplasm in a fat-tail gecko, endolymphatic sac carcinoma in a tokay gecko, thyroid carcinomas in two species of knob-tail gecko, a chromatophoroma in a day gecko and melanophoroma, spindle cell sarcoma, oviductal carcinoma, squamous cell carcinoma, rhabdomyosarcoma, and fibrosarcoma in leopard geckos (Mikaelian et al. 2000; Hadfield et al. 2012; Heckers et al. 2012; Boyer et al. 2013; Rovira et al. 2014; Sander et al. 2015; Kubiak et al. 2020).

14.4.1.10 Autotomy

Autotomy is a defensive mechanism seen in many gecko species, where the tail is detached at a pre-existing intravertebral region of weakness known as a fracture plane (Delorme et al. 2012). Ongoing muscular contractions cause the detached tail to twitch, distracting the predator and allowing the gecko to escape.

Autotomy has long been identified to result from immobilisation or rough handling of the tail, or trauma from a cagemate or other animal (Woodland 1920). The remaining stump will bleed very little but appears as an open wound. Surgical closure or excessive interference at the stump will hinder regeneration. The gecko should be moved onto paper towel to keep the wound clean and housed separately until the tail has regenerated. Feeding of crickets should be avoided as these may cause further trauma to the open wound. Although the gecko has lost a large lipid store, there is no apparent increase in metabolic demands during tail regeneration and increased food quantity does not appear necessary (Congdon et al. 1974). The tail will regrow over a period of four to eight weeks and lacks the transverse indented bands and tubercles of the original tail (Delorme et al. 2012). A similar regrowth is seen following surgical amputation of the tail (Delorme et al. 2012).

14.4.2 Infectious Conditions

14.4.2.1 Endoparasites

14.4.2.1.1 Helminths Oxyurids (pinworms) are frequently found on faecal examination of geckos and are rarely overtly pathogenic (Reese et al. 2004). They should only be treated if clinical signs or high burdens are present. Diarrhoea, weight loss, anorexia, and reduced growth are consistent with excessive oxyurid loads. Treatment is fenbendazole.

14.4.2.1.2 Cryptosporidia *Cryptosporidium saurophilum* has been associated with intestinal epithelial hypertrophy in leopard geckos in particular, but also in Giant day geckos, sand geckos (*Chondrodactylus angulifer*), and house geckos (*Hemidactylus turcicus*) (Upton and Barnard 1987; Upton et al. 1989; Taylor et al. 1999). Clinical signs include abdominal distension, failure to grow, diarrhoea, and weight loss. Less commonly, glossitis and cloacitis may be seen (Boyer et al. 2013). Mortality in epizootics can vary from 50 to 100% (Coke and Tristan 1998; Koudela and Modry 1998). Subclinically infected animals become carriers, capable of shedding infectious oocysts and may develop clinical disease if immunosuppressed in future (Deming et al. 2008; Boyer et al. 2013). Diagnosis is by demonstration of the oocysts on flotation or acid-fast staining of faeces, detection of Cryptosporidial DNA in faeces using PCR, or identification of organism and associated inflammation on intestinal histopathology. A single negative faecal sample is not reliable for confirming uninfected status as animals with a low level of infection can test negative however, in infected animals with marked weight loss oocyst shedding is high and false negatives are less likely (Deming et al. 2008).

Emaciated geckos (those having lost 50% body weight) should be euthanased due to intractable progression (Coke and Tristan 1998; Deming et al. 2008). For animals with less advanced disease, clinical recovery to a carrier status appears possible in some cases (Deming et al. 2008). Paromomycin and hyperimmune bovine colostrum reduce clinical signs and oocyst shedding but do not eliminate infection (Coke and Tristan 1998; Graczyk et al. 1999; Pantchev et al. 2008). Asymptomatic cagemates or recovered animals should be considered as likely infected and kept in isolation from uninfected animals.

14.4.2.1.3 Protozoal Enteritis Soft, unformed stools, or those with undigested food are abnormal and protozoan colitis is a common cause in leopard geckos (Boyer et al. 2013). Microscopy of fresh faecal samples may show motile protozoa, such as Trichomonads and metronidazole is used for treatment. Trichomonads have also been associated with subcutaneous and ocular lesions in geckos and a higher dose of metronidazole is used for these atypical lesions (Miller et al. 1994).

The amoeba *Entamoeba invadens* has been associated with large intestinal necrosis in tokay geckos (Brannian and Greve 1987), and intestinal pathology in crested geckos (Mayer and Donnelly 2013). Metronidazole can be used for therapy.

14.4.2.1.4 Pentastomes Pentastomes are worm-like arthropod parasites of the respiratory tract of reptiles, birds, and mammals (Paré 2008). *Raillietiella gehyrae, R. frenatus* and *R. affinis* have all been reported in tokay geckos (Reese et al. 2004). Pulmonary infection was identified in 30% of tokay geckos undergoing post-mortem in one zoo collection but pathogenicity appeared low (Brannian and Greve 1987). Infection is also reported in wild house geckos (*Hemidactylus turcicus, H. frenatus, H. platyurus, Gecko monarchus*), four-clawed gecko (*Gehyra mutilate*), mourning geckos, the Northern dtella (*Gehyra australis*), knob-tailed geckos (*Nephrurus laevissimus*), and Standings day geckos (*Phelsuma standingi*) (Bursey and Goldberg 1999; Barton 2007; Paré 2008). This genus of pentastomids is not known to have zoonotic potential (Reese et al. 2004). Faecal flotation to demonstrate eggs, and microscopy of respiratory secretions to demonstrate all life stages, can be used for ante-mortem diagnosis and adults may be found on gross post-mortem examination (Paré 2008). Medical therapy appears unsuccessful, with fenbendazole, praziquantel, and ivermectin at standard doses proving ineffective in a tokay gecko, though high dose ivermectin therapy appeared successful in a tokay gecko and Standings day geckos without apparent toxicity (Micinilio 1996; Wright 1997). In larger hosts, surgical or endoscopic removal of adult pentastomes is possible (Paré 2008).

14.4.2.2 Dermatitis

Primary dermatitis appears uncommon though a small number of cases of fungal dermatitis have been reported. Primary fungal ulcerative dermatitis associated with the *Chrysosporium* anamorph of *Nannizziopsis vriesii* has been described in leopard geckos (Toplon et al. 2013), and in the common New Zealand gecko (*Hoplodactylus maculatus*) associated with a *Paecilomyces* species. The *Paecilomyces* infection progressed to a fatal mycotic pneumonia and sepsis (Cork and Stockdale 1994). *Mucor ramosissimus* was isolated in an outbreak of fungal dermatitis in Marlborough green geckos (*Naultinus manukanus*) concurrently affected by enteric protozoal parasitism and exposed to humidity extremes (Gartrell and Hare 2005).

Dermatitis may also be a consequence of dysecdysis, excessive exposure to UV lighting or thermal injury and identification and resolution of cause as well as management of any secondary infection are necessary. Trauma from companions is not uncommon, and tends to present with crescentic wounds that typically heal with minimal intervention (Figure 14.14). Scarring may theoretically result from dermal injury, with consequent dysecdysis of affected areas. However, in leopard geckos, even apparently severe or full-thickness defects heal with regeneration of skin structures and pigmentation, and without production of vascular granulation tissue, fibrosis, or scarring (Peacock et al. 2015). Tail injuries may result in autotomy.

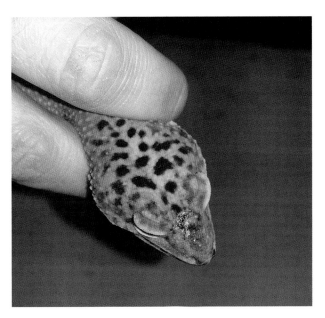

Figure 14.14 Bite injury to head from companion, note the typical crescent shape of wound corresponding to maxillary dentition.

14.4.2.3 Viral Infections

Co-infection with Cryptosporidia and adenovirus have been reported in a Tokay gecko and leopard geckos, associated with wasting (Wellehan et al. 2004). In the same study, fat-tail geckos with wasting had eublepharid adenovirus 1 isolated (without evident cryptosporidiosis) and the role of this virus in disease requires further characterisation.

A reovirus has been linked to syncytial cell enteropathy and hepatopathy, with clinical signs of weight loss, sepsis, gastric and hepatic necrosis in juvenile leopard geckos (Garner et al. 2009).

Granulomatous lesions affecting the tongue and liver have been associated with a ranavirus in a leaf-tailed gecko (Marschang et al. 2005).

14.5 Imaging

Radiography is commonly used to evaluate bone density and injury, intestinal foreign bodies and the reproductive system (Figure 14.15). Occasionally it is used to help differentiate osteomyelitis from other causes of digital swelling such as articular gout. Due to patient size and lack of natural contrast, survey radiography has limited value for visceral assessment and the dorsoventral view is most frequently used (Figure 14.16). Intra-coelomic injection of air has been suggested to improve visualisation of

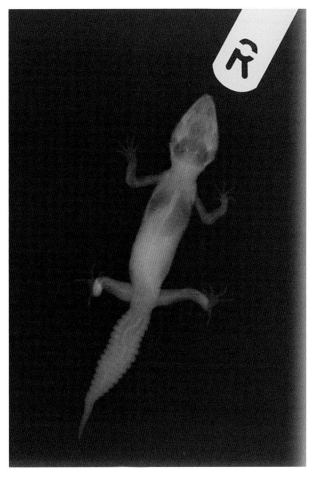

Figure 14.15 Advanced NSHP in a leopard gecko with loss of bone density (Source: photo courtesy of Kate Everett).

abnormal structures (Hernandez-Divers 2006) but is likely to cause pain to the patient and carries a risk of significant complications. Females of species with endolymphatic sacs will demonstrate marked mineralisation of the cervical region.

Ultrasonographic anatomy has been described in leopard geckos, using a 13–18 MHz linear array transducer (Cojean et al. 2018b). This was found to be useful to visualise the caudal lungs, liver, intestinal tract, coelomic vasculature, reproductive tract and brain. Ovarian follicles appear hypoechoic, and homogenous echogenic follicles are associated with degeneration or infection (Kophamel et al. 2018). Individuals in shed cannot be assessed reliably as ecdysis results in acoustic shadowing (Cojean et al. 2018b). The heart is in the pectoral girdle and is not easily visualised for echocardiography though the author has identified and treated a pericardial effusion by percutaneous drainage in one leopard gecko using an approach through the left axilla.

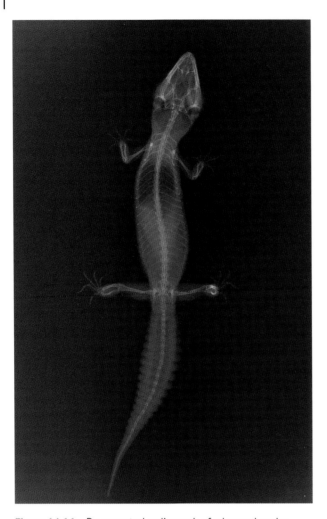

Figure 14.16 Dorsoventral radiograph of a leopard gecko -
note the lack of soft tissue detail and improved bone density
when compared to Figure 14.15 (Source: photo courtesy of
Manor vets).

14.6 Preventative Health Measures

Preventative health measures are limited in geckos – in most cases focusing mainly on intestinal parasite screening and maintaining good standards of husbandry to reduce incidence of many of the common diseases. Faecal parasitology in clinically well patients should be carried out every six months as many parasites have direct life cycles and burdens can accumulate over time. In individuals or groups with previous known parasite burdens then this should be carried out every three months. New animals should also undergo parasite screening and in leopard geckos this should include *C. saurophilum* PCR (or acid-fast staining as a cheaper but less sensitive technique).

In one study evaluating *Salmonella* presence in 110 tokay geckos, a prevalence of 31–73% was identified across three groups with 17 different serotypes found (Smith et al. 2012). Given the zoonotic potential, and increased detection of reptile-associated serotypes, particularly in young children (Olsen et al. 2001), screening pet reptiles appears a sensible precaution. However, shedding is infrequent, complicating detection, and antibiotic treatment is not advisable. It is often more practical to advise owners to assume their pet reptile carries *Salmonella* and is intermittently shedding bacteria in faeces and to be vigilant with hygiene rather than screen on a routine basis.

Formulary

	Dose	Route	Frequency of administration	Comments
Anaesthetic agents				
Alfaxalone	15 mg/kg	IM		Leopard geckos: IM injection results in more reliable sedation and shorter duration (21 minutes) than SC injection. Additional anaesthesia (e.g. isoflurane) and analgesia necessary for surgical procedures (van den Heuvel 2017)
	10–30 mg/kg	SC		Leopard geckos: Variable sedation, higher doses more reliable but result in prolonged sedation of over 120 mins (Doss et al. 2017)
Ketamine; diazepam	60 mg/kg; 1 mg/kg	IM		Tokay geckos (Primaditya 2012)
Ketamine; diazepam; isoflurane	5 mg/kg; 1 mg/kg; 2–5%	IM; IM; inhalation		New Caledonian giant gecko (*Rhacodactylus leachianus*): pre-medication followed by isoflurane for maintenance (Kophamel et al. 2018)

(Continued)

	Dose	Route	Frequency of administration	Comments
Dexmedetomidine; midazolam	0.1 mg/kg; 1 mg/kg	SC		Leopard geckos: Moderate sedation. Reversal with 1 mg/kg atipamezole and 0.05 mg/kg flumazenil can hasten recovery (Doss et al. 2017)
Alfaxalone; midazolam	15 mg/kg; 1 mg/kg	SC		Leopard geckos: Moderate sedation, recovery can be prolonged especially if flumazenil reveral not used (Doss et al. 2017)
Isoflurane	5% for induction, 1–3% for maintenance	inhalation		Induction can be prolonged
Analgesia				
Morphine	5–10 mg/kg	SC, IM	q24h	Based on bearded dragon dose (Sladky et al. 2008)
Tramadol	10 mg/kg	IM/PO	q24h	Leopard geckos: decreased response to painful stimulus seen (van den Heuvel 2017)
Meloxicam	0.3 mg/kg	SC/PO	q24h	Anecdotal dose, no evidence of efficacy (Cojean et al. 2018a)
Carprofen	4 mg/kg	SC	q24h	New Caledonian giant gecko (*Rhacodactylus leachianus*) (Kophamel et al. 2018)
Lidocaine	2 mg/kg			Extrapolated from other reptile species (Schumacher and Yelen 2006). Dilution of commercial preparations is often necessary for accurate dosing of small patients.
Antibiotics				
Trimethoprim-sulfa	30 mg/kg	PO	q24 h for 7 d	(Jenkins 1991)
Enrofloxacin	10 mg/kg	IM, SC, PO	q24h	Injectable preparations can result in localised inflammation (Gibbons et al. 2013)
Oxytetracycline	6–10 mg/kg	PO, IM	q24h	Long-acting injectable preparations can result in localised inflammation (Gibbons et al. 2013)
Ceftazidime	20–40 mg/kg	IM	q2–3d	Keep frozen and out of light once reconstituted (Gibbons et al. 2013)
Chloramphenical	40 mg/kg	PO, SC, IM	q24h	(Jenkins 1991)
Antiparasitic agents				
Fenbendazole	50 mg/kg	PO	q24h for 3–5 days	Nematode infestations (Klingenberg 2007)
Paromomycin	50–800 mg/kg	PO	q24h	To manage Cryptosporidiosis, oocyst shedding and clinical signs reduced whilst on treatment. Recurrence after cessation of therapy (Coke and Tristan 1998)
	100 mg/kg	PO	q24h for 7 days, then q84h for 72 days	To manage Cryptosporidiosis, oocyst shedding and clinical signs reduced whilst on treatment but infection not eliminated (Pantchev et al. 2008)
Hyperimmune bovine colostrum	1–3% bodyweight	PO	q1wk	For reducing shedding of cryptosporidiosis (Graczyk et al. 1999)
Nitazoxanide	q24 hr. for 5 days, then 50 mg/kg q24 hr. for 23 days	PO		For cryptosporidiosis (Wellehan 2013)
Ivermectin	0.2 mg/kg	PO/SC	q2wks	For nematodes (Boyer 1998)
	1 mg/kg	PO	Two doses two weeks apart	Tokay and day geckos, used for pentastomiasis treatment, significant potential for toxicity at high dose used (Micinilio 1996; Wright 1997)

(*Continued*)

(Continued)

	Dose	Route	Frequency of administration	Comments
Metronidazole	20 mg/kg	PO	q48h for 10 days	For diarrhoea associated with protozoa. Can be extended to 20 day course if protozoa still present in faeces (Boyer et al. 2013)
	40–200 mg/kg	PO	q2wks	For trichomoniasis of soft tissues (Miller et al. 1994)
Miscellaneous				
Calcium gluconate	100 mg/kg	SC, IM	q6–24h	Management of hypocalcaemia (Gibbons et al. 2013)
Oxytocin	1–5 U/kg	IM	repeat after 1hr. if unsuccessful	(Divers 1996) Used for uterine inertia in the absence of egg adherence, egg deformity or oviductal pathology
Oral calcium and vitamin D (ZolcalD)	1 ml/kg	PO	daily	For supplementation of hypocalcaemic animals
Pentobarbitone	60–100 mg/kg	Intracardiac/IC		For euthanasia, pithing required after cardiac arrest
Tricaine methanesulfonate (MS222)	250–500 mg/kg of dilute solution (1%) for sedation, followed by second injection of 8–12.5 g/kg (50% solution) once sedated	IC		For euthanasia. MS-222 should be buffered to a neutral pH with bicarbonate before use. Cardiorespiratory activity ceased 30–60s after the second injection (Conroy et al. 2009)

References

Allen, M.E., Oftedal, O.T., and Ullrey, D.E. (1993). Effect of dietary calcium concentration on mineral composition of fox geckos (*Hemidactylus garnoti*) and Cuban tree frogs (*Osteopilus septentrionalis*). *Journal of Zoo and Wildlife Medicine* 24 (2): 118–128.

Andrews, R.M. and Pough, F.H. (1985). Metabolism of squamate reptiles: allometric and ecological relationships. *Physiological Zoology* 58 (2): 214–231.

Barker, D., Fitzpatrick, M.P., and Dierenfeld, E.S. (1998). Nutrient composition of selected whole invertebrates. *Zoo Biology*: Published in affiliation with the American Zoo and Aquarium Association 17 (2): 123–134.

Barton, D.P. (2007). Pentastomid parasites of the introduced Asian house gecko, *Hemidactylus frenatus* (Gekkonidae), in Australia. *Comparative Parasitology* 74 (2): 254–259.

Bertelsen, M.F. (2007). Squamates (snakes and lizards). In: Zoo Animal and Wildlife Immobilization and Anesthesia (eds. G. West, D. Heard and N. Caulkett), 233–243. Ames, IA: Blackwell Publishing.

Bonney, C.H., Hartfiel, D.A., and Schmidt, R.E. (1978). *Klebsiella pneumoniae* infection with secondary hypopyon in tokay gecko lizards. *Journal of the American Veterinary Medical Association* 173 (9): 1115.

Boyer, T.H. (1998). Essentials of Reptiles: A Guide for Practitioners: An Update to a Practitioner's Guide to Reptilian Husbandry and Care, 1–253. Lakewood, CO: AAHA Press.

Boyer, T.H., Garner, M.M., Reavill, D.R. et al. (2013). Common problems of leopard geckos (Eublepharis macularius). Proceedings of the Association of Reptilian and Amphibian Veterinarians conference, Indianapolis, IN: 17–25.

Brannian, R.E. and Greve, J.H. (1987). Diseases and parasites of a captive population of Tokay geckos. Proceedings of the First International Conference on Zoological and Avian Medicine. AAV-AAZV: 481–486.

Brown, S.G. and Duffy, P.K. (1992). The effects of egg-laying site, temperature, and salt water on incubation time and hatching success in the gecko *Lepidodactylus lugubris*. *Journal of Herpetology* 26 (4): 510–513.

Brown, S.G. and O'Brien, J. (1993). Pseudosexual and dominance behaviour: their relationship to fecundity in the unisexual gecko, *Lepidodactylus lugubris*. *Journal of Zoology* 231 (1): 61–69.

Brown, S.G. and Sakai, T.J.Y. (1988). Social experience and egg development in the parthenogenic gecko, *Lepidodactylus lugubris*. *Ethology* 79 (4): 317–323.

Bursey, C. and Goldberg, S. (1999). *Skrjabinodon piankai* sp. n.(Nematoda: Pharyngodonidae) and other helminths of geckos (Sauria: Gekkonidae: Nephrurus spp.) from

Australia. *Journal of the Helminthological Society of Washington* 66 (2): 175–179.

Carman, E.N., Ferguson, G.W., Gehrmann, W.H. et al. (2000). Photobiosynthetic opportunity and ability for UV-B generated vitamin D synthesis in free-living house geckos (*Hemidactylus turcicus*) and Texas spiny lizards (*Sceloporus olivaceous*). *Copeia* 2000 (1): 245–250.

Cojean, O., Lair, S., and Vergneau-Grosset, C. (2018a). Evaluation of β-carotene assimilation in leopard geckos (*Eublepharis macularius*). *Journal of Animal Physiology and Animal Nutrition* 102 (5): 1411–1418.

Cojean, O., Vergneau-Grosset, C., and Masseau, I. (2018b). Ultrasonographic anatomy of reproductive female leopard geckos (*Eublepharis macularius*). *Veterinary Radiology and Ultrasound* 59 (3): 333–344.

Coke, R.L. and Tristan, T.E. (1998). Cryptosporidium infection in a colony of leopard geckos, *Eublepharis macularius*. In: Proceedings of the 5th Annual Conference of the Association of Reptilian and Amphibian Veterinarians (eds. M.W. Frahm and L.C. Boyer), 157–163. Kansas City, MO: University Press.

Congdon, J.D., Vitt, L.J., and King, W.W. (1974). Geckos: adaptive significance and energetics of tail autotomy. *Science* 184 (4144): 1379–1380.

Conroy, C.J., Papenfuss, T., Parker, J. et al. (2009). Use of tricaine methanesulfonate (MS222) for euthanasia of reptiles. *Journal of the American Association for Laboratory Animal Science* 48 (1): 28–32.

Cork, S.C. and Stockdale, P.H.G. (1994). Mycotic disease in the common New Zealand gecko (*Hoplodactylus maculatus*). *New Zealand Veterinary Journal* 42 (4): 144–147.

Cuellar, O. and Kluge, A.G. (1972). Natural parthenogenesis in the gekkonid lizard *Lepidodactylus lugubris*. *Journal of Genetics* 61 (1): 14.

Delorme, S.L., Lungu, I.M., and Vickaryous, M.K. (2012). Scar-free wound healing and regeneration following tail loss in the leopard gecko, *Eublepharis macularius*. *The Anatomical Record: Advances in Integrative Anatomy and Evolutionary Biology* 295 (10): 1575–1595.

Deming, C., Greiner, E., and Uhl, E.W. (2008). Prevalence of cryptosporidium infection and characteristics of oocyst shedding in a breeding colony of leopard geckos (*Eublepharis macularius*). *Journal of Zoo and Wildlife Medicine* 39 (4): 600–608.

DeNardo, D.F. and Helminski, G. (2001). The use of hormone antagonists to inhibit reproduction in the lizard, *Eublepharus macularius*. *Journal of Herpetological Medicine and Surgery* 11 (3): 4–7.

Di Giuseppe, M., Martínez-Silvestre, A., Luparello, M. et al. (2017). Post-ovulatory dystocia in two small lizards:

leopard gecko (*Eublepharis macularius*) and crested gecko (*Correlophus ciliatus*). *Russian Journal of Herpetology* 24 (2): 128–132.

Divers, S.J. (1996). Medical and surgical treatment of preovulatory ova stasis and postovulatory egg stasis in oviparous lizards. *Proceedings of the Association of Reptilian and Amphibian Veterinarians* 1996: 119–123.

Divers, S. (1999). Administering fluid therapy to reptiles. *Exotic DVM* 1 (2): 5–10.

Divers, S.J. and Cooper, J.E. (2000). Reptile hepatic lipidosis. *Seminars in Avian and Exotic Pet Medicine* 9 (3): 153–164.

Donoghue, S. (2006). Nutrition. In: Reptile Medicine and Surgery, 2e (ed. D. Mader), 282. St. Louis, MO: Saunders Elsevier.

Doss, G.A., Fink, D.M., Sladky, K.K. et al. (2017). Comparison of subcutaneous dexmedetomidine–midazolam versus alfaxalone–midazolam sedation in leopard geckos (*Eublepharis macularius*). *Veterinary Anaesthesia and Analgesia* 44 (5): 1175–1183.

Fink, D.M., Doss, G.A., Sladky, K.K. et al. (2018). Effect of injection site on dexmedetomidine-ketamine induced sedation in leopard geckos (*Eublepharis macularius*). *Journal of the American Veterinary Medical Association* 253 (9): 1146–1150.

Gabor, L.J. (2005). Nutritional degenerative myopathy in a population of captive bred *Uroplatus phantasticus* (satanic leaf-tailed geckoes). *Journal of Veterinary Diagnostic Investigation* 17 (1): 71–73.

Gamble, T. (2010). A review of sex determining mechanisms in geckos (Gekkota: Squamata). *Sexual Development* 4 (1–2): 88–103. https://doi.org/10.1159/000289578.

Garner, M.M., Lung, N.P., and Murray, S. (1999). Xanthomatosis in geckos: five cases. *Journal of Zoo and Wildlife Medicine* 30 (3): 443–447.

Garner, M.M., Farina, L.L., and Wellehan, J.F.X. (2009). Reovirus-associated syncytial cell enteropathy and hepatopathy in leopard geckos (Eublepharis macularius). *Proceedings of the Association of Reptilian and Amphibian Veterinarians*: 8–15.

Garrick, D. (2008). Body surface temperature and length in relation to the thermal biology of lizards. *Bioscience Horizons* 1 (2): 136–142.

Gartrell, B.D. and Hare, K.M. (2005). Mycotic dermatitis with digital gangrene and osteomyelitis, and protozoal intestinal parasitism in Marlborough green geckos (*Naultinus manukanus*). *New Zealand Veterinary Journal* 53 (5): 363–367.

Gibbons, P., Klaphake, E., and Carpenter, J.W. (2013). Reptiles. In: Exotic Animal Formulary, 4e (eds. J.W. Carpenter and C.J. Marion), 83–182. St Louis, MO: Saunders.

Gould, A., Molitor, L., Rockwell, K. et al. (2018). Evaluating the physiologic effects of short duration ultraviolet B radiation exposure in leopard geckos (*Eublepharis macularius*). *Journal of Herpetological Medicine and Surgery* 28 (1): 34–39.

Graczyk, T.K., Cranfield, M.R., and Bostwick, E.F. (1999). Hyperimmune bovine colostrum treatment of moribund leopard geckos (*Eublepharis macularius*) infected with cryptosporidium sp. *Veterinary Research* 30 (4): 377–382.

Griffing, A.H., Sanger, T.J., Matamoros, I.C. et al. (2018). Protocols for husbandry and embryo collection of a parthenogenetic gecko, *Lepidodactylus lugubris* (Squamata: Gekkonidae). *Herpetological Review* 49 (2): 230–235.

Gutzke, W.H.N. and Crews, D. (1988). Embryonic temperature determines adult sexuality in a reptile. *Nature* 332 (6167): 832.

Hadfield, C.A., Clayton, L.A., Clancy, M.M. et al. (2012). Proliferative thyroid lesions in three diplodactylid geckos: *Nephrurus amyae, Nephrurus levis*, and *Oedura marmorata*. *Journal of Zoo and Wildlife Medicine* 43 (1): 131–140.

Hall, A.J. and Lewbart, G.A. (2006). Treatment of dystocia in a leopard gecko (*Eublepharis macularius*) by percutaneous ovocentesis. *The Veterinary Record* 158 (21): 737–739.

Heckers, K.O., Aupperle, H., Schmidt, V. et al. (2012). Melanophoromas and iridophoromas in reptiles. *Journal of Comparative Pathology* 146 (2): 258–268.

Hernandez-Divers, S.J. (2006). Reptiles radiology: techniques, tips and pathology. *Proceedings of the North American Veterinary Conference* 20: 1626–1630.

van den Heuvel, M.W.J. (2017). Repeated measurement comparison of different protocols for anesthesia and analgesia consisting of Alfaxalone, Meloxicam, and Butorphanol or Tramadol IM in Leopard Geckos (*Eublepharis macularius*). Master's thesis, University of Utrecht.

Hochleithner, C. and Holland, M. (2014). Ultrasonography. In: Current Therapy in Reptile Medicine and Surgery (eds. D.R. Mader and S.J. Divers), 107–127. St. Louis, MO: Elsevier/Saunders.

Jenkins, J.R. (1991). Medical management of reptile patients. *The Compendium on Continuing Education for the Practicing Veterinarian* 13: 980–988.

Klaphake, E. (2010). A fresh look at metabolic bone diseases in reptiles and amphibians. *The Veterinary Clinics of North America. Exotic Animal Practice* 13 (3): 375–392.

Klingenberg, R.J. (2007). Understanding Reptile Parasites: From the Experts at Advanced Vivarium Systems. Advanced Vivarium Systems, Inc.

Knotek, Z., Cermakova, E., and Oliveri, M. (2017). Reproductive medicine in lizards. *The Veterinary Clinics of North America. Exotic Animal Practice* 20 (2): 411–438.

Kophamel, S., Lebens, M., Gunther, P. et al. (2018). Lipogranulomatous oophoritis in a Leach's giant gecko (*Rhacodactylus leachianus*). *Wiener Tierärztliche Monatsschrift* 105 (3–4): 73–80.

Koudela, B. and Modry, D. (1998). New species of *Cryptosporidium* (Apicomplexa: Cryptosporidiidae) from lizards. *Folia Parasitologica* 45 (2): 93–100.

Kratochvíl, L. and Frynta, D. (2007). Phylogenetic analysis of sexual dimorphism in eye-lid geckos (Eublepharidae): the effects of male combat, courtship behaviour, egg size, and body size. In: Sex, Size and Gender Roles (eds. D.J. Fairbairn, W.U. Blanckenhorn and T. Szekely), 154–162. New York: Oxford University Press.

Kroenlein, K.R., Sleeman, J.M., Holladay, S.D. et al. (2008). Inability to induce tympanic squamous metaplasia using organochlorine compounds in vitamin A-deficient red-eared sliders (*Trachemys scripta elegans*). *Journal of Wildlife Diseases* 44 (3): 664–669.

Kubiak, M., Denk, D., and Stidworthy, M.F. (2020). Retrospective review of neoplasms of captive lizards in the United Kingdom. *Veterinary Record* 186 (1): 28–28.

LaDage, L.D., Gutzke, W.H., Simmons, R.A. et al. (2008). Multiple mating increases fecundity, fertility and relative clutch mass in the female leopard gecko (*Eublepharis macularius*). *Ethology* 114 (5): 512–520.

Le Souëf, A.T., Barry, M., Brunton, D.H. et al. (2015). Ovariectomy as treatment for ovarian bacterial granulomas in a Duvaucel's gecko (*Hoplodactylus duvaucelii*). *New Zealand Veterinary Journal* 63 (6): 340–344.

Leary, S., Underwood, W., Anthony, R. et al. (2013). Captive amphibians and reptiles. In: AVMA Guidelines for the Euthanasia of Animals: 2013 Edition, 76–78. Schaumburg, IL: American Veterinary Medical Association.

Loew, E.R. (1994). A third, ultraviolet-sensitive, visual pigment in the Tokay gecko (*Gekko gekko*). *Vision Research* 34 (11): 1427–1431.

Marschang, R.E., Braun, S., and Becher, P. (2005). Isolation of a ranavirus from a gecko (*Uroplatus fimbriatus*). *Journal of Zoo and Wildlife Medicine* 36 (2): 295–300.

Martinez-Jimenez, D. and Hernandez-Divers, S.J. (2007). Emergency care of reptiles. *The Veterinary Clinics of North America. Exotic Animal Practice* 10 (2): 557–585.

Mayer, J. and Donnelly, T.M. (2013). Entamoebiasis. In: Clinical Veterinary Advisor (eds. J. Mayer and T.M. Donnelly), 100–101. St. Louis, MO: W.B. Saunders.

McBride, M. and Hernandez-Divers, S.J. (2004). Nursing care of lizards. *The Veterinary Clinics of North America. Exotic Animal Practice* 7 (2): 375–396.

Micinilio, J. (1996). Ivermectin for the treatment of pentastomids in a Tokay gecko, *Gekko gecko*. *Bulletin of the Association of Reptilian and Amphibian Veterinarians* 6 (2): 5–6.

Mikaelian, I., Lynch, S., Harshbarger, J.C. et al. (2000). Malignant chromatophoroma in a day gecko (*Phelsuma madagarescencis grandis*). *Exotic Pet Practice* 5 (10): 1–2.

Miller, H.A., Frye, F.L., and Graig, T.M. (1994). Trichomonas associated with ocular and subcutaneous lesions in geckos. Proceedings of the Annual Conference of the American Association of Zoo Veterinarians: 124–126.

Millichamp, N.J., Jacobson, E.R., and Wolf, E.D. (1983). Diseases of the eye and ocular adnexae in reptiles. *Journal of the American Veterinary Medical Association* 183 (11): 1205–1212.

Music, M.K. and Strunk, A. (2016). Reptile critical care and common emergencies. *The Veterinary Clinics of North America. Exotic Animal Practice* 19 (2): 591–612.

Olsen, S.J., Bishop, R., Brenner, F.W. et al. (2001). The changing epidemiology of *Salmonella*: trends in serotypes isolated from humans in the United States, 1987–1997. *The Journal of Infectious Diseases* 183 (5): 753–761.

Pantchev, N., Rueschoff, B., Kamhuber-Pohl, A. et al. (2008). Kryptosporidiose-Therapie bei Leopardgeckos (*Eublepharis macularius*) mit Azithromycin (Zithromax®) und Paromomycinsulfat (Humatin®)–Fallbeispiele und Literaturübersicht. *Kleintierpraxis* 10 (2): 95–104.

Paré, J.A. (2008). An overview of pentastomiasis in reptiles and other vertebrates. *Journal of Exotic Pet Medicine* 17 (4): 285–294.

Peacock, H.M., Gilbert, E.A., and Vickaryous, M.K. (2015). Scar-free cutaneous wound healing in the leopard gecko, *Eublepharis macularius. Journal of Anatomy* 227 (5): 596–610.

Primaditya, F.M. (2012). Profil Lama Anestesi Dari Penggunann Ketamin Secara Tunggal, Kombinasi Ketamin-Xylazin, Dan Ketamin-Diazepam Pada Tokek (Gekko gecko). Doctoral dissertation, Universitas Airlangga.

Radtkey, R.R., Donnellan, S.C., Fisher, R.N. et al. (1995). When species collide: the origin and spread of an asexual species of gecko. *Proceedings of the Royal Society of London B: Biological Sciences* 259 (1355): 145–152.

Reavill, D.R. and Griffin, C. (2014). Common pathology and diseases seen in pet store reptiles. In: Current Therapy in Reptile Medicine and Surgery (eds. D.R. Mader and S.J. Divers), 13–19. St. Louis, MO: Elsevier.

Redrobe, S. (2004). Anaesthesia and analgesia. In: BSAVA Manual of Reptiles, 2e (eds. S. Girling and P. Raiit), 131–146. Quedgeley: BSAVA.

Reese, D.J., Kinsella, J.M., Zdziarski, J.M. et al. (2004). Parasites in 30 captive Tokay Geckos, *Gekko gecko. Journal of Herpetological Medicine and Surgery* 14 (2): 21–25.

Rovira, A.I., Holzer, T.R., and Credille, K.M. (2014). Systemic Mastocytosis in an African fat-tail gecko (*Hemitheconyx caudicinctus*). *Journal of Comparative Pathology* 151 (1): 130–134.

Sabath, M.D. (1981). Gekkonid lizards of Guam, Mariana Islands: reproduction and habitat preference. *Journal of Herpetology* 15 (1): 71–75.

Sander, S.J., Ossiboff, R.J., Stokol, T. et al. (2015). Endolymphatic sac carcinoma in situ in a tokay gecko (*Gekko gecko*). *Journal of Herpetological Medicine and Surgery* 25 (3–4): 82–86.

Schmidt, R.E. and Toft, J.D. (1981). Ophthalmic lesions in animals from a zoologic collection. *Journal of Wildlife Diseases* 17 (2): 267–275.

Schumacher, J. and Yelen, T. (2006). Anaesthesia and analgesia. In: Reptile Medicine and Surgery (ed. D.R. Mader), 442–452. St Louis, MO: Elsevier.

Sladky, K.K., Kinney, M.E., and Johnson, S.M. (2008). Analgesic efficacy of butorphanol and morphine in bearded dragons and corn snakes. *Journal of the American Veterinary Medical Association* 233 (2): 267–273.

Smith, K.F., Yabsley, M.J., Sanchez, S. et al. (2012). Salmonella isolates from wild-caught Tokay geckos (*Gekko gecko*) imported to the US from Indonesia. *Vector Borne and Zoonotic Diseases* 12 (7): 575–582.

Stevens, Y. (2008). Sperm competition in leopard geckos, Eublepharis macularius. Does mating order affect paternity? http://edepot.wur.nl/320482 (accessed 27 November 2018).

Taylor, M.A., Geach, M.R., and Cooley, W.A. (1999). Clinical and pathological observations on natural infections of cryptosporidiosis and flagellate protozoa in leopard geckos (*Eublepharis macularius*). *Veterinary Record* 145 (24): 695–699.

Thorogood, J. and Whimster, I.W. (1979). The maintenance and breeding of the leopard gecko. *International Zoo Yearbook* 19 (1): 74–78.

Toplon, D.E., Terrell, S.P., Sigler, L. et al. (2013). Dermatitis and cellulitis in leopard geckos (*Eublepharis macularius*) caused by the *Chrysosporium* anamorph of *Nannizziopsis vriesii. Veterinary Pathology* 50 (4): 585–589.

Trifonov, V.A., Giovannotti, M., O'Brien, P.C. et al. (2011). Chromosomal evolution in Gekkonidae. I. Chromosome painting between *Gekko* and *Hemidactylus* species reveals phylogenetic relationships within the group. *Chromosome Research* 19 (7): 843–855.

Uetz, P. (2009). The TIGR Reptile Database. http://www.reptile-database.org vol 2008 (accessed 23 December 2019).

Upton, S.J. and Barnard, S.M. (1987). Two new species of coccidia (Apicomplexa: Eimeriidae) from Madagascar gekkonids. *The Journal of Protozoology* 34 (4): 452–454.

Upton, S.J., McAllister, C.T., Freed, P.S. et al. (1989). *Cryptosporidium* spp. in wild and captive reptiles. *Journal of Wildlife Diseases* 25 (1): 20–30.

Viets, B.E., Tousignant, A., Ewert, M.A. et al. (1993). Temperature-dependent sex determination in the leopard gecko, *Eublepharis macularius*. *Journal of Experimental Zoology* 265 (6): 679–683.

de Vosjoli, P. (2004). The Leopard Gecko Manual. Irvine, CA: Advanced Vivarium Systems Inc.

de Vosjoli, P., Viets, B., Tremper, R. et al. (1998). The Leopard Gecko Manual, 85. Escondido, CA: Advanced Vivarium Systems.

Wangen, K., Kirshenbaum, J., and Mitchell, M.A. (2013). Measuring 25-hydroxyvitamin D levels in leopard geckos exposed to commercial ultraviolet B lights. Proceedings of the Association of Reptilian and Amphibian Veterinarians: 42.

Webb, A.R. and Holick, M.F. (1988). The role of sunlight in the cutaneous production of vitamin D3. *Annual Review of Nutrition* 8 (1): 375–399.

Wellehan, J. (2013). Cryptosporidiosis. In: Clinical Veterinary Advisor: Birds and Exotic Pets (eds. J. Mayer and T. Donelly), 89–90. St. Louis, MO: Elsevier Saunders.

Wellehan, J.F., Johnson, A.J., Harrach, B. et al. (2004). Detection and analysis of six lizard adenoviruses by consensus primer PCR provides further evidence of a reptilian origin for the atadenoviruses. *Journal of Virology* 78 (23): 13366–13369.

Wiggans, K.T., Sanchez-Migallon Guzman, D., Reilly, C.M. et al. (2018). Diagnosis, treatment, and outcome of and risk factors for ophthalmic disease in leopard geckos (*Eublepharis macularius*) at a veterinary teaching hospital: 52 cases (1985–2013). *Journal of the American Veterinary Medical Association* 252 (3): 316–323.

Woodland, W.N.F. (1920). Memoirs: some observations on caudal autotomy and regeneration in the gecko (*Hemidactylus flaviviridis*, Rppel), with notes on the tails of *Sphenodon* and *Pygopus*. *Journal of Cell Science* 2 (257): 63–100.

Wright, K. (1997). Ivermectin for treatment of pentastomids in the Standing's day gecko, *Phelsuma standingi*. *Bulletin of the Association of Reptilian and Amphibian Veterinarians* 7 (1): 5.

15

Chameleons
Marie Kubiak

The Chameleonidae family comprises over 200 species, predominantly originating from Africa with scant extension into Southern Asia and Europe (Uetz and Hošek 2018). They are differentiated from other lizards by their zygodactylous feet, long, extendable tongue, rotating eye turrets, and often striking appearance. Many species have the ability to change skin colouration based on endocrine, environmental, and social cues for the purposes of communication, blending into surroundings, or thermoregulation. Although popular as pets, particularly the veiled chameleon upon which this chapter will focus, these are difficult species to maintain well in captivity and should be avoided by inexperienced reptile keepers. Biological parameters of selected chameleon species are given in Table 15.1.

Many species are declining in the wild and all chameleon species are listed on CITES Appendix II (except *Brookesia perarmata*), resulting in monitoring and restrictions to international trade. Other than veiled chameleons (*Chamaeleo calyptratus*) and, to a lesser extent panther chameleons (*Furcifer pardalis*), which rely on captive bred individuals for the pet trade, the majority of chameleons are taken from wild populations. As such, restricting international trade restricts availability of individuals for the pet trade. *B. perarmata* is listed on CITES appendix I, effectively prohibiting international trade to protect native populations. Conversely, chameleons can be invasive species in suitable climates with both veiled and Jacksons chameleons (*Chamaeleo jacksonii*) in Hawaii, and veiled and Oustalet's chameleons (*Furcifer oustaleti*) in Florida establishing breeding wild populations and posing a threat to native fauna (Kraus et al. 2012; Chiaverano et al. 2014; Smith et al. 2016).

The Carolina anole (*Anolis carolinensis*) is occasionally incorrectly referred to as 'The American chameleon' but belongs to the family Dactyloidae and is distinct from the true chameleons.

15.1 Husbandry

The majority of chameleons are solitary in the wild with defined territories, and adults can be aggressive to conspecifics so should be housed separately. Some species, such as Jackson's and Panther chameleons, can be kept as breeding pairs or small groups of females with a single male though the large sizes of enclosures required for group housing are often impractical for private keepers (de Vosjoli 1990). Bearded pygmy chameleons (*Rieppeleon brevicaudatus*) can be maintained in pairs. Juveniles often tolerate crèche rearing given sufficient space.

Wooden vivaria are not recommended as poor ventilation and porous walls alongside the necessarily high humidity can predispose to bacterial and fungal proliferation. Tall glass vivaria with large vented areas for airflow, or mesh screened enclosures are preferred. Their arboreal lifestyle requires vertical as well as horizontal space, with branches and planting at multiple levels. Live plants are ideal for maintaining stable humidity, and an aesthetic display. Enclosure size for veiled chameleons should be a minimum of 60 cm wide, 60 cm deep and 90 cm high for a single animal but larger naturally planted enclosures should be encouraged as these will provide a wider variety of microhabitats and stimulation for animals. Larger species, such as panther chameleons require enclosures of at least 90 × 90 × 90 cm. Adjacent enclosures should be separated by solid visual barriers but care must be taken not to compromise ventilation.

A substrate of soil, coconut fibre, or peat will maintain humidity and allow plant growth. Particulate substrates such as gravel or bark chips are best avoided as these can adhere to the tongue if feeding attempts are inaccurate, resulting in tongue or oral trauma, and potential ingestion and obstruction of the intestinal tract. Females require a

Handbook of Exotic Pet Medicine, First Edition. Edited by Marie Kubiak.
© 2021 John Wiley & Sons Ltd. Published 2021 by John Wiley & Sons Ltd.
Companion website: www.wiley.com/go/kubiak/exotic_pet_medicine

Table 15.1   Biological parameters of selected chameleon species.

Species	Lifespan in captivity	Adult weight	Body length (including tail)	Breeding strategy	Gestation length	Incubation length	Sexual maturity	Clutch/ brood size
Veiled or Yemen chameleon (*Chameleo calyptratus*)	Females 2–3 years, males 5–6 years	Female 90–120 g, males 90–200 g	Males 35–60 cm, females 25–35 cm	Oviparous	20–30 days (retention of sperm can lead to a second clutch after a further 90–120 days)	170–220 days	4–6 months	15–85
Panther chameleon (*Furcifer pardalis)*	Females 2–3 years, males 5–10 years	Female 60–100 g, Male 140–190 g	Males 40–55 cm, females <35 cm	Oviparous	20–35 days	8–12 months	8–12 months	12–46
Jackson's chameleon (*Trioceros jacksonii*)	5–10 years	80–200 g	23–33 cm	Ovoviviparous	7–9 months (retention of sperm can lead to a second brood after a further 3 months)	N/A	9–12 months	20–30
Bearded pygmy chameleon (*Rieppeleon brevicaudatus*)	1–3 years	no data	5–8 cm	Oviparous	unknown	45–90 days	unknown	up to 9

deep substrate for egg laying and this should be provided in a contained receptacle, such as a plant pot, to allow stable tunnel formation, consistent temperatures and humidity around eggs, and to avoid disrupting plants when removing eggs. Substrate should be spot-cleaned daily, or invertebrates (such as millipedes, woodlice, and springtails) used as biological cleaners.

Tropical species require higher environmental temperatures than their montane equivalents. Daytime basking opportunities can be provided using an overhead heat lamp, outside the enclosure where a mesh ceiling is present or, if placed within the enclosure, a guard cage must be placed around the lamp to avoid direct contact. Constant basking opportunity is required during the day and lamps should be positioned to provide the appropriate temperature at the highest branch. Branches must be securely fixed under the basking source to provide a stable support for the acrobatic lateral basking seen in chameleons. In gravid females, extended basking times may be seen (Figure 15.1), with some animals attaining an inverted position to maximise exposure of the ventrum to the heat source (de Vosjoli 1990). Ambient temperatures are best achieved by heating the room to a suitable temperature as infra-red lamps, ceramic lamps, and heat mats all provide focal heat. It is advisable to provide a cooler period in winter to mimic seasonal variation and stimulate normal reproductive cycles in breeding chameleons. Cold chameleons will appear dark, remain under available heat sources, and reduce

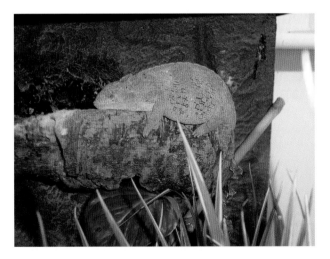

Figure 15.1   Gravid females will bask for prolonged periods, as with this heavily gravid Johnston's chameleon.

activity and feeding. Chameleons kept at excessively high temperatures will demonstrate hyperactivity, light colouration, and oral gaping (de Vosjoli 1990). Temperatures and basic husbandry requirements are detailed in Table 15.2.

Ultraviolet light (including both UV-A and UV-B wavelengths) should be provided during the daytime, with a photoperiod of 13 hours in the summer and 10 hours in the winter. UV lights should be replaced every 6–12 months, or as required based on UV-B output (measured as UV index) regularly using a handheld meter (Baines et al. 2016). Chameleons are able to visualise UV-A (Bowmaker et al. 2005) and it is

Table 15.2 Environmental parameters of selected chameleon species.

Species	Daytime ambient temperature (°C)	Daytime basking temperature (°C)	Night temperature (°C)	Ultraviolet lighting	Humidity	Diet
Veiled or Yemen chameleon (*Chameleo calyptratus*)	22–26	28–33	18–25	UV Index 1.0–2.6	50–75%	Crickets, locusts, silkworms, waxworms, cockroaches and soldierfly larvae for adults, calcium supplement at each feed, multivitamin supplement once/twice weekly; fruitflies, subadult crickets and moulted (white) mealworms for juveniles, multivitamin and calcium supplement daily. Adults may take small amounts of fruit or vegetables
Panther chameleon (*Furcifer pardalis*)	23–28	30–34	17–25	UV Index 1.0–2.6	60–70%	Invertebrates as for veiled chameleons, plus mealworms and neonatal mice can be offered sparingly to animals in low body condition
Jackson's chameleon (*Trioceros jacksonii*)	20–24	28–30	12–18	UV Index 0.7–2.6	50–60%	Varied invertebrates as for veiled chameleons
Bearded pygmy chameleon (*Rieppeleon brevicaudatus*)	15–25	22–25, very sensitive to higher temperatures	15–22	UV Index 0.1–1.0	60–80%	Pinhead crickets, hatchling cockroaches, fruitflies, silkworms

believed that visualisation of ultraviolet light is important in food selection, communication, and selecting basking sites. UV-B light is important for endogenous synthesis of Vitamin D for calcium homeostasis and panther chameleons have been shown to be able to self-regulate in the presence of UV-B lighting, by altering basking behaviour depending on circulating vitamin D levels (Karsten et al. 2009).

Humidity is crucial for maintaining chameleon health and is difficult to consistently manage optimally. Chameleons require higher humidity than many more commonly kept reptile species and will rarely drink from bowls, preferring to drink droplets from leaves or décor. As such, chronic dehydration is a common debilitating factor in many disease processes. Environmental humidity and drinking opportunities must be maintained at all times using a combination of automatic misters or foggers, overhead drip systems, waterfalls, and manual spraying.

Chameleons are predominantly insectivores and a variety of appropriately sized food items should be offered, which themselves have been fed a varied vegetable diet. Juveniles and dwarf species will feed twice daily and adults of larger species may feed as infrequently as twice a week, Chameleons can be habituated to feed from a bowl, usually placed at height in their enclosure, but foraging should be encouraged in healthy animals to maintain activity and normal feeding responses. Injuries can occur from prey bites to debilitated, inactive chameleons but these are uncommon and are not seen as a primary concern. Food should dusted with a calcium powder at each feed, and with a supplement containing vitamins A and D once or twice weekly.

15.2 Breeding

Veiled chameleons are seasonal breeders in the wild but will breed year round in captivity. Females of this species demonstrate colour changes, from a dark green/brown to a lighter green with blue spots dorsally, that is associated with receptive behaviour towards males (Annis 1995). These colour changes correlate with sex hormone cycles, and an interval of 112–152 days is seen between receptive phases (Kummrow et al. 2010a). When blue colouration is noted females can be introduced into the cage of the male and the male should approach and initiate copulation which is repeated several times through the day. It is advisable to remove the female after no more than eight hours to prevent aggression (Diaz et al. 2015). One to twenty four hours after mating, orange markings develop and females darken to brown when a male approaches and are no longer-receptive (Annis 1995). If mating is unsuccessful, the female can be reintroduced to the male three to seven days after the initial attempt (Diaz et al. 2015). Oviposition occurs when the oestrogen: progesterone ratio decreases with eggs tending to be laid 21–30 days after mating but retained sperm can also result in subsequent clutches with a 90–120 days interval (Stahl 1997). Captive females can lay three to four clutches annually (Kummrow et al. 2010a) but this level of productivity is highly debilitating. The female will dig a vertical tunnel to lay 15–85 eggs (Schmidt 2001). Occasionally further eggs may be laid after a few days (Diaz et al. 2015). These eggs have shells of a leathery texture. Females may lay infertile eggs in the absence of a male and these are smaller and often discoloured.

In all oviparous species of chameleon, incubation period is long compared to most other lizards with duration typically within the range 180–365 days. Incubation of veiled chameleon eggs takes approximately 200 days at 26 °C (Diaz et al. 2015), higher temperatures or a peak in humidity towards the end of incubation can shorten incubation time. This prolonged incubation is due to embryonic immaturity at the time of lay and an extended diapause of 60–80 days following egg laying (Andrews and Donoghue 2004). This is an adaptation to wild conditions, allowing nesting when predation risk is low, and hatching when food supply is plentiful.

Chameleons exhibit no parental care and artificial incubation with stable temperatures and humidity is preferred to leaving eggs within the substrate. Eggs should be placed 1–2 cm apart in a moist substrate, such as vermiculite, in the incubator and not rotated. The container should be weighed and humidity maintained by adding water to the substrate to maintain the original weight.

In ovoviviparous species of chameleon, mating is followed by a long first gestation period before young are born within thin membranes. Subsequent births may be at shorter intervals as multiple broods can be developing simultaneously at different stages using retained sperm from the previous mating (Davison 1997).

15.2.1 Neonatal Care

Neonates of oviparous species should remain in the incubator for 24 hours to resorb remaining yolk sac prior to transfer to a rearing enclosure under similar conditions to those for adults. Neonates of ovoviviparous species can move into a rearing tank immediately. Neonates can remain in small groups until four months of age when they reach maturity to facilitate normal behavioural development, and then should be housed individually (Ballen et al. 2014; Diaz et al. 2015). They should be fed twice daily, and preferably kept on a solid substrate such as paper towels to avoid substrate ingestion (Stahl 1997).

Sex determination of embryos is currently poorly understood. Andrews (2005) reports that the sex of offspring of both veiled and panther chameleons is independent of egg incubation temperature, unlike temperature dependent sex determination seen in many other lizard families. This is

supported by identification of an XX/XY sex chromosome system in veiled chameleons, ZZ/ZW in Oustalet's chameleon (*F. oustaleti*) and a complex Z1Z1Z2Z2/Z1Z2W system in panther chameleons (Rovatsos et al. 2015; Nielsen et al. 2018). However, Ballen et al. (2016) found hatchling sex ratios altered with interaction between egg size and incubation temperature in veiled chameleons. This suggests that sex determination may be more complex than genetics alone but the interactions described have not been shown to be consistent so should be interpreted cautiously.

15.3 Clinical Evaluation

15.3.1 History-Taking

A detailed history is essential for identifying the contribution of husbandry to potential disease in chameleons. Enclosure design, humidity, drinking water provision, temperature, lighting, and diet are particularly important. Reproductive status, presence of other chameleons, quarantine provision, and previous medical concerns should also be discussed.

15.3.2 Handling

Many chameleons will tolerate an initial visual examination whilst static on an arm or branch, but palpation and oral examination necessitates restraint. This is best accomplished in medium-large species by using the second and third fingers of the handler's dominant hand to restrain the head and prevent bites, whilst the rest of the hand gentle surrounds the body. Chameleons will resent restraint less if permitted to continue to grip onto a small branch with their feet.

15.3.3 Sex Determination

In some species, including veiled and slender chameleons (*Chamaeleo gracilis*), males are easily differentiated by the tarsal spur on the caudal aspect of the hind feet, and this is present from hatching (Figure 15.2). A larger cephalic casque and bilateral swellings of the hemipenes within the tail base are seen in adult males of most chameleon species (Figure 15.3) (Diaz et al. 2015). Females are smaller and lack these features (Figure 15.4).

15.3.4 Clinical Examination

A clinical examination should include a thorough evaluation of the skin, long bones, joints, and oral cavity. The mouth is often opened as a defensive display on handling, or can be opened using gentle consistent traction on the intermandibular skin fold in larger species. The mandibles should be gentle compressed lateromedially to assess for

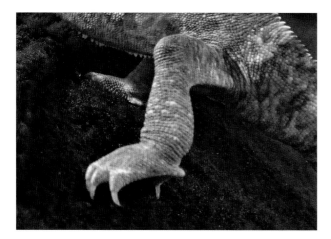

Figure 15.2 Tarsal spur on the caudal aspect of the foot in a male veiled chameleon (*Source:* photo courtesy of Sarah Pellett).

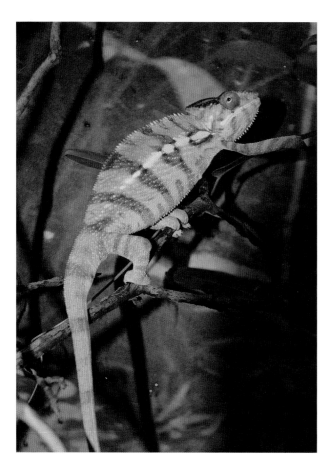

Figure 15.3 Male panther chameleon with larger casque and hemipene swellings at tail base (*Source:* Courtesy of Drayton Manor Park Zoo).

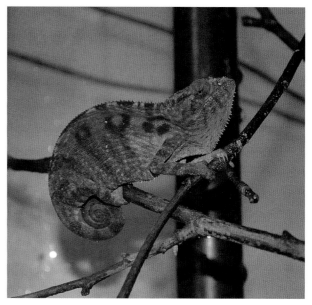

Figure 15.4 Female panther chameleon, note the minimal adornments and flat tail base (*Source:* Courtesy of Drayton Manor Park Zoo).

15.4 Basic Techniques

15.4.1 Sample Collection

Faecal samples are often passed during transport or examination, but it is sensible to request owners bring a recent sample from the individual animal to the consultation. A warm water bath or enema may also encourage defaecation.

Blood samples are most commonly collected from the ventral coccygeal vein and 0.5–0.8% of bodyweight can be taken (Cannon 2003). The chameleon is held upright with its back against the handler to allow the sampler access to the ventral tail. The vein is located on the midline, just ventral to the coccygeal vertebrae and the sample can be collected at any point of the tail (though the proximal 3 cm is best avoided in males to avoid inadvertent trauma to the more lateral hemipenes). A 23–27G needle attached to a 1 ml syringe is inserted between scales at a 90° angle to the skin, and advanced until the vertebrae are contacted. The needle is then incrementally withdrawn until blood flows into the hub. Once sufficient sample is obtained, the needle is withdrawn and manual pressure applied for 30–60 seconds, or a bandage placed for 1–2 minutes. Both heparin and EDTA can be used as anticoagulants for samples.

15.4.2 Nutritional Support

Short periods of anorexia may be normal relating to follicular activity or pre-laying changes in females, and in males exposed to females. Intervention should be considered for anorexia in excess of seven days duration or in an unwell

softening of the bone, in a healthy chameleon there should be minimal flexibility. Palpation of the coelomic cavity in a normal chameleon should only identify poorly differentiated soft tissue; presence of discrete masses or a bloated appearance require further investigation.

animal if weight loss results, or in an obese animal at high risk of hepatic lipidosis. Insects with biting mouth parts should not be left in an enclosure with non-feeding animals as debilitated chameleons are vulnerable to injury from such prey, particularly crickets.

In a dehydrated animal, rehydration should be the priority before nutritional replacement to support renal function and avoid electrolyte abnormalities associated with re-feeding syndrome.

Liquidised invertebrates, commercial liquid feeds for omnivores or insectivores, or a purine-based carnivore diet mixed with an equal proportion of herbivore diet are suitable for short-term nutritional support. Liquid can be syringed onto the lips, or gently into the mouth in small quantities. Larger volumes can be administered by gavage tube with the animal firmly restrained and a rubber tube passed down the oesophagus into the distal oesophagus or stomach. However, this method risks damage to the delicate tongue and hyoid apparatus and placement of an oesophageal feeding tube is preferred where repeat feeds are likely to be needed.

15.4.3 Fluid Therapy

Fluid requirements are approximately 20 ml/kg/day (Gibbons 2009). If the gastrointestinal tract is not compromised, oral fluids can be administered by the same methods as nutritional support.

Parenteral rehydration with warmed normal saline is often tolerated better than repeat force feeding of electrolyte solutions. Subcutaneous injections of fluid boluses are easily given over the flanks where loose skin is present and can be useful in gradual rehydration of noncritical patients. Intracoelomic fluids are poorly absorbed and risk visceral trauma so are best avoided.

Intravenous fluid therapy is difficult to achieve repeatedly though off the needle boluses of fluids can be given into the ventral coccygeal vein. Intraosseous fluid administration is often easier to manage, with placement of a hypodermic or spinal needle into the femur or tibia in patients with radiographically confirmed normal bone density. A needle is inserted via the greater trochanter (or tibial tuberosity) under sterile conditions and secured in place with tissue glue and adhesive bandage to allow repeated small boluses of fluids to be administered. Analgesia is mandatory for patients with intraosseous catheters in place.

15.4.4 Anaesthesia

Fasting prior to anaesthesia is not required but it is prudent to avoid feeding on the day of the anaesthesia.

Analgesia is often overlooked as overt signs of pain may not be shown. Where pain may be a consequence of illness or intervention, analgesia should be given. There is a lack of robust pharmacokinetic and pharmacodynamics data and analgesic doses are typically extrapolated from other reptile species. Pre-medication with analgesia is recommended for painful procedures and morphine or methadone are most frequently administered prior to procedures. Peri-operative fluid therapy is also advisable to support renal perfusion.

Anaesthesia is best induced using an intravenous agent such as alfaxalone or propofol into the ventral tail vein as chameleons can breath-hold for long periods and inhalation of volatile agents results in a slow and unpredictable induction (Figure 15.5). The patient can then be intubated using a 1–2 mm endotracheal tube, or 14–18 G intravenous cannula attached to an endotracheal tube connector and maintained on a volatile inhalant anaesthetic in oxygen. Intermittent positive pressure ventilation will be required to maintain anaesthesia and oxygenation. If unilateral lung inflation is noted, the tube may have been advanced too far and should be gently withdrawn until bilateral inflation is demonstrated.

On recovery, ventilation should change from oxygen to room air to normalise circulating oxygen levels and hasten the return of spontaneous ventilation (Odette et al. 2015). Once breathing without assistance the reptile can be extubated and transferred to a pre-warmed recovery area and be maintained at 24–30 °C until mobile. Once the patient is able to move and climb to regulate their own temperature, they can be returned to a vivarium with standard temperature gradients.

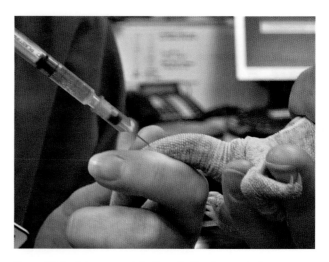

Figure 15.5 Intravenous injection of alfaxalone to induce anaesthesia in a veiled chameleon.

15.4.5 Euthanasia

In the conscious chameleon, intravenous injection of 400 mg/kg pentobarbitone via the ventral tail vein is straightforward and results in rapid loss of consciousness and cardiac activity. Pithing is necessary to cause cessation of brainstem activity and typically involves passing a metal rod or large needle into the brainstem through the skull or roof of the mouth. This is often not cosmetically acceptable for pets and can be technically challenging. The author prefers to inject 100 mg/kg pentobarbitone through the foramen magnum into the brainstem in the unconscious animal as an alternative.

15.4.6 Hospitalisation Requirements

Chameleons should be kept away from hospitalised predatory mammals, birds, and reptiles, in a warm, quiet area of the hospital. Hospital enclosures should provide the temperature, humidity, lighting, and space requirements for the species, but often enrichment and display aspects are sacrificed to allow good hygiene. Paper substrate and fixed plastic climbing apparatus replace soil and plants, and manual water spraying is sufficient if carried out every two to four hours. For chameleons with mobility compromise, deep substrate and low climbing apparatus are preferred. Careful management of heating is needed to ensure basking opportunities are available for animals that are temporarily unable to climb, and that there is no potential for hyperthermia in less mobile individuals. Handling should be minimised as chameleons are easily stressed and do not gain any benefit from human contact.

15.5 Common Medical and Surgical Conditions

15.5.1 Non-specific Debilitation

Many chameleons present as acute deteriorations of chronic conditions and the original disease process or causative management deficiencies may not be initially evident. Loss of body condition or muscle mass, dehydration, enophthalmia, dark colouration, weak foot and tail grip, or injury from prey insects are common but non-specific secondary concerns. Prognosis in these cases is typically guarded.

Initial first aid involves rehydration, provision of suitable environmental conditions (with temperatures and humidity maintained at the high end of the species range), and treatment of any injuries. Further investigation to determine underlying health conditions, typically comprising

blood sample collection, faecal parasitology, and imaging, can be carried out promptly as anaesthesia is not necessary. Chronic renal compromise, nutritional secondary hyperparathyroidisim, and reproductive pathology are common findings, but any chronic or advanced disease process can present in a similar fashion.

15.5.1.1 Nutritional Secondary Hyperparathyroidism (NSHP)

This remains a common syndrome in captive chameleons, and results from disruption to calcium homeostasis. It most commonly presents as fibrous osteodystrophy with long bone bowing (particularly affecting the radius and tibia), distortion of the casque or mandible, and pathological fractures. Dystocia, tremors, anorexia, seizures, inability to retract the tongue, generalised weakness, and paralysis may also be seen (Klaphake 2010). Total serum calcium levels of <2.3 mmol/l are supportive of NSHP in growing veiled chameleons (Hoby et al. 2010) though levels may be normal in mild/moderate cases due to ongoing liberation of calcium from bone. Ionised calcium levels are preferred as protein bound calcium included in total calcium values is inactive. Phosphorus and alkaline phosphatase levels are commonly increased in NSHP due to ongoing demineralisation of bone. Radiography is valuable in confirming diagnosis and determining prognosis (Figure 15.6). In severe cases, where multiple limbs are affected or mandibular distortion prevents normal feeding, euthanasia is advisable.

Treatment of mild–moderate cases is appropriate where return to normal mobility and feeding is possible. Therapy includes provision of oral vitamin D and calcium, assist feeding, appropriate analgesia, and long-term husbandry correction.

Provision of artificial ultraviolet light in the UV-B wavelength enables endogenous vitamin D synthesis and enhances breeding success in Panther chameleons (Ferguson et al. 1996, 2005). However, in veiled chameleons, provision of UV-B lighting alone was found to be insufficient to prevent NSHP, and solely dietary supplementation with Vitamin D was even less effective (Hoby et al. 2010). Daily supplementation of livefood with calcium and Vitamin A, independent of UV-B exposure, appeared to prevent NSHP but the optimal combination is supplementation of food with calcium, vitamins A and D and provision of UV-B lighting (Hoby et al. 2010; Haxhiu et al. 2014).

15.5.2 Vitamin A Deficiency

Commercially bred insects are a poor source of Vitamin A and additional supplementation is needed for captive

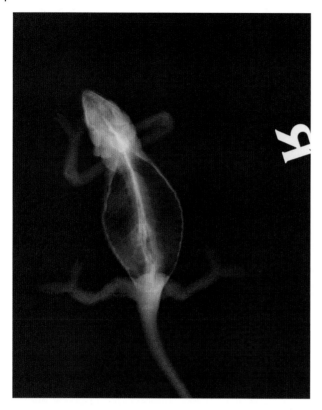

Figure 15.6 NSHP in a veiled chameleon, note the lack of mineralisation of bone and poorly distinct pathological fractures of both femurs (*Source:* Courtesy of Manor vets).

chameleons. Supplements should contain Vitamin A, rather than beta carotene precursors and insect prey should also be fed with a retinol rich diet (50–100 IU/g) prior to using them as a food source (Stahl 1997). Vitamin A is important for breeding, vision, growth, and immunocompetence as in other reptiles but there has also been a link identified in panther chameleons between low dietary Vitamin A and nutritional secondary hyperparathyroidism (NSHP) (Ferguson et al. 1996). Skin lesions, hemipene impaction, periocular swelling, ocular discharge, temporal gland impactions (at the commissures of the mouth), cervical oedema, respiratory disease, weakness, neurological symptoms, and metabolic bone disease-like symptoms are all additional recognised consequences of deficiency in vitamin A in chameleons (Ferguson et al. 1996; Hoby et al. 2010). Diagnosis is made based on nutrition provided, clinical examination, and exclusion of other causes. Liver biopsy for Vitamin A assay may be used as a confirmatory test but invasive testing is rarely justified.

Parenteral vitamin A replacement is most effective but injectable solutions are highly concentrated and typically combined with other vitamins or minerals at inappropriate levels. Overdose is easily inadvertently achieved and causes disruption to enteric absorption of Vitamin D with associ-

ated NSHP, as well as similar clinical signs to Vitamin A deficiency. Oral Vitamin A supplements are slower to result in improvements but are potentially safer and readily available. Long-term dietary and husbandry improvements are necessary to prevent recurrence. Ferguson (1994) reports that 37.51 U of vitamin A given orally seems to be adequate for female panther chameleons, but higher levels (1–2 IU/g bodyweight weekly) may be required for growing or breeding animals (Ferguson 1994; Ferguson et al. 1996).

15.5.3 Renal Disease

Chronic renal disease is reported to be one of the most common causes of death in captive chameleons (Stahl 2003). Vitamin A deficiency, chronic dehydration, chronic bacterial infection, intoxication, hyperparathyroidism, and excessive vitamin D supplementation have been postulated as potential factors (Kramer 2006). Anorexia, weight loss, dehydration, lethargy, and weakness may be seen but are non-specific changes common to a variety of causes. Biochemistry commonly shows elevation of uric acid and phosphorus (>3.23 mmol/l), and a calcium:phosphorus ratio of 1.5 : 1 or lower (Stahl 2003; Selleri and Hernandez-Divers 2006) which fail to normalise with fluid therapy. Aspartate aminotransferase, creatinine phosphokinase, and lactate dehydrogenase are often elevated but are non-specific, though a marked increase in Aspartate aminotransferase in the absence of soft tissue trauma is supportive of a diagnosis of renal disease (Suedmeyer 1995). Glomerular disease may lead to renal loss of albumin and hypoalbuminaemia (Hernandez-Divers et al. 2005). Haemoconcentration and anaemia may both be present, complicating interpretation of packed cell volume (PCV) (Selleri and Hernandez-Divers 2006). Surgical or endoscopic biopsy can be used to categorise the renal pathology and target therapy but non-specific fibrosis is often identified and invasive procedures should be avoided in animals where prognosis is evidently poor. Iohexol clearance tests can be used to evaluate renal function in reptiles, and the protocol described for green iguanas is likely suitable for chameleons. 75 mg/kg iohexol is administered by intravenous injection into the ventral tail vein, with 0.5 ml blood collected for Iohexol assay at 4, 8, and 24 hours after administration to determine glomerular filtration rate (GFR) (Hernandez-Divers et al. 2005; Selleri and Hernandez-Divers 2006). Samples need to be stored and transferred on ice to a suitable laboratory. The mean GFR in green iguanas with normal hydration status was found to be 16.56 ± 3.90 ml/kg/h and this is the baseline recommended for chameleons in the absence of family-specific data. Reduction in GFR has been demonstrated in iguanas with renal disease, proportional to the severity of renal pathology (Hernandez-Divers et al. 2005). Urinalysis is rarely useful due to post-renal modifications of urine and contamination of samples with faeces in the cloaca, though cytology may occasionally highlight casts or pathogens (Selleri and Hernandez-Divers 2006).

Treatment options comprise rehydration and diuresis with fluid therapy as well as correction of electrolyte disturbances and reduction of circulating uric acid and these are detailed in the formulary. Where phosphorus exceeds 5 mmol/l or calcium:phosphorus ratio is <1, response to treatment is unlikely and euthanasia should be advised.

Renal cysts have been reported in a veiled chameleon with clinical presentation relating to the large size of the cysts rather than renal dysfunction (Zwart 2006).

15.5.4 Neoplasia

Chameleons appear over-represented with neoplastic disease compared to most other reptile families, with panther chameleons in particular identified as significantly more likely to be diagnosed with neoplasia than other lizard species (Kubiak et al. 2020). Squamous cell carcinomas are the most common neoplastic entity and a multicentric form is recognised in chameleons (Abou-Madi and Kern 2002; Garner et al. 2004; Kubiak et al. 2020). Intralesional carboplatin therapy appeared to induce regression in carcinomas in one panther chameleon but other treatment options have not been explored (Johnson et al. 2016). Chromatophoromas have been reported in veiled chameleons as slow growing pigmented dermal masses with metastasis and local recurrence common after excision (Reavill et al. 2004; Lewis et al. 2015). Poorly defined mesenchymal neoplasms have also been reported in small numbers. Two hepatomas have been diagnosed histologically in flap-necked chameleons (*Chamaeleo dilpeis*) and single cases of hepatic carcinoma, biliary adenocarcinoma, biliary adenoma, lymphoid leukaemia, liposarcoma, and melanoma are described in various species (Garner et al. 2004; Schmid-Brunclik et al. 2007; Kubiak et al. 2020).

15.5.5 Stomatitis/Dental Disease

Stomatitis is uncommonly seen as a primary infection of the lips, gingiva, and tongue. Animals may demonstrate anorexia, facial swelling, and an inability to close the mouth or use the tongue. For mild–moderate lesions with minimal necrosis, swabs of lesions can be cultured to guide antibiotic therapy. For severe lesions, gentle debridement of lesions under anaesthesia, collection of biopsy samples for culture, and a combination of topical and systemic antimicrobial therapy is preferred.

Dental disease and osteomyelitis are more common. Chameleons have acrodont dentition, with teeth lacking roots but fused together and set superficially but firmly within the mandible and maxilla (Dosedělová et al. 2016). An inappropriate soft diet, oral trauma, or poor hygiene predispose to bacterial proliferation on and around the teeth. Osteomyelitis is a common sequel as the infections extend into the adjacent mandible and maxilla. Gingival regression, tartar, loss of teeth, gingivitis, and facial abscessation may be identified on examination. Debridement of lesions, systemic antibiotic therapy based on microbial culture, oral disinfectants, and dietary modification are necessary (Stahl 1997). For advanced osteomyelitis, prognosis is guarded to poor so radiography is recommended to assess severity prior to starting treatment.

Fungal periodontal osteomyelitis was associated with loss of teeth, an open wound on the mandible and loss of lingual soft tissues in a panther chameleon (Heatley et al. 2001).

15.5.6 Ophthalmic Disease

Exophthalmia may occur with expansion of the globe, conjunctiva, or retrobulbar tissues. Globular expansion may be a consequence of uveitis, panophthalmitis, or glaucoma but is uncommon (Coke and Couillard 2002). Conjunctivitis may be associated with contact with irritant plant saps (e.g. Ficus), pathogen accumulation due to poor hygiene or ventilation, Vitamin A deficiency, or foreign body presence – most frequently seen in gravid females digging in substrate (Coke and Couillard 2002). Physiological ocular flushing to clear suspected foreign material can be induced by simulating heavy rainfall with a shower or watering system. Excess water is voluntarily taken in and flushed through the choana, nasolacrimal duct, and conjunctival sac (Coke and Couillard 2002). Alternatively a soft nasolacrimal cannula can be placed in the palpebral aperture to gently irrigate the cornea and conjunctival fornix with isotonic ocular flush.

Retrobulbar swelling is most frequently a consequence of abscessation or cellulitis. This may be a primary infection, or secondary to stomatitis tracking along the nasolacrimal duct, haematogenous spread of infection from a distant site, or local traumatic injury. Debridement may be necessary alongside systemic antibiotic therapy (ideally based on culture of an aspirate or flush of the lesion). *Pseudomonas* species appear common opportunistic pathogens with periocular infections (Schumacher et al. 1996; Abou-Madi and Kern 2002). Rarely parasitic causes, such as aberrant larval migration of the intestinal nematode *Hexametra angusticaecoides* or *Foleyella* filarioid worms, are responsible (Thomas et al. 1996; Coke 1997). A single case of retrobulbar venous distension associated with suspected cardiac failure has been described in a juvenile veiled chameleon (Buhler et al. 2009), and a bee sting has been associated with short-term periocular swelling in a Southern dwarf chameleon (*Bradypodion ventrale*) (Bustard 1963).

Ocular neoplasia appears uncommon, but squamous cell carcinoma of periocular skin has been reported in a veiled chameleon, with surgical resection apparently successful in resolving the lesion (Abou-Madi and Kern 2002).

Visual compromise will affect feeding ability in chameleons and hand-feeding or assist feeding may be necessary during recovery.

15.5.7 Respiratory Disease

Bacterial infections of the respiratory system are common in the veiled chameleon, and carry a guarded prognosis (Stahl 1997). Clinical signs may include dyspnoea, open mouth breathing, tacky oral mucus, or facial swelling associated with sinus distension. Ocular discharge or swelling may also be seen in chronic cases. Samples for bacteriology can be aspirated from swellings, or by tracheal/lung lavage under anaesthesia. Gram-negative opportunistic pathogens such as *Pseudomonas*, *Aeromonas*, *Klebsiella* and *Proteus* species are often isolated (Stahl 1996). Systemic antibiotics, nebulisation, Vitamin A supplementation, and debridement or lavage of sinus lesions may be used and recovery can take six to eight weeks. Environmental hygiene, enclosure temperatures, ventilation, and vitamin A content of diet should be evaluated and modified where necessary.

Veiled chameleons have salt glands within the nares and small quantities of white, crystalline nasal discharge should not be confused with abnormal discharges (Stahl 1997).

15.5.8 Fungal Dermatitis and Granulomatous Disease

Metarhizium granulomatis (formerly *Chamaeleomyces granulomatis*) is a recently documented primary fungal pathogen of chameleons. Infection can result in dermatitis, glossitis, pharyngitis, synovitis, and endophthalmitis or disseminated granulomatous disease (Figure 15.7) (Sigler et al. 2010; Schmidt et al. 2012; Pfaff et al. 2015). Outbreaks can occur in groups of chameleons but individual cases may be spread over many months (Sigler et al. 2010). Vertical transfer may be a mode of transmission where ovarian or oviductal granulomas are present (Sigler et al. 2010). Confirmed infections have been predominantly

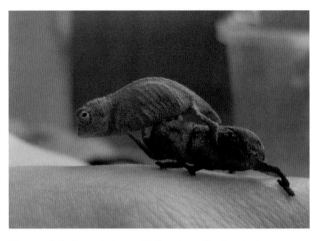

Figure 15.7 Fungal dermatitis in a juvenile Bearded pygmy chameleon – note the black discolouration of the skin in the affected animal.

reported in veiled chameleons but infection has also been identified in one panther and one carpet chameleon, and suspected in Jackson's chameleons (Sigler et al. 2010; Pfaff et al. 2015). Diagnosis is by fungal culture or PCR performed on swabs collected from visible lesions or on tissue samples. Histopathology of the typical 1–3 mm white granulomas demonstrates wide, smooth conidia forming chains, and easily fragmented hyphae (Sigler et al. 2010). Treatment is based on isolate sensitivity results as resistance to multiple antifungal agents has been reported (Schmidt et al. 2012).

Metarhizium viride (formerly *Paecilomyces viridis*) has been reported to cause a similar presentation of localised or disseminated granulomatous disease in veiled, panther and carpet chameleons (Segretain et al. 1964; Schmidt et al. 2017).

The *Chrysosporium* anamorph of *Nannziopsis vriesii* has not been reported as a natural infection in chameleons but has been experimentally shown to cause active infections with resulting dermatitis and granulomatous inflammation in veiled chameleons with compromised epidermal integrity (Paré et al. 2006). A related fungus, now classified as *Nannizziopsis dermatitidis,* has been reported, with one paper describing three cases in a Jackson's, a Parson's (*C. parsonii*) and a Jewel chameleon (*C. lateralis*) (Paré et al. 1997; Sigler et al. 2013).

Other cases of fungal dermatitis include *Mucor circinelloides* in a two-lined chameleon (*C. bitaeniatus*) and a common chameleon (*C. chamaeleon*), two cases of *Fusarium oxysporum* in flap-necked chameleons and an *Aspergillus* sp. in a Jackson's chameleon (Austwick and Keymer 1981; Frye 1981; Zwart and Schroder 1985). Yeast infections have also been reported, with *Candida*

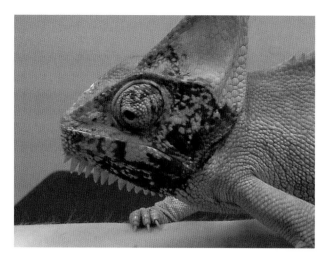

Figure 15.8 Photodermatitis in a veiled chameleon due to a malfunctioning ultraviolet light emitting excessive short wavelength light.

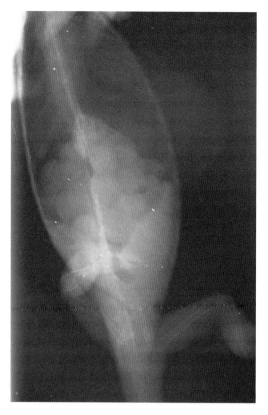

Figure 15.9 Large numbers of circular soft tissues densities in the mid-coelom of this veiled chameleon consistent with ovarian follicles.

guillermondii in a Fischer's chameleon (*C. fischeri*) and a Jackson's chameleon and an unidentified species in a Meller's chameleon (*C. melleri*) (Austwick and Keymer 1981; Zwart and Schroder 1985).

Non-fungal dermatitis may also occasionally be seen as a consequence of thermal insult, exposure to inappropriate intensity or wavelength of UV light (Figure 15.8), traumatic injury, parasitism or opportunistic bacterial infection but is rarely reported in chameleons.

15.5.9 Follicular Stasis

This is the failure to ovulate or resorb ovarian follicles (Pimm 2013) and is a common clinical syndrome in veiled chameleons. Causative factors are not fully understood, but may include the absence of a male at the appropriate stage of the female reproductive cycle, environmental factors such as absence of seasonal changes, lack of a laying site or excess corticosterone in stressed animals (Pimm 2013).

Follicular stasis typically results in coelomic distension, inappetance, and lethargy but these can be difficult to differentiate from physiological changes in a heavily gravid animal resulting in late presentation for treatment in the majority of cases. Radiography can indicate presence of large numbers of follicles (Figure 15.9), but differentiation from eggs may not be obvious in all cases. Using ultrasound examination to obtain more information on follicles is valuable in differentiation of normal reproductive activity from a pathological status. Table 15.3 details differing characteristics of normal follicles, abnormal follicles, and

ovulated eggs based on data published by Pimm (2013), though absolute differentiation is not always straightforward. Persistence of follicles >8 mm for more than three weeks or presence of follicles of variable echogenicity has been suggested as indicative of follicular stasis (Pimm 2013). Additionally presence of mature sized follicles in an animal showing lethargy, distension, and anorexia is highly suspicious.

A decreasing oestrogen:progesterone ratio appears important in triggering ovulation in veiled chameleons (Licht et al. 1984; Amey and Whittier 2000; Kummrow et al. 2010b). However, attempts to induce ovulation of retained follicles using progesterone and GnRH depot formulations have been unsuccessful (Pimm 2013). Surgical removal of the ovaries is the recognised treatment for this condition (Figure 15.10) and is carried out as described for bearded dragons in Chapter 13, though a paracostal approach can be used as an alternative to a paramedian incision. The paracostal incision is made between ribs or behind the last rib, for access to the ovaries. This avoids the ventral abdominal vein but risks trauma to the smaller intercostal vessels. Additionally access may be limited by inflation of caudal lung fimbriae (thin

Table 15.3 Characteristics used to differentiation normal follicles, abnormal follicles and eggs on ultrasonographic examination (Pimm 2013).

	Normal follicle	Retained follicle	Egg
Distribution	Clustered in mid coelom	Clustered in mid coelom	Wider distribution through mid and caudal coelom, less marked clustering – dispersed along oviducts
Size	Mature follicles: average 1.01×0.85 cm with a maximum of 1.04×0.95 cm,	May be size of mature follicles or enlarged. Small atretic follicles may be present simultaneously.	1.27×0.8 cm, maximum of 1.46×0.97 cm
Shape	Spherical, ratio of length: width <1.27 strongly indicates follicle	Spherical or irregular, ratio not established	Ovoid, ratio of length: width >1.56 strongly indicates egg
Persistence	12–18 weeks gradual enlargement to mature size prior to ovulation	Remain on follicle indefinitely, mature sized follicles considered abnormal if retained >3wks	3–5 weeks prior to oviposition
Ultrasonic appearance	Hypoechoic	Variable echogenicity, some hyperechoic follicles often present	More hyperechoic, shell often poorly delineated
Radiographic appearance	Poorly defined soft tissue densities in mid coelom	Poorly defined soft tissue densities in mid coelom	More defined soft tissues densities in mid and caudal coelom, often with more radiodense border

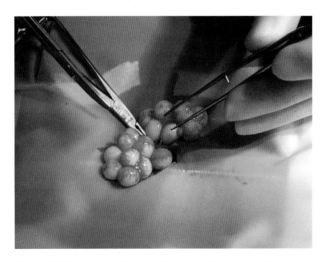

Figure 15.10 Paramedian incision to perform ovariectomy. Note the abnormally increased vascularity over the follicles consistent with oophoritis.

walled extension of lungs, similar to air sacs in birds), limited retraction of the ribs and position of coelomic viscera in some cases. Bilateral paracostal incisions may be needed in some cases to access both ovaries.

15.5.10 Dystocia

'Egg binding' is the description of retention of eggs beyond the length of a normal gestation, whereas dystocia is the failure to lay fully formed eggs. Dystocia has been associated with drought in wild common chameleon and in captivity is associated with poor or excessive body condition,

lack of a proper nesting site, the presence or absence of a male at the correct time of the cycle, oversized eggs, and hypocalcaemia (Backues and Ramsay 1994; Stahl 1997; Cuadrado et al. 2002; Kramer 2006; Sykes 2010). Retained eggs can cause localised inflammation, facilitate opportunistic bacterial colonisation, and rupture can lead to acute yolk coelomitis (Rivera 2008).

Affected animals may present as clear cases with straining, digging, and attempted oviposition attempts, or with non-specific debilitation. A presumptive diagnosis can be made based on failure of oviposition at the expected time post-copulation, and is confirmed with radiographic or ultrasound demonstration of mature eggs (Figure 15.11). Medical management can be attempted at an early stage and where eggs are confirmed to be of normal size and shape. Calcium administration, followed by arginine vasotocin or oxytocin can be used to induce oviposition (Rivera 2008) It is however important to be aware that radiographically normal retained eggs can be adhered to the oviduct wall and induced contractions may potentially result in oviductal rupture. Most chameleons present in an advanced stage of disease and fail to respond. In these cases surgical intervention is necessary, with salpingotomy to remove eggs or, preferably, ovariosalpingectomy to remove the entire reproductive tract and prevent future recurrence. This is carried out as for other lizard species (see Chapter 13) though a paracostal approach can be used in the laterally compressed chameleon as an alternative to the paramedian approach.

Preventative measures have been limited to prophylactic surgical removal of the ovaries (or ovaries and oviducts).

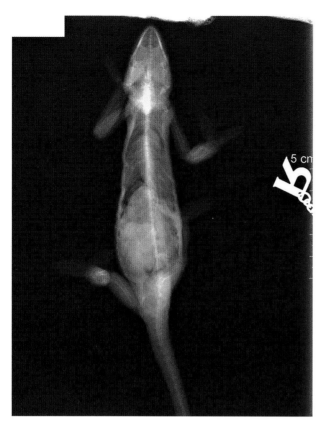

Figure 15.11 A presumptive diagnosis of dystocia was made with eggs visible on the radiograph of this veiled chameleon with lethargy, anorexia and weakness 40 days after a known mating. NSHP is also present.

Deslorelin has been trialled but does not appear to suppress reproductive activity in veiled chameleons (Knotek 2014).

15.5.11 Hemipene Prolapse

One or both hemipenes may prolapse through the vent in response to local trauma, inflammation, or infection. Vitamin A deficiency has also been associated with hemipene prolapse in panther and veiled chameleons (Stahl 1997; Ferguson et al. 1996), due to impaction of hemipene pockets by debris secondary to squamous metaplasia of the epithelial lining. Prolapsed hemipenes can be differentiated from intestinal or cloacal prolapse by their linear shape and origin caudal to the vent aperture. Where the hemipenes remain vital, they should be kept moist using water-soluble lubricants and swelling reduced using compresses, hyperosmotic glucose solutions, and systemic anti-inflammatory agents. They can then be inverted and replaced into the pocket within the tail base under sedation. A cruciate suture over the hemipene opening can be placed temporarily to allow swellings to fully resolve without recurrence of prolapse. Where tissue is devitalised, amputation under anaesthesia is indicated and this is carried out by placement of a transfixing ligature of fine, long-lasting absorbable suture material (such as 4–0 polydioxanone) at the hemipene base, followed by sharp dissection of the free end. As urination occurs independently of the hemipene, only reproductive function is compromised by hemipene amputation. Where Vitamin A deficiency or infection is present, these factors need addressing concurrently.

15.5.12 Endoparasites

Oxyurid worms and coccidia are commonly identified in chameleons. Flagellates, amoeba, and other nematodes may be present in wild caught chameleons and are rare in captive bred individuals.

Oxyurids (pinworms) have low pathogenicity and are rarely of clinical significance though increased numbers are common in debilitated animals. They are identified by their asymmetrical appearance, with one convex and one flattened side. Treatment is only necessary if clinical signs such as ill thrift or diarrhoea are present.

Coccidia of the genera *Isospora, Eimeria* and *Choleoeimeria* are recognised as parasites of chameleons (Modry and Koudela 1995; Modry et al. 1997, 2000, 2001). Clinical signs may include anorexia, diarrhoea, regurgitation, and haemorrhagic enteritis (Mader 2006). High mortality rates have been observed in juvenile chameleons (Modry and Koudela 1998). Diagnosis is made by observation of oocysts on direct smears of faecal material, or preferably using faecal flotation techniques. Treatment of infected animals, using toltrazuril or sulphonamides, and cleaning and disinfection of the environment are necessary (Cervone et al. 2016).

Cryptosporidiosis has been identified in a panther chameleon, and Johnston's chameleons (*Trioceros johnstonii*) (Klingenberg 1996a; Kubiak, unpublished data). This parasite is chronically debilitating and has no successful treatment. Animals should be screened by microscopy of faeces using acid-fast staining techniques, or PCR prior to movement into a collection to avoid introducing infected animals.

Foleyella filarial nematodes are seen in wild caught chameleons, with *F. furcata* and *F. brevicauda* commonly seen in Madagascan species (Brygoo 1963). *Foleyella* adults are found in subcutaneous swellings and within the lungs and coelomic cavity (Bartlett 1987). Female worms release large numbers of microfilariae into blood but lack of suitable arthropod intermediate hosts means that infected chameleons in temperate climes are end-stage hosts (Brygoo 1960; Schacher and Khalil 1968). Most infections are asymptomatic but heavy infestations can result in organ damage or toxaemia secondary to widespread tissue necrosis. Medical treatment can result in endotoxic shock as dead nematodes

and microfilaria break down simultaneously. Surgical removal of adults via small skin incisions over evident swellings or at coelomic endoscopy is preferred.

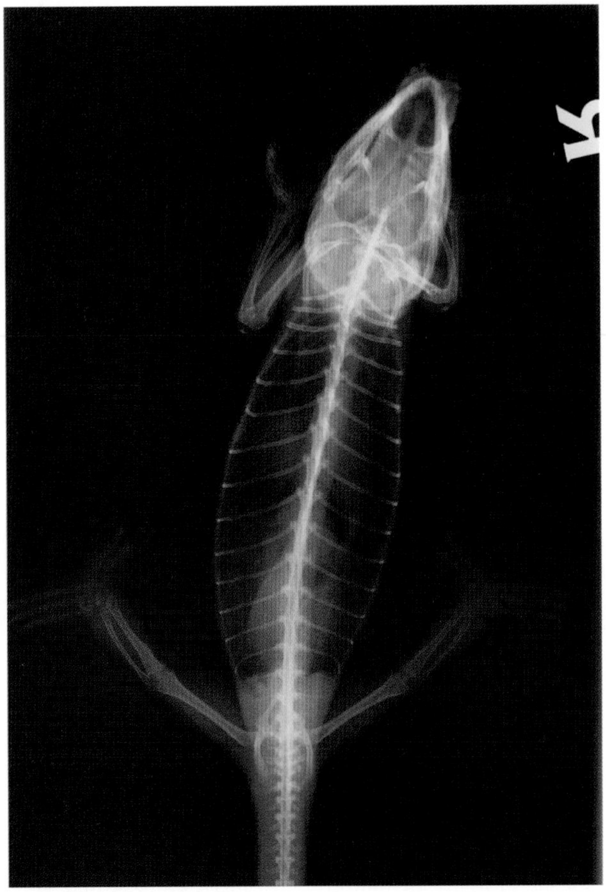

15.6 Preventative Health Measures

15.6.1 Neutering Technique

Prophylactic neutering may be of benefit to female veiled chameleons given the high incidence of follicular stasis and associated mortality. A bilateral ovariectomy is carried out via a paracostal or paramedian incision. The ovaries in acyclic animals appear as small clusters of follicles <1 mm in diameter, and are located against the dorsal body wall. All follicles must be successfully removed otherwise ovarian regeneration may result with resumption of egg production. There is no need to remove the oviducts in a prophylactic ovariectomy.

15.7 Radiographic Imaging

Radiographic positioning is challenging in the conscious chameleon as they are highly active and resent restraint. Use of a horizontal beam whilst allowing chameleons to perch on a branch is often successful. Dorsoventral and laterolateral views are commonly used for survey radiography, or investigation of specific concerns (Figures 15.12 and 15.13).

The soft tissues are superimposed and poorly defined but radiography is valuable for identifying alterations in bone density or structure (Figure 15.6), and investigating respiratory infections, reproductive pathology (Figures 15.9 and 15.11) or gastrointestinal pathology. Ultrasound evaluation is preferred for thorough reproductive assessment of female chameleons.

Figure 15.12 Dorsoventral view of a veiled chameleon, note the clearly defined bones (*Source:* Courtesy of Manor vets).

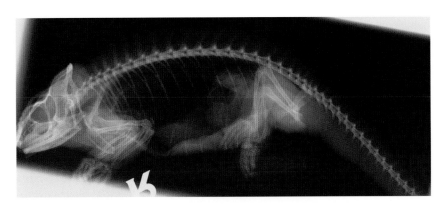

Figure 15.13 Laterolateral view of veiled chameleon, stomach, respiratory tract and liver are distinguishable but soft tissue contrast is often poor (*Source:* Courtesy of Manor vets).

Formulary

Medication	Dose	Dosing interval	Additional comments
Anaesthesia			
Isoflurane	3–5% induction 1–3% maintenance		(Jenkins 2006). Breath-holding and prolonged induction are common, injectable agents are preferred.
Propofol	5–10 mg/kg IV or IO	10–25 mins anaesthesia	(Kramer 2006), can be extended by maintenance with a volatile agent
Alfaxalone	5 mg/kg IV	5–10 mins anaesthesia	(Knotek et al. 2011), can be extended by maintenance with a volatile agent. Higher doses required if IM injection used
Analgesia			
Morphine	1–5 mg/kg	q24h	Extrapolated from data in other lizard species (Sladky and Mans 2012)
Methadone	3–5 mg/kg	q24h	Extrapolated from data in other lizard species (Sladky and Mans 2012)
Butorphanol	2 mg/kg SC		Used as pre-medicant (Knotek et al. 2011), no evidence for analgesia
Meloxicam	0.2 mg/kg SC PO	q24h	Extrapolated from data in other lizard species (Divers et al. 2010) No evidence of analgesia, presumed anti-inflammatory effect. Use with caution in dehydrated animals, or where renal disease may be present.
Tramadol	10 mg/kg PO	q 48–72h	Extrapolated from data in other reptile species (Sladky and Mans 2012)
Antibiotics			
Ceftazidime	20–40 mg/kg IM, SC, IV	q24–48h	(Stahl 1997) Note the shorter dosing interval compared to other reptiles
Enrofloxacin	5–10 mg/kg PO, IM	q24h	Can cause soft tissue necrosis when injected (Carpenter 2013)
Metronidazole	20–50 mg/kg PO, SC	q24–48h	(Carpenter 2013)
Amikacin	50 mg/10 ml saline for nebulisation	30mins nebulisation q12h	Useful for pneumonia. Can be given systemically at 5 mg/kg IM, then 2.5 mg/kg q72h but is nephrotoxic (Carpenter 2013)
Trimethoprim/sulfadiazine	20–30 mg/kg PO, SC	q24h	(Klingenberg 1996b)
Itraconazole	10 mg/kg PO	q24h for 21 days	For fungal infections (Paré et al. 2006)
Voriconazole	10 mg/kg PO	q24h for 28 days	For fungal infections (Schmidt 2016)
Terbinafine	5 mg/kg PO	q24h for 10 weeks	For fungal infections (Schmidt et al. 2017)
Antiparasitics			
Fenbendazole	50 mg/kg PO	q 2 wks for two doses	(de Vosjoli 1990) For nematodes
Metronidazole	40–60 mg/kg PO	q 7–14 d for 2–3 doses	For flagellates and amoeba (Stahl 1997)
Ivermectin	0.08 mg/kg IM, SC, PO	q 10–14d	Avoid use in wild caught or debilitated chameleons (le Berre 1995)
Toltrazuril	5–7 mg/kg	q24h for 2–3 doses	Toltrazuril was effective for treatment of *Eimeria*, not for *Choleoeimeria* where sulphonamides are preferred (Modry and Sloboda 2004)

(Continued)

(Continued)

Medication	Dose	Dosing interval	Additional comments
Renal disease			
Isotonic or hypotonic fluids	20–25 ml/kg/d	In divided doses	Preferably given by IV or IO administration initially, and SC and PO once rehydrated
Calcium gluconate	50–100 mg/kg IM, SC	q6–12h	Used where hypocalcemia is present or calcium phosphorous ratio is 1:1 or lower (Selleri and Hernandez-Divers 2006)
Aluminium hydroxide	15–45 mg/kg PO	q24–48h	Phosphate binder (Selleri and Hernandez-Divers 2006)
Trimethoprim/ sulfadiazine	30 mg/kg PO	q24–48hrs	Use where a bacterial component is suspected, once hydration is corrected
Furosemide	2–5 mg/kg IV, IM	q24h	Exerts diuresis at tubules (Selleri and Hernandez-Divers 2006)
Allopurinol	20 mg/kg PO	q 24h	Decreases uric acid formation (Selleri and Hernandez-Divers 2006)
Probenecid	2–4 mg/kg PO	q24h	Increases uric acid excretion (Selleri and Hernandez-Divers 2006)
Miscellaneous			
Calcium gluconate	100 mg/kg IM, SC	q6h	used to induce oviposition (Knotek et al. 2017)
Oxytocin	5–10 IU IM	repeated q12–24h	
Arginine Vasotocin	0.5–1.0 ug/kg IM	q12–24h	More reliable than oxytocin, less readily available (Stahl 1997)
Vitamin A	66 000 IU/kg PO	q 7 d × 2 doses	For treatment of clinical deficiency (Stahl 1997)

References

Abou-Madi, N. and Kern, T.J. (2002). Squamous cell carcinoma associated with a periorbital mass in a veiled chameleon (*Chamaeleo calyptratus*). *Veterinary Ophthalmology* 5 (3): 217–220.

Amey, A.P. and Whittier, J.M. (2000). Seasonal patterns of plasma steroid hormones in males and females of the bearded dragon lizard, *Pogona barbata*. *General and Comparative Endocrinology* 117 (3): 335–342.

Andrews, R.M. (2005). Incubation temperature and sex ratio of the veiled chameleon (*Chamaeleo calyptratus*). *Journal of Herpetology* 39 (3): 515–518.

Andrews, R.M. and Donoghue, S. (2004). Effects of temperature and moisture on embryonic diapause of the veiled chameleon (*Chamaeleo calyptratus*). *Journal of Experimental Zoology Part A: Comparative Experimental Biology* 301 (8): 629–635.

Annis, J.M. (1995). Veiled chameleon (*Chamaeleo calyptratus*) natural history, captive management, and breeding. In: *Care and Breeding of Panther, Jackson's, Veiled, and Parson's Chameleons* (eds. P. deVosjoli and G. Ferguson), 77–99. Santee: Advanced Vivarium Systems, Inc.

Austwick, P.K.C. and Keymer, I.F. (1981). Fungi and actinomycetes. In: *Diseases of the Reptilia*, vol. 1 (eds. J.E. Cooper and O.F. Jackson), 193–231. London, UK: Academic Press, Harcourt Brace Jovanovich.

Backues, K.A. and Ramsay, E.C. (1994). Ovariectomy for treatment of follicular stasis in lizards. *Journal of Zoo and Wildlife Medicine* 25 (1): 111–116.

Baines, F., Chattell, J., Dale, J. et al. (2016). How much UV-B does my reptile need? The UV-tool, a guide to the selection of UV lighting for reptiles and amphibians in captivity. *Journal of Zoo and Aquarium Research* 4 (1): 42–63.

Ballen, C., Shine, R., and Olsson, M. (2014). Effects of early social isolation on the behaviour and performance of juvenile lizards, *Chamaeleo calyptratus*. *Animal Behaviour* 88: 1–6.

Ballen, C.J., Shine, R., Andrews, R.M. et al. (2016). Multifactorial sex determination in chameleons. *Journal of Herpetology* 50 (4): 548–551.

Bartlett, C.M. (1987). The reptilian filarioid genus *Foleyella* Seurat, 1917 (Onchocercidae: Dirofilariinae) and its relationship to other dirofilariine genera. *Systematic Parasitology* 9 (1): 43–56.

Bowmaker, J.K., Loew, E.R., and Ott, M. (2005). The cone photoreceptors and visual pigments of chameleons. *Journal of Comparative Physiology A* 191 (10): 925–932.

Brygoo, E.R. (1960). Evolution de *Foleyella furcata* (von Linstow, 1899) chez *Culex fatigans* Wiedemann, 1828. *Archives de l'Institut Pasteur de Madagascar* 28: 129–138.

Brygoo, E.R. (1963). Contribution à la connaissance de la Parasitologie des Caméléons malgaches-(2e partie). *Annales de Parasitologie Humaine et Comparée* 38 (4): 525–739.

Buhler, I., Reese, S., and Hoffmann, I. (2009). Bilateral periocular swelling due to nutritional vitamin imbalance in a Veiled Chameleon (*Chameleo calyptratus*). *Veterinary Ophthalmology* 12 (Abstracts): 4.

Bustard, H.R. (1963). Growth, sloughing, feeding, mating, gestation, life-span, and poor health of chamaeleons in captivity. *Copeia* 1963 (4): 704–706.

Cannon, M.J. (2003). Husbandry and veterinary aspects of the bearded dragon (*Pogona* spp.) in Australia. *Seminars In Avian and Exotic Pet Medicine* 12 (4): 205–214.

Carpenter, J.W. (2013). Exotic animal formulary (Ed. 4). *Journal of Exotic Pet Medicine* 22: 308–309.

Cervone, M., Fichi, G., Lami, A. et al. (2016). Internal and external parasitic infections of pet reptiles in Italy. *Journal of Herpetological Medicine and Surgery* 26 (3–4): 122–130.

Chiaverano, L.M., Wright, M.J., and Holland, B.S. (2014). Movement behavior is habitat dependent in invasive Jackson's chameleons in Hawaii. *Journal of Herpetology* 48 (4): 471–479.

Coke, R.L. (1997). *Hexametra* transmission between wild-caught panther chameleons (*Chamaeleo pardalis*) and captive-born veiled chameleons (*Chamaeleo calyptratus*). Proceedings of the Annual Conference of the Association of Reptilian and Amphibian Veterinarians. Houston. 25–27.

Coke, R.L. and Couillard, N.K. (2002). Ocular biology and diseases of Old World chameleons. *The Veterinary Clinics of North America. Exotic Animal Practice* 5 (2): 275–285.

Cuadrado, M., Díaz-Paniagua, C., Quevedo, M.A. et al. (2002). Hematology and clinical chemistry in dystocic and healthy post-reproductive female chameleons. *Journal of Wildlife Diseases* 38 (2): 395–401.

Davison, L.J. (1997). *Chameleons: Their Care and Breeding*. Surrey, Canada: Hancock House Publishing.

de Vosjoli, P. (1990). *The General Care and Maintenance of True Chameleons. Part I Husbandry*. Lakeside: The Herpetological Library.

Diaz, R.E., Anderson, C.V., Baumann, D.P. et al. (2015). Captive Care, Raising, and Breeding of the Veiled Chameleon (Chamaeleo calyptratus). *Cold Spring Harbor Protocols* 2015 (10): 087718.

Divers, S., Papich, M., McBride, M. et al. (2010). Pharmacokinetics of Meloxicam following intravenous and oral administration in green iguanas (*Iguana iguana*). *American Journal of Veterinary Research* 71 (11): 1277–1283.

Dosedělová, H., Štěpánková, K., Zikmund, T. et al. (2016). Age-related changes in the tooth–bone interface area of acrodont dentition in the chameleon. *Journal of Anatomy* 229 (3): 356–368.

Ferguson, G.W. (1994). Old World chameleons in captivity: growth, maturity, and reproduction of Malagasy panther chameleons (*Chamaeleo pardalis*). In: *Captive Management and Conservation of Amphibians and Reptiles* (eds. J. Murphy, K. Adler and J.T. Collins), 323–331. Hays, KS: The Society for the Study of Amphibians and Reptiles.

Ferguson, G.W., Gehrmann, W.H., Chen, T.C. et al. (2005). Vitamin D-content of the eggs of the panther chameleon *Furcifer pardalis*: its relationship to UVB exposure/vitamin D-condition of mother, incubation and hatching success. *Journal of Herpetological Medicine and Surgery* 15 (4): 9–13.

Ferguson, G.W., Jones, J.R., Gehrmann, W.H. et al. (1996). Indoor husbandry of the panther chameleon *Chamaeleo [Furcifer] pardalis*: effects of dietary vitamins A and D and ultraviolet irradiation on pathology and life-history traits. *Zoo Biology* 15 (3): 279–299.

Frye, F.L. (1981). *Biomedical and Surgical Aspects of Captive Reptile Husbandry*. Malabar, FL: Veterinary Medicine Publishing Co.

Garner, M.M., Hernandez-Divers, S.M., and Raymond, J.T. (2004). Reptile neoplasia: a retrospective study of case submissions to a specialty diagnostic service. *The Veterinary Clinics of North America. Exotic Animal Practice* 7 (3): 653–671.

Gibbons, P.M. (2009). Critical care nutrition and fluid therapy in reptiles. Proceedings of the 15th Annual International Veterinary Emergency and Critical Care Symposium, Chicago, IL 91–94.

Haxhiu, D., Hoby, S., Wenker, C. et al. (2014). Influence of feeding and UVB exposition on the absorption mechanisms of calcium in the gastrointestinal tract of veiled chameleons (*Chamaeleo calyptratus*). *Journal of Animal Physiology and Animal Nutrition* 98 (6): 1021–1030.

Heatley, J.J., Mitchell, M.A., Williams, J. et al. (2001). Fungal periodontal osteomyelitis in a chameleon, *Furcifer pardalis*. *Journal of Herpetological Medicine and Surgery* 11 (4): 7–12.

Hernandez-Divers, S.J., Stahl, S.J., Stedman, N.L. et al. (2005). Renal evaluation in the healthy green iguana (*Iguana iguana*): assessment of plasma biochemistry, glomerular filtration rate, and endoscopic biopsy. *Journal of Zoo and Wildlife Medicine* 36 (2): 155–168.

Hoby, S., Wenker, C., Robert, N. et al. (2010). Nutritional metabolic bone disease in juvenile veiled chameleons

(*Chamaeleo calyptratus*) and its prevention–3. *The Journal of Nutrition* 140 (11): 1923–1931.

Jenkins, J.R. (2006). *Common Conditions of the Chameleon*. Birmingham UK: British Small Animal Veterinary Congress.

Johnson, J.G. III, Naples, L.M., Chu, C. et al. (2016). Cutaneous squamous cell carcinoma in a panther chameleon (*Furcifer pardalis*) and treatment with carboplatin implantable beads. *Journal of Zoo and Wildlife Medicine* 47 (3): 931–934.

Karsten, K.B., Ferguson, G.W., Chen, T.C. et al. (2009). Panther chameleons, *Furcifer pardalis*, behaviorally regulate optimal exposure to UV depending on dietary vitamin D3 status. *Physiological and Biochemical Zoology* 82 (3): 218–225.

Klaphake, E. (2010). A fresh look at metabolic bone diseases in reptiles and amphibians. *Veterinary Clinics: Exotic Animal Practice* 13 (3): 375–392.

Klingenberg, R.J. (1996a). Enteric cryptosporidiosis in a Colony of indigo snakes, *Drymarchon corais* spp., a panther chameleon, *Chamaeleo pardalis*, and a Savannah monitor, *Varanus examthematicus*. *Bulletin of the Association of Reptilian and Amphibian Veterinarians* 6 (1): 5–9.

Klingenberg, R.J. (1996b). Therapeutics. In: *Reptile Medicine and Surgery* (ed. D.R. Mader), 299–321. Philadelphia: WB Saunders.

Knotek, Z. (2014). Reproductive strategies in captive female veiled chameleons. Proceedings of the UPAV/AAVAC/ARAV Conference, Cairns, 22–24 April: 127–130.

Knotek, Z., Cermakova, E., and Oliveri, M. (2017). Reproductive medicine in lizards. *Veterinary Clinics: Exotic Animal Practice* 20 (2): 411–438.

Knotek, Z., Hrda, A., Kley, N. et al. (2011). August. Alfaxalon anaesthesia in veiled chameleon (Chamaeleo calyptratus). Proceedings of the 18th Annual Conference of the Association of Reptilian and Amphibian Veterinarians, Seattle: 179-181.

Kramer, M. (2006). Veterinary Management of Chameleons Proceedings of the Western Veterinary Conference, Las Vegas, NV, 23 February.

Kraus, F., Medeiros, A., Preston, D. et al. (2012). Diet and conservation implications of an invasive chameleon, *Chamaeleo jacksonii* (Squamata: Chamaeleonidae) in Hawaii. *Biological Invasions* 14 (3): 579–593.

Kubiak, M., Denk, D., and Stidworthy, M. (2020). Retrospective review of neoplasms of captive lizards in the United Kingdom. *Veterinary Record* 186: 28.

Kummrow, M.S., Smith, D.A., Crawshaw, G. et al. (2010a). Characterization of fecal hormone patterns associated with the reproductive cycle in female veiled chameleons (*Chamaeleo calyptratus*). *General and Comparative Endocrinology* 168 (3): 340–348.

Kummrow, M.S., Mastromonaco, G.F., Crawshaw, G. et al. (2010b). Fecal hormone patterns during non-ovulatory reproductive cycles in female veiled chameleons (*Chamaeleo calyptratus*). *General and Comparative Endocrinology* 168 (3): 349–355.

le Berre, F. (1995). *The New Chameleon Handbook*, 138. Hauppauge, NY: Barron's Educational Series, Inc.

Lewis, N., Martinson, S., Wadowska, D. et al. (2015). Malignant mixed chromatophoroma with cutaneous, pulmonary, and testicular metastases in a veiled chameleon (*Chamaeleo calyptratus*). *Journal of Herpetological Medicine and Surgery* 25 (1–2): 16–20.

Licht, P., Millar, R., King, J.A. et al. (1984). Effects of chicken and mammalian gonadotropin-releasing hormones (GnRH) on in vivo pituitary gonadotropin release in amphibians and reptiles. *General and Comparative Endocrinology* 54 (1): 89–96.

Mader, D.R. (ed.) (2006). *Reptile Medicine and Surgery*, 2e. St. Louis, MO: Saunders (Elsevier Inc.).

Modry, D. and Koudela, B. (1995). Description of *Isospora jaracimrmani* sp. n. (Apicomplexa: Eimeriidae) from the Yemen chameleon, *Chamaeleo calyptratus* (Sauria: Chamaeleonidae). *Folia Parasitologica* 42: 313–316.

Modry, D. and Koudela, B. (1998). Isosporan infections of *Chamaeleo calyptratus* represent growing problem for its breeding in captivity. *Reptile and Amphibian Magazine* 54: 38–41.

Modry, D., Koudela, B., and Volf, J. (1997). Four new species of *Isospora* Schneider, 1881 (Apicomplexa: Eimeriidae) from reptiles from the islands of Seychelles. *Systematic Parasitology* 37 (1): 73–78.

Modry, D., Šlapeta, J.R., and Koudela, B. (2000). Six new species of coccidia (Apicomplexa: Eimeriidae) from east African chameleons (Sauria: Chamaeleonidae). *Journal of Parasitology* 86 (2): 373–379.

Modry, D., Šlapeta, J.R., and Koudela, B. (2001). *Eimeria hajeki* n. sp.(Apicomplexa: Eimeriidae), a new coccidian parasite of the pygmy chameleon, *Rampholeon temporalis* (Matschie, 1892)(Reptilia: Chamaeleonidae) from Usambara Mountains, Tanzania. *Journal of Parasitology* 87 (5): 1104–1105.

Modry, D. and Sloboda, M. (2004). Control of coccidiosis in chameleons using toltrazuril – results of an experimental trial. In: *Proceedings of the 7th International Symposium on Pathology and Medicine in Reptiles and Amphibians*, 93. Berlin: Edition Chimaira.

Nielsen, S.V., Banks, J.L., Diaz, R.E. Jr. et al. (2018). Dynamic sex chromosomes in Old World chameleons (Squamata: Chamaeleonidae). *Journal of Evolutionary Biology* 31 (4): 484–490.

Odette, O., Churgin, S.M., Sladky, K.K. et al. (2015). Anesthetic induction and recovery parameters in bearded dragons (*Pogona vitticeps*): comparison of isoflurane delivered in 100% oxygen versus 21% oxygen. *Journal of Zoo and Wildlife Medicine* 46 (3): 534–540.

Paré, J.A., Coyle, K.A., Sigler, L. et al. (2006). Pathogenicity of the *Chrysosporium* anamorph of *Nannizziopsis vriesii* for veiled chameleons (*Chamaeleo calyptratus*). *Sabouraudia* 44 (1): 25–31.

Paré, J.A., Sigler, L., Hunter, D.B. et al. (1997). Cutaneous mycoses in chameleons caused by the *Chrysosporium* anamorph of *Nannizziopsis vriesii* (Apinis) Currah. *Journal of Zoo and Wildlife Medicine* 28 (4): 443–453.

Pfaff, M., Schmidt, V., Plenz, B. et al. (2015). Examination on the occurence, clinical appearence and the detection of *Chamaeleomyces* sp.in clinically diseased chameleons. *Berliner und Münchener Tierärztliche Wochenschrift* 128 (1–2): 39–45.

Pimm, R. (2013). Characterization of Follicular Stasis in a Colony of Female Veiled Chameleons (Chamaeleo calyptratus). Doctoral dissertation. University of Guelph.

Reavill, D.R., Schmidt, R.E., and Stevenson, R. (2004). Malignant chromatophoromas in three veiled chameleons (*Chamaeleo calyptratus*). Proceedings of the Association of Reptilian and Amphibian Veterinarians: 131–133.

Rivera, S. (2008). Health assessment of the reptilian reproductive tract. *Journal of Exotic Pet Medicine* 17 (4): 259–266.

Rovatsos, M., Pokorná, M.J., Altmanová, M. et al. (2015). Female heterogamety in Madagascar chameleons (Squamata: Chamaeleonidae: *Furcifer*): differentiation of sex and neo-sex chromosomes. *Scientific Reports* 5: 13196.

Schacher, J.F. and Khalil, G.M. (1968). Development of *Foleyella philistinae* Schacher and Khalil, 1967 (Nematoda: Filarioidea) in *Culex pipiens molestus* with notes on pathology in the arthropod. *The Journal of Parasitology* 54 (5): 869–878.

Schmid-Brunclik, N., Stefka, S.C., Madeleine, K.B. et al. (2007). Liposarcoma in a veiled chameleon, *Chamaeleo calyptratus*. *Journal of Herpetological Medicine and Surgery* 17 (4): 132–135.

Schmidt, V., Klasen, L., Schneider, J. et al. (2017). Characterisation of *Metarhizium viride* mycosis in veiled chameleons (*Chamaeleo calyptratus*), panther chameleons (*Furcifer pardalis*) and inland bearded dragons (*Pogona vitticeps*). *Journal of Clinical Microbiology* 55 (3): 832–843.

Schmidt, V., Plenz, B., Pfaff, M. et al. (2012). Disseminated systemic mycosis in veiled chameleons (*Chamaeleo calyptratus*) caused by *Chamaeleomyces granulomatis*. *Veterinary Microbiology* 161 (1–2): 145–152.

Schmidt, W. (2001). *Chamaeleo calyptratus: The Yemen Chameleon*. Munster: Matthias Schmidt Publications.

Schumacher, J., Pellicane, C.P., Heard, D.J. et al. (1996). Periorbital abscess in a three-horned chameleon (*Chamaeleo jacksonii*). *Veterinary and Comparative Ophthalmology* 6 (1): 30–33.

Segretain, G., Fromentin, H., Destombes, P. et al. (1964). *Paecilomyces viridis* nov. sp., dimorphic fungus, agent of a generalized mycosis in *Chamaeleo lateralis* gray. *Comptes Rendus de l'Académie des Sciences* 259: 58–261.

Selleri, P. and Hernandez-Divers, S.J. (2006). Renal diseases of reptiles. *Veterinary Clinics: Exotic Animal Practice* 9 (1): 161–174.

Sigler, L., Gibas, C.F.C., Kokotovic, B. et al. (2010). Disseminated mycosis in veiled chameleons (*Chamaeleo calyptratus*) caused by *Chamaeleomyces granulomatis*, a new fungus related to *Paecilomyces viridis*. *Journal of Clinical Microbiology* 48 (9): 3182–3192.

Sigler, L., Hambleton, S., and Paré, J.A. (2013). Molecular characterization of reptile pathogens currently known as members of the *Chrysosporium* anamorph of *Nannizziopsis vriesii* (CANV) complex and relationship with some human-associated isolates. *Journal of Clinical Microbiology* 51 (10): 3338–3357.

Sladky, K.K. and Mans, C. (2012). Clinical analgesia in reptiles. *Journal of Exotic Pet Medicine* 21 (2): 158–167.

Smith, D., Vinci, J., Anderson, C.V. et al. (2016). Observations on nesting and clutch size in *Furcifer oustaleti* (Oustalet's chameleon) in South Florida. *Southeastern Naturalist* 15 (sp8): 75–88.

Stahl, S. (1996). Veterinary management of Old World chameleons. In: *Advances in Herpetoculture* (ed. P. Strimple), 151–160. International Herpetological Symposium.

Stahl, S.J. (1997). Captive management, breeding, and common medical problems of the veiled chameleon (*Chamaeleo calyptratus*). In: *Proceedings of the Association of Reptilian and Amphibian Veterinarians*, 29–40. Houston, TX: ARAV.

Stahl, S.J. (2003). Pet lizard conditions and syndromes. *Seminars in Avian and Exotic Pet Medicine* 12 (3): 162–182.

Suedmeyer, W.K. (1995). Hypocalcemia and hyperphosphatemia in a green iguana, *Iguana iguana*, with concurrent elevation of serum glutamic oxalic transaminase. *Bulletin of the Association of Reptilian and Amphibian Veterinarians* 5 (3): 5–6.

Sykes, J.M. (2010). Updates and practical approaches to reproductive disorders in reptiles. *Veterinary Clinics: Exotic Animal Practice* 13 (3): 349–373.

Thomas, C.L., Artwohl, J.E., Pearl, R.K. et al. (1996). Swollen eyelid associated with *Foleyella* sp infection in a chameleon. *Journal of the American Veterinary Medical Association* 209 (5): 972–973.

Uetz, P. and Hošek, J. (eds.) (2018). The reptile database. http://www.reptile-database.org (accessed 9 August 2018).

Zwart, P. (2006). Renal pathology in reptiles. *The Veterinary Clinics of North America. Exotic Animal Practice* 9 (1): 129–159.

Zwart, P. and Schroder, H.D. (1985). Mykosen. In: *Handbuch der Zookrankheiten*, vol. 1 (eds. R. Ippen, H.D. Schroder and K. Elze), 349–366. Berlin, Germany: Akademie Verlag.

16

Corn Snakes
Marie Kubiak

Corn snakes (*Pantherophis guttatus*, previously *Elaphe guttata* [Utiger et al. 2002]), are a medium-sized non-venomous colubrid snake, from the Colubrinae subfamily which also includes the morphologically similar rat snakes and king snakes. Corn snakes originate from South Eastern USA but are highly adaptive, living in forest, semi-desert, and grassland habitats, and even populating urban areas (Burbrink 2002). This adaptive capacity has led to invasive populations in Brazil, Australia, South Africa, Spain, Hawaii, and on several Caribbean islands, with implications for native biodiversity (Burbrink 2002; Fonseca et al. 2014).

Keeping of corn snakes is restricted or prohibited in some regions, though there are no restrictions currently in the UK (Fisher and Csurhes 2009; Fonseca et al. 2014; Worthington-Hill et al. 2014). This species is abundant in the wild and has the conservation status of 'least concern' (Echternacht and Hammerson 2016). Corn snakes are very popular as companion animals and their docile nature, moderate size and tolerance of a range of environmental conditions make them one of the more suitable pet snake species for novice keepers (Fisher and Csurhes 2009; Gaspar and Dulman 2014; Worthington-Hill et al. 2014). Hybridisation and development of varying colour patterns ('morphs') has maintained interest from herpetoculturists. Wild types are orange with darker saddles and a black and white chequered ventrum (Figure 16.1) (Werler and Dixon 2004). Albino, amelanistic, and anerythristic variants have been selectively bred (Figure 16.2) (Bartlett et al. 2001). Selected biological parameters of corn snakes are given in Table 16.1.

16.1 Husbandry

16.1.1 Enclosure

Corn snakes are solitary animals and are best kept singly to avoid conflict and competition for resources. A wooden vivarium is suitable for this species, maintaining visual barriers and thermal insulation, but these may need adapting with secure vents to provide adequate ventilation. Minimum enclosure length should allow the snake to stretch out fully, with enclosure length equating to the snout-vent length of the snake, with height and width at least 1/3 of this value. This should be considered an absolute minimum standard with the largest possible space provided to achieve the greatest range of microclimates available and allow a wide range of behaviours. Corn snakes are an active, engaging species when provided with adequate space. Although primarily terrestrial they also climb well, with juveniles observed to spend significant amounts of time resting at height (Mattison 2006; Nail 2008). Adequate enclosure height with secure branches, or other structures, are recommended to allow this normal behaviour as well as providing sufficient floorspace for terrestrial activity.

16.1.2 Heating

Corn snakes are active at night in warm conditions, and in colder periods they become diurnal or brumate in refugia (Gibbons and Dorcas 2005; Jose 2006). Ambient temperature should be maintained above 18 °C day and night utilising central heating or a thermostatically controlled heat source

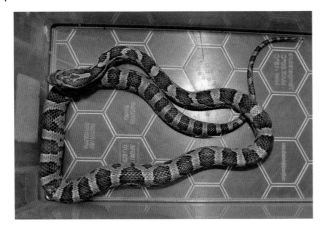

Figure 16.1 Normal or wild morph (pattern) of a corn snake.

Table 16.1 Selected biological parameters of corn snakes.

Lifespan	15–25 years
Length	90–170 cm
Adult weight	800–1000 g
Daytime temperature range	21–29 °C
Night temperatures	18–24 °C
Humidity	30–70%
Clutch size	1–50 (20–25 typical)
Incubation length	90–100 days at 26 °C, 60–65 days at 29.5 °C

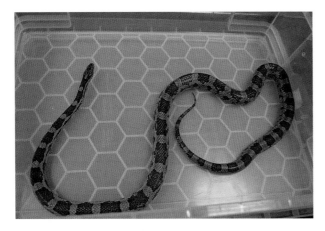

Figure 16.2 Anerythristic morph of a corn snake, note the absence of red pigmentation.

such as a ceramic bulb or heat pad. A secondary heat source such as an overhead bulb or ceramic heater (protected to prevent direct contact) should provide a focal, thermostatically-controlled, warm area at one end of the tank during the day (Figure 16.3) (Roark and Dorcas 2000). The resulting thermal gradient throughout the enclosure allows the snake to self-regulate temperature according to physiological status, with higher temperatures selected after feeding or when reproductively active (Roark and Dorcas 2000; Bontrager et al. 2006). Inadequate temperatures reduce speed of digestion and have been associated with regurgitation and refusal of feeds in juvenile corn snakes (Sievert et al. 2005).

16.1.3 Lighting

Corn snakes on an appropriate diet will receive their calcium and Vitamin D requirements from food so will survive without ultraviolet-B (UV-B) lighting (Gaspar and Dulman 2014). However, they are able to synthesise Vitamin

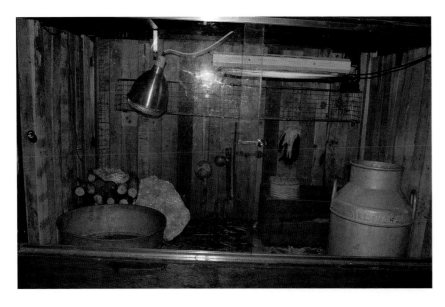

Figure 16.3 Enclosure for a corn snake, note the guarded heat lamp, UV lighting, and multiple recluse areas (*Source*: photo courtesy of Drayton Manor Park Zoo).

D on exposure to UV-B light (Acierno et al. 2008), suggesting that they have evolved to utilise UV-B exposure. Full spectrum lighting is of additional benefit as reptiles' vision extends into the UV spectrum and UV-A remains important for social and behavioural cues (Brames 2007). Increased activity has been observed in juvenile corn snakes exposed to low level UV light, compared to juveniles kept without UV lighting, similar to studies of other snake species (Bellamy and Stephen 2007; Nail 2008). High output UV lighting however led to more reclusive behaviour in juvenile corn snakes and may be aversive (Nail 2008). This suggests that a low output UV-A and UV-B source is preferable, with areas of shade, and is likely to be beneficial in vitamin D synthesis and stimulating activity and normal behaviours.

16.1.4 Feeding

Corn snakes are carnivores that feed opportunistically, striking and using constriction to incapacitate small mammals, but will also take reptiles, birds, or amphibians. Individuals can take prey of up to 45% of their body weight (Crocker-Buta and Secor 2014), but they have a tendency for obesity in captivity. Frozen–thawed rats or mice, equating to a feed of 15–20% of the snake's mass, can be offered every two weeks and reduced to every four weeks in winter (Gaspar and Dulman 2014; Stahlschmidt et al. 2017). Frozen mice and rats of various sizes can be obtained from pet shops, and live feeding should be avoided due to prey welfare concerns and the potential for injury to the snake. Owners may opt to feed in a separate enclosure to avoid stimulating an aggressive feeding response when opening the vivarium, or to prevent substrate being ingested with the food.

A large water bowl allows for drinking and bathing and is readily used by this species.

16.1.5 Substrate

Aspen shavings and similar fine wood shavings are generally suitable, though cedar and pine should be avoided due to potential presence of toxic or irritant constituents (Mitchell 2004). Soil and leaf litter are also potential alternatives, but should be purchased from a clean source, or sterilised prior to use to avoid introduction of fungal pathogens. Planted vivaria are rarely successful as corn snakes will use the substrate and disrupt plant stability and root formation.

Newspaper and paper towel are suitable for quarantine and hospitalisation purposes, but not for long-term maintenance as they do not permit microclimates to be established within substrate, limiting selection of appropriate temperature and humidity zones.

16.1.6 Breeding

Corn snakes are oviparous seasonal breeders. The breeding season in corn snakes is relatively long for snakes, at six to seven months in March–September (Fahrig et al. 2007). Cooling animals to induce brumation can be used to mimic seasonal changes and induce reproductive activity. No food is offered, temperatures are gradually reduced to 10–12 °C and lighting withdrawn for two to three months prior to return to normal conditions (Stahl 2002; Oliveri et al. 2018). Reproductive receptivity would then be expected to be seen once the female has completed a successful shed (Stahl 2002). Males evaginate one hemipene into the cloaca of a receptive female and a small volume of semen moves along a groove in the hemipene (Funk 1996; Fahrig et al. 2007). Repeat matings occur and oblong, leathery-shelled eggs (Figure 16.4) are laid by the female approximately 6 weeks later, usually preceded by a shed 7–14 days prior (Stahl 2002; Blackburn and Flemming 2009). A clutch can be up to 50 eggs, and these are laid within a 24 hour period (Stahl 2002). Incubated eggs hatch after 90–100 days at 26 °C, and 60–65 days at 29.5 °C (Stahl 2002; Blackburn and Flemming 2009). Females are able to retain sperm for future ovulations (Oliveri et al. 2018). The sex of colubrids is genetically determined and not dependent on incubation temperature (Bull 1980).

Neonates have an egg tooth, enabling them to 'pip' by slicing the egg shell. They should be left in the incubator for 12–24 hours prior to movement to individual enclosures, where they are maintained under similar conditions to adults. Substrate of paper towel is preferred until the yolk sac is fully resorbed.

Semen collection and artificial insemination has been successfully carried out in corn snakes but there is no need for assisted techniques in this species currently (Fahrig et al. 2007; Oliveri et al. 2018).

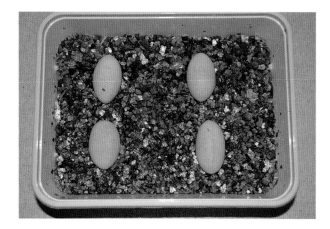

Figure 16.4 Corn snake eggs prepared for artificial incubation (*Source*: photo courtesy of Drayton Manor Park Zoo).

16.2 Clinical Evaluation

16.2.1 History-Taking

Husbandry assessment remains crucial, with inappropriate temperatures, poor ventilation, and inactivity (e.g. due to small enclosure size) common concerns. Overfeeding may also be a concern with excess adipose deposits common, and lipomas over-represented in this species (Garner et al. 2004).

16.2.2 Handling

Docile animals can be handled without significant restraint, lifting the snake at two points, supporting both the cranial and caudal ends. It is always acceptable to ask an owner to remove a snake from its travel bag or tub as they will be familiar with its temperament – most will happily oblige. If they are not willing then it is prudent to approach the snake more cautiously. Once out, supporting the head and neck with one hand and wrapping the lower body and tail around the same arm will help keep the snake still and give a free hand for examination. This is safe in this species as corn snakes are not large enough to cause human harm – if the snake is nervous and demonstrates constriction, gently unwind from the tail tip.

Corn snakes may occasionally show defensive behaviours if a threat is perceived (Werler and Dixon 2004). A coiled posture is assumed, with the head elevated and the neck flexed in an S-shape, ready to strike. The tail tip may also vibrate rapidly. If a snake presents these behaviours, removing any stressors and allowing time for it to settle is advisable prior to handling. Where this is not possible, placing a towel over the snake and gently grasping the animal just behind the head through the towel will immobilise the head and prevent bites. Once restrained, the opposing hand can be passed under the towel to restrain the head and allow the towel to be removed for examination (Figure 16.5). Some animals will pass urates, faeces, or express the musk glands on restraint (Werler and Dixon 2004).

16.2.3 Sex Determination

Males tend to have broader tail bases (just caudal to the vent) but lack any additional external features so probing is generally required to confirm presence or absence of hemipenes. The two inverted hemipenes in males form sulci caudal to the vent that extend for a distance equivalent to six or more scales on the overlying skin. Females have only shallow scent glands in this position that equate to two to four scales in length (Mitchell 2004). A lubricated sexing probe

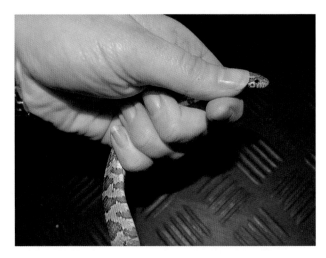

Figure 16.5 Immobilisation of the head using the thumb behind the occiput and index finger encircling the neck. Used to restrain a fractious animal, or for examination of the head.

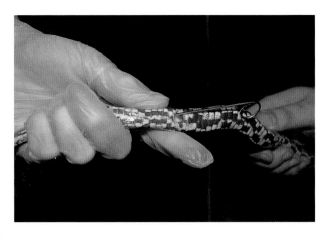

Figure 16.6 Probing to determine sex. In females a probe will pass a short distance into the scent glands, in males the hemipene sulci result in the probe passing a greater distance.

can be passed from the vent caudally, and the depth the probe will pass determines the sex of the animal (Figure 16.6).

Applying pressure to the hemipene region to exteriorise the hemipene is known as 'popping' and can be used in juveniles but is not recommended for adults due to potential traumatic injury (Stahl 2002).

16.2.4 Clinical Examination

A systematic examination from head to tail is necessary, with assessment including examination of the spectacles (clear, fused eyelids), nares, oral cavity, skin, and vent, and palpation of the entire coelomic cavity.

Dermatitis, stomatitis, abnormal respiratory secretions or noise, masses, cardiomegaly, and fluid distention of the intestinal tract are regularly identified in this species.

16.3 Basic Techniques

16.3.1 Sample Collection

Small blood samples are preferentially collected from the ventral tail vein. A 23–25G needle is inserted on the ventral midline between scales approximately 5 cm caudal to the vent. Aspiration using a 1 ml syringe yields a slow flow of blood (Bush and Smeller 1978) and pre-heparinising the syringe will avoid premature clotting of samples. Larger samples are collected from the heart and pre-heparinisation of the syringe should not be used for this site. The snake is restrained by an assistant and the pulsatile motion of the heart is identified on the ventral aspect of the snake, around 1/5 of the snout-vent length of the snake (Divers 2008). The heart is immobilised by compressing the coelom with the thumb of the non-dominant hand cranial to the heart. The inserted needle is angled craniodorsally at a 45° angle between scales at the level of the apex of the heart, and advanced into the ventricle (de la Navarre 2006). Gentle aspiration yields pulsatile flow of blood. Pressure is applied to the site for 30–60 seconds on needle withdrawal.

Lithium heparin is preferred as the anticoagulant for haematology and biochemistry as EDTA may lyse cells, altering measured parameters (Cray and Zaias 2004). Nucleated erythrocytes necessitate manual haematology on a stained blood smear (Cray and Zaias 2004).

Faecal samples may be passed by animals on handling, or a cloacal flush can be carried out using warmed saline to gain a dilute sample (de la Navarre 2006). Flotation techniques are commonly used to concentrate and enhance detection of coccidial oocysts or nematode ova. Direct microscopy to identify flagellates is recommended for animals with gastrointestinal symptoms.

16.3.2 Nutritional Support

Anorexia is a normal response to low temperatures and reproductive activity, and may also be seen in some individuals at shed periods. Both males and females in active breeding stages, and females prior to oviposition, will stop feeding. Physiological anorexia should not be accompanied by an appreciable change in body weight or condition.

Scent is a key part of feeding stimulation in corn snakes, with visual cues of low value (Worthington-Hill et al. 2014). Freshly killed rodents, different rodent species with a novel scent (such as gerbils or hamsters), or warmed, opened carcasses may stimulate non-feeding snakes.

Anorexia is common to many disease processes in corn snakes. Snakes can tolerate prolonged periods with lack of food so nutritional support is rarely necessary and successful management of the primary disease will often be sufficient

to restart feeding. Chronic disease with advanced weight loss, or chronic disease in juveniles, may justify assist feeding. Rehydration is necessary first to avoid electrolyte aberrations associated with refeeding syndrome (Mans and Braun 2014). Commercial exotic carnivore liquid feeds are readily available and are administered by orogastric gavage using a flexible feeding tube (Mans and Braun 2014). The lubricated tube is gently passed to approximately 1/4 of the distance from the snout to the vent in order to access the stomach. Volumes recommended range from 2 to 10% of bodyweight and will depend on the animal's clinical status and growth stage, though lower volumes are typically used (Calvert 2004). Alternatively, volume fed can be calculated more precisely using body weight (W, in kg):

$$\text{Weekly energy requirement}\left(kJ\right) = 180 \times W^{0.98}$$

As an example, an adult corn snake weighing 900 g requires 162 kJ weekly, and this can be divided into two assist feeds per week. Daily feeds are not necessary and are likely to increase patient stress. Where long-term assist feeding is expected, a pharyngostomy tube can be surgically placed to facilitate regular feeding.

16.3.3 Fluid Therapy

Fluid requirements approximate 25 ml/kg/day and warmed isotonic crystalloid fluids are suitable (Maclean and Raiti 2004). Oral fluids are rarely sufficient alone to improve hydration status but may be used alongside other routes. Subcutaneous fluids are used commonly for gradual rehydration, with small volumes given at multiples sites over the epaxial muscles (Gibbons 2009). Intravenous routes allow for rapid rehydration but are rarely used due to the need for surgical placement of jugular catheters using a cut-down technique. Bolus administration of fluids is possible but challenging using the tail vein in larger animals. Intracoelomic fluids have been used historically due to ease of administration of large volumes, however there is potential for laceration of viscera, induction of coelomitis, reduction in lung expansion, and poor uptake so this route is not recommended.

Weight gain, resumption of urination, and resolution of tachycardia indicate a positive response to rehydration (Gibbons 2009). Elevations in PCV, uric acid, and total protein are often seen in dehydrated patients and will resolve with successful rehydration.

16.3.4 Anaesthesia

Volatile agents alone are rarely suitable for induction in snakes as breath holding and cardiac shunting of blood from the pulmonary to the systemic circulation results, uptake of anaesthetic gases is low and metabolic acidosis may result (Leary et al. 2013; Jakobsen et al. 2017). Administration of a high concentration of oxygen in inspired gas will also induce respiratory depression, slowing induction and recovery (Mosley 2005). Intravenous or intracardiac propofol has been the preferred choice for induction (Mosley 2005), but more recently alfaxalone has become available and can be administered by intravenous, intracardiac, or intramuscular routes. When administered by intramuscular injection in snakes, injection into the cranial half of the body has been shown to produce better sedation than injection into the caudal body. Duration of anaesthesia is around 40 minutes when given by the cranial intramuscular route at 20 mg/kg (James et al. 2018), though intravenous administration appears to result in quicker onset and shorter duration of action. Ketamine combinations with alpha-2 agonists or benzodiazepines have been used in reptiles but give less predictable depth of anaesthesia and recovery is often prolonged (Bertelsen 2014).

Volatile agents are good options for maintenance of anaesthesia, though ventilation is often required as apnoea and respiratory depression are common in anaesthetised snakes. Intubation is straightforward – the mouth is opened and the glottis is readily visible, caudal to the tongue sheath (Figure 16.7). A long endotracheal tube (or modified dog urinary catheter) is advanced to approximately 15–20% of snout-vent length and positioning confirmed with observation of body wall movement on ventilation. Snakes should be kept within their preferred thermal range throughout procedures to facilitate metabolism of medication and avoid a prolonged recovery.

For recovery, ventilating with room air rather than pure oxygen may speed return to spontaneous ventilation (Mosley 2005). Once making conscious movements, animals can be extubated and maintained in a pre-heated enclosure providing ambient temperatures around 25 °C, with no focal heat as this may result in thermal injury from prolonged exposure. Once mobile, animals can return to their normal enclosure.

Analgesia is complicated by the lack of data on effective agents, and information is often extrapolated though perception of pain and analgesic effects may vary significantly between reptile species (Sladky et al. 2008). Current recommendations for analgesia are included in the formulary. The butorphanol dose found to reduce response to a pain stimulus in corn snakes was very high at 20 mg/kg and may cause respiratory depression (Sladky et al. 2008) or produce lack of response due to sedative rather than analgesic effects. Administration of butorphanol at this dose has resulted in fatalities (Sladky and Mans 2012). Morphine, even at high doses, did not consistently affect the response to a nociceptive stimulus in corn snakes despite being a good analgesic in other reptile species (Sladky et al. 2008; Sladky and Mans 2012). Non-steroidal anti-inflammatory drugs, particularly meloxicam, are widely used in reptile patients but no data on analgesia effect is available (Sladky and Mans 2012). Much more work is needed in reptiles to determine the most effective analgesic regimens and species-specific doses.

16.3.5 Euthanasia

This is best achieved by administering 100 mg/kg pentobarbitone by intracardiac injection, or intracoelomic injection of 500 mg/kg in small individuals (Leary et al. 2013). Sedation or anaesthesia prior to injection is recommended, to avoid discomfort. Decapitation, freezing and blunt trauma are not suitable methods.

(a) (b)

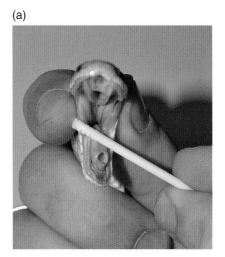 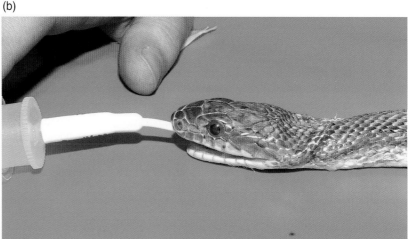

Figure 16.7 (a) The glottis is clearly evident within the mouth, facilitating endotracheal intubation. (b) Intubation of a corn snake for maintenance of anaesthesia. Note the skin tenting indicating pronounced dehydration (*Source*: Photo courtesy of Sergio Silvetti).

The reptile brain is able to withstand oxygen deprivation for prolonged periods and so once unconscious, destruction of the brainstem using pithing is advisable to prevent recovery (Leary et al. 2013). This involves passing a metal rod or large needle into the brain through the roof of the mouth and physically destroying the tissue.

16.3.6 Hospitalisation Requirements

Snakes should be hospitalised away from domestic pets to avoid stress to smaller prey species from snakes, and to snakes from larger animals.

Vivaria with appropriate heating and lighting should be available for clinics seeing reptile patients. This should be easily disinfected, with disposable cardboard box hides and paper towel substrate often used for short-term housing of patients.

It is often preferable to maintain recovering patients within temperature gradients towards the top end of their thermal range, to optimise immune function and healing potential but this may not be appropriate for all patients, and hydration and clinical status should be considered.

16.4 Common Medical and Surgical Conditions

16.4.1 Anorexia

Failure to feed is a non-specific sign of ill health in corn snakes, but can also been seen as a physiological response in some circumstances. Protracted anorexia (over two months), anorexia associated with loss of body condition or weight, or anorexia in an animal that is clinically unwell merits veterinary assessment. Table 16.2 details some common causes of anorexia.

In all cases a review of husbandry and a thorough clinical examination should be carried out to narrow the differential diagnoses and guide treatment. Where a pathological cause is suspected, but is unclear, further diagnostics including haematology, biochemistry, radiography, and ultrasonography are often valuable. Nutritional support may be applied after rehydration, where significant loss of body condition has occurred but correction of the primary process to enable self-feeding to return is preferred where body condition is not critical.

16.4.2 Dysecdysis

The outer keratinised portion of skin is shed in a single piece every three to four months in adults, and this process is termed ecdysis. Growing juveniles shed more frequently at every three to eight weeks (Penning 2012). Low temperatures, ill health, and malnutrition may extend the shedding cycle, whereas ectoparasitism, dermatitis, or endocrine disease may increase shedding frequency (Harkewicz 2002). Disruption to the shedding process, including incomplete or protracted ecdysis, is termed dysecdysis. Inappropriate humidity, dehydration, dermal injury, inflammation or scarring, and debilitation are common factors in dysecdysis. Retained areas of skin may cause irritation or act as a nidus for infection. If the distal tail is affected then progressive contraction of unshed skin can cause avascular necrosis of the tail tip (Harkewicz 2002). Soaking the snake in tepid water for 20–30 minutes can aid in atraumatic removal of retained skin using a damp towel or forceps. Shed skin should not be forcefully removed as this may damage the underlying skin.

In snakes, the eyelids are replaced by a clear skin layer, termed the spectacle (van Doorn and Sivak 2013). The spectacles may be retained in dysecdysis, giving a dull appearance to the eye. This can be seen with generalised dysecdysis, or with localised irritation, such as periocular snake mite infestation. Applying hypromellose drops repeatedly over a 30 minute period may aid in separating the old and new spectacle at the periphery, allowing gentle removal with a cotton bud or forceps. Forceful removal can damage the new spectacle, with exposure of the cornea and potential for permanent eye damage. If the spectacle is not readily removed then correcting causative factors and leaving it to be cast at the next shed is recommended.

Hyperthyroidism is described as a cause of increased frequency of ecdysis in corn snakes, due to primary hyperthyroidism, or hyperthyroidism secondary to pituitary pathology (Whiteside and Gamer 2001; Harkewicz 2002). However, convincing evidence of clinical hyperthyroidism is lacking and reports suggests that hyperthyroidism should reduce rather than increase the frequency of ecdysis (Chiu and Lynn 1970; Chiu et al. 1983; Hunt 2015). Serum thyroxine levels can be assessed in cases of atypical ecdysis frequency, the normal range for free T4 in this species is reported to be 0.45–6.06 nmol/l (Greenacre et al. 2001).

16.4.3 Dermatitis

Dermatitis may present as increased shedding frequency, localised skin retention, alteration of pigmentation, swelling, abscessation, exudative ulceration, or sloughing of tissue (Hoppmann and Barron 2007). Thermal, chemical, bacterial, and fungal causes are well recognised.

Thermal burns are a major differential for dermal injury in pet snakes (Hoppmann and Barron 2007). It has been hypothesised that snakes process thermal stimuli differently to other animals, with a reduced response to noxious thermal stimuli seen (Sladky et al. 2008). This may explain

Table 16.2 Common causes of anorexia in corn snakes.

Cause of anorexia	Action
Environmental	
Low or fluctuating temperatures	Review temperatures and improve heat provision. If animals are undergoing an intentional cooling period prior to raising temperatures in order to induce breeding then a reduction in appetite is expected.
Stressors	Assess for potential stressors (e.g. co-habiting with larger corn snake, excessive handling, constant light exposure) and resolve
Inappropriate prey offered	Prey of inappropriate size, of too low temperature or of unfamiliar appearance or scent may not stimulate a normal feeding response. Offer food of correct size, and of a familiar type that has been warmed to approximately 37 °C. If unsuccessful and the snake is clinically well, try novel, strongly scented items such as hamsters, or freshly killed rodents.
Overfeeding	Review feeding schedule and quantity fed, as well as body condition of snake. Reduce food if overweight or fed excessively
Newly acquired snakes	Newly acquired animals, or those recently moved into a new enclosure may temporarily become anorexic. Avoid handling or excess interference for first few weeks of acclimatisation and continue to offer food. Captive bred corn snakes rarely undergo significant anorexia following changes in circumstance.
Physiological	
Breeding season	Both male and female snakes may become anorexic when reproductively active. Males may become more active. Soft swelling of the mid-coelom may be seen in pre-ovulatory females. Continue to offer food and monitor condition and body weight as these should remain stable.
Gravid female prior to oviposition	Female snakes will reduce food intake when gravid and may become completely anorexic (Gregory et al. 1999). Offer food once oviposition has been completed.
Seasonal response	Even if temperatures remain stable other changes, such as external photoperiod, may be perceived by snakes and induce a reduction in feeding in winter. This is uncommon and can be countered by raising usual environmental temperatures by 2 °C.
Ecdysis	It is common for snakes to refuse food when shedding. Animals will have a blue-grey colour to the skin, which is often most prominent over the eyes. Feeding should resume once shedding has been completed.
Medical	
Orofacial disease	Stomatitis, traumatic injury, respiratory disease or reduced vision may disrupt normal feeding cues and prehension of food. Physical examination will aid detection and feeding should resume once the primary concern is resolved.
Debiliation or disease	Anorexia is a common, non-specific symptom in an unwell snake and can be difficult to differentiate from environmental and physiological causes in the early stages. Weight loss or presence of clinical signs of illness support suspicion of a health concern. Clinical examination may identify the cause, but in many cases haematology, biochemistry, imaging and specific pathogen screens may be required to identify the cause.

the failure of snakes to move away from malfunctioning or inappropriate heat sources, resulting in contact burns that can be extensive. No external damage may be seen immediately after thermal insult and most snakes only present days later once sloughing of damaged tissues commences. Open wounds may result over a large area of the body surface with potential for significant loss of fluid and protein in exudates, and opportunistic infection. All cases require analgesia and replacing substrate with paper towel or a bare vivarium floor temporarily will aid in keeping traumatised areas clean.

First degree burns are superficial, affecting only the epidermis with erythema and blistering often resulting (Mader 2002). Topical treatment such as silver sulphasalazine or zinc oxide will aid healing, with resolution of lesions in a four- to six-week period.

Second degree burns are associated with necrosis of the epidermis and damage to the deeper dermis. Swelling, blistering, discoloration of skin, and exudative lesions are seen. Systemic antibiotic therapy and topical treatments are necessary for these cases (Harkewicz 2002) but scarring can result. Adhesive sterile dressings can be placed over injuries to prolong action of topical agents and protect the wound (Mader 2002). Maintaining snakes at the top end of their temperature gradient will accelerate healing (Smith et al. 1988). Fluid therapy requirements will depend on the area of the burn and the fluid losses sustained.

Third degree burns have full thickness skin damage with sloughing of skin across the lesion. Fluid therapy is necessary as losses can be significant. Daily bandage changes, systemic and topical antibiotics, and multimodal analgesia are necessary for management of these cases in the first days to weeks of treatment, with ongoing medical therapy and less frequent bandage changes required for the four to six month healing period (Mader 2002). Significant scarring will result and may interfere with ecdysis.

Bacterial or fungal infections are rarely primary concerns, but follow insult to skin integrity such as a burn or bite from prey, or chronic husbandry deficiency such as excessive or insufficient humidity, low environmental temperatures, obesity, unsanitary conditions, or malnutrition (Harkewicz 2002; Hoppmann and Barron 2007). Where substrate is consistently wet or heavily contaminated, the ventrum is most commonly affected and may appear erythematous and develop vesicles or ulceration (Hoppmann and Barron 2007). The underlying cause should be corrected. Skin lesions should be cultured to guide therapy, and antimicrobials, analgesia, topical disinfectants, and debridement and subsequent protection of affected areas using bandaging considered based on severity of lesions. Fungal lesions may require biopsy for confirmation of diagnosis (Hoppmann and Barron 2007).

Primary fungal pathogens are uncommon in captive animals, but *Ophidiomyces ophiodiicola* (formerly *Chrysosporium ophiodiicola*) is an emerging disease in wild and captive snake populations and has been reported in colubrid snakes (Allender et al. 2015). Infection in most snakes affects the head and ventral scales with caseation and crusts but the one clinical case reported in a corn snake presented with a subcutaneous nodule (Sigler et al. 2013). *O. ophiodiicola* has also been demonstrated to cause disease in experimentally infected corn snakes (Lorch et al. 2015). Infected animals in this study developed oedema, crusting, and hyperpigmentation of scales, increased ecdysis frequency and dysecdysis but appeared able to clear the fungal infection following ecdysis (Lorch et al. 2015). For clinical cases, biopsy for fungal culture and histology is recommended, with treatment comprising systemic and topical antifungals. *O. ophiodiicola* appears poorly responsive to itraconazole and ketoconazole therapy, and voriconazole has been associated with death of snakes at 5 mg/kg (Rajeev et al. 2009; Sigler et al. 2013;

Lindemann et al. 2017). Terbinafine has been demonstrated to be effective *in vitro*, and reaches expected therapeutic levels in cottonmouths (*Agkistrodon piscivorous*) with nebulisation or placement of a subcutaneous implant (Kane et al. 2017). Based on the study findings, 30 minutes nebulisation daily using a 2 mg/ml terbinafine solution was recommended as a potential treatment. Oral and topical terbinafine formulations are commercially available but no dosing schedules have been determined. Exposure of spores for 2 minutes to 3% bleach, or for 10 minutes to 70% ethanol or quaternary ammonium products have been shown to be effective for disinfection, but chlorhexidine and propiconazole were ineffective (Rzadkowska et al. 2016).

16.4.4 Respiratory Disease

In snakes, the right lung is a simple sac, lined with respiratory epithelium cranially and avascular non-respiratory epithelium caudally, resulting in a relatively small surface area for gas exchange (Schumacher 2003). The left lung is vestigial in colubrids. Clinical respiratory disease is common in pet snakes but in the author's experience, respiratory disease is less common in colubrid snakes than larger, sedentary boids. Clinical signs include nasal discharge, audible respiratory noise, presence of secretions in the oral cavity, stomatitis, dyspnoea, open mouth breathing, elevation of the head and neck, and cyanosis (Schumacher 2003). Disease is often advanced by the time of overt symptoms and presentation. Radiography is of limited value for mild–moderate disease but may show abscess formation, fluid accumulation, or increased radiodensity of the lung in advanced cases. Computed tomography is of higher sensitivity for lesions and is preferred for diagnosing and monitoring respiratory disease but is not as readily available. Ultrasonography may identify increases in fluid or soft tissue and facilitate collection of aspirate samples for culture or cytology (Schumacher 2003). Endoscopy of the trachea is limited by patient size, but swabs can often be collected for culture and PCR diagnostics for upper respiratory tract diseases. Tracheal and lung wash samples are advisable to determine specific pathogen presence in lower respiratory tract disease (Murray 2005). Percutaneous surgical endoscopic access to the lung can be utilised for sample collection or topical therapy of focal lesions.

Bacteria, particularly gram-negative organisms, are commonly isolated from respiratory cases and may be primary pathogens, opportunistic invaders, or co-infections.

Viral respiratory pathogens reported in corn snakes include ophidian paramyxovirus, reovirus, and adenovirus (Abbas et al. 2011). These viruses may be present in clinical cases, asymptomatic animals, or as part of mixed infections (Abbas et al. 2011), so a positive result should be interpreted in accordance with the animal's clinical status. For paramyxovirus, demonstration of a rising titre is recommended to confirm active infection (Jacobson and Origgi 2002). It is unknown if snakes with static antibody levels have cleared infection or remain permanently infected, though a small proportion of corn snakes experimentally infected with paramyxovirus appeared able to clear infection (Pees et al. 2016). Supportive care may allow recovery in less severe cases. These viruses are highly infectious and can spread within and between collections readily, emphasising the importance of biosecurity, quarantine, and targeted screening of new animals.

Non-infectious respiratory disease is uncommon but may include penetrating injuries, neoplasia, or exposure to irritant gases or aerosols.

Treatment of respiratory disease involves targeted therapy for the primary cause where possible, husbandry improvements, and supportive measures. The lack of a diaphragm, reliance on skeletal muscles for air movement, and lack of a developed mucocilary system means that respiratory secretion clearance is poor in snakes. Fluid therapy, nebulisation, encouraging activity, coupage and drainage of secretions by elevating the mid body above the head may aid clearance of debris in lower respiratory tract disease. Maintaining animals at the top end of their thermal range will aid immune function and maintaining a high humidity level may decrease secretion viscosity, enhancing clearance.

16.4.5 Cardiac Disease

A detailed description of cardiac anatomy and physiology in snakes is beyond the scope of this chapter but major differences will be mentioned. Cranially there are two atria, and caudally a single ventricle, subdivided by a muscular ridge – the vertical septum. The thin-walled sinus venosus, is located dorsal to the right atrium and receives blood from the systemic circulation, contracting prior to atrial contraction to aid filling of the right atrium (Farrell et al. 1998; Jensen et al. 2014). During respiration, the ventricle is functionally divided by the vertical septum to function as a bi-chambered heart, in an equivalent way to mammals. When apnoeic, parasympathetic tone increases resulting in bradycardia and increased pulmonary resistance. Under these conditions blood from the right side of the heart is shunted across the ventricle and a significant proportion of the blood re-enters the systemic circulation, bypassing the pulmonary circulation (Bogan 2017). This reduces cardiac activity when oxygen is unavailable, but maintains perfusion to the systemic circulation.

Cardiac disease may present with regurgitation, anorexia, lethargy, weight loss, peripheral oedema, cyanosis, open mouth breathing, or a discrete swelling (Figure 16.8) (Kik and Mitchell 2005; Beaufrère et al. 2016). Assessment should take place with the snake at an appropriate temperature as cardiac function can alter with hyper- or hypothermia. The cardiac position can be localised on examination by placing the snake in dorsal recumbency and visualising a pulsatile region approximately 20–23% along the length of the body of the snake (Divers 2008). Auscultation with a stethoscope is unrewarding, but Doppler ultrasonic probes can be useful in assessing for alterations in heart sounds (Kik and Mitchell 2005; Mitchell 2009). In another colubrid, the yellow rat snake (*Elaphe obsoleta quadrivitatta*), creatine kinase rises with myocardial damage and may be useful in supporting a diagnosis of cardiomyopathy (Ramsay and Dotson 1995). For electrocardiography (ECG), lead II is most frequently used. The negative lead is placed one to two heart lengths cranial to the heart on the right, the positive lead placed on the left, approximately 60–75% along the body and the neutral lead placed on the right, opposite the positive lead (Kik and Mitchell 2005; Bogan 2017). The trace has P and T waves and a QRS complex, similar to that seen in mammals but amplitude may be lower, hindering interpretation (Kik and Mitchell 2005). An additional 'SV' wave may been seen prior to the P wave, reflecting depolarisation of the sinus venosus (Martinez-Silvestre et al. 2003). ECG interpretation is not yet well described in snakes and caution should be exercised when making a diagnosis based on an ECG alone.

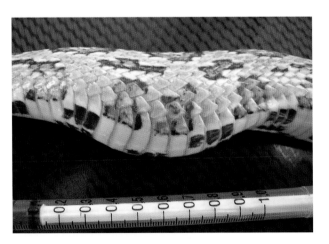

Figure 16.8 Pronounced pulsatile swelling in the cranial coelom indicative of cardiomegaly. Cardiac disease appears common in colubrid snakes.

Radiography, particularly the laterolateral view of the cranial-mid body, may support cardiac disease, with cardiomegaly, hepatomegaly, pulmonary oedema, vascular mineralisation, or ascites potential findings (Mitchell 2009). Echocardiography may be hampered by poor acoustic coupling but soaking the snake in warm water prior to scanning and using large volumes of coupling gel will aid image quality. A ventral approach is advised, directly over the heart (Schilliger et al. 2006). Potential pathology that can be detected includes pericardial effusion, alterations in valve function or anatomy, parasite presence, neoplasia, or mineralisation of tissues (Bogan 2017). Chamber dilation or thickening of the myocardium may be suspected on echocardiography, but objective assessment is not possible due to a lack of normal values for this species. Cardiomegaly has been reported in this species but prevalence is undetermined (Kik and Mitchell 2005). The author has seen a disproportionately high prevalence of dilated cardiomyopathy in corn and rat snakes, but no evident primary cause has been identified. Treatment for cardiac disease is extrapolated from therapy in domestic mammals though dosing regimens are not validated.

16.4.6 Stomatitis

Oral examination is readily achieved in a restrained snake by gently passing a flat card or blunt probe into the mouth from the diastema at the rostral tip to open the mouth. There are six rows of teeth, two mandibular and four maxillary, with teeth continuously shed and replaced (Mehler and Bennett 2003). The tongue sheath and trachea are identifiable as projections from the floor of the oral cavity.

Petechiation, cyanosis, tacky oral secretions, mucosal inflammation, loss of multiple teeth, haemorrhage, or anatomical asymmetry indicate further evaluation is necessary (Mehler and Bennett 2003). Rostral trauma associated with rubbing on, or colliding with, enclosure walls is uncommon in this species.

Stomatitis or 'mouth rot' is a common reason for presentation of captive snakes, and encompasses gingivitis, glossitis, palatitis, and cheilitis from bacterial, fungal, and viral causes. Symptoms may include hyperptyalism, anorexia, dysphagia, loss of teeth, and an irregular appearance to gingiva. Gram-negative bacteria are most commonly isolated from stomatitis cases but there is a significant overlap with commensal bacteria, suggesting external factors may influence development of clinical disease (Rosenthal and Mader 1996). In chronic cases there can be local extension of infection to the nasolacrimal duct, subspectacular space,

facial bones, or upper respiratory tract, or distant spread as bacterial emboli or septicaemia. Treatment involves targeted antibiotic therapy based on culture results from lesions, irrigation of lesions using topical antiseptics, and analgesia. Radiographs are useful to determine prognosis and to guide surgical debridement of necrotic or abscessated areas in advanced cases (Mehler and Bennett 2003). For poorly responsive cases histopathology, with particular focus on neoplasia or mycobacteria, and viral screening is advisable.

Ophidian paramyxovirus can result in stomatitis but respiratory and neurological symptoms are more pronounced (Hyndman 2012). Fungal or parasitic stomatitis is rare in captive snakes (Mehler and Bennett 2003).

16.4.7 Ophthalmic Disease

Retained spectacles are the most common ophthalmic abnormality identified in snakes, followed by subspectacular abscess, ocular trauma, and cataracts (Hausmann et al. 2013). Feeding of live prey was found to be a significant cause of ophthalmic trauma and is best avoided.

Subspectacular abscess formation is commonly a consequence of bacterial stomatitis extending along the nasolacrimal duct into the subspectacular space. Colubrid snakes appear more likely to suffer from this condition than other snake families (Hausmann et al. 2013). Animals present with apparent opaque distension of the subspectacular space. The subspectacular space measures approximately 0.14 mm in normal corn snakes (Hollingsworth et al. 2007), but can be increased dramatically with accumulation of purulent material. Systemic antibiotics and anti-inflammatory agents are administered and a 30° wedge resection of the ventral spectacle carried out for drainage and ongoing topical therapy (Cullen et al. 2000). Recurrence is common and may require repeat surgical intervention (Hausmann et al. 2013). Culture of material collected at surgery is advised to guide antibiotic therapy. *Staphylococcus* spp., *Salmonella arizonae* and *Pseudomonas aeruginosa* have been cultured from four cases of subspectacular infections, all presumed to be opportunistic pathogens (Hausmann et al. 2013).

Occasionally an obstruction of the nasolacrimal duct leads to sterile distension of the subspectacular space and treatment involves drainage of the fluid and management of the inflammatory process causing the obstruction. Untreated, these cases can progress to subspectacular abscess formation.

Cataracts have been reported in other colubrids (Martin et al. 1994; Daltry 2006), but appear rare in corn snakes. Phacoemulsification has been used successfully in the closely related Texas rat snake (Ledbetter et al. 2017).

16.4.8 Gastrointestinal Disease

Routine parasite assessment of faecal samples is advisable annually for clinically well snakes, and at presentation for animals presenting for any illness, ideally including testing for Cryptosporidia.

Cryptosporidium coccidia are a significant cause of gastrointestinal disease in reptiles, with *Cryptosporidium serpentis* recognised as the predominant snake pathogen and *Cryptosporidium varanii* (syn. *Cryptosporidium saurophilum*) predominating in lizards, with other species less commonly identified (Xiao et al. 2004; Pavlasek and Ryan 2008; Richter et al. 2011). Oocysts are shed in the faeces of infected animals and remain viable for over a year (Jenkins et al. 1997). Ingestion results in release of sporozoites in the intestinal tract which migrate into the gastric epithelial cells to replicate in snakes (Greiner 2003). Released merozoites can directly infect other epithelial cells and repeat this process, or form gametes to generate oocysts (Greiner 2003). Clinical signs in snakes include regurgitation, gastric distension, weight loss, anorexia, diarrhoea, and incomplete digestion of food (Richter et al. 2011). Chronic gastritis with mucosal hypertrophy, hyperaemia, cobblestone appearance, reduced prominence of rugal folds, and luminal reduction may be noted on endoscopy or post-mortem examination (Cimon et al. 1996; Bercier et al. 2017). Cryptosporidiosis is typically a chronic disease of adult animals, though one case in a one-year-old corn snake has been reported. In this case, the snake was concurrently infected with adenovirus and it was hypothesised that immunosuppression was a contributing factor to disease development (Mahapatra et al. 2013). Biliary tract cryptosporidiosis and associated cholecystitis has been reported in corn snakes with concurrent intestinal cryptosporidiosis, with no clinical signs of biliary disease (Cimon et al. 1996). A case of oesophageal-gastric-duodenal double compounded intussusception has also been reported as a suspected consequence of cryptosporidiosis in a corn snake (Bercier et al. 2017).

Oocysts are very small and almost transparent so identification on faecal sample flotation can be insensitive. Acid-fast staining of samples can increase sensitivity (Greiner 2003). PCR can be performed on faecal samples, gastric wash samples, gastric biopsy, or regurgitated food items and shows greater sensitivity (Yimming et al. 2016). Speciation of cryptosporidia detected by any test is important as *Cryptosporidium parvum* and *Cryptosporidium muris* from rodent prey can be present within the intestinal tract following a feed as incidental findings (Greiner 2003). A high detection rate of Cryptosporidia has been reported in corn snakes in one study, with 25% of samples testing positive on PCR (Richter et al. 2011). Interestingly of the 27 positive samples, 17 were *C. varanii*, one was a similar lizard genotype and the other 9 samples did not achieve a species level diagnosis. In this study it was not determined whether these infections were associated with clinical disease, though other reports suggest that both natural and experimental infection of corn snakes with *C. varanii* does not appear to result in clinical disease (Xiao et al. 2004; Plutzer and Karanis 2007). Other studies have demonstrated a predominance of *C. serpentis*, or incidental findings of *C. parvum* and *C. muris*, in corn snakes with a positive *Cryptosporidium* PCR (Xiao et al. 2004; Yimming et al. 2016).

Treatment of infected animals is unlikely to be successful so it is important to quarantine and test new animals prior to introduction into a collection. Weekly testing over a 30 day period has been recommended (Greiner 2003). Halofuginone, spiramycin, and paromomycin have been trialled in snakes but were unsuccessful (Graczyk et al. 1996). Hyperimmune bovine colostrum, has been shown to reduce clinical signs and oocyst shedding in snakes with no side effects, but convincing evidence of clearance of infection is lacking (Graczyk et al. 1998). Complete disinfection of enclosures of infected animals is difficult, as the recommended methods of heat treatment, ammonia-based disinfectants, dessication, and prolonged exposure to ultraviolet light will significantly reduce numbers, but not eliminate viable oocysts (King and Monis 2007).

Other endoparasites appear uncommon pathogens in corn snakes. *Eimeria* oocysts and *Ophiostrongylus* ova have been identified as co-infections in corn snakes with clinical Cryptosporidiosis (Cimon et al. 1996). Unspecified strongylids were identified in 40% of corn snakes in one study but a wider survey of colubrid snakes found a much lower overall parasitic prevalence with low numbers (<3.3%) testing positive for *Kalicephalus*, ascarids, heterakids, *Rhabdias*, Strongyloides, oxyurids, and *Balantidium* and moderate numbers (7.4%) positive for *Nyctotherus* (Pasmans et al. 2008; Rataj et al. 2011). Some protozoa may be commensal, but the author has seen clinical signs in colubrid snakes of gas distension of the intestinal tract, foul-smelling liquid faeces, and anorexia in association with high numbers of flagellated motile protozoa on faecal microscopy. Treatment with metronidazole resolves symptoms effectively.

16.4.9 Reproductive Pathology

Dystocia is common in snakes, and inciting factors include a lack of a suitable nesting site, social stressors, dehydration, malnutrition, obesity, pathology of the reproductive tract, renomegaly, and oversized or malformed eggs (DeNardo 2006; Sykes 2010). Presenting signs include failure to complete oviposition of a clutch of eggs, prolonged unproductive straining, oviductal prolapse, or non-specific signs such as lethargy and anorexia in an animal beyond the expected date of oviposition (Sykes 2010). Eggs are relatively large and are often visible and palpable along the ventral surface of the caudal coelom, as a series of soft swellings. Gentle palpation may identify abnormally shaped or sized eggs, but care should be taken as the oviduct is thin and highly fragile (Stahl 2002). Imaging can be used to confirm numbers of eggs present as some, notably the smaller infertile eggs ('slugs') may not be as readily palpated. If all eggs appear normal in structure then medical therapy using calcium and oxytocin can be considered. This is not appropriate if oviposition started more than 72 hours previously as response will be poor and there is a higher likelihood of adhesion of eggs to the oviduct wall, risking oviductal rupture (Stahl 2002). Arginine vasotocin is more effective than oxytocin but is not currently commercially available (Millichamp et al. 1983).

An alternative to medical therapy is manual removal, or 'milking' of eggs, but this typically requires sedation and carries a significant risk of oviductal trauma so is often not an appropriate approach (DeNardo 2006). Eggs are progressively pushed caudally and out of the cloaca by running a thumb firmly in short strokes along the ventral aspect of the snake. If large eggs are not able to be fully exteriorised, the contents may be aspirated through the vent once the egg is visualised, enabling collapse and easier passage. This is often useful where one oversized egg is preventing oviposition of following eggs. Manual removal should not be carried out after oxytocin therapy as this increases the potential for oviductal rupture (Millichamp et al. 1983).

Percutaneous aspiration is an alternative to enable passage of large eggs. Under sterile conditions a wide gauge needle is inserted, between the first and second row of lateral scales, into the egg (Stahl 2002). The egg contents are aspirated and the snake will then normally pass the collapsed egg within 24 hours (Stahl 2002). There is a risk of ongoing leakage of egg contents into the oviduct and the coelom, resulting in salpingitis or coelomitis, particularly with incomplete deflation. Chronically retained eggs tend to have solid contents and cannot be aspirated (Stahl 2002) and adhesed eggs will not progress.

Surgery is preferred if medical therapy, egg manipulation, or ovocentesis has failed, or where adhesion to the oviduct wall is suspected based on chronicity of signs or immobility of one or more eggs (Lock 2000). General anaesthesia is required, and a lateral coeliotomy is carried out. The skin is

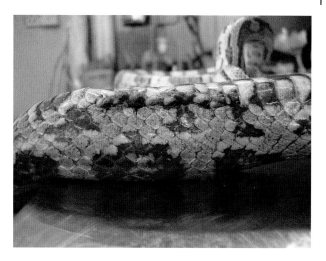

Figure 16.9 Use of everting horizontal mattress sutures for skin closure following salpingotomy.

prepared with a dilute iodine solution, and gently scrubbed between scales using a soft brush. The incision is made directly over the egg, two rows of scales dorsal to the gastric scales with the incision following the scale margins (Bercier et al. 2017). The ribs are transected and the coelomic membrane sharply dissected to visualise the egg within the oviduct. An incision is made in the thin oviduct wall and the egg removed. Additional eggs may be manipulated through the same incision, but often multiple skin and oviduct incisions are necessary to remove all eggs. The oviduct is then closed with a continuous inverting pattern using a 4.0–5.0 long-lasting absorbable suture material such as polydioxanone and the process repeated for the contralateral oviduct, through the same skin incisions. If a prolapse, salpingitis, or oviductal rupture is present, salpingectomy and removal of the ipsilateral ovary is advisable but requires multiple incisions in order to ligate associated vessels and remove all tissues (Lock 2000). An everting pattern such as horizontal mattress sutures, or skin staples, is used for skin closure (Figure 16.9) and sutures or staples are removed at six to eight weeks post-surgery.

16.4.10 Neoplasia

A wide range of case reports of neoplasia have been published for this species, with many affecting young adult snakes of one to five years of age. These are listed in Table 16.3. In the majority of cases a visible swelling is identified (Figure 16.10), though for an oviductal carcinoma, mucopurulent salpingitis without an overt mass was the primary finding (Pereira and Viner 2008).

Table 16.3   Reported neoplasms in corn snakes.

Neoplasm	Age	Comments	Reference
Subcutaneous lipomas	Various	Reported to be over-represented in corn snakes	Frye (1994), Reavill and Schmidt (2003), Garner et al. (2004), Dietz et al. (2016)
Infiltrative lipoma	Adult; 12 yr	Initial fine needle aspiration (FNA) indicative of lipoma in both cases	Burkert et al. (2002), Pinto et al. (2018)
Cardiac haemangioma	3 yr	Associated with atrial wall	Stumpel et al. (2012)
Iridophoroma	22 yr	No metastasis	Muñoz-Gutiérrez et al. (2016)
Malignant mixed chromatophoroma	17 yr	Metastasised	Muñoz-Gutiérrez et al. (2016)
Renal adenoma	Adult	Died 3 m post-surgery	Jacobson et al. (1986)
Renal cell carcinoma	8 yr	Amelanistic, anerythristic morph. Metastasised to contralateral kidney, liver, and lung 3 months after nephrectomy	Barten et al. (1994)
Renal adenocarcinoma	5 yr	Metastasised to contralateral kidney 1.5 months after excision	Kao et al. (2016)
Oviductal adenocarcinoma	Adult	No distinct mass, oviduct distended by mucopurulent material	Pereira and Viner (2008)
Ovarian undifferentiated carcinoma	6 yr	9 × 4 cm mass	Petterino et al. (2006)
Pulmonary adenocarcinoma	>1.5 yr	No age given, only time on display	Catão-Dias and Nichols (1999)
Adrenal adenocarcinoma	>11 yr	No age given, only time on display	Catão-Dias and Nichols (1999)
Cloacal adenocarcinoma	>5 yr	No age given, only time on display	Catão-Dias and Nichols (1999)
Intestinal adenocarcinoma		Reported as common in corn snakes, one case with metastasis to liver	Garner (2005)
Colonic adenocarcinoma	3 yr	Multinodular mass at junction of colon and cloaca	Latimer and Rich (1998)
Rhabdomyosarcoma		Retrovirus identified in neoplasm	Lunger et al. (1974)
Leiomycosarcoma	>9 yr	Duodenal	Catão-Dias and Nichols (1999)
Fibrosarcoma	12 yr	Suspected invasion into ribs and spine	McNulty and Hoffman (1995)
Metastatic chondrosarcoma	2 yr	Mandibular primary with metastases in the heart, lung, kidney, pancreas, eye	Schmidt and Reavill (2012)
Vertebral chondrosarcoma		Three cases arising from vertebral articulations, metastasis noted in one case	Dawe et al. (1980), Garner et al. (1995), Garner (2005)
Splenic haemangiosarcoma	Adult	Died 1.5 m post-surgery	Tuttle et al. (2006)
Myeloid leukaemia	>7.5 yr	Multiple organs affected	Catão-Dias and Nichols (1999)

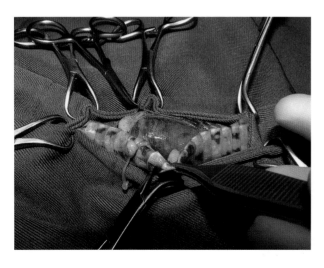

Figure 16.10   Exploratory coeliotomy for investigation of caudal coelomic mass. An intestinal adenocarcinoma was confirmed on histology (Source: Photo courtesy of Sergio Silvetti).

16.4.11 Neurological Disease

Symptoms of neurological disease in snakes include tremors, seizures, incoordination, blindness, opisthotonus, behavioural changes, obtundation and a failure to feed (Fleming et al. 2003; Mariani 2007). Differential diagnoses include toxin exposure (e.g. nicotine, permethrin), thermal injury, severe renal or hepatic disease, physical trauma, malnutrition, adverse response to medication, viral infection (e.g. Ophidian Paramyxovirus, Ophidian reovirus), bacterial infection of the central nervous system, or hypothermia (Mariani 2007). A case series of three corn snakes with clinical signs and histological findings consistent with the viral Inclusion disease of boids has been reported (Fleming et al. 2003). The report concluded that a similar viral cause may be responsible for the disease in corn snakes but no virus was able to be identified.

16.4.12 Renal Disease

In snakes, the right kidney is located cranial to the left and both have a clear overlapping lobular structure. The primary waste product is uric acid, which is expelled as a white paste with small quantities of clear liquid, and can be post-renally modified limiting the value of urinalysis. Renal compromise may result in anorexia, gout, convulsions, and uncoordinated movements (Divers 2008) but appears uncommon in snakes with only one report of non-neoplastic renal pathology in a corn snake. Giant cell nephritis was described by Zwart (2006), with palpable renal enlargement noted on examination, and histology of the swollen kidneys demonstrating interstitial aggregations of multinucleate giant cells.

16.4.13 Ectoparasitism

Mites are a common finding in captive snakes (Harkewicz 2002). The snake mite (*Ophionyssus natricis*) causes localised irritation, disruption to skin shedding and may act as a vector for pathogens (Harkewicz 2002). Affected snakes may demonstrate an increased frequency of shedding, increased bathing, and adult mites can be observed on the skin, particularly in skin folds around the eyes and mouth (Harkewicz 2002). Ivermectin or fipronil are preferred for treatment. Permethrins can be used but there are reports of toxicity in snakes (Brooks et al. 1998; Whitehead 2010), and the author has seen multiple cases of neurological symptoms in juvenile corn snakes treated with over the counter permethrin sprays that resolved with supportive treatment.

16.5 Preventative Health Measures

No routine vaccinations or parasite treatments are recommended. For new animals, a clinical examination, faecal parasite screen, and husbandry review are advisable. Virology screens should be considered based on risk analysis from the originating collection, and size and type of collection the animal is introduced into. For a single pet animal an exhaustive diagnostic panel is rarely appropriate, but if an animal is being introduced into a large, multi-species or high value collection then there is justification to perform a wider array of pre-movement testing and maintain a longer quarantine period of at least six months. Owners should keep good records detailing feeding and shedding schedules and annual faecal parasitology is a sensible precaution.

16.6 Imaging

Radiography is of particular value for skeletal lesions, uric acid depositions, mineralisation of soft tissues, gastrointestinal foreign bodies, dystocia, effusions, and organomegaly (de la Navarre 2006). However, radiography is insensitive in identification of lower respiratory tract pathology (Schumacher 2003) and the coelomic soft tissues offer poor contrast. Contrast studies using barium have been described to enhance detail, but transit time can be in excess of 72 hours (Banzato et al. 2013).

Ultrasonography has been used to assess reproductive status of female corn snakes, with 8–12 MHz linear transducers used to visualise ovarian follicles. The left ovary is found at a distance of 64–75% along the snout-vent length (SVL), and the right ovary is 70–80% SVL (Divers 2008). Pre-ovulatory follicles have a round, uniform hyperechoic appearance in comparison to previtellogenic, hypoechoic follicles (Oliveri et al. 2018). Ocular ultrasonography is also reported in corn snakes, with ultra-high frequency probes necessary (Hollingsworth et al. 2007). Echocardiography is valuable for subjective assessment of cardiac anatomy and contractility but no reference ranges for measurements have been documented for this species. The liver (30–50% SVL) and intestinal tract (stomach 48–58% SVL [Divers 2008]) can also be assessed readily using ultrasonography.

Nuclear scintigraphy, using ^{99m}Tc-MAG$_3$ provides high quality images of the kidneys in corn snakes and may be a valuable tool in the future given the limitations of other methods of imaging (Sykes IV et al. 2006).

Formulary

Medication	Dose	Dosing interval	Additional comments
Anaesthesia			
Alfaxalone	20 mg/kg IM		Inject into cranial half of body, gives 40 mins anaesthesia (James et al. 2018)
Alfaxalone	5–10 mg/kg IV, IC		Fast onset, 15–20 mins anaesthesia
Propofol	5–10 mg/kg IV, IC		IV access may not be feasible in all individuals, use lower dose for intracardiac route (Bennett et al. 1998; Stahl 2002)
Isoflurane	2–3% inhaled		Induction may be prolonged. Useful for maintenance at 1–2% (Bertelsen et al. 2005)
Sevoflurane	4–5% inhaled		Induction may be prolonged. Useful for maintenance at 2–3% (Bertelsen et al. 2005)
Medetomidine and ketamine	0.15 mg/kg and 10 mg/kg IM, IV		Useful for sedation, can be partially reversed with atipamezole but recovery may be prolonged (Mosley 2005; Bertelsen 2014)
Analgesia			
Butorphanol	10 mg/kg SC, IM	q24h	Demonstrated to reduce response to thermal stimulus in one study at 20 mg/kg (Sladky et al. 2008), but respiratory depression possible and this high dose is not advisable (Sladky and Mans 2012)
Morphine	1–5 mg/kg SC, IM	q24h	Effective analgesia in other reptile species. Analgesic efficacy inconsistent in this species (Sladky and Mans 2012)
Tramadol	5–10 mg/kg SC, IM, PO	q48h	Extrapolated from other reptile species (Baker et al. 2011)
Meloxicam	0.2–0.3 mg/kg IV, IM, SC, PO	q24–48h	Presumed anti-inflammatory effects (Sladky and Mans 2012)
Antibiotics			
Oxytetracycline	6–10 mg/kg PO, IM, SC	q24h	Injectable preparations can result in localised inflammation (Gibbons et al. 2013)
Azithromycin	10 mg/kg PO	q2–7 days	Based on royal python (*Python regius*) dose (Coke et al. 2003)
Ceftazidime	20 mg/kg IM, IV	q 48–72h	Used for gram-negative bacterial infections. Third generation cephalosporin, should not be first line antibiotic choice
Enrofloxacin	5–10 mg/kg PO, IM, SC	q24h	Injectable preparations can cause tissue necrosis (Gibbons et al. 2013). Fluoroquinolones should not be first line antibiotics.
Terbinafine	2 mg/ml solution, nebulisation	30 mins nebulisation daily	To treat fungal dermatosis, including *Ophidiomyces ophiodiicola* (Kane et al. 2017)
Antiparasitics			
Metronidazole	100 mg/kg PO	Two doses, 2 weeks apart	Flagellates (Scullion and Scullion 2009)
Fenbendazole	25 mg/kg PO	Weekly for up to four treatments	Amoebae, flagellates and enteric helminths (Funk and Diethelm 2006)
Paromomycin	300–360 mg/kg PO	q48h for 2 weeks	For Cryptospodiosis, does not eliminate disease in corn snakes (Paré and Barta 1997)
Hyperimmune bovine colostrum	10 ml/kg PO	Weekly for 6 weeks	For Cryptosporidiosis, reduced clinical signs and shedding (Graczyk et al. 1998)
Ivermectin	200 ug/kg SC, IM	repeat after 2 wks	Snake mites (Harkewicz 2002)

(Continued)

Medication	Dose	Dosing interval	Additional comments
Ivermectin	5 mg/l dilution topically on animals and equipment	repeat after 2 wks	Snake mites (Harkewicz 2002)
Fipronil (0.29% spray)	2 ml/kg topically	q 7–10 days	For ectoparasites, spray or wipe on snake in a well-ventilated space, wash off after 5 mins (Fitzgerald and Vera 2006)
Miscellaneous			
Furosemide	2–5 mg/kg IM	q24h	Diuretic for cardiac cases, variable efficacy across species, no data in corn snakes (Selleri and Hernandez-Divers 2006; Bogan 2017)
Pimobendan	0.2 mg/kg PO	q24h	Extrapolated from lizard dose (Jepson 2009). For dilative cardiomyopathy or congestive heart failure
Allopurinol	20 mg/kg PO	q24h	Decreases uric acid synthesis in renal compromise (Selleri and Hernandez-Divers 2006)
Probenecid	2–4 mg/kg PO	q24h	Increases uric acid excretion, for renal compromise (Selleri and Hernandez-Divers 2006)
Methimazole	2 mg/kg PO	q24h	For hyperthyroidism (Harkewicz 2002)
Thyroxine	0.025 mg/kg PO	q1–5 days	For hypothyroidism (Hunt 2015)
Oxytocin	5–20 iu/kg IM	Start at lower end, repeat with higher dose 6–12 hrs later for maximum of 3 doses	For dystocia (Stahl 2002)
Barium 25%	25 ml/kg PO		For gastrointestinal contrast studies (Banzato et al. 2013)

References

Abbas, M.D., Marschang, R.E., Schmidt, V. et al. (2011). A unique novel reptilian paramyxovirus, four atadenovirus types and a reovirus identified in a concurrent infection of a corn snake (*Pantherophis guttatus*) collection in Germany. *Veterinary Microbiology* 150 (1–2): 70–79.

Acierno, M.J., Mitchell, M.A., Zachariah, T.T. et al. (2008). Effects of ultraviolet radiation on plasma 25-hydroxyvitamin D3 concentrations in corn snakes (*Elaphe guttata*). *American Journal of Veterinary Research* 69 (2): 294–297.

Allender, M.C., Raudabaugh, D.B., Gleason, F.H. et al. (2015). The natural history, ecology, and epidemiology of *Ophidiomyces ophiodiicola* and its potential impact on free-ranging snake populations. *Fungal Ecology* 17: 187–196.

Baker, B.B., Sladky, K.K., and Johnson, S.M. (2011). Evaluation of the analgesic effects of oral and subcutaneous tramadol administration in red-eared slider turtles. *Journal of the American Veterinary Medical Association* 238 (2): 220–227.

Banzato, T., Hellebuyck, T., Van Caelenberg, A. et al. (2013). A review of diagnostic imaging of snakes and lizards. *Veterinary Record* 173 (2): 43–49.

Barten, S.L., Davis, K., Harris, R.K. et al. (1994). Renal cell carcinoma with metastases in a corn snake (*Elaphe guttata*). *Journal of Zoo and Wildlife Medicine* 25 (1): 123–127.

Bartlett, P.P., Griswold, B., and Bartlett, R.D. (2001). Corn snake. In: *Reptiles, Amphibians, and Invertebrates: An Identification and Care Guide* (eds. P.P. Bartlett, B. Griswold and R.D. Bartlett), 41–42. Hauppage, NY: Barron's Educational Series.

Beaufrère, H., Schilliger, L., and Pariaut, R. (2016). Cardiovascular system. In: *Current Therapy in Exotic Pet Practice* (eds. M.A. Mitchell and T.N. Tully), 151–220. St. Louis, MO: Elsevier.

Bellamy, T. and Stephen, I. (2007). The Effect of Ultra-Violet B (UVB) Illumination and Vitamin D3 on the Activity, Behaviour and Growth Rate of the Juvenile Jamaican Boa Epicrates subflavus. Master's dissertation. University of London, United Kingdom.

Bennett, R.A., Schumacher, J., Hedjazi-Haring, K. et al. (1998). Cardiopulmonary and anesthetic effects of propofol administered intraosseously to green iguanas. *Journal of the American Veterinary Medical Association* 212 (1): 93–98.

Bercier, M., Zoll, W., Rosenberg, J.F. et al. (2017). Gastric intussusceptions in a red corn snake (*Pantherophis guttatus*) associated with Cryptosporidiosis. *Case Reports in Veterinary Medicine* 2017: 4270904.

Bertelsen, M.F. (2014). Squamates (snakes and lizards). In: *Zoo Animal and Wildlife Immobilization and Anesthesia*, 2e (eds. G. West, D. Heard and N. Caulkett), 351–363. Chichester, UK: Wiley.

Bertelsen, M.F., Mosley, C., Crawshaw, G.J. et al. (2005). Inhalation anesthesia in Dumeril's monitor (*Varanus dumerili*) with isoflurane, sevoflurane, and nitrous oxide: effects of inspired gases on induction and recovery. *Journal of Zoo and Wildlife Medicine* 36 (1): 62–68.

Blackburn, D.G. and Flemming, A.F. (2009). Morphology, development, and evolution of fetal membranes and placentation in squamate reptiles. *Journal of Experimental Zoology Part B: Molecular and Developmental Evolution* 312 (6): 579–589.

Bogan, J.E. Jr. (2017). Ophidian cardiology – a review. *Journal of Herpetological Medicine and Surgery* 27 (1–2): 62–77.

Bontrager, L.R., Jones, D.M., and Sievert, L.M. (2006). Influence of meal size on postprandial thermophily in cornsnakes (*Elaphe guttata*). *Transactions of the Kansas Academy of Science* 109 (3): 184–190.

Brames, H. (2007). Aspects of light and reptilian immunity. *Iguana* 14 (1): 19–23.

Brooks, J.E., Savarie, P.J., and Johnston, J.J. (1998). The oral and dermal toxicity of selected chemicals to brown tree snakes (*Boiga irregularis*). *Wildlife Research* 25 (4): 427–435.

Bull, J.J. (1980). Sex determination in reptiles. *The Quarterly Review of Biology* 55 (1): 3–21.

Burbrink, F.T. (2002). Phylogeographic analysis of the cornsnake (*Elaphe guttata*) complex as inferred from maximum likelihood and Bayesian analyses. *Molecular Phylogenetics and Evolution* 25 (3): 465–476.

Burkert, B.A., Tully, T.N., Nevarez, J. et al. (2002). Infiltrative lipoma in a corn snake, *Elaphe guttata guttata*. *Journal of Herpetological Medicine and Surgery* 12 (3): 33–35.

Bush, M. and Smeller, J. (1978). Blood collection and injection techniques in snakes. *Veterinary Medicine, Small Animal Clinician* 73 (2): 211–214.

Calvert, I. (2004). Nutritional problems. In: *BSAVA Manual of Reptiles* (eds. S.J. Girling and P. Raiti), 289–308. Gloucester, UK: British Small Animal Veterinary Association.

Catão-Dias, J.L. and Nichols, D.K. (1999). Neoplasia in snakes at the National Zoological Park, Washington, DC (1978–1997). *Journal of Comparative Pathology* 1 (120): 89–95.

Chiu, K.W. and Lynn, W.G. (1970). The role of the thyroid in skin-shedding in the shovel-nosed snake, *Chionactis occipitalis*. *General and Comparative Endocrinology* 14: 467–474.

Chiu, K.W., Leung, M.S., and Maderson, P.F.A. (1983). Thyroid and skin-shedding in the rat snake (*Ptyas korros*). *The Journal of Experimental Zoology* 225 (3): 407–410.

Cimon, K.Y., Oberst, R.D., Upton, S.J. et al. (1996). Biliary cryptosporidiosis in two corn snakes (*Elaphe guttata*). *Journal of Veterinary Diagnostic Investigation* 8 (3): 398–399.

Coke, R.L., Hunter, R.P., Isaza, R. et al. (2003). Pharmacokinetics and tissue concentrations of azithromycin in ball pythons (*Python regius*). *American Journal of Veterinary Research* 64 (2): 225–228.

Cray, C. and Zaias, J. (2004). Laboratory procedures. *The Veterinary Clinics of North America. Exotic Animal Practice* 7 (2): 487–518.

Crocker-Buta, S.P. and Secor, S.M. (2014). Determinants and repeatability of the specific dynamic response of the corn snake, *Pantherophis guttatus*. *Comparative Biochemistry and Physiology Part A: Molecular & Integrative Physiology* 169: 60–69.

Cullen, C.L., Wheler, C., and Grahn, B.H. (2000). Diagnostic ophthalmology. Bullous spectaculopathy in a king snake. *The Canadian Veterinary Journal* 41 (4): 327.

Daltry, J.C. (2006). The effect of black rat *Rattus rattus* control on the population of the Antiguan racer snake *Alsophis antiguae* on Great Bird Island, Antigua. *Conservation Evidence* 3: 30–32.

Dawe, C.J., Small, J.D., Banfield, W.G. et al. (1980). Chondrosarcoma of a corn snake (*Elaphe guttata*) and nephroblastoma of a rainbow trout (*Salmo gairdneri*) in cell culture. In: *The Comparative Pathology of Zoo Animals* (eds. R. Montali and G. Migaki), 603–612. Washington, DC: Smithsonian Institute Press.

DeNardo, D. (2006). Dystocias. In: *Reptile Medicine and Surgery*, 2e (ed. D. Mader), 787–792. St. Louis, MO: Elsevier Inc.

Dietz, J., Heckers, K.O., Aupperle, H. et al. (2016). Cutaneous and subcutaneous soft tissue tumours in snakes: a retrospective study of 33 cases. *Journal of Comparative Pathology* 155 (1): 76–87.

Divers, S. (2008). Snake radiology: the essentials. Proceedings of the North American Veterinary Conference, 19–23 January, Orlando, FL: 1772–1774.

van Doorn, K. and Sivak, J.G. (2013). Blood flow dynamics in the snake spectacle. *Journal of Experimental Biology* 216 (22): 4190–4195.

Echternacht, A. and Hammerson, G.A. (2016). *Pantherophis guttatus*. The IUCN Red List of Threatened Species 2016: e.T63863A71740603. http://dx.doi.org/10.2305/IUCN.UK.2016-3.RLTS.T63863A71740603.en. (accessed 29 November 2018).

Fahrig, B.M., Mitchell, M.A., Eilts, B.E. et al. (2007). Characterization and cooled storage of semen from corn snakes (*Elaphe guttata*). *Journal of Zoo and Wildlife Medicine* 38 (1): 7–12.

Farrell, A.P., Gamperl, A.K., and Francis, E.T.B. (1998). Comparative aspects of heart morphology. In: *Biology of the Reptilia*, vol. 19 (Morphology G) (eds. C. Gans and A.S. Gaunt), 375–424. Ithaca, NY: Society for the Study of Amphibians and Reptiles.

Fisher, P.L. and Csurhes, S. (2009). *Pest Animal Risk Assessment: American Corn Snake Elaphe guttata.* Brisbane: Queensland Primary Industries and Fisheries.

Fitzgerald, K.T. and Vera, R. (2006). Acariasis. In: *Reptile Medicine and Surgery*, 2e (ed. D.R. Mader), 728. St. Louis, MO: Saunders, Elsevier.

Fleming, G.J., Heard, D.J., Jacobson, E.R. et al. (2003). Cytoplasmic inclusions in corn snakes, *Elaphe guttata*, resembling inclusion body disease of boid snakes. *Journal of Herpetological Medicine and Surgery* 13 (2): 18–22.

Fonseca, É., Marques, R., and Tinôco, M.S. (2014). New records of *Pantherophis guttatus* (Squamata: Colubridae) in the state of Bahia, an alien species to Brazil. *Salamandra* 50: 241–244.

Frye, F.L. (1994). *Reptile Clinician's Handbook: A Compact Clinical and Surgical Reference*. Malabar, FL: Krieger Publishing Company.

Funk, R.S. (1996). Biology: snakes. In: *Reptile Medicine and Surgery* (ed. D.R. Mader), 39–46. Philidelphia, PA: W. B. Saunders Co.

Funk, R.S. and Diethelm, G. (2006). Reptile formulary. In: *Reptile Medicine and Surgery*, 2e (ed. D.R. Mader), 1119–1139. St. Louis, MO: Saunders Elsevier.

Garner, M.M. (2005). Trends in reptilian neoplasia: a diagnostian's perspective. Proceedings of the North American Veterinary Conference, 8–12 January, Orlando, FL: 1278–1280

Garner, M.M., Collins, D., and Joslin, J. (1995). Vertebral chondrosarcoma in a corn snake. Proceedings of Annual Conference AAZV, August: 332–333.

Garner, M.M., Hernandez-Divers, S.M., and Raymond, J.T. (2004). Reptile neoplasia: a retrospective study of case submissions to a specialty diagnostic service. *Veterinary Clinics: Exotic Animal Practice* 7 (3): 653–671.

Gaspar, C. and Dulman, O.M. (2014). Observations regarding the accommodation and feeding of leisure reptiles. *Lucrari Stiintifice, seria Medicină Veterinară* 57 (3–4): 260.

Gibbons, P.M. (2009). Critical care nutrition and fluid therapy in reptiles. Proceedings of the 15th Annual International Veterinary Emergency & Critical Care Symposium: 91–94.

Gibbons, J.W. and Dorcas, M.E. (2005). *Snakes of the Southeast*. Athens, GA: University of Georgia Press.

Gibbons, P., Klaphake, E., and Carpenter, J.W. (2013). Reptiles. In: *Exotic Animal Formulary*, 4e (eds. J.W. Carpenter and C.J. Marion), 83–182. St. Louis, MO: Saunders.

Graczyk, T.K., Cranfield, M.R., and Hill, S.L. (1996). Therapeutic efficacy of halofuginone and spiramycin treatment against *Cryptosporidium serpentis* (Apicomplexa: Cryptosporidiidae) infections in captive snakes. *Parasitology Research* 82 (2): 143–148.

Graczyk, T.K., Cranfield, M.R., Helmer, P. et al. (1998). Therapeutic efficacy of hyperimmune bovine colostrum treatment against clinical and subclinical *Cryptosporidium serpentis* infections in captive snakes. *Veterinary Parasitology* 74 (2–4): 123–132.

Greenacre, C.B., Young, D.W., Behrend, E.N. et al. (2001). Validation of a novel high sensitivity radioimmunoassay procedure for measurement of total thyroxine concentration in psittacine birds and snakes. *American Journal of Veterinary Research* 62 (11): 1750–1754.

Gregory, P.T., Crampton, L.H., and Skebo, K.M. (1999). Conflicts and interactions among reproduction, thermoregulation and feeding in viviparous reptiles: are gravid snakes anorexic? *Journal of Zoology* 248 (2): 231–241.

Greiner, E.C. (2003). Coccidiosis in reptiles. *Seminars in Avian and Exotic Pet Medicine* 12 (1): 49–56.

Harkewicz, K.A. (2002). Dermatologic problems of reptiles. *Seminars in Avian and Exotic Pet Medicine* 11 (3): 151–161.

Hausmann, J.C., Hollingsworth, S.R., Hawkins, M.G. et al. (2013). Distribution and outcome of ocular lesions in snakes examined at a veterinary teaching hospital: 67 cases (1985–2010). *Journal of the American Veterinary Medical Association* 243 (2): 252–260.

Hollingsworth, S.R., Holmberg, B.J., Strunk, A. et al. (2007). Comparison of ophthalmic measurements obtained via high-frequency ultrasound imaging in four species of snakes. *American Journal of Veterinary Research* 68 (10): 1111–1114.

Hoppmann, E. and Barron, H.W. (2007). Dermatology in reptiles. *Journal of Exotic Pet Medicine* 16 (4): 210–224.

Hunt, C. (2015). Thyroid adcnocarcinoma in a Gartcr snakc (Thamnophis marcianus). Proceedings of BVZS Spring meeting, Loughborough, UK: 38.

Hyndman, T. (2012). Paramyxoviruses in Australian snakes. Doctoral dissertation, Murdoch University, https://researchrepository.murdoch.edu.au/id/eprint/10648 (accessed 15 April 2019).

Jacobson, E.R. and Origgi, F. (2002). Use of serology in reptile medicine. *Seminars in Avian and Exotic Pet Medicine* 11 (1): 33–45.

Jacobson, E.R., Long, P.H., Miller, R.E. et al. (1986). Renal neoplasia of snakes. *Journal of the American Veterinary Medical Association* 189 (9): 1134–1136.

Jakobsen, S.L., Williams, C.J., Wang, T. et al. (2017). The influence of mechanical ventilation on physiological parameters in ball pythons (*Python regius*). *Comparative Biochemistry and Physiology Part A: Molecular and Integrative Physiology* 207: 30–35.

James, L.E., Williams, C.J., Bertelsen, M.F. et al. (2018). Anaesthetic induction with alfaxalone in the ball python (*Python regius*): dose response and effect of injection site. *Veterinary Anaesthesia and Analgesia* 45 (3): 329–337.

Jenkins, M.B., Anguish, L.J., Bowman, D.D. et al. (1997). Assessment of a dye permeability assay for determination of inactivation rates of *Cryptosporidium parvum* oocysts. *Applied and Environmental Microbiology* 63 (10): 3844–3850.

Jensen, B., Boukens, B., Wang, T. et al. (2014). Evolution of the sinus venosus from fish to human. *Journal of Cardiovascular Development and Disease* 1 (1): 14–28.

Jepson, L. (2009). *Exotic Animal Medicine: A Quick Reference Guide*. London, UK: WB Saunders.

Jose, S. (2006). Resident snakes common in other habitats. In: *The Longleaf Pine Ecosystem: Ecology, Silviculture, and Restoration* (eds. S. Jose, E.J. Jokela and D.L. Miller), 172–173. New York: Springer.

Kane, L.P., Allender, M.C., Archer, G. et al. (2017). Pharmacokinetics of nebulized and subcutaneously implanted terbinafine in cottonmouths (*Agkistrodon piscivorus*). *Journal of Veterinary Pharmacology and Therapeutics* 40 (5): 575–579.

Kao, C.F., Chen, J.L., Tsao, W.T. et al. (2016). A renal adenocarcinoma in a corn snake (*Pantherophis guttatus*) resembling human collecting duct carcinoma. *Journal of Veterinary Diagnostic Investigation* 28 (5): 599–603.

Kik, M.J. and Mitchell, M.A. (2005). Reptile cardiology: a review of anatomy and physiology, diagnostic approaches, and clinical disease. *Seminars in Avian and Exotic Pet Medicine* 14 (1): 52–60.

King, B.J. and Monis, P.T. (2007). Critical processes affecting *Cryptosporidium* oocyst survival in the environment. *Parasitology* 134 (3): 309–323.

Latimer, K.S. and Rich, G.A. (1998). Colonic adenocarcinoma in a corn snake (*Elaphe guttata guttata*). *Journal of Zoo and Wildlife Medicine: Official Publication of the American Association of Zoo Veterinarians* 29 (3): 344–346.

Leary, S., Underwood, W., Anthony, R. et al. (2013). *AVMA Guidelines for the Euthanasia of Animals: 2013 Edition*. Schaumburg, IL: American Veterinary Medical Association.

Ledbetter, E.C., de Matos, R., Riedel, R.M. et al. (2017). Phacoemulsification of bilateral mature cataracts in a Texas rat snake (*Elaphe obsoleta lindheimeri*). *Journal of the American Veterinary Medical Association* 251 (11): 1318–1323.

Lindemann, D.M., Allender, M.C., Rzadkowska, M. et al. (2017). Pharmacokinetics, efficacy, and safety of voriconazole and itraconazole in healthy cottonmouths (*Agkistrodon piscivorus*) and massasauga rattlesnakes (*Sistrurus catenatus*) with snake fungal disease. *Journal of Zoo and Wildlife Medicine* 48 (3): 757–766.

Lock, B.A. (2000). Reproductive surgery in reptiles. *The Veterinary Clinics of North America. Exotic Animal Practice* 3 (3): 733–752.

Lorch, J.M., Lankton, J., Werner, K. et al. (2015). Experimental infection of snakes with *Ophidiomyces ophiodiicola* causes pathological changes that typify snake fungal disease. *MBio* 6 (6) https://doi.org/10.1128/mBio.01534-15.

Lunger, P.D., Hardy, W.D. Jr., and Clark, F. (1974). C-type virus particles in a reptilian tumor. *Journal of the National Cancer Institute* 52 (4): 1231–1235.

Maclean, B. and Raiti, P. (2004). Emergency care. In: *BSAVA Manual of Reptiles* (eds. S.J. Girling and P. Raiti), 65–66. Gloucester, UK: British Small Animal Veterinary Association.

Mader, D. (2002). Treating burns in reptiles, Proceedings TUFTS Animal Expo, Boston, MA.

Mahapatra, D., Reinhard, M., and Naikare, H.K. (2013). Adenovirus and cryptosporidium co-infection in a corn snake (*Elaphae guttata guttata*). *Journal of Zoo and Wildlife Medicine* 44 (1): 220–224.

Mans, C. and Braun, J. (2014). Update on common nutritional disorders of captive reptiles. *Veterinary Clinics: Exotic Animal Practice* 17 (3): 369–395.

Mariani, C.L. (2007). The neurologic examination and neurodiagnostic techniques for reptiles. *The Veterinary Clinics of North America. Exotic Animal Practice* 10 (3): 855–891.

Martin, J.C., Schelling, S.H., and Pokras, M.A. (1994). Gastric adenocarcinoma in a Florida indigo snake (*Drymarchon corais couperi*). *Journal of Zoo and Wildlife Medicine* 25 (1): 133–137.

Martinez-Silvestre, A., Mateo, J.A., and Pether, J. (2003). Electrocardiographic parameters in the Gomeran giant lizard, *Gallotia bravoana*. *Journal of Herpetological Medicine and Surgery* 13 (3): 22–26.

Mattison, C. (2006). *Snake – The Essential Visual Guide to the World of Snakes*. New York: DK Publishing.

McNulty, E. and Hoffman, R. (1995). Fibrosarcoma in a corn snake, *Elaphe guttata*. *Bulletin of the Association of Reptilian and Amphibian Veterinarians* 5 (3): 7–8.

Mehler, S.J. and Bennett, R.A. (2003). Oral, dental, and beak disorders of reptiles. *The Veterinary Clinics of North America. Exotic Animal Practice* 6 (3): 477–503.

Millichamp, N.J., Lawrence, K., Jacobson, E.R. et al. (1983). Egg retention in snakes. *Journal of the American Veterinary Medical Association* 183 (11): 1213.

Mitchell, M.A. (2004). Snake care and husbandry. *The Veterinary Clinics of North America. Exotic Animal Practice* 7 (2): 421–446.

Mitchell, M.A. (2009). Reptile cardiology. *The Veterinary Clinics of North America. Exotic Animal Practice* 12 (1): 65–79.

Mosley, C.A. (2005). Anesthesia and analgesia in reptiles. *Seminars in Avian and Exotic Pet Medicine* 14 (4): 243–262.

Muñoz-Gutiérrez, J.F., Garner, M.M., and Kiupel, M. (2016). Cutaneous chromatophoromas in captive snakes. *Veterinary Pathology* 53 (6): 1213–1219.

Murray, M.J. (2005). Pneumonia and lower respiratory tract diseases. In: *Reptile Medicine and Surgery*, 2e (ed. D.R. Mader), 865–877. St. Louis, MO: Saunders.

Nail, A. (2008). Does exposure to UVB light influence the growth rates and behaviour of hatchling Corn Snakes, *Pantherophis guttatus*? BI6154–Dissertation at Reaseheath College.

de la Navarre, B.J. (2006). Common procedures in reptiles and amphibians. *Veterinary Clinics: Exotic Animal Practice* 9 (2): 237–267.

Oliveri, M., Bartoskova, A., Spadola, F. et al. (2018). Method of semen collection and artificial insemination in snakes. *Journal of Exotic Pet Medicine* 27 (2): 75–80.

Paré, J.A. and Barta, J.R. (1997). Treatment of cryptosporidiosis in Gila monsters (*Heloderma suspectum*) with paromomycin. *Proceedings of the Association of Reptilian and Amphibian Veterinarians*: 23.

Pasmans, F., Blahak, S., Martel, A. et al. (2008). Introducing reptiles into a captive collection: the role of the veterinarian. *The Veterinary Journal* 175 (1): 53–68.

Pavlasek, I. and Ryan, U. (2008). *Cryptosporidium varanii* takes precedence over *C. saurophilum*. *Experimental Parasitology* 118 (3): 434–437.

Pees, M., Neul, A., Müller, K. et al. (2016). Virus distribution and detection in corn snakes (*Pantherophis guttatus*) after experimental infection with three different ferlavirus strains. *Veterinary Microbiology* 182: 213–222.

Penning, D.A. (2012). Growth rates and prey-handling behavior of hatchling corn snakes *Pantherophis guttatus* (Colubridae). Doctoral dissertation, University of Central Missouri.

Pereira, M.E. and Viner, T.C. (2008). Oviduct adenocarcinoma in some species of captive snakes. *Veterinary Pathology* 45 (5): 693–697.

Petterino, C., Bedin, M., Podestà, G. et al. (2006). Undifferentiated tumor in the ovary of a corn snake (*Elaphe guttata guttata*). *Veterinary Clinical Pathology* 35 (1): 95–100.

Pinto, F.F., Craveiro, H., Marrinhas, C. et al. (2018). What is your diagnosis? Multiple masses in a corn Snake (*Pantherophis guttatus*). *Veterinary Clinical Pathology*: 1–3. https://doi.org/10.1111/vcp.12687.

Plutzer, J. and Karanis, P. (2007). Molecular identification of a *Cryptosporidium saurophilum* from corn snake (*Elaphe guttata guttata*). *Parasitology Research* 101 (4): 1141–1145.

Rajeev, S., Sutton, D.A., Wickes, B.L. et al. (2009). Isolation and characterization of a new fungal species, *Chrysosporium ophiodiicola*, from a mycotic granuloma of a black rat snake (*Elaphe obsoleta obsoleta*). *Journal of Clinical Microbiology* 47 (4): 1264–1268.

Ramsay, E.C. and Dotson, T.K. (1995). Tissue and serum enzyme activities in the yellow rat snake (*Elaphe obsoleta quadrivitatta*). *American Journal of Veterinary Research* 56 (4): 423–428.

Rataj, A.V., Lindtner-Knific, R., Vlahović, K. et al. (2011). Parasites in pet reptiles. *Acta Veterinaria Scandinavica* 53 (1): 33.

Reavill, D. and Schmidt, R. (2003). Lipomas in corn snakes (Elaphe guttata guttata): a series of four cases. Proceedings of the Annual Conference of the Association Reptilian and Amphibian Veterinarians.

Richter, B., Nedorost, N., Maderner, A. et al. (2011). Detection of *Cryptosporidium* species in feces or gastric contents from snakes and lizards as determined by polymerase chain reaction analysis and partial sequencing of the 18S ribosomal RNA gene. *Journal of Veterinary Diagnostic Investigation* 23 (3): 430–435.

Roark, A.W. and Dorcas, M.E. (2000). Regional body temperature variation in corn snakes measured using temperature-sensitive passive integrated transponders. *Journal of Herpetology* 34 (3): 481–485.

Rosenthal, K.L. and Mader, D.R. (1996). Special topics: microbiology. In: *Reptile Medicine and Surgery* (ed. D.R. Mader), 119–125. Philadelphia: WB Saunders.

Rzadkowska, M., Allender, M.C., O'Dell, M. et al. (2016). Evaluation of common disinfectants effective against *Ophidiomyces ophiodiicola*, the causative agent of snake fungal disease. *Journal of Wildlife Diseases* 52 (3): 759–762.

Schilliger, L., Tessier, D., Pouchelon, J.L. et al. (2006). Proposed standardization of the two-dimensional echocardiographic examination in snakes. *Journal of Herpetological Medicine and Surgery* 16 (3): 76–87.

Schmidt, R.E. and Reavill, D.R. (2012). Metastatic chondrosarcoma in a corn snake (*Pantherophis guttatus*).

Journal of Herpetological Medicine and Surgery 22 (3): 67–69.

Schumacher, J. (2003). Reptile respiratory medicine. *The Veterinary Clinics of North America. Exotic Animal Practice* 6 (1): 213–231.

Scullion, F.T. and Scullion, M.G. (2009). Gastrointestinal protozoal diseases in reptiles. *Journal of Exotic Pet Medicine* 18 (4): 266–278.

Selleri, P. and Hernandez-Divers, S.J. (2006). Renal diseases of reptiles. *Veterinary Clinics: Exotic Animal Practice* 9 (1): 161–174.

Sievert, L.M., Jones, D.M., and Puckett, M.W. (2005). Postprandial thermophily, transit rate, and digestive efficiency of juvenile cornsnakes, *Pantherophis guttatus*. *Journal of Thermal Biology* 30 (5): 354–359.

Sigler, L., Hambleton, S., and Paré, J.A. (2013). Molecular characterization of reptile pathogens currently known as members of the *Chrysosporium* anamorph of *Nannizziopsis vriesii* complex and relationship with some human-associated isolates. *Journal of Clinical Microbiology* 51 (10): 3338–3357.

Sladky, K.K. and Mans, C. (2012). Clinical anesthesia in reptiles. *Journal of Exotic Pet Medicine* 21 (1): 17–31.

Sladky, K.K., Kinney, M.E., and Johnson, S.M. (2008). Analgesic efficacy of butorphanol and morphine in bearded dragons and corn snakes. *Journal of the American Veterinary Medical Association* 233 (2): 267–273.

Smith, D.A., Barker, I.K., and Allen, O.B. (1988). The effect of ambient temperature and type of wound on healing of cutaneous wounds in the common garter snake (*Thamnophis sirtalis*). *Canadian Journal of Veterinary Research* 52 (1): 120.

Stahl, S.J. (2002). Veterinary management of snake reproduction. *Veterinary Clinics: Exotic Animal Practice* 5 (3): 615–636.

Stahlschmidt, Z.R., French, S.S., Ahn, A. et al. (2017). A simulated heat wave has diverse effects on immune function and oxidative physiology in the corn snake (*Pantherophis guttatus*). *Physiological and Biochemical Zoology* 90 (4): 434–444.

Stumpel, J.B.G., Del-Pozo, J., French, A. et al. (2012). Cardiac hemangioma in a corn snake (*Pantherophis guttatus*). *Journal of Zoo and Wildlife Medicine* 43 (2): 360–366.

Sykes, J.M. (2010). Updates and practical approaches to reproductive disorders in reptiles. *Veterinary Clinics: Exotic Animal Practice* 13 (3): 349–373.

Sykes, J.M. IV, Schumacher, J., Avenell, J. et al. (2006). Preliminary evaluation of 99mTechnetium diethylenetriamine pentaacetic acid, 99mTechnetium dimercaptosuccinic acid, and 99mTechnetium mercaptoacetyltriglycine for renal scintigraphy in corn snakes (*Elaphe guttata guttata*). *Veterinary Radiology & Ultrasound* 47 (2): 222–227.

Tuttle, A.D., Harms, C.A., Van Wettere, A.J. et al. (2006). Splenic hemangiosarcoma in a corn snake, *Elaphe guttata*. *Journal of Herpetological Medicine and Surgery* 16 (4): 140–143.

Utiger, U., Helfenberger, N., Schätti, B. et al. (2002). Molecular systematics and phylogeny of Old and New World ratsnakes, *Elaphe* Auct., and related genera (Reptilia, Squamata, Colubridae). *Russian Journal of Herpetology* 9 (2): 105–124.

Werler, J.E. and Dixon, J.R. (2004). Corn snake. In: *Texas Snakes: Identification, Distribution and Natural History* (eds. J.E. Werler, J.R. Dixon and R. Levoy), 107–111. Austin, TX: University of Texas Press.

Whitehead, M. (2010). Permethrin toxicity in exotic pets. *The Veterinary Record* 166 (10): 306.

Whiteside, D.P. and Gamer, M.M. (2001). Thyroid adenocarcinoma in a crocodile lizard, *Shinisaurus crocodilurus*. *Journal of Herpetological Medicine and Surgery* 11 (1): 13–16.

Worthington-Hill, J.O., Yarnell, R.W., and Gentle, L.K. (2014). Eliciting a predatory response in the eastern corn snake (*Pantherophis guttatus*) using live and inanimate sensory stimuli: implications for managing invasive populations. *International Journal of Pest Management* 60 (3): 180–186.

Xiao, L., Ryan, U.M., Graczyk, T.K. et al. (2004). Genetic diversity of *Cryptosporidium* spp. in captive reptiles. *Applied and Environmental Microbiology* 70 (2): 891–899.

Yimming, B., Pattanatanang, K., Sanyathitiseree, P. et al. (2016). Molecular identification of *Cryptosporidium* species from pet snakes in Thailand. *The Korean Journal of Parasitology* 54 (4): 423.

Zwart, P. (2006). Renal pathology in reptiles. *The Veterinary Clinics of North America. Exotic Animal Practice* 9 (1): 129–159.

17

Boas and Pythons
Joanna Hedley

Boas and pythons are two of the most popular groups of non-venomous snakes kept in captivity, ranging in size from dwarf boas of only 30–60 cm in length, up to the Green anaconda (*Eunectes murinus*) and Reticulated python (*Python reticulatus*) which may reach over 8 m. However, despite considerable variation in size, lifestyle, and external appearance, all these snakes share a number of common anatomical characteristics. Both boas and pythons possess a vestigial pelvic girdle and hind limbs (seen externally as small spurs either side of the cloaca). Unlike many other snakes, most also have a left lung which can be up to 75% as large as the right lung.

Pythons can be differentiated from boas by several external features. Although both types of snakes can have heat-sensing pits (labial pits) lining the upper lip, in pythons these pits are positioned centrally in the scales, as opposed to boas where the pits are positioned between the scales if present. A python also possesses extra postfrontal bones and premaxillary teeth, whereas a boa lacks these. Finally, examination of the tail reveals an undivided subcaudal scute in a boa, compared to divided scutes in a python.

Biological and environmental parameters of commonly kept boa and python species are listed in Table 17.1.

17.1 Boas

The taxonomy of boas (Table 17.2) can be confusing due to a recent reclassification (Pyron et al. 2014), but currently boas can be divided into the following subfamilies as defined by the Reptile Database (Uetz et al. 2017). The natural habitat and lifestyle can vary considerably according to species as shown by the following examples;

- **Boa constrictors (*Boa constrictor* and *Boa imperator*)**

The Boa constrictor (often known as the Common or Red tailed boa) (Figure 17.1) originates from Central and South America, where it is found throughout a variety of habitats from dense rainforest to drier lowlands. It lives a moderately arboreal lifestyle and is mostly crepuscular or nocturnal, but appears very adaptable and is often found around human habitats where rodent prey is plentiful. A number of subspecies exist and reclassification is ongoing. The two most common boas kept in captivity are *Boa constrictor constrictor* and *Boa imperator* (previously *B. c imperator*). Both grow into large snakes, often at least 2–3 m in length and can live for 20–30 years in captivity.

- **Emerald tree boa (*Corallus caninus*)**

The Emerald tree boa as its name implies, lives an arboreal lifestyle, originating from the rainforests of South America where it is active at night. Juveniles have a distinctive brick-red to orange appearance, before gradually changing colour over a period of 12 months to the classic emerald green. In captivity, these snakes can be difficult to keep due to the challenges of mimicking their high humidity natural environment without compromising on temperature range or ventilation. They also appear easily stressed and have the reputation of a more aggressive temperament than some other boas.

- **Green anaconda (*Eunectes murinus*)**

The Green anaconda is found in the wetlands of South America where it lives a nocturnal lifestyle. The eyes and nares have a dorsal position on the anaconda's head allowing them to lie almost completely submerged to ambush prey. With a potential adult weight of >200 kg, the Green anaconda is the heaviest snake in the world and can overpower large prey animals including deer, wild pigs, and even caiman. These snakes can be challenging to keep in captivity due to their size and unpredictable nature.

Table 17.1 Biological parameters of selected species.

	Average adult weight	Average adult length	Average lifespan (years)	Geographical range	Lifestyle	Habitat	Preferred temperature range (°C)	Preferred humidity (%)	Feeding interval for adult
Boa constrictor (*Boa constrictor*)	10–25 kg	1.5–4 m	25–30	Central and South America	Terrestrial, semi-arboreal	Rainforest, lowlands	26–32	50–80	q2–3 weeks
Emerald tree boa (*Corallus caninus*)	1.5–2 kg	1.5–2 m	15–20	South America	Arboreal	Rainforest	25–35	60–80	q10 days–3 weeks
Green anaconda (*Eunectes murinus*)	50–75 kg but can reach >200 kg	5–6 m	20–25	South America	Mostly aquatic	Wetlands	26–32	60–90	q2–6 weeks
Rosy boa (*Lichanura trivirgata*)	300–600 g	60–120 cm	20–30	California, Arizona, and Mexico	Terrestrial	Desert, arid scrubland	25–30	30–50	q7–10 days
Reticulated python (*Python reticulatus*)	60–90 kg	3–6 m but can reach >7 m	15–25	South East Asia	Arboreal, terrestrial	Grasslands, rainforest, wetlands	26–32	50–80	q2–4 weeks
Royal python (*Python regius*)	1.3–1.8 kg	1–1.5 m	20–30	Central and Western Africa	Mostly terrestrial	Grasslands, forest	24–32	50–80	q10–14 days
Carpet python (*Morelia spilota*)	8–10 kg	1.5–3 m	15–25	New Guinea, Indonesia, Australia	Semi-arboreal	Rainforests, woodland	26–32	40–60	q2–3 weeks
Green tree python (*Morelia viridis*)	1.1–1.6 kg	1.2–1.8 m	15–20	New Guinea, Indonesia, Australia	Arboreal	Rainforest	24–32	40–70	q10 days–3 weeks

Table 17.2 Taxonomy of boas.

Family Boidae

Subfamily Boinae (Boas)	'True' boas including the Boa constrictor (*Boa constrictor*), Emerald tree boa (*Corallus caninus*), Rainbow boa (*Epicrates cenchria*) and Anacondas (*Eunectes* spp.)
Subfamily Ungaliophiinae	Dwarf boas
Subfamily Erycinae	Sand boas
Subfamily Calabariinae	African burrowing python (*Calabaria reinhardtii*)
Subfamily Candoiinae	South Pacific boas
Subfamily Sanziniinae	Madagascan ground and tree boas
Subfamily Charininae	Rosy boa (*Lichanura trivirgata*) and rubber boas (*Charina* spp.)
Family Bolyeriidae	Round Island Boas
Family Tropidophiidae	Another group of dwarf boas

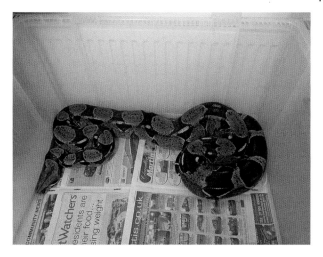

Figure 17.1 Common boa.

● Rosy boa (*Lichanura trivirgata*)

The Rosy boa is a small- to medium-sized boa recognised by its pattern of three wide black, brown, or orange stripes running along the body. Found throughout California, Arizona, and Mexico, mostly in desert or arid scrubland habitats, it lives a nocturnal lifestyle and rests the majority of the day hidden between rocks and crevices. As a smaller snake, predators are a significant threat, but unlike more aggressive boids, its defence tactic is to curl up in a ball with its head in the centre. Rosy boas therefore tend to make fairly docile pets in captivity although can be shy if unused to handling.

Boas are typically viviparous, giving birth to live young. Breeding seasons may be altered in captivity and gestation periods can vary according to species and external temperatures. However, examples for some of the common pet species are listed in Table 17.3.

17.2 Pythons (Family Pythonidae)

Pythons are found throughout the Old World in varying habitats and genera commonly kept are listed in Table 17.4 (Pyron et al. 2014). As with boas, natural habitat and lifestyle can vary considerably according to species as shown by the following examples.

● Royal python (*Python regius*)

Royal or ball pythons originate from Central and Western Africa, where they can be found in grasslands and forest habitats. They live a mostly terrestrial, nocturnal lifestyle, curling into a ball when threatened by predators such as

Table 17.3 Breeding information for selected boa species.

	Average gestation period (months)	Typical breeding season	Comments
Boa constrictor (*Boa constrictor*)	4–8	October–February	(Ross and Marzec 1990). Parthenogenesis reported (Booth et al. 2010)
Emerald tree boa (*Corallus caninus*)	6–7	January–June	(Ross and Marzec 1990)
Green anaconda (*Eunectes murinus*)	6–7	March–July	(Ross and Marzec 1990). Parthenogenesis reported (O'Shea et al. 2016)
Rosy boa (*Lichanura trivirgata*)	4–6	March–April	(Ross and Marzec 1990)
Brazilian Rainbow boa (*Epicrates cenchria cenchria*)	4–5	February–May	Parthenogenesis reported (Kinney et al. 2013)

Table 17.4   Python genera maintained in captivity.

Antaresia	Children's pythons
Apodora	Papuan python (*A. papuana*)
Aspidites	Black headed python (*A. melanocephalus*) and Woma (*A. ramsayi*)
Bothrochilus	Bismarck ringed python (*B. boa*)
Leiopython	White lipped python
Liasis	Water pythons
Morelia	Tree pythons including the Carpet python (*M. spilota*) and Green tree python (*M. viridis*)
Python	'True' pythons including the Royal python (*P. regius*), Reticulated python (*P. reticulatus*)

humans (Figure 17.2). They only grow to 1–1.5 m in length and are popular pets due to their manageable size and docile nature. Initially most individuals in the pet trade were wild-caught, but in subsequent years 'ranching' became more popular. This involves capture of gravid female snakes from their natural environment, and maintaining them in captivity until their eggs are laid. Eggs are then incubated and juveniles exported to the international market. Both capture of wild snakes and ranching methods carry significant welfare and health concerns. Nowadays, captive breeding supplies the majority of the pet population in the UK, with a huge demand for breeding numerous colour mutations or 'morphs'. Popular morphs include albino, leucistic, jungle, pinstripe, and spider varieties. Such specific breeding is associated with its own set of problems, in particular various genetic disorders. A classic example would be that of 'wobble syndrome' in the spider morph. Affected snakes may be seen with tremors, torticollis, ataxia, and reduced righting reflex and signs appear to be exaggerated during periods of increased activity such as feeding. Exact prevalence is uncertain, but it has been suggested that all individuals of this morph are affected to some degree (Rose and Williams 2014).

Reticulated python (*Python reticulatus*)

The Reticulated python originates from South East Asia, and is the longest snake species in the world with recorded lengths of over 9 m. Habitats are variable ranging from grasslands to rainforest, although they are often associated with rivers and lakes and are excellent swimmers. They naturally prey on a variety of mammals and birds in the wild and may be found around human habitats at times. In captivity, their size and unpredictable nature should not be underestimated.

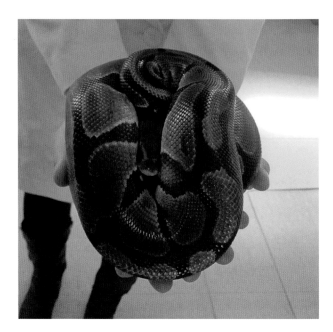

Figure 17.2   Royal or ball python demonstrating defensive behaviour.

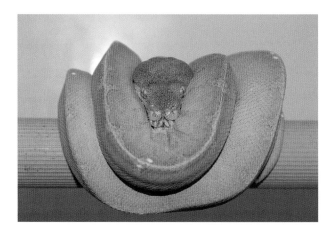

Figure 17.3   Green tree python (*Source:* Photo courtesy of Chris Mitchell).

Green tree python (*Morelia viridis*)

The Green tree python (Figure 17.3) originates from the rainforests of New Guinea, Indonesia, and Northern Australia, where it is active at night. Despite sharing a remarkably similar appearance and lifestyle to that of the South American Emerald tree boa, the two species have evolved completely separately to fit into their ecological niches. Green tree pythons can be distinguished from boas by differences in their heat sensing pits; green tree pythons only have pits within the first rostral scales, whereas in the boas they lie between the scales all along the upper lip. The juveniles of both species take time to develop the bright green adult colouration, but in green tree pythons the

Table 17.5 Breeding parameters for common python species (Ross and Marzec 1990).

	Typical breeding season	Oviposition	Incubation period (days)
Reticulated python (*Python reticulatus*)	September–November	December–May	86–95
Royal python (*Python regius*)	September–February	March–June	56–64
Carpet python (*Morelia spilota*)	December–March	March–June	49–72
Green tree python (*Morelia viridis*)	August–January	November–May	39–65
Burmese python (*Python molurus*)	November–February	February–May	58–63

hatchlings can have a bright yellow colouration which is never seen in the juvenile boas.

Pythons are oviparous; they reproduce by laying eggs. Breeding seasons may be altered in captivity and both gestation periods and incubation periods can vary according to species and external temperatures. Examples for some of the common pet species are listed in Table 17.5.

17.3 Husbandry

Boas and pythons need to be kept in a secure enclosure, adequate for their size. Whilst there are no legal minimum space requirements in UK, it is recommended that snakes are at least able to stretch out completely. This may be difficult to ensure for some of the larger snake species if kept in standard commercial vivaria or rack systems. Supervised exercise time in a secure room is therefore particularly encouraged for those snakes in smaller set ups. For terrestrial species (e.g. Kenyan Sand boa, *Eryx colubrinus*), the enclosure should be long and wide, whereas height is more important for the arboreal species (e.g. Emerald Tree Boa). Concerns are often raised that younger snakes or particularly shy species may be anxious in a large space. There is however, no evidence for this in either wild or captive snakes as and as long as plenty of hide areas are provided, enclosures should be as large as possible.

The enclosure itself should be well-ventilated, but also insulated to avoid excessive temperature fluctuation. This balance can be difficult to achieve especially in species which require a higher level of humidity. A primary background heat source should be used to provide a general minimum temperature. This may be a heat mat, ceramic heat source, reptile radiator, or background room heating. A secondary heat source such as a basking lamp can then be placed at one end of the enclosure to create a temperature gradient, allowing the snake to move to its chosen temperature within a set range. This secondary heat source should be turned off at night, mimicking the natural temperature decrease. Heat sources should be controlled by a thermostat and maximum and minimum temperatures carefully monitored. Care should be taken to protect the snake from direct contact with the heat source to avoid burn injuries, for example by placing a heat mat on the external wall of the enclosure rather than the floor, or applying a guard around the lamp. Each species will have a slightly different natural temperature range (see Table 17.1) and this should be replicated in captivity.

Many boa and python species are crepuscular or nocturnal and ultraviolet (UV) light requirements have not been established (Hedley and Eatwell 2013). However addition of a UVA/B light has been suggested to have behavioural benefits even if snakes are only emerging from hide areas at dawn and dusk when UV levels are less intense. Photoperiods should ideally mimic those in the wild (on average 12 hours light per day) and output of lights should be monitored weekly or lights changed regularly according to manufacturer's guidelines. Care should be taken to avoid higher intensity lights and give the opportunity to hide as many of these snake species will not naturally be exposed to strong sunlight in the wild (Gardiner et al. 2009).

The enclosure may need to be sprayed or misted multiple times over the course of a day to maintain humidity levels and these should be monitored using a hygrometer. For those species requiring particularly high humidity levels, automated misting systems can be useful.

On the floor, substrate should be provided which should be easy to clean and non-irritating. The ideal choice will depend on the species; whether they need a dry or humid environment and how much they exhibit burrowing behaviour. Aromatic substrates such as cedar chip should always be avoided due to risks of respiratory and skin irritation. The enclosure should be spot cleaned whenever urates or faeces are passed, in addition to regular substrate changes and cleaning using a reptile-specific disinfectant. Finally, appropriate furniture should be provided to allow hiding areas at both the hotter and cooler ends, in addition to opportunities to bask, burrow, or climb depending on species preference.

Natural diet may vary depending on species, but all boas and pythons eat whole prey. In captivity this is generally replicated by the feeding of pre-killed rodents, or rabbits for the larger individuals. It is important that these food animals are themselves healthy and in good nutritional status. If frozen, they should be defrosted properly and warmed before being fed. Owners may choose to feed their snake in a separate enclosure so that snakes do not associate the opening of their vivarium door with food being placed inside. This minimises the risk of accidental owner injury and also avoids the risk of inadvertent substrate ingestion for the snake. However, more nervous individuals may not feed in less familiar surroundings so routines may need to be adapted accordingly. The feeding of live vertebrate prey is never recommended, as it results in a highly stressful death for the prey species and also puts the snake at risk of injuries from rodent attack.

Feeding frequency will depend on snake size, age, reproductive status, and activity levels. Obesity is a commonly seen problem in captivity as wild lifestyles are generally less sedentary and food availability is less reliable. Recommendations vary from every one to two weeks for smaller boas or pythons to every one to two months for larger individuals. Although snakes can physically ingest extremely large food items, ideally they should be fed prey of a size that is approximately the width of the widest part of the snake's body.

Species should not be mixed, due to varying husbandry requirements, the potential for aggression, and potential susceptibility to pathogens that may be carried asymptomatically by another species. However if mixing is necessary, only those from the same geographical origins should be kept together to minimise potential for differing husbandry requirements or exposure to novel pathogens (Varga 2004).

17.4 Clinical Evaluation

17.4.1 History-Taking

In addition to a full medical history, an extensive husbandry and diet assessment should always be collected, as many health concerns can be secondary to environmental or nutritional deficits. Husbandry questionnaires can be useful to ensure no details are missed. If the owner keeps records of feeding, weights, or shedding or has photos of the enclosure these should also be provided.

17.4.2 Handling

Small boa or python species can easily be handled by one person, but for larger snakes of over 5 ft, at least two handlers will be necessary. Well-handled snakes can usually be gently scooped out of their enclosure. The snake should be held so that its body is fully supported. Larger more aggressive snakes may require a snake hook for initial capture. The head should then be restrained and the rest of the body supported. Salmonellosis is a potential zoonotic risk, so protective gloves may be considered and good hygiene is vital.

17.4.3 Sex Determination

Male and female boas and pythons may be distinguished by their external appearance once mature. Males usually have a longer thinner tail with larger cloacal spurs, whereas females have a shorter broader tail and smaller spurs. However, cloacal probing is usually used to confirm gender more objectively. A small well-lubricated blunt metal snake sexing probe is inserted into the cloaca towards the tail. In a male snake, this probe should pass into the hemipene pocket to a depth of six or more scales, whereas in a female the probe will pass fewer than six scales.

17.4.4 Clinical Examination

Clinical examination should ideally begin with indirect observation of the snake within its enclosure or transport container if possible. If the individual's behaviour is a concern, owners should be encouraged to bring in videos of their snake displaying the abnormal behaviour. Respiratory rate and effort can be observed, although are likely to vary depending on external temperature and stress levels. Locomotion and neurological status can also be assessed.

Next a full head to tail examination can be performed. Eyes should be assessed to check that the spectacles are clear and smooth. Nares should be checked for any signs of discharge. The face should appear symmetrical. Examination of the oral cavity may be performed at this point or left until later in the procedure as it is often resented by the snake. A thin folded layer of paper or card may be inserted into the diastema at the rostral extent of the mouth and used as a gag to encourage the snake to open its mouth. The mucous membranes, dentition, and the glottis may then be fully assessed. Auscultation can be challenging in snakes as sounds may not transmit well via a standard stethoscope. However the apex beat of the heart may be visualised externally on the ventral body wall and a Doppler probe can be used to listen to the heart beat if there are any concerns. The ventral surface of the snake may then be palpated for any masses or swellings. The skin should be thoroughly examined for any lesions such as burns or other traumatic injuries or mites. The cloaca should be checked for any prolapses. All snakes should be weighed at every examination.

17.5 Basic Techniques

17.5.1 Sample Collection

Blood samples can be taken from the ventral tail vein or via cardiocentesis. The ventral tail vein is preferred, but is a blind technique and the short broad tail of many boas and pythons can make this more challenging than in other snake species. Cardiocentesis may be performed following observation of the apex beat or by using a Doppler probe to locate the heart (Figure 17.4). Although generally considered a 'safe' technique, sampling can be resented and cardiac tamponade has been reported leading to death in one case (Isaza et al. 2004; Selleri and Girolamo 2012). Therefore, sedation may be considered to minimise stress and movement, especially if other diagnostics are also due to be performed. Blood volume of a reptile is approximately 5–8% of bodyweight so 0.5 ml blood per 100 g bodyweight can be safely taken. Blood should be placed into a heparin tube if only a small sample is available and submitted to a laboratory that is experienced in interpreting reptile samples. Manual haematology is necessary as nucleated erythrocytes cause erroneous results in automated counts. Interpreting both haematology and biochemistry results can be challenging, due at least in part to the lack of data for many species, and the wide variation in 'reference ranges' for others. Many of the 'reference ranges' are in fact based on small sample sizes, and sometimes a mixture of both clinically normal and subclinically abnormal speci-mens. Results may also be affected by a number of variables including age, sex, reproductive status, temperature, season, nutritional status, and stress. Serial blood sampling may therefore be necessary to identify significant variations for an individual.

Faecal samples may be collected and checked for endoparasites including *Cryptosporidium* if there is any suspicion of gastrointestinal disease. Faecal culture and sensitivity may be considered in select cases, but is not routinely performed as results are often unhelpful. Many snakes have been found to carry *Salmonella* spp. as part of their commensal intestinal flora and although this has potential zoonotic implications, it rarely seems to cause a problem for the snake unless intestinal integrity is compromised.

17.5.2 Fluid Therapy

Fluid requirements for snakes are generally considered to be lower than for mammals of the same weight, due to their lower metabolic rate. Volumes of 15–30 ml/kg/day are recommended and fluid types are similar to those used in mammals. Fluids are normally administered only once or twice daily as absorption is slow and handling may be stressful. The following routes can be considered:

Bathing – some snakes may choose to drink when placed in a warm water bath and allowed to almost completely submerge. Care should be taken to ensure the snake is able to hold its head up and bathing should be supervised.

Oral route – fluids may be administered via a lubricated stomach tube (a urinary catheter or similar soft flexible tube can be used). The tube should be pre-measured to the level of the stomach (located approximately half way between head and vent), the mouth gently opened using an atraumatic gag and the tube gently passed caudally with the snake supported in an upright position. Initially a smaller volume is administered and if tolerated then larger volumes up to 3% body weight can be given.

Subcutaneous route – snakes have minimal subcutaneous space so large volumes cannot be given by this route. Absorption is best when administered via the lateral sinuses, which are located between the epaxial muscles dorsally and the ribs ventrally. Warming fluids or adding hyaluronidase also appears to increase absorption.

Intravenous route – intravenous jugular catheterisation is possible, but requires general anaesthesia for a cut down technique for placement so is not routinely performed.

17.5.3 Nutritional Support

If clinically well snakes are not eating voluntarily, a full review of the environment and feeding strategies should

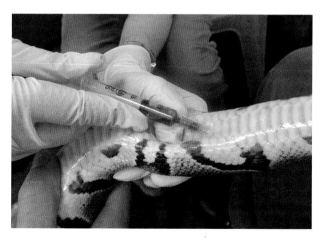

Figure 17.4 Cardiocentesis for collection of a blood sample.

however be considered to encourage the snake to start eating again. Tricks can include;

- Ensuring that the snake is completely undisturbed when presented with food – many snakes will not eat when observed
- Varying the time of day that food is presented – pythons are naturally more likely to eat at night time
- Feeding in a separate small dark secluded hide, pillow case or similar, within the vivarium. Pythons are ambush predators, feeding on rodents who pass into their burrows in the wild
- Varying the food type or size e.g. albino rodents are not always perceived as a recognisable food source and brown rats may be better accepted
- Feeding recently killed prey or moving the prey in front of the snake using long forceps can stimulate interest.

Royal pythons have a reputation for poor appetites and can be difficult to get feeding consistently in captivity. Traditionally this was more of a problem in wild-caught individuals who were more nervous in their new captive environment and did not appear to recognise the unfamiliar laboratory rodent prey offered. However even with captive bred individuals appetite can be variable. This may be due to stress, seasonal changes, overfeeding, or potentially underlying disease. It is therefore important to maintain accurate feeding and weight records. If maintaining weight and otherwise clinically well, a short period of anorexia may not be a cause for concern.

Adult boas and pythons can survive for long periods without eating but if beginning to lose weight will eventually need nutritional support. Animals should always be hydrated prior to feeding to prevent any risks of refeeding syndrome. There are various powdered food types specifically available for exotic carnivore species. Alternatively cat or dog recovery formulas may be used in the short-term. These may be mixed with water and administered by stomach tube as for fluids. Volumes and frequencies will depend on individual's weight and the manufacturer's guidelines. However, multiple repeat force feeding should be avoided if possible as the stress of frequent interventions may discourage the snake from eating voluntarily. Every effort should be made to try to encourage voluntary eating.

17.5.4 Anaesthesia

Anaesthesia of boas and pythons can be a time-consuming process. Pre-anaesthetic stabilisation is vital, with the patient warmed to an appropriate temperature, rehydrated, and any underlying diseases addressed if possible. Ideally the snake should also not have been fed for at least three days prior to the anaesthetic as regurgitation is possible.

Analgesia should always be provided for any potentially painful procedure. Unfortunately pain in snakes can be difficult to recognise and consequently the efficacy of analgesics is currently uncertain. Feeding behaviour has been suggested as a potential method of assessing pain in royal pythons, but there are many other factors that may also affect failure to eat including the temperament of certain royal pythons who can be known for their variable feeding habits (James et al. 2017). Any change from the individual's normal behaviour, whether that be appetite, activity levels, or temperament should therefore be taken into account when trying to assess level of potential pain.

Due to the lack of data regarding analgesic efficacy, multimodal analgesia is usually recommended. Pre-operative administration of meloxicam has been evaluated in royal pythons and although no side-effects were reported, no evidence of actual analgesic effect was established (Olesen et al. 2008). NSAIDS may however be used for their anti-inflammatory properties, as snakes have been shown to possess both COX-1 and COX-2 enzymes (Sadler et al. 2016). Opioids have also been evaluated, both kappa and full mu agonists, but again no evidence of analgesic effect has been proven in boid or python species. Mu agonists appear the most clinically useful in other reptile groups and it is thought that transdermal fentanyl patches may have some use for delivering fentanyl to the bloodstream in snakes at what is generally considered to be clinically effective in other species (Darrow et al. 2016). However again, no actual evidence of analgesic effect has been established at this stage (Kharbush et al. 2017). More recent research has evaluated the effect of dexmedetomidine on ball pythons (Bunke et al. 2018). Results appear promising with dexmedetomidine causing increased noxious thermal withdrawal latency without causing excessive sedation. However, use in clinical cases has not yet been evaluated. Finally although efficacy is uncertain, local anaesthetics should also be considered for any surgical procedures as physiologically their mode of action should be similar to that in other species.

Following stabilisation, sedation or general anaesthesia may be performed. Gaseous induction within a chamber is an option for very small patients, but ideally injectable agents are preferred prior to the administration of gaseous agents to provide a faster, less stressful induction and more stable anaesthetic. Drugs may be administered either via the intramuscular (Figure 17.5) or intravenous route (ventral tail vein). Intracardiac administration of propofol has been reported, but other routes are preferable if possible (McFadden et al. 2011a). Propofol and alfaxalone are two of the most commonly used anaesthetic agents and usually provide sufficient sedation to allow intubation. Alternatively combinations of sedatives such as alpha-2

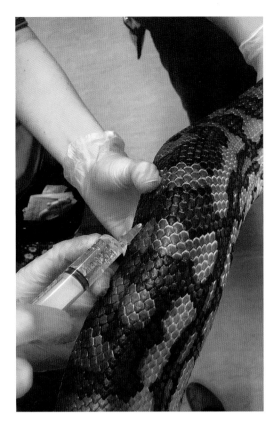

Figure 17.5   Intramuscular injection of alfaxalone for sedation.

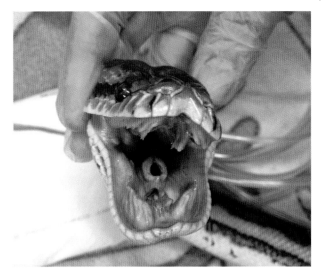

Figure 17.6   The glottis is readily visualised for intubation, the smaller and more rostral tongue sheath should be avoided.

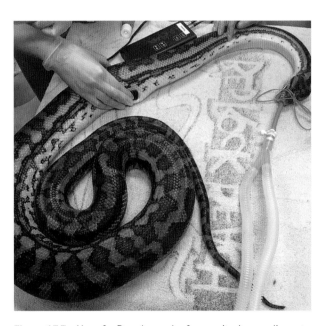

Figure 17.7   Use of a Doppler probe for monitoring cardiac rate and rhythm under anaesthesia.

agonists or midazolam plus ketamine may be administered via intramuscular injection, although effects appear more variable. Intubation is usually straightforward as the glottis can be easily visualised (Figure 17.6). Long, narrow uncuffed endotracheal tubes (or adapted urinary catheters) should be used to avoid tracheal damage. Once intubated, snakes may then be maintained on gaseous anaesthesia with isoflurane or sevoflurane most commonly used.

Intermittent positive pressure ventilation is usually required (either manually or mechanically) as spontaneous ventilation relies on active muscle movements which are suppressed under general anaesthesia. Initially high concentrations of gaseous agents (4–5% isoflurane or 6–8% sevoflurane) and higher than normal respiratory rates are likely to be necessary to ensure surgical anaesthesia. However, once the appropriate depth of anaesthesia has been established by lack of response to surgical stimulation, both ventilation rates and gaseous agent concentrations can be reduced. Response to changes in anaesthetic concentration are slow, so anaesthetic gas may be turned off prior to the end of the procedure to avoid a prolonged recovery. When ventilating, care should be taken not to overinflate the lungs. Depth of each ventilation should be visually observed, compared to normal breathing movements, and pressures kept <10–15 mmHg.

Anaesthetic monitoring can be challenging especially if controlling ventilation, as many of the monitoring devices used on other species are unreliable in snakes. Heart rate and rhythm can be monitored by taping a Doppler probe over the heart (Figure 17.7) or by watching the apex beat. Temperature can be monitored using a deep cloacal probe, but due to their poikilothermic nature, an anaesthetised snake's temperature is likely to be close to that of the room temperature which should be kept warm (~25–30 °C) throughout the procedure. Depth of anaesthesia can be difficult to assess as heart rate often does not change, but a positive reaction to tail pinch usually indicates a reduction in anaesthetic depth as snakes tend to recover tail first. Alternatively running a hand firmly down the side of the snake may elicit a reaction if at a light plane of anaesthesia (the Bauchstreich response) (Redrobe 2004).

Additional monitoring aids such as pulse oximetry or capnography may be used to help establish trends, but absolute figures are unlikely to be accurate. Oscillometric blood pressure monitoring has been evaluated in various boa and python species with a cuff placed around the tail immediately distal to the vent. Measurements were however found to be unreliable when compared to direct blood pressure recording (Chinnadurai et al. 2009). Unfortunately direct blood pressure monitoring involves cut down methods to cannulate a large artery so is not likely to be practical in most cases.

Recovery from anaesthesia can often be prolonged due to a snake's slow metabolic rate. Unlike mammals, the respiratory drive is thought to be more sensitive to hypoxia (which stimulates respiratory rate) rather than hypercapnia (which stimulates tidal volume) (Redrobe 2004). Recovering snakes are therefore usually ventilated with room air rather than 100% oxygen. Increasing temperature will also increase tidal volume, so maintaining a suitable environmental temperature and additional warming aids such as the use of a hairdryer can be helpful. However care should be taken not to warm the animal excessively without providing adequate ventilation as oxygen demand will increase with temperature. Care should also be taken to avoid burn injuries caused by aggressive heating in the immobile animal. Extubation should only occur when normal voluntary breathing is occurring and jaw tone has returned. Anaesthetic monitoring should be continued until the animal is consistently moving around and can be returned to their enclosure.

17.5.5 Euthanasia

Euthanasia should ideally be performed by an intravenous overdose of an anesthetic agent (e.g. pentobarbitone) (Leary et al. 2013). If intravenous access is not possible, the intracardiac route should be used ideally following sedation or anaesthesia. Complete death (as defined by loss of brainstem activity) may be difficult to confirm, so once the animal appears to have lost all reflexes and the heart beat is no longer audible using a Doppler probe, pithing should be performed to destroy the brain. This may be either via the oral cavity or occipital route.

17.5.6 Hospitalisation Requirements

Snakes should be housed in a secure vivarium which can be easily cleaned between patients. Plastic vivaria with newspaper substrate are often favoured in a clinical setting. Temperature range and humidity should be controlled as

appropriate for the species. A hide should be provided and this may either be a disposable cardboard box or one from the home setting that will be familiar to the snake. Arboreal species require secure raised branch structures.

Inpatients should be examined and weighed daily, although treatment frequencies may need to be minimised if animals are not accustomed to frequent handling.

17.6 Common Medical and Surgical Conditions

Boas and pythons can be presented to the veterinary clinic for a variety of reasons, but clinical signs are often non-specific, for example, lethargy or anorexia. Behavioural changes such as anorexia may occur naturally at certain times of year, during periods of reproductive activity (Table 17.5) or ecdysis. These normal patterns must be differentiated from anorexia as a sign of underlying disease. Long periods of anorexia however, may lead to weight loss and predispose to hepatic lipidosis in previously obese individuals (Simpson and Langenburg 2006). A detailed history, physical examination, and diagnostic work up are, therefore, often necessary to establish the underlying problem.

17.6.1 Stomatitis

Stomatitis is a common problem in captive boas and pythons and often associated with respiratory infections. Owners may have noticed facial swellings or gingival discolouration (Figure 17.8), or alternatively reluctance to feed may be the only clinical sign. Predisposing factors include suboptimal environmental temperatures, poor hygiene, or trauma. Inflammation and secondary infection then occur, in particular an overgrowth of commensal Gram negative bacteria such as *Pseudomonas, Aeromonas, Proteus* and *Escherichia coli*, and a variety of anaerobes (Draper et al. 1981; Stewart 1990; Steeil et al. 2013). On clinical examination, gingival mucosa may appear inflamed or discoloured and excess mucus can be visualised within the oral cavity. A sample should be taken from the oral cavity for bacterial and fungal culture and sensitivity to guide antimicrobial choice. If swelling appears severe, further investigations such as radiography and biopsy for histopathology may also be necessary. Atypical infections such as *Mycobacterium chelonei* may initially present as stomatitis and a number of different oral tumours have also been reported in various boa and python species (Quesenberry et al. 1986; Thompson et al. 2015). Treatment usually involves a combination of topical and systemic antibiotics in addition to correcting any underlying husbandry deficits. Anti-inflammatories should be considered as this is

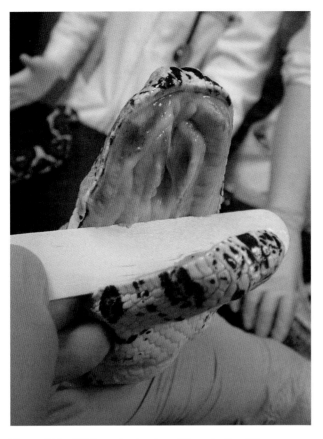

Figure 17.8   Mild–moderate stomatitis, note the diffuse gingival oedema and focal erythema.

tomography (CT) is particularly useful to avoid superimposition of skeletal structures allowing more subtle lesions to be detected (Pees et al. 2007). Microbiology samples may be collected via a tracheal wash or performed endoscopically (as described later). Treatment usually involves a prolonged course of systemic antimicrobial therapy (from two weeks up to several months). Nebulisation can also be effective in combination with systemic treatment.

Tracheal obstructions should be considered in dyspnoeic patients that fail to respond to standard therapeutics. Obstructions may occur following ongoing infections, or in royal pythons, tracheal chondromas should be considered as a potential differential (Penner et al. 1997; Drew et al. 1999). Masses may be detected by radiography or CT, although tracheoscopy is necessary to obtain samples for histopathology. Surgical resection of the affected portion of the trachea and subsequent anastomosis has been reported to have successful outcomes in some cases (Diethelm et al. 1996). Alternatively, proliferative tracheitis associated with bacterial infections may also result in partial or complete obstructions. Saccular lung cannulation may be required to allow ventilation and can be maintained in place for one to two weeks until the tracheal pathology has been resolved (Myers et al. 2009).

17.6.3   Cardiac Conditions

Cardiac disease is not uncommon in boas and pythons and may be seen in association with respiratory or systemic signs. A variety of pathologies including endocarditis, myocarditis, and restrictive cardiomyopathy have all been reported, ultimately resulting in congestive heart failure (Rishniw and Carmel 1999; Schilliger et al. 2003; Wernick et al. 2015; Schilliger et al. 2016). Alternatively, congenital defects can also be found (Jensen and Wang 2009). Diagnosis can be challenging as minimal clinical signs are evident until disease is advanced. Owners may report lethargy, anorexia, weight loss, or dyspnoea. Auscultation using a standard stethoscope is limited, but on clinical examination, an enlarged heart may be visualised. Radiography can be used to rule out other more common problems and to assess cardiac size. The administration of barium into the oesophagus can help highlight the cardiac silhouette but size may vary post-prandially (Zerbe et al. 2011). Echocardiography however is the diagnostic tool of choice for cardiac disease and standard techniques have been reported for performing an echocardiographic examination in boas and pythons (see Section 17.7). If cardiac disease is detected, treatment options are similar to those for dogs and cats, but efficacy and dose regimens of medications are not known in reptiles. In theory, frusemide should have limited effect in reptiles, as its main site of

potentially a very painful condition. Supportive feeding may also be required, especially if the animal has not eaten for some time.

17.6.2   Respiratory Conditions

Respiratory infections can often be seen in association with stomatitis, or as a sole concern. Owners may report wheezing, clicking sounds, bubbles from the mouth or nares, or have seen the snake resting in abnormal postures, often stretched out. Alternatively, lethargy and anorexia may be the only clinical signs. Inadequate temperatures, poor hygiene, and poor ventilation may all predispose to the overgrowth of commensal bacteria or fungi within the respiratory tract. However, atypical bacterial infections such as mycobacteriosis, fungal pathogens, or viral infections such as ophidian paramyxovirus or nidovirus should also be considered, especially if a new snake has been added to the collection in recent months (Hernandez-Divers and Shearer 2002; Miller et al. 2004; Uccellini et al. 2014). The diagnostic approach may include imaging to establish location and extent of disease and sampling for cytology, culture, and sensitivity and viral screens. Computed action, the loop of Henlé is absent. However, in practice it does appear useful for reducing oedema. Unfortunately treatment is often just palliative before euthanasia becomes necessary.

17.6.4 Neurological Conditions

Neurological problems in boas and pythons can occur for a variety of reasons and obtaining a definitive diagnosis pre-mortem can be challenging. Neurological examination and diagnostic tests can be difficult to perform or interpret due to anatomical and physiological limitations, as well as patient size or temperament. There are however two significant viral infections that may be associated with neurological signs in these species; Ophidian paramyxovirus (oPMV) and arenavirus (the aetiological agent for inclusion body disease [IBD]). Other viruses such as Sunshine virus are also emerging as potential pathogens in pythons which may become more significant (Hyndman et al. 2012).

oPMV may result in a variety of neurological signs including torticollis, stargazing, a reduced righting reflex, and eventually death. Respiratory and gastrointestinal signs may also be seen (Orós et al. 2001). Alternatively, some individuals appear totally asymptomatic. Transmission is mainly by direct contact with respiratory secretions but also potentially via snake mites. Diagnosis has historically been based on repeat serological testing or post-mortem examination. Nowadays however PCR testing of choanal or cloacal swabs is preferred. Treatment is supportive only so euthanasia should be considered for clinically affected animals.

IBD may result in neurological signs similar to oPMV and is prevalent in captive boas and pythons (Chang et al. 2016). However in boas, neurological signs usually only occur at the terminal stage of disease, often following a period of regurgitation and gradual weight loss. In pythons, neurological signs can be seen at an early stage and the disease appears to progress more quickly. The exact aetiology was unknown until recently, but appears to be due to an arenavirus (Hetzel et al. 2013). Diagnosis has historically been based on histopathology with biopsies taken from multiple organs to increase the chances of detecting the characteristic intracytoplasmic inclusion bodies. Liver, kidney, and oesophageal tonsil biopsies are the best ante-mortem samples or alternatively brain and pancreas post-mortem. A PCR test is now available to screen for arenavirus infection from a blood sample and an oesophageal swab. As with paramyxovirus, treatment is supportive only and euthanasia should be considered.

In younger snakes, congenital abnormalities can also be seen. 'Wobble syndrome' appears relatively common in spider morphs of royal pythons. A caudal coiling syndrome

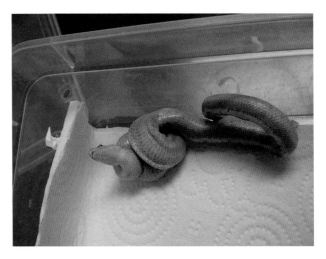

Figure 17.9 Congenital coiling deformity in a rosy boa.

has also been described in hatchling boa constrictors (Fitzgerald et al. 1990) and has been seen by the author in rosy boas (Figure 17.9). Under anaesthesia, the coils could be straightened out, but in conscious animals the muscles contracted to permanently coil in the caudal half. The condition appears progressive with no effective treatment and the pathogenesis not fully understood.

17.6.5 Reproductive Disease

Both pre- and post-ovulatory dystocia may be seen in boas and pythons, although post-ovulatory dystocia is the most common presentation, especially in oviparous pythons. Predisposing factors include lack of a suitable nesting site, stress, inappropriate nutrition, or other underlying disease. Snakes may appear lethargic, anorexic, or begin to pass eggs but not complete parturition. If the process has not been completed within 48–72 hours, dystocia is suspected. Eggs may often be palpable or even visible in the caudal third of the body as soft oval masses. Treatment may be as simple as correcting any underlying stressors in the environment, and providing a warm, secluded nesting area. Warm water bathing may also be useful. However, often by the time animals are presented, more invasive treatment is required. One option is sedation and manual manipulation of eggs to gently ease them out of the cloaca. There are however, risks to this approach with oviduct prolapse or rupture being a possible consequence. If possible, saline insufflation of the oviduct and removal of the eggs under endoscopic guidance is preferred. After the procedure the oviduct can then be examined again to confirm there has been no iatrogenic trauma. Alternatively in some cases, surgical removal of the eggs or whole reproductive tract may be necessary via a standard coeliotomy approach as described later (Patterson and Smith 1979).

Boas are ovoviviparous and give birth to fully formed neonates. Signs of dystocia may be less pronounced. Radiography of snakes with clinical signs, or that have exceeded the expected gestation period, can help with assessment. The foetuses should be individually coiled within their membranes but with dystocia membrane rupture often occurs with foetal uncoiling evident on radiographs (Figure 17.10). Caesarian section is necessary in this situation (Figure 17.11).

17.6.6   Skin Conditions

The structure of a snake's skin is vastly different to that of mammals or birds with skin being regularly shed in one piece throughout an individual's life (ecdysis). Dysecdysis (difficulty shedding) generally occurs secondary to husbandry deficits such as inappropriate environmental temperatures or humidity, or malnutrition. Alternatively, it may be seen secondary to dermatological disease such as ectoparasites, bacterial or fungal infections, or traumatic injuries (White et al. 2011). Treatment is usually fairly simple and involves increasing environmental humidity, warm water baths, and gentle manipulation of retained skin with a wet cotton bud to aid removal. Retained skin should never be pulled off with excessive force as underlying tissues may be easily damaged. Problem areas (e.g. areas of scarring or retained spectacles) may need treatment over several consecutive sheds.

Snake mites (*Ophionyssus natricis*) are the most common ectoparasite seen and will infest any snake species. They can be particularly hard to eliminate as mites do not spend their entire life cycle on the snake, but have several resting non-feeding stages (Wozniak and DeNardo 2000). Owners may physically see mites on their snake or in the environment. Mites are a brown-black colour and are commonly found between scales especially around the eyes, mouth,

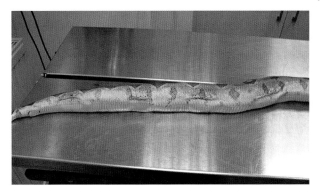

Figure 17.11   Multiple incisions required for caesarean section to remove foetuses from the snake shown in Figure 17.10.

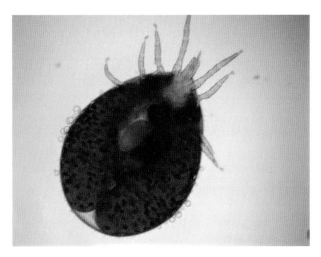

Figure 17.12   *Ophionyssus natricis* mite.

and cloaca. Identification of mites on a tape strip confirms diagnosis (Figure 17.12). In the environment they may be found in dark moist places such as wood décor or vivarium joints. Alternatively, snakes may be noted to spend more time soaking in the water bowl, presumably to relieve

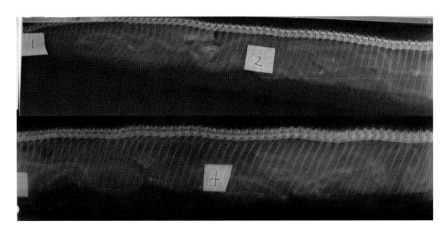

Figure 17.10   Lateral radiographs of a boa with prolonged gestation. Note the uncoiling of foetuses consistent with membrane rupture and dystocia.

irritation caused by the mites. As well as dysecdysis, mites can also cause more serious problems such as anaemia and have been suggested to be involved in the transmission of some infectious diseases (e.g. oPMV). Various treatments are available although fipronil and ivermectin are the most common choices. Care should be taken to avoid overdosage, especially when treating smaller individuals. Concurrent treatment of the environment is vital to prevent recontamination, although infections can be difficult to eliminate especially from wooden vivaria. All substrate should be discarded and replaced with paper which can be changed daily. All cage furniture should also be discarded if it cannot be completely cleaned and disposable hides such as cardboard boxes used until the infection has cleared. Vivaria may be treated with the same parasiticides as those used on the animal, but should be allowed to air fully before the reptile is returned to this environment. Alternatively predatory mites may be used as a form of biological control, for example in collections where chemical treatment is undesirable (Schilliger et al. 2013).

Burns are another common dermatological presentation, either due to the use of inappropriate heat devices in the vivarium or a device malfunction (Figure 17.13). All heat-ing devices should be well protected from direct contact with snakes who often appear poor at perceiving thermal pain (especially if the rest of their body is not warm), so will not move away from excessive heat. Burns can consequently be deep and extensive. Burn injuries should be gently washed under cool water and analgesia provided. If superficial, then application of a topical treatment (e.g. silver sulphadiazine) may be sufficient, but if deeper then thorough flushing, topical and systemic antibiotic treatment, and bandaging may be necessary. Fluid loss from a burn can be significant so rehydration should be considered. Secondary infection is common so antibiotic cover should also be provided and substrate changed to clean paper that will minimise contamination of any open wounds. Healing can be prolonged and scarring is likely.

17.6.7 Musculoskeletal Conditions

Proliferative spinal osteopathy is associated with new bone formation and bridging of vertebrae and has been reported in a variety of species, although often the exact cause is difficult to establish. Suggested aetiologies include bacterial or viral infection, trauma, hypovitaminosis D, hypervitaminosis A, neoplasia, or prolonged inactivity (Fitzgerald and Vera 2006). Snakes may be presented with limited movement or visible spinal swellings. Bony proliferation may be seen on radiography, although advanced imaging modalities will provide more information and can be particularly helpful to plan sites to biopsy (Di Girolamo et al. 2014; Hedley and Volk 2015). Samples should be submitted for both culture and histopathology. Antimicrobial treatment and analgesics may provide some palliative support, but this is often a progressive condition and euthanasia may need to be considered.

Spinal problems such as osteoarthrosis or osteoarthritis often occur in older individuals and may present in similar fashion but pathology remains localised to a small area.

17.6.8 Ocular Conditions

A variety of ocular conditions are encountered in boas and pythons, including retained spectacles, pseudobuphthalmos, subspectacular abscesses, trauma, cataracts, congenital microophthalmia and anophthalmia (Hausmann et al. 2013; Da Silva et al. 2015). In one study, *Epicrates* spp. appeared to have a higher prevalence of ocular lesions than other species, in particular retained spectacles, although the reason for this was unclear (Hausmann et al. 2013).

Generally principles of ophthalmological examination, diagnostics, and treatment are similar to those in other species, although the presence of the spectacle may limit visualisation of the posterior eye and effects of topical

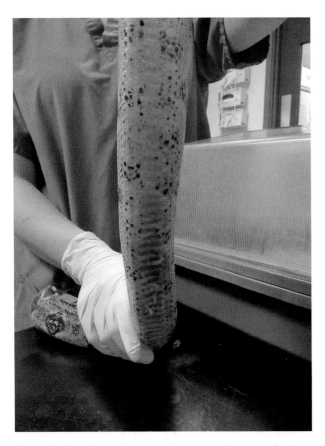

Figure 17.13 First degree burn in a common boa associated with direct contact with a malfunctioning heat source.

treatments. The spectacle is a clear layer of skin which covers and protects the cornea and is shed regularly along with the rest of the skin during ecydsis. A narrow corneospectacular space exists between the cornea and overlying spectacle and subspectacular abscesses can occur either secondary to a penetrating wound or by infection ascending the lacrimal duct. The eye will appear opaque and enlarged (Figure 17.14). Abscesses may be drained under general anaesthesia by excising a small part of the spectacle. The lacrimal duct may also be cannulated. Alternatively, pseudobuphthalmos may also present as enlargement or protrusion of the globe.

Retained spectacles occur in snakes in association with dysecdysis (Figure 17.15). Predisposing factors such as poor husbandry or mites should therefore be corrected. Increasing humidity and soaking with warm water may help to loosen spectacles. Alternatively, various tear

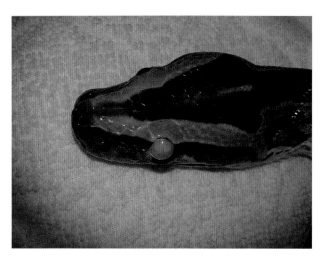

Figure 17.14   Subspectacular abscess in a Burmese python.

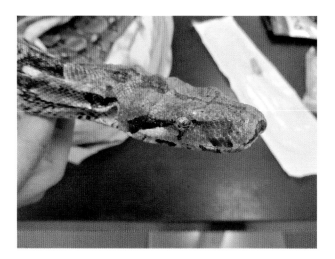

Figure 17.15   Retained spectacle in a common boa with concurrent dehydration.

replacement drops or contact lens solutions have been used. Once loosened the spectacle may be rolled away from the cornea gently with a damp cotton bud. If this is not possible, excessive force should not be used as it is easy to damage the delicate cornea beneath. Instead husbandry should be improved and the spectacle may be lost at the subsequent shed, or removal can be attempted again. If spectacles are retained for consecutive sheds despite conservative treatment, a general anaesthetic may be necessary for the spectacle to be carefully removed.

17.6.9   Surgical Considerations

In snakes, the standard coeliotomy approach is at the lateral margin of the body between the first and second row of lateral scales counting upwards from the ventral scutes. Due to the elongated layout of the internal organs, multiple organs may not be easily accessible from a small incision and a good knowledge of surgical anatomy is necessary in order to plan the most appropriate incision site along the snake's length. Multiple incisions may be preferred, if for example taking biopsies of more than one organ, or removing eggs from the length of the oviduct. The incision is made in the soft tissues between the scales, following the line of the scales. Radiosurgery or laser surgery may be considered to minimise haemorrhage, but are associated with more inflammatory response than a simple scalpel incision (Hodshon et al. 2013). Visibility within the coleomic cavity may be limited and the use of good lighting, retractors and magnifying loupes can help minimise tissue trauma.

Following surgery, wound healing is slow and the nature of a snake's inelastic skin causes wound edges to naturally invert. Everting patterns such as horizontal mattress sutures are therefore recommended. Tissue glue appears associated with the least inflammatory reaction so can be used to close small superficial wounds. Polyglactin 910 (Vicryl®) and chromic gut appear to be associated with the most inflammatory changes, so monofilament suture types are recommended (McFadden et al. 2011b). Even suture types which would be completely absorbed in mammals remain present for more than 90 days following surgery. Skin sutures should not be removed until at least six weeks post-surgery and ideally also after one cycle of ecdysis has occurred.

17.7   Imaging

Plain radiographs may be obtained without the need for sedation. The snake can be positioned either within a box or tube or directly on the x-ray plate. Dorsoventral and laterolateral (preferably using a horizontal beam) views should be taken. Positioning may not always be ideal, but obvious findings such as significant skeletal abnormalities, eggs or foreign bodies should be detected. Images may however be limited by poor contrast and superimposition of the ribs and spine. Multiple images will also be required to examine the whole length of the snake for survey radiographs. For larger or less compliant individuals, chemical restraint is likely to be necessary, especially for diagnostic images of the head or lungs. Contrast radiography should be considered for evaluation of the gastrointestinal system. Barium sulphate can be administered via an oesophageal tube at 15–25 ml/kg and highlights the oesophagus and stomach well, although distribution throughout the intestines can vary (Banzato et al. 2012a).

Ultrasound can be performed without sedation and will provide helpful information about coelomic structures. A probe size of ~ 7.5 mHz is ideal for medium-larger snakes and a dorsolateral approach to probe placement with the snake in normal ventral recumbency is recommended for visualisation of most organs. Normal ultrasonographic anatomy of coelomic organs has been described in several boid and python species (Isaza et al. 1993; Banzato et al. 2012b). The liver, gall bladder, stomach, pancreas, intestines, and kidneys should all be identifiable. Spleen, gonads, and hemipenes may also be visualised and some authors suggest ultrasound to be the preferred method of gender determination if probing is not possible (Gnudi et al. 2009). A higher frequency probe (10 mHz) and some experience with this technique would however be needed.

Echocardiography has been well described in both boas and pythons due to the variety of cardiac disorders reported in these species. A standard examination technique is recommended with the snake restrained in dorsal recumbency for a ventral approach. The right and left intercostal approaches can also be used to provide additional information. A good knowledge of normal snake anatomy is vital to interpret normal and abnormal findings. Both cardiac anatomy and the echocardiographic procedure are well-described by Schilliger et al. (2006). Normal images and dimensions are available for some species, but body mass, body length, and sex may affect cardiac measurements (Snyder et al. 1999; Conceição et al. 2014). It should be noted that cardiac dimensions will also fluctuate depending on how recently the snake has fed, so physiologic changes should be considered when interpreting measurements (Zerbe et al. 2011).

Advanced imaging techniques such as CT and magnetic resonance imaging (MRI) are increasingly being used in reptile medicine as they become more widely available. Both techniques will eliminate many of the limitations of radiography by avoiding superimposition of skeletal structures and allowing accurate reconstruction of the animal's anatomy. CT is particularly useful for imaging of the res-

piratory and skeletal systems, in addition to certain soft tissue structures such as follicles which are readily visualised (Pees et al. 2009; Banzato et al. 2011). Usually snakes are sedated or anaesthetised for the procedure, but images obtained from a curled snake can be reconstructed using curved multiplanar reformatting (MPR) software to yield clinically useful information (Hedley et al. 2014). MRI in contrast is more useful for evaluation of soft tissue structures, but will require chemical restraint, due to the length of procedure and sensitivity to motion artefacts.

Endoscopy can be a helpful technique for further evaluation of the gastrointestinal tract, respiratory system, or other coelomic structures. Sedation or general anaesthesia is generally necessary to provide complete immobilisation and analgesia should be administered for any invasive procedures. Rigid endoscopes are used most commonly, with a 2.7 mm scope usually the most versatile for multiple different species. However, flexible endoscopes of similar sizes can also be helpful for evaluation of the respiratory tract or the gastrointestinal tract in smaller species. The length of scope compared to snake size will be the main limiting factor as to how much of the gastrointestinal tract can be evaluated via either the oral or cloacal approach. The respiratory tract may be accessed either via the trachea or a surgical approach via the air sac (Jekl and Knotek 2006). Samples may be obtained via this route for culture, cytology or histopathology (Stahl et al. 2008).

Coelioscopy is less commonly performed as multiple entry sites would be necessary to examine all major organs. Snakes also have more diffuse coelomic fat than other reptiles and insufflation can be more challenging. If a targeted endoscopic approach of one organ or region is required, the position of the desired organ should be identified (via another imaging modality if necessary) and a small incision may be made between the first and second rows of lateral scales, similar to a surgical coeliotomy approach. The endoscope may then be directed either between the ribs in larger snakes, or just medial to the ribs in smaller species (Divers 2010).

17.8 Preventative Health Measures

Signs of disease in snakes can be subtle until problems are advanced. Owners should therefore be advised to keep accurate records of weights, feeding, and shedding so that any changes are noticed at an early stage. Annual physical examinations are recommended for all boas and pythons with further disease screening if indicated.

All individuals should be quarantined when entering a new snake collection and observed for any signs of disease. The progression of infectious diseases in snakes is often slow, therefore a minimum period of three months is recommended, although longer periods for up to 12 months have been suggested in certain situations (Lock and Wellehan 2015). During this time period, a full physical examination should be performed, plus any relevant disease screening. This may vary depending on the collection, but faecal parasitology (including acid-fast stain for *Cryptosporidium*), arenavirus, and paramyxovirus screening should be considered (Varga 2004). Microchipping if desired may be performed in the left flank anterior to the cloaca (BVZS 2017). Tissue glue should be applied over the needle entry site.

17.9 Formulary

Research into pharmacokinetics and pharmacodynamics is limited in snakes, but some drugs have been studied in certain python species. Where, species specific information is unknown, dosages are extrapolated from that available for other snakes or reptiles. Suggested dose rates for commonly used drugs are listed in the formulary.

Formulary

Medication	Dose	Dosing interval	Comments
Sedatives/anaesthetics			
Alfaxalone	<9 mg/kg IV		Based on study involving a variety of snake species including carpet pythons (Scheelings et al. 2011)
Propofol	5 mg/kg IV		(Meredith 2015)
Medetomidine and Ketamine	0.1–0.2 mg/kg (Me); 20–30 mg/kg (K) IM		(Meredith 2015)
Midazolam and Ketamine	0.2–0.8 mg/kg (Mi); 20–30 mg/kg (K) IM		(Meredith 2015)
Analgesia			
Morphine	1 mg/kg IM one-off		Anecdotal dose with no proven effect
Meloxicam	0.2 mg/kg SC, IM	q24h	Anecdotal dose with no proven effect
Lidocaine	1–2 mg/kg		as local infusion/nerve block (Meredith 2015)
Meloxicam	0.1–0.5 mg/kg PO, SC, IM	q24–48h	(Meredith 2015)
Antibiotics			
Ceftazidime	20 mg/kg	q72h	Based on study involving a variety of snake species (Lawrence et al. 1984)
Piperacillin	100 mg/kg IM	q48h	Based on pharmacokinetic study in blood pythons (Hilf et al. 1991a)
Enrofloxacin	10 mg/kg loading dose, then 5–10 mg/kg IM	q48h	Based on study in Burmese pythons (Young et al. 1997)
Marbofloxacin	10 mg/kg s.c., i.m., p.o. q48h		Based on studies in royal pythons (Coke et al. 2006; Hunter et al. 2007)
Amikacin	3.48 mg/kg IM	q 6 days (q72h for *Pseudomonas*)	Based on studies in royal pythons (Johnson et al. 1997)
Gentamicin	Most snakes: 2.5 mg/kg IM	q72h	(Hilf et al. 1991b; Meredith 2015)
	Blood pythons: 2.5 mg/kg IM then 1.5 mg/kg	q96h	
Azithromycin	10 mg/kg PO	q3d for skin infections; q5d for respiratory tract infections; q7d for liver and kidney infections	Based on studies in royal pythons (Coke et al. 2003; Hunter et al. 2003)
Metronidazole	100 mg/kg PO	repeat after 14 days	(Meredith 2015)

(Continued)

(Continued)

Medication	Dose	Dosing interval	Comments
Anti-parasitic agents			
Fenbendazole	50–100 mg/kg PO 20–25 mg/kg PO	Once q24h for 3–5 days	(Holt and Lawrence 1982)
Fipronil	Spray on to cloth first then wipe over surface of reptile	q7–14d until negative for ectoparasites.	(Meredith 2015) Beware of use in debilitated reptiles, those which have recently shed their skin and in small species where overdosage and toxicity may occur
Ivermectin	0.2 mg/kg SC, PO Environmental control for snake mites (*Ophionyssus natricis*) at dilution of 5 mg/l water sprayed in enclosure	repeat in 10–14 days until negative for ectoparasites q7–10d	Accurate dosage is particularly important in small individuals where overdosage and toxicity may occur

References

Banzato, T., Russo, E., Di Toma, A. et al. (2011). Evaluation of radiographic, computed tomographic, and cadaveric anatomy of the head of boa constrictors. *American Journal of Veterinary Research* 72 (12): 1592–1599.

Banzato, T., Russo, E., Finotti, L. et al. (2012a). Development of a technique for contrast radiographic examination of the gastrointestinal tract in ball pythons (*Python regius*). *American Journal of Veterinary Research* 73 (7): 996–1001.

Banzato, T., Russo, E., Finotti, L. et al. (2012b). Ultrasonographic anatomy of the coelomic organs of boid snakes (*Boa constrictor imperator, Python regius, Python molurus molurus* and *Python curtus*). *American Journal of Veterinary Research* 73 (5): 634–645.

Booth, W., Johnson, D.H., Moore, S. et al. (2010). Evidence for viable, non-clonal but fatherless Boa constrictors. *Biology Letters* 7 (2): 253–256.

Bunke, L.G., Sladky, K.K., and Johnson, S.M. (2018). Antinociceptive efficacy and respiratory effects of dexmedetomidine in ball pythons (*Python regius*). *American Journal of Veterinary Research* 79 (7): 718–726.

British Veterinary Zoological Society (BVZS) (2017). Microchipping Guidelines. https://www.bvzs.org/members/guidelines (accessed 22 July 2017).

Chang, L., Fu, D., Stenglein, M.D. et al. (2016). Detection and prevalence of boid inclusion body disease in collections of boas and pythons using immunological assays. *The Veterinary Journal* 218: 13–18.

Chinnadurai, S.K., Wrenn, A., and DeVoe, R.S. (2009). Evaluation of noninvasive oscillometric blood pressure monitoring in anesthetized boid snakes. *Journal of the American Veterinary Medical Association* 234 (5): 625–630.

Coke, R.L., Hunter, R.P., Isaza, R. et al. (2003). Pharmacokinetics and tissue concentrations of azithromycin in ball pythons (*Python regius*). *American Journal of Veterinary Research* 64 (2): 225–228.

Coke, R.L., Isaza, R., Koch, D.E. et al. (2006). Preliminary single-dose pharmacokinetics of marbofloxacin in ball pythons (*Python regius*). *Journal of Zoo and Wildlife Medicine* 37 (1): 6–10.

Conceição, M.E.B., Monteiro, F.O., Andrade, R.S. et al. (2014). Effect of biometric variables on two-dimensional echocardiographic measurements in the red-tailed boa (*Boa constrictor constrictor*). *Journal of Zoo and Wildlife Medicine* 45 (3): 672–677.

Da Silva, M.A.O., Bertelsen, M.F., Wang, T. et al. (2015). Unilateral microphthalmia or anophthalmia in eight pythons (Pythonidae). *Veterinary Ophthalmology* 18 (s1): 23–29.

Darrow, B.G., Myers, G.E., KuKanich, B. et al. (2016). Fentanyl transdermal therapeutic system provides rapid systemic fentanyl absorption in two ball pythons (*Python regius*). *Journal of Herpetological Medicine and Surgery* 26 (3): 94–99.

Di Girolamo, N., Selleri, P., Nardini, G. et al. (2014). Computed tomography–guided bone biopsies for evaluation of proliferative vertebral lesions in two boa constrictors (*Boa constrictor imperator*). *Journal of Zoo and Wildlife Medicine* 45 (4): 973–978.

Diethelm, G., Stauber, E., and Tillson, M. (1996). Tracheal resection and anastomosis for an intratracheal chondroma in a ball python. *Journal of the American Veterinary Medical Association* 209 (4): 786–788.

Divers, S. (2010). Reptile diagnostic endoscopy and endosurgery. *The Veterinary Clinics of North America. Exotic Animal Practice* 13 (2): 217–242.

Draper, C., Walker, R., and Lawler, H. (1981). Patterns of oral bacterial infection in captive snakes. *Journal of the American Veterinary Medical Association* 179 (11): 1223–1226.

Drew, M.L., Phalen, D.N., Berridge, B.R. et al. (1999). Partial tracheal obstruction due to chondromas in ball pythons (*Python regius*). *Journal of Zoo and Wildlife Medicine* 30 (1): 151–157.

Fitzgerald, K. and Vera, R. (2006). Spinal osteopathy. In: *Reptile Medicine and Surgery*, 2e (ed. D. Mader), 906–912. St. Louis: Saunders Elsevier.

Fitzgerald, S.D., Janovitz, E.B., Burnstein, T. et al. (1990). A caudal coiling syndrome associated with lymphocytic epaxial perineuritis in newborn boa. *Journal of Zoo and Wildlife Medicine* 21 (4): 485–489.

Gardiner, D.W., Baines, F.M., and Pandher, K. (2009). Photodermatitis and photokeratoconjunctivitis in a ball python (*Python regius*) and a blue-tongue skink (*Tiliqua spp.*). *Journal of Zoo and Wildlife Medicine* 40 (4): 757–766.

Gnudi, G., Volta, A., Di Ianni, F. et al. (2009). Use of ultrasonography and contrast radiography for snake gender determination. *Veterinary Radiology and Ultrasound* 50 (3): 309–311.

Hausmann, J.C., Hollingsworth, S.R., Hawkins, M.G. et al. (2013). Distribution and outcome of ocular lesions in snakes examined at a veterinary teaching hospital: 67 cases (1985–2010). *Journal of the American Veterinary Medical Association* 243 (2): 252–260.

Hedley, J. and Eatwell, K. (2013). The effects of UV light on calcium metabolism in ball pythons (*Python regius*). *Veterinary Record* 173 (14): 345.

Hedley, J. and Volk, H. (2015). Surgical treatment of a vertebral lesion in a reticulated python (*Python reticulatus*). In: *British Veterinary Zoological Society Conference*, 50. Loughborough: BVZS.

Hedley, J., Eatwell, K., and Schwarz, T. (2014). Computed tomography of ball pythons (*Python regius*) in curled recumbency. *Veterinary Radiology and Ultrasound* 55 (4): 380–386.

Hernandez-Divers, S.J. and Shearer, D. (2002). Pulmonary mycobacteriosis caused by *Mycobacterium haemophilum* and *M marinum* in a royal python. *Journal of the American Veterinary Medical Association* 220 (11): 1661–1663.

Hetzel, U., Sironen, T., Laurinmäki, P. et al. (2013). Isolation, identification, and characterization of novel arenaviruses, the etiological agents of boid inclusion body disease. *Journal of Virology* 87 (20): 10918–10935.

Hilf, M., Swanson, D., Wagner, R. et al. (1991a). Pharmacokinetics of piperacillin in blood pythons (*Python curtus*) and in vitro evaluation of efficacy against aerobic gram-negative bacteria. *Journal of Zoo and Wildlife Medicine* 22: 199–203.

Hilf, M., Swanson, D., Wagner, R. et al. (1991b). A new dosing schedule for gentamicin in blood pythons (Python curtus): a pharmacokinetic study. *Research in Veterinary Science* 50 (2): 127–130.

Hodshon, R.T., Sura, P.A., Schumacher, J.P. et al. (2013). Comparison of first-intention healing of carbon dioxide laser, 4.0-MHz radiosurgery, and scalpel incisions in ball pythons (*Python regius*). *American Journal of Veterinary Research* 74 (3): 499–508.

Holt, P.E. and Lawrence, K. (1982). Efficacy of fenbendazole against the nematodes of reptiles. *Veterinary Record* 110 (13): 302–304.

Hunter, R.P., Koch, D.E., Coke, R.L. et al. (2003). Azithromycin metabolite identification in plasma, bile, and tissues of the ball python (*Python regius*). *Journal of Veterinary Pharmacology and Therapeutics* 26 (2): 117–121.

Hunter, R.P., Koch, D.E., Coke, R.L. et al. (2007). Identification and comparison of marbofloxacin metabolites from the plasma of ball pythons (*Python regius*) and blue and gold macaws (*Ara ararauna*). *Journal of Veterinary Pharmacology and Therapeutics* 30 (3): 257–262.

Hyndman, T.H., Shilton, C.M., Doneley, R.J. et al. (2012). Sunshine virus in Australian pythons. *Veterinary Microbiology* 161 (1–2): 77–87.

Isaza, R., Ackerman, N., and Jacobson, E.R. (1993). Ultrasound imaging of the coelomic structures in the boa constrictor (*Boa constrictor*). *Veterinary Radiology and Ultrasound* 34 (6): 445–450.

Isaza, R., Andrews, G.A., Coke, R.L. et al. (2004). Assessment of multiple cardiocentesis in ball pythons (*Python regius*). *Journal of the American Association for Laboratory Animal Science* 43 (6): 35–38.

James, L.E., Williams, C.J., Bertelsen, M.F. et al. (2017). Evaluation of feeding behavior as an indicator of pain in snakes. *Journal of Zoo and Wildlife Medicine* 48 (1): 196–199.

Jekl, V. and Knotek, Z. (2006). Endoscopic examination of snakes by access through an air sac. *Veterinary Record* 158 (12): 407.

Jensen, B. and Wang, T. (2009). Hemodynamic consequences of cardiac malformations in two juvenile ball pythons (*Python regius*). *Journal of Zoo and Wildlife Medicine* 40 (4): 752–756.

Johnson, J.H., Jensen, J.M., Brumbaugh, G.W. et al. (1997). Amikacin pharmacokinetics and the effects of ambient temperature on the dosage regimen in ball pythons (*Python regius*). *Journal of Zoo and Wildlife Medicine* 28 (1): 80–88.

Kharbush, R.J., Gutwillig, A., Hartzler, K.E. et al. (2017). Antinociceptive and respiratory effects following application of transdermal fentanyl patches and assessment of brain μ-opioid receptor mRNA expression in ball pythons. *American Journal of Veterinary Research* 78 (7): 785–795.

Kinney, M.E., Wack, R.F., Grahn, R.A. et al. (2013). Parthenogenesis in a Brazilian Rainbow Boa (*Epicrates cenchria cenchria*). *Zoo Biology* 32 (2): 172–176.

Lawrence, K., Muggleton, P.W., and Needham, J.R. (1984). Preliminary study on the use of ceftazidime, a broad spectrum cephalosporin antibiotic, in snakes. *Research in Veterinary Science* 36 (1): 16–20.

Leary, S., Underwood, M.W., Anthony, R. et al. (2013). *AVMA Guidelines for the Euthanasia of Animals: 2013 Edition*. Schaumburg, IL: American Veterinary Medical Association.

Lock, B. and Wellehan, J. (2015). Ophidia (snakes). In: *Fowler's Zoo and Wild Animal Medicine*, 8e (eds. R. Miller and M. Fowler), 60–74. St. Louis. MO: Elsevier Saunders.

McFadden, M.S., Bennett, R.A., Reavill, D.R. et al. (2011a). Clinical and histologic effects of intracardiac administration of propofol for induction of anesthesia in ball pythons (*Python regius*). *Journal of the American Veterinary Medical Association* 239 (6): 803–807.

McFadden, M.S., Bennett, R.A., Kinsel, M.J. et al. (2011b). Evaluation of the histologic reactions to commonly used suture materials in the skin and musculature of ball pythons (*Python regius*). *American Journal of Veterinary Research* 72 (10): 1397–1406.

Meredith, A. (2015). *BSAVA Small Animal Formulary: Part B: Exotic Pets*. Gloucester, UK: BSAVA.

Miller, D.L., Radi, Z.A., Stiver, S.L. et al. (2004). Cutaneous and pulmonary mycosis in green anacondas (*Euncectes murinus*). *Journal of Zoo and Wildlife Medicine* 35 (4): 557–561.

Myers, D., Wellehan, J., and Isaza, R. (2009). Saccular lung cannulation in a ball python (*Python regius*) to treat a tracheal obstruction. *Journal of Zoo and Wildlife Medicine* 40 (1): 214–216.

Olesen, M.G., Bertelsen, M.F., Perry, S.F. et al. (2008). Effects of preoperative administration of butorphanol or meloxicam on physiologic responses to surgery in ball pythons. *Journal of the American Veterinary Medical Association* 233 (12): 1883–1888.

Orós, J., Sicilia, J., Torrent, A. et al. (2001). Immunohistochemical detection of ophidian paramyxovirus in snakes in the Canary Islands. *Veterinary Record* 149 (1): 21–23.

O'Shea, M., Slater, S., Scott, R. et al. (2016). *Eunectes murinus* (green anaconda) reproduction / facultative parthenogenesis. *Herpetological Review* 47: p73.

Patterson, R.W. and Smith, A. (1979). Surgical intervention to relieve dystocia in a python. *Veterinary Record* 104 (24): 551–552.

Pees, M.C., Kiefer, I., Ludewig, E.W. et al. (2007). Computed tomography of the lungs of Indian pythons (*Python molurus*). *American Journal of Veterinary Research* 68 (4): 428–434.

Pees, M., Kiefer, I., Thielebein, J. et al. (2009). Computed tomography of the lung of healthy snakes of the species *Python regius, Boa constrictor, Python reticulatus, Morelia viridis, epicrates cenchria,* and *Morelia spilota. Veterinary Radiology and Ultrasound* 50 (5): 487–491.

Penner, J.D., Jacobson, E.R., Brown, D.R. et al. (1997). A novel *Mycoplasma sp.* associated with proliferative tracheitis and pneumonia in a Burmese python (*Python molurus bivittatus*). *Journal of Comparative Pathology* 117 (3): 283–288.

Pyron, R.A., Reynolds, R.G., and Burbrink, F.T. (2014). A taxonomic revision of boas (*Serpentes: Boidae*). *Zootaxa* 3846 (2): 249–260.

Quesenberry, K., Jacobson, E.R., Allen, J.L. et al. (1986). Ulcerative stomatitis and subcutaneous granulomas caused by *Mycobacterium chelonei* in a boa constrictor. *Journal of the American Veterinary Medical Association* 189 (9): 1131.

Redrobe, S. (2004). Anaesthesia and analgesia. In: *Manual of Reptiles* (eds. S. Girling and P. Raiti), 131–146. Gloucester: BSAVA.

Rishniw, M. and Carmel, B. (1999). Atrioventricular valvular insufficiency and congestive heart failure in a carpet python. *Australian Veterinary Journal* 77 (9): 580–583.

Rose, M.P. and Williams, D.L. (2014). Neurological dysfunction in a ball python (*Python regius*) colour morph and implications for welfare. *Journal of Exotic Pet Medicine* 23 (3): 234–239.

Ross, R. and Marzec, G. (1990). *The Reproductive Husbandry of Pythons and Boas*. Stanford, CA: Institiute for Herpetological Research.

Sadler, R.A., Schumacher, J.P., Rathore, K. et al. (2016). Evaluation of the role of the cyclooxygenase signaling pathway during inflammation in skin and muscle tissues of ball pythons (*Python regius*). *American Journal of Veterinary Research* 77 (5): 487–494.

Scheelings, T.F., Baker, R.T., Hammersley, G. et al. (2011). A preliminary investigation into the chemical restraint with alfaxalone of selected Australian squamate species. *Journal of Herpetological Medicine and Surgery* 21 (63): 63–67.

Schilliger, L., Vanderstylen, D., Piétrain, J. et al. (2003). Granulomatous myocarditis and coelomic effusion due to *Salmonella enterica arizonae* in a Madagascar Dumerili's boa (*Acrantophis dumerili*). *Journal of Veterinary Cardiology* 5 (1): 43–45.

Schilliger, L., Vanderstylen, D., Piétrain, J. et al. (2006). Proposed standardization of the two-dimensional echocardiographic examination in snakes. *Journal of Herpetological Medicine and Surgery* 16 (3): 76–87.

Schilliger, L.H., Morel, D., Bonwitt, J.H. et al. (2013). *Cheyletus eruditus* (Taurrus®): an effective candidate for the biological control of the snake mite (*Ophionyssus natricis*). *Journal of Zoo and Wildlife Medicine* 44 (3): 654–659.

Schilliger, L., Chetboul, V., Damoiseaux, C. et al. (2016). Restrictive cardiomyopathy and secondary congestive heart failure in a McDowell's carpet python (*Morelia spilota mcdowelli*). *Journal of Zoo and Wildlife Medicine* 47 (4): 1101–1104.

Selleri, P. and Girolamo, N. (2012). Cardiac tamponade following cardiocentesis in a cardiopathic boa constrictor imperator (*Boa constrictor imperator*). *Journal of Small Animal Practice* 53 (8): 487.

Simpson, M. and Langenburg, J. (2006). Hepatic lipidosis in a black-headed python (*Aspidites melanocephalus*). *Veterinary Clinics of North America. The Veterinary Clinics of North America. Exotic Animal Practice* 9 (3): 589–598.

Snyder, P.S., Shaw, N.G., and Heard, D.J. (1999). Two-dimensional echocardiographic anatomy of the snake heart (*Python molurus bivittatus*). *Veterinary Radiology & Ultrasound* 40 (1): 66–72.

Stahl, S.J., Hernandez-Divers, S.J., Cooper, T.L. et al. (2008). Evaluation of transcutaneous pulmonoscopy for examination and biopsy of the lungs of ball pythons and determination of preferred biopsy specimen handling and fixation procedures. *Journal of the American Veterinary Medical Association* 233 (3): 440–445.

Steeil, J., Schumacher, J., Hecht, S. et al. (2013). Diagnosis and treatment of a pharyngeal squamous cell carcinoma in a Madagascar ground boa (*Boa madagascariensis*). *Journal of Zoo and Wildlife Medicine* 44 (1): 144–151.

Stewart, J. (1990). Anaerobic bacterial infections in reptiles. *Journal of Zoo and Wildlife Medicine* 21 (2): 180–184.

Thompson, K.A., Campbell, M., Levens, G. et al. (2015). Bilaterally symmetrical oral amelanotic melanoma in a boa constrictor (*Boa constrictor constrictor*). *Journal of Zoo and Wildlife Medicine* 46 (3): 629–632.

Uccellini, L., Ossiboff, R.J., de Matos, R.E. et al. (2014). Identification of a novel nidovirus in an outbreak of fatal respiratory disease in ball pythons (*Python regius*). *Virology Journal* 11 (1): 144.

Uetz, P., Freed, P., and Hošek, J. (eds.) (2017). The Reptile Database. http://www.reptile-database.org (accessed 22 July 2017).

Varga, M. (2004). Captive maintenance and welfare. In: *Manual of Reptiles* (eds. S. Girling and P. Raiti), 6–17. Gloucester: BSAVA.

Wernick, M.B., Novo-Matos, J., Ebling, A. et al. (2015). Valvulopathy consistent with endocarditis in an Argentine boa (*Boa constrictor occidentalis*). *Journal of Zoo and Wildlife Medicine* 46 (1): 124–129.

White, S.D., Bourdeau, P., Bruet, V. et al. (2011). Reptiles with dermatological lesions: a retrospective study of 301 cases at two university veterinary teaching hospitals (1992–2008). *Veterinary Dermatology* 22 (2): 150–161.

Wozniak, E. and DeNardo, D. (2000). The biology, clinical significance and control of the common snake mite, *Ophionyssus natricis*, in captive reptiles. *Journal of Herpetological Medicine and Surgery* 10 (3): 4–10.

Young, L., Schumacher, J., and Papich, M. (1997). Disposition of enrofloxacin and its metabolite ciprofloxacin after intramuscular injection in juvenile Burmese pythons (*Python molurus bivittatus*). *Journal of Zoo and Wildlife Medicine* 28 (1): 71–79.

Zerbe, P., Glaus, T., Clauss, M. et al. (2011). Ultrasonographic evaluation of postprandial heart variation in juvenile Paraguay anacondas (*Eunectes notaeus*). *American Journal of Veterinary Research* 72 (9): 1253–1258.

18

Mediterranean Tortoises

Sarah Brown

Mediterranean tortoises predominantly belong to the genus *Testudo*. These tortoises are native to areas of southern Europe, northern Africa, and the Middle East and many species are considered vulnerable in the wild, with *Testudo kleinmanni* deemed critically endangered (The IUCN Red List 2017). Their taxonomic classification has been extremely challenging and is still subject to change. Despite the many apparent divergent lineages and subspecies, in practical terms, their husbandry and dietary needs will be similar. Biological parameters of Mediterranean tortoises are listed in Table 18.1. In-depth species and subspecies identification is beyond the scope of this chapter but a brief summary is detailed in Table 18.2.

In the United Kingdom, classically, the tortoises kept as pets have been *Testudo* species (usually *T. graeca*, *T. hermanni*, or *T. marginata*), which were wild-caught and imported to the UK until the early 1980s (Türkozan et al. 2008). The wild-caught tortoises that are still alive now present to veterinary practice as a geriatric population with geriatric issues, such as renal disease and reproductive disorders, often compounded by chronic suboptimal environmental and dietary provision.

This trade was banned in 1984, and now the sale of tortoises is regulated under the Convention on International Trade in Endangered Species (CITES). Of the Mediterranean tortoise species, *T. kleinmanni* is listed under Appendix I, whereby trade is illegal. The remainder of the species are listed under Appendix II where trade or commercial use is allowed under DEFRA licence (an 'Article 10' certificate (Gov.uk 2013), although *Testudo horsfieldi* do not currently require licencing for trade.

There has been a surge in numbers of captive-bred juvenile tortoises, particularly *T. horsfieldi*, in the UK (Türkozan et al. 2008). These are presenting to veterinary practice with a separate set of health issues compared to the geriatric population, such as metabolic bone disease (MBD) and accelerated growth. They are often bred in large farms in continental Europe and are then brought to UK pet shops for sale, and so infectious disease outbreaks and endoparasitism are more common, compounded by the stress of overcrowding and travel.

18.1 Husbandry

Many clinical presentations in tortoises are due, at least in part, to inadequate husbandry and dietary provision, so the clinician should be familiar with the species' natural history and captive requirements. There is still a tendency in the UK to keep tortoises, particularly those wild-caught individuals entering the pet trade prior to the 1984 ban, outdoors year-round without supplemental heat or ultraviolet (UV) light provision, or indoors with inappropriate heat and UV light. Diets offered are often suboptimal and hibernation is frequently poorly managed. As reptiles are often slow to develop clinical disease and survive for relatively long periods with suboptimal management, it can be very difficult for keepers to accept that changes should be made. Veterinary staff play an important role in client education, and care should be taken to work with the keeper to improve compliance. Many medical conditions are compounded by poor environment and nutrition, and treatment plans that do not take husbandry and diet into account are less likely to succeed.

The temperate climate in many regions, including the UK, is not suitable for Mediterranean tortoise species to live outdoors all year round without supplemental heat and UV light provision. Accommodation will vary with age and group sizing, but should usually comprise an indoor enclosure, e.g. a tortoise table (an open-topped enclosure with side walls to prevent escape) or enclosed vivarium with appropriate heat and UVB lamps, and an outdoor enclosure

Handbook of Exotic Pet Medicine, First Edition. Edited by Marie Kubiak.
© 2021 John Wiley & Sons Ltd. Published 2021 by John Wiley & Sons Ltd.
Companion website: www.wiley.com/go/kubiak/exotic_pet_medicine

Table 18.1   Basic data: Mediterranean tortoises.

Adult size	Species-dependent. From 10–12 cm carapace length (*T. kleinmanni*) to 24–40 cm (*T. marginata*). Usually reach adult size by 10–15 years old. Females generally larger than males.
Lifespan	50–100 years
Social nature	Solitary. Can be kept in groups but monitor for aggression.
Diet	Herbivorous
Environmental Temperatures	POTZ (Preferred Optimal Temperature Zone) 20–32 °C PBT (Preferred Body Temperature) 26–30 °C. Heliotherms – will need a basking spot.
Need for ultra-violet lighting?	Yes, preferred UV Index range of 1.0–2.6 (Baines et al. 2016)
Potential to hibernate?	Most have the biological capacity to hibernate, depending on environmental conditions. *F. nabeulensis* and *T. kleinmanni* do not hibernate (Highfield 1996).
Conservation Status	Many species considered vulnerable in the wild, with *T. kleinmanni* considered critically endangered. All species are listed under CITES Appendix II apart from *T. kleinmanni* which is on Appendix I.

available in good, warm weather. Conservatories or greenhouses can be adapted to provide appropriate accommodation, with heat lamps and full spectrum lighting, but care should be taken that temperatures do not move out of the desired range in seasonal extremes. Outdoor enclosures must be secure and 'escape-proof', with no access for wildlife, dogs, or other pets.

Tortoise tables have the advantages of improved space and ventilation over vivaria and are generally preferred, but it can be more difficult to maintain the appropriate temperature range if the ambient room temperature is low.

Mediterranean tortoises are adapted to relatively arid or semi-arid environments, so excessive humidity is to be avoided.

18.1.1   Heat Provision

Mediterranean tortoises bask in the sun to thermoregulate, and to expose themselves to UV light. The ultra-violet B (UVB) range of wavelengths is essential for tortoises to synthesise endogenous vitamin D3. This in turn allows adequate uptake of calcium in the diet. Captive environments should aim to provide the species' preferred optimum temperature zone (POTZ – the range of temperatures at which normal physiological functions can occur) and adequate exposure to appropriate UV light (Baines et al. 2016). *The importance of adequate heat and UVB provision cannot be over-stated.* The photoperiod for wild tortoises will vary from approximately 14 hours in summer to 10–12 hours in winter.

Heat can be provided by a lamp at one end, creating a temperature gradient across the enclosure which allows the tortoise to thermoregulate and select its preferred temperature appropriate for its physiological status at that time. Mediterranean tortoises are heliotherms (daylight basking reptiles) (Meek 1984) and are adapted to absorb heat from an overhead source, such as a lamp. The temperature under the heat lamp (at tortoise level) should be approximately 32–35 °C, with a background temperature

Table 18.2   Mediterranean tortoise species identification (Ernst and Barbour 1989; Highfield 1996; Jessop 2009; IUCN 2017).

Testudo (Agrionemys) horsfieldi (Horsfield's tortoise, Russian/Afghan/Steppe tortoise)	Four claws on forefeet (all other *Testudo* species have five). A small tortoise with small, indistinct spurs on tail tip and on thighs.
Testudo hermanni	Horny spur on end of tail and no thigh spurs. The subspecies taxonomy is controversial.
Testudo graeca (complex)	The 'spur-thigh complex' is a very heterogenous group, all characterised by caudal spurs on the thighs and a hinged caudal plastron. There is marked variation within the group and identification of species and subspecies is still controversial.
Testudo ibera	Considered as a separate species within the 'spur-thigh complex'
Furculachelys nabeulensis (Tunisian tortoise)	Small and delicate, often with pale skin. Important to differentiate from other spur-thighed tortoises as this does not hibernate.
Testudo marginata	Flared marginal scutes and three or more pairs of plastral triangular markings.
Testudo weissingeri	Originally considered a dwarf population of *T marginata*, but some consider it a separate species.
Testudo kleinmanni	Small and delicate with one pair of triangular plastral markings. No thigh spur. Does not hibernate.

of 20–25 °C at the cooler end. The night-time temperature should ideally not drop below 18 °C (McArthur and Barrows 2004). The basking lamp may be a spotlight, tungsten, or mercury vapour bulb. Ceramic lamps which give out radiant heat but no visible light can also be useful to supplement heat provision, e.g. at night, independently of the bright basking spot. Red lamps are not recommended. Selection of an appropriate wattage of basking bulb along with thermostats and timers should be used to make sure that the enclosure does not overheat, and that a circadian cycle is provided. It should be noted that combined heat and UV sources, such as mercury vapour bulbs, should not be controlled via a thermostat as this may result in the light source turning off intermittently leading to a disrupted photoperiod. Maximum-minimum thermometers within the enclosure are also useful but must be reliable and regularly checked. Heat mats are not recommended and have been associated with excessive plastron growth rate and increased incidence of gastrointestinal issues, in the author's experience. If heat mat use cannot be avoided, they can be placed on the sides of an enclosure so as to give radiant heat rather than be in direct contact with the tortoise. Hides should be provided within the enclosure at both hot and cool ends.

18.1.2 Ultra-Violet Light Provision

Provision of appropriate ultraviolet light is essential as herbivorous tortoises gain little vitamin D from dietary sources. UV radiation cannot pass through glass and is reduced by mesh, so any lamps will need to be situated within the enclosure. UV radiation drops off quickly with increased distance and so the lamp should be suspended at an appropriate height to allow adequate UVB exposure (usually 30–45 cm above the carapace, but this will vary with manufacturer and lamp output). The lamps are usually placed near the basking spot so as to permit heat and UVB exposure concurrently to mimic sunlight. Most lights are rated according to percentage UVB output. Mediterranean tortoises usually require lights rated as 5.0 or 8.0 (Jepson 2014). UV output from lamps varies and will decline over time, and so these lamps will need to be regularly monitored using a handheld metre, and replaced when UV output falls below a UV index of 1.0 (Baines et al. 2016). If owners are not monitoring the light output, the UVB exposure of the animal is unknown. Owners will often elect to replace unmonitored lamps every 8–12 months to attempt to maintain UVB exposure.

18.1.3 Substrate

Mediterranean tortoises burrow and dig, creating microclimates within the substrate and an enclosure should provide opportunity for this. Substrate selection can be difficult as ingestion of particulate substrates such as wood chippings may cause issues, whilst other substrates can be dusty or harbour microorganisms. In the author's experience, a 2:1 topsoil/playground sand mix can allow digging and formation of microclimates within the enclosure, but give adequate drainage and minimise issues with ingestion. Enclosures should be cleaned out regularly and faeces removed as soon as possible.

18.1.4 Water Provision

Water should always be provided in a shallow dish. Bathing of the tortoise in shallow warm water for 10–15 minutes once or twice a week is also recommended to allow drinking, encourage urination and defaecation and allow uptake of fluid into the bladder (see Section 18.4.2).

18.1.5 Diet

Mediterranean tortoises are herbivores, requiring high fibre, calcium-rich, low-protein, and low-fat diets. The calcium: phosphorus ratio should be at least 1.5–2:1 (Scott 1996). Wild chelonian diets will tend to have a higher Ca:P ratio of at least 4:1 (Highfield 1994). Incorrect dietary provision is the cause of many health issues for tortoises, such as MBD and accelerated growth.

Green, leafy foods should provide the bulk of the diet such as grasses, dandelion leaves, watercress, and sowthistle. Lettuce leaves are a good source of water, but are not nutritionally complete. A wide variety of leafy greens should be offered with daily calcium supplementation. Flowers such as dandelions and nasturtiums are usually readily eaten. Wild foraging or allowing tortoises to graze freely can be a useful method of sourcing suitable foods such as sowthistle or clovers (Highfield 2000). Seed mixes can be bought, allowing suitable plants for Mediterranean tortoises to be grown in a home or garden environment.

Some vegetables can be given in moderation in addition to leafy greens. Cucumbers can be a good fluid source, whilst grated carrot and peppers provide a source of vitamin A. Beans and pulses are generally to be avoided as protein levels are relatively high and the phytic acid they contain may bind calcium, reducing its bioavailability. Brassicas such as broccoli and cabbage contain goitrogens which may induce hypothyroidism if fed exclusively. Spinach and rhubarb leaves contain oxalic acid which may bind calcium and reduce its bioavailability (Innis 1994). Some common garden plant species, including Rhododendron, daffodil, and buttercup species, are toxic and should be completely avoided. Fruit is not recommended as a dietary component.

A small amount of food is generally offered twice a day as tortoises tend to graze rather than eat a large amount of food in one meal. Juveniles are prone to overfeeding with resultant accelerated growth problems if offered excessive quantities or high calorie foods. In indoor enclosures, feeding from a bowl or tile will help to reduce the risk of substrate ingestion. Food placed directly under a heat source will desiccate rapidly.

Pelleted diets have become available for tortoises. These are usually too high in protein and too low in fibre and fluid for herbivorous *Testudo* species. The author has seen many growth issues in juvenile tortoises fed a primarily pelleted diet and as such does not recommend them.

Occasionally in the wild, Mediterranean tortoises may eat high protein meals, e.g. carrion if found, to supplement their nutritionally poor wild diet. However, the feeding of high protein meals (e.g. dog or cat food), whilst often very palatable to tortoises, is not advised in captivity as the excess protein can have serious impacts on growth and renal function.

18.1.6 Supplementation

Calcium supplementation is advised, particularly for juveniles and for females of reproductive age. It is important, in conjunction with adequate heat and UVB light provision, to help prevent MBD. This is best supplied as a commercial calcium salt supplement typically provided daily on food, with a multi-vitamin preparation containing vitamins D_3 and A once a week, though individual commercial product recommendations may vary from this schedule. Some keepers may use cuttlefish, limestone powder, or eggshells as supplementation but calcium availability of these items may be inconsistent.

18.1.7 Social and Species Groupings

Mediterranean tortoises are not 'social' animals, and indeed are often solitary in the wild, with large home ranges. Males in particular can be territorial and aggressive towards other males and to females housed with them. Bites are often given to the legs, head, and caudal carapace. Keeping tortoises in pairs or groups can be stressful to some individuals, particularly if the enclosure size is relatively small. No more than one male should be kept in an enclosure, with one male to two or more females in a mixed sex grouping. Tortoises of very different sizes should not be kept together. Any introductions should be made after a quarantine period of at least six months.

Different species of tortoises should not be mixed in captivity due to the variation between species in susceptibility to infectious pathogens, different behaviours (particularly relating to courtship and mating), and variation in husbandry conditions required.

18.2 Hibernation

Due to tortoises' inability to maintain their body temperature independently of the temperature of their environment, a number of *Testudo* species found in temperate areas have developed the ability to hibernate during the cold winter months. Some *Testudo* species, primarily those with ranges extending into North Africa, hibernate in parts of their natural range and remain active through the winter in others. Hibernation conserves energy and enables the tortoise to cope through periods of natural food shortage. It is important to note that *Furculachelys nabeulensis* (Tunisian tortoise) and *T kleinmanni* do not hibernate in the wild, and so should not be hibernated in captivity.

Species from regions with very hot summers will aestivate through the hot periods. Indeed, some species such as *T. horsfieldi* may do both, avoiding the long winters and very hot, arid summers.

Hibernation is triggered by a reduction in ambient temperature, decreasing photoperiod, and decreasing light intensity. In captivity artificial manipulation of temperature and photoperiod, and careful monitoring before, during and after hibernation is vital. Some keepers choose not to hibernate their tortoises at all, but 'overwinter' them by maintaining them at warm temperatures. It is difficult to predict the long-term effect of this as it is only relatively recently that large numbers of juvenile *Testudo* tortoises have been kept in captivity, but it is proposed that persistent non-hibernation of hibernating species could cause growth problems, disruption to reproduction, and potential hepatic and metabolic dysfunction (Highfield 1996).'Hibernating' tortoises in a low ambient temperature enclosure, such as at room temperature is not acceptable, as the metabolic rate will not drop to hibernation levels and so a protracted state of catabolism will be maintained with subsequent metabolic catastrophe. Suitable conditions must be provided to properly hibernate tortoises to avoid detrimental effects.

18.2.1 Hibernation of Juvenile Tortoises

There is some debate on this matter, with some keepers performing short, controlled hibernation from the first year, with others not hibernating them until at least three to four years old. Juvenile tortoises would hibernate in the wild and cease growing for this period, and it does appear that accelerated growth and early maturity may be linked with lack of hibernation (Highfield 1996; author observation).

18.2.2 Hibernation Duration

Testudo species would rarely hibernate for longer than 12 weeks in the wild, allowing a long summer period to recover before the next winter hibernation period. However, if left to hibernate according to the UK climate, most would start hibernation in late October and not wake until April. This extended hibernation results in a prolonged negative energy balance and gives insufficient time to recover before the next hibernation period. Many tortoises will survive this approach in the medium-term but become physiologically weakened each year, eventually leading to post-hibernation health problems.

The recommended maximum length of hibernation is 12 weeks for a healthy adult tortoise, so hibernation will need to be actively ended by warming the tortoise prior to Spring, or hibernation onset delayed by maintaining higher temperatures and longer photoperiod through winter.

18.2.3 Hibernation Preparation

Most keepers prepare for hibernation in early Autumn but a health check-up in late summer is advisable so that fitness prior to hibernation can be assessed. The tortoise should be weighed and measured and faecal parasite evaluation carried out. An underweight or ill tortoise should not be hibernated but instead 'overwintered' with appropriate heat and UVB light provision.

Once an individual is deemed fit enough to hibernate, a pre-hibernation period can be planned. During this time the tortoise should be exposed to a reduced photoperiod and gradually reducing temperatures, dropping by approximately 5 °C per week (McArthur and Barrows 2004). For the three to four weeks prior to hibernation the tortoise should be bathed daily to encourage rehydration and defaecation, and fasted to ensure that there is no food present in the gastrointestinal tract during hibernation. Once the ambient temperature is down to 10–15 °C and the tortoise is inactive, it can be transferred to the hibernation accommodation.

18.2.4 Hibernation Accommodation

The ideal hibernation temperature is 5 °C (Highfield 1996), with a range of 3–7 °C. Temperatures higher then this will lead to activity and catabolism and temperatures lower than this will risk ice crystal formation with potential brain and ocular damage.

Fridges are ideal hibernation enclosures, provided that temperature control is reliable. The fridge should not be used for human food due to potential zoonotic risk. The door should be opened daily to allow air change and inspection of the tortoise. Maximum-minimum thermometers can be used to allow accurate and simple monitoring of internal fridge temperature.

Insulated boxes inside a cool building can also be used provided there is a stable, appropriate temperature and

adequate monitoring of both hibernation conditions and duration. Air holes should be kept to a minimum and the chamber carefully placed to avoid touching external walls. There should be no risk of rodent access and temperature monitoring must be carried out.

Outdoor hibernation is not advised due to the risk of frost damage, flooding, temperature fluctuations, and rodent or other predator damage.

The tortoise may be handled during hibernation without disturbing hibernation and inspection should check for nasal discharge, plastron erythema, and any skin damage. Tortoises should be weighed twice weekly, and if they lose more than 5% of the pre-hibernation weight then they should be woken up and hibernation abandoned. Most tortoises will lose less than 2% of their bodyweight during hibernation (Chitty and Raftery 2013). If the tortoise has urinated it should be woken up as its fluid reservoir will not be recouped. After waking at any point, tortoises should never be returned to hibernation.

18.2.5 Waking from Hibernation

Tortoises only enter or remain in hibernation whilst the temperature is within a certain range – as the temperature rises above 10 °C, the metabolic rate returns to normal and hibernation comes to an end. Upon awakening, tortoises should be checked for signs of disease such as stomatitis, nasal discharge, dermal swellings, or wounds.

Tortoises should be provided with a basking lamp and UVB light in an indoor enclosure, and should be bathed twice daily in shallow warm water to encourage drinking, urination, and defaecation. The environmental temperature should be gradually increased to the normal range over the first 24 hours. Succulent, palatable foods such as cucumber or fruit can be offered initially, and the diet then changed back to a higher fibre balance. Appetite, urination, and defaecation should be monitored closely by the keeper, and if the tortoise is not eating or urinating within a week of waking, veterinary attention should be sought.

At waking, tortoises will normally have a low white blood cell count and high urea levels. This combination of immunosuppression and dehydration means that the tortoise is very vulnerable, particularly if basic husbandry requirements such as heat and fluid provision are not met.

18.3 Clinical Evaluation

18.3.1 History Taking

Due to the limitations of clinical examination in tortoises, and the influence of diet and husbandry on their health, history-taking is disproportionately important compared to other species and should be thorough. A questionnaire for the owner to fill out prior to the consultation can be a useful way of gathering information. The owner can be asked to bring photographs of the tortoise's enclosure at home. A checklist for history taking is provided in Figure 18.1.

18.3.2 Handling

Gloves should be worn when handling tortoises, and changed between individuals. This is to avoid the potential for zoonotic infection (e.g. Salmonellosis) and cross-infection between tortoises (particularly for different species).

Examination may be limited if the tortoise withdraws into its shell. Most tortoises will retreat if approached from above, so approach from behind and below. Lightly touching the tail or carefully tilting the tortoise forward may encourage the tortoise to extend its head and forelimbs. The head can then be restrained with a thumb and forefinger and the mouth opened with the other hand. In smaller, more intractable individuals, e.g. *T. horsfieldi*, a blunt dental hook can be inserted under the upper jaw and the head gently drawn forwards and out. Care must be taken to avoid trauma from the probe. Rotating the dental probe sideways allows the beak to be opened using the probe as a gag (Figure 18.2). The forelimbs may be restrained along the sides of the body to allow access to the head, but care should be taken as forceful handling can lead to proximal limb fractures.

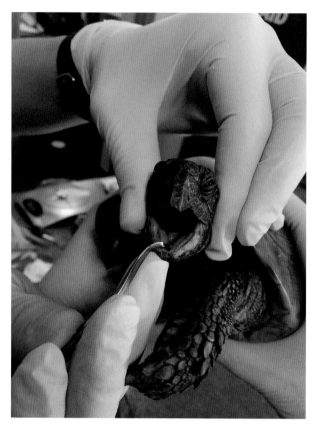

Figure 18.2 Oral examination using a blunt hook (*Source: Courtesy of Sarah Brown*).

Care should be taken when handling potentially gravid females as if held upside down eggs may be displaced into the bladder, requiring surgical removal (Barrows et al. 2004).

HISTORY	**ENVIRONMENT**	**REPRODUCTIVE DATA**
• Date	• Method of heat provision?	• When were eggs last laid?
• Client identification	• Max, min and average daytime/night time temps?	• Kept in isolation or as part of group?
• Animal identification / microchip number		• Last contact with opposite sex?
• Species (common and scientific names)	• How is humidity varied and monitored?	• Breeding history
• Sex and age	• What type of ultra-violet lighting is provided?	**DISEASE CONTROL**
• Reason for presentation		• Quarantine programme? How long?
KEEPER/COLLECTION DETAILS	What is the photoperiod?	• What disinfectants are used?
• Captive-bred or wild-caught?	**NUTRITION**	• When did this tortoise last meet a new chelonian?
• Appropriate CITES licence available?	• Describe diet.	• Any other reptiles in the household?
• Duration of ownership?	• Does food vary with season?	
• Previous ownership details?	• Is any mineral or vitamin supplement offered?	**HIBERNATION**
• Disease history and any previous veterinary treatment?		• Hibernated?
	• How is food prepared?	• When?
HOUSING	• Is water provided/changed/filtered?	• How?
• Indoors, outdoors or both?	• How often is the tortoise bathed?	• What post hibernation management is offered?
• Diagram / photo / description	**OBSERVATIONS**	
• Size of enclosure	• Appetite?	**DISEASE HISTORY**
• Substrate used?	• Activity and mobility?	• Any previous illness or treatment
	• Urine output?	
	• Faecal output?	

Figure 18.1 Checklist for history taking.

18.3.3 Sex Determination

The sex of Mediterranean tortoises is determined by egg incubation temperature, rather than chromosomes so DNA sexing is not possible. Ultrasonography or coelioscopy may be used to assess sex, but the former is sometimes unreliable, and the latter invasive. The presence of calcified eggs on radiography will confirm that the individual is female. Usually sex assessment is made on visual inspection (Table 18.3). Mediterranean tortoise species are sexually dimorphic, although the differences may not be obvious in juveniles or in individuals with aberrant growth (e.g. accelerated growth or MBD). Physical size rather than age appears to be the trigger for sexual maturity in tortoises. Captive tortoises tend to grow faster than wild counter-parts, due often to higher food availability, and may attain sexual maturity earlier. For example, wild *T. graeca* will mature at 12–15 years of age, whereas captive individuals may mature in 5–7 years (Highfield 1996).

18.3.4 Clinical Examination

The tortoise should be observed at rest to assess its demeanour and alertness before a systematic clinical examination. It should be borne in mind that cooling during transport to the veterinary practice may affect behaviour and clinical presentation. A checklist for clinical examination of Mediterranean tortoises is provided in Figure 18.4.

A record of weight and body dimensions should be part of any individual health assessment. The tortoise should be weighed at each examination, and if hospitalised, at the same time each day. Tortoises' large bladders will form a significant component of weight so if emptied, will show as a weight reduction. Length is best measured as straight carapace length (SCL; Figure 18.5). The Jackson ratio curve of weight/length has been used historically by keepers and vets as part of health assessments of *T. graeca* and *T. hermanni* (Jackson 1980). This is now felt to be less useful as many healthy captive tortoises will differ from the 'normal' cited by the ratio, due to variation in body size and shape within subspecies, seasonal variation in body fat levels, and differing gastrointestinal and bladder contents (Barrows et al. 2004; Chitty and Raftery 2013).

Table 18.3 Sex differentiation using external features in Mediterranean tortoises.

Male	Female
• Longer, thicker tail, often carried sideways (Figure 18.3a)	• Short tail (Figure 18.3b)
• Slit-like vent situated more distally (beyond carapacial rim)	• Rounded vent orifice situated more proximally (at or cranial to carapacial rim)
• Concave plastron	• Flatter plastron
• Males usually smaller than females of the same species	• Females usually larger than males of the same species

(a)   (b)

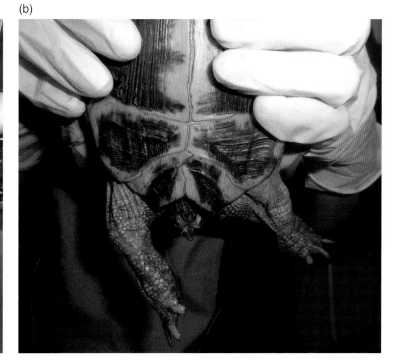

Figure 18.3   (a) Male *T. hermanni* – note the long tail and concave plastron (*Source:* Courtesy of Sarah Brown). (b) Female *T. horsfieldi* – note the shorter tail and flattened plastron (*Source:* Courtesy of Sarah Brown).

HEAD:

Eyes

Check menace and pupillary reflexes if possible. Check for swellings, discharges, corneal lesions, cataracts, foreign bodies, etc.
Sunken eyes can indicate severe dehydration
Compare both eyes
Closed eyes may not be primary disease issue

Beak and Jaw

Overgrowth?
Instability?
Flexibility?

Oral Cavity

Mucous membrane colour (normally pink): pallor? cyanosis? congestion? Yellow colouration is a normal finding
Stomatitis: discharge, ulceration and petechiae
Pus protruding into pharynx from ear abscessation?
Swellings around neck and chin?

Nares

Normally symmetrical, patent with no discharge
Any discharge is abnormal
Erosions, softness and depigmentation often noted with upper respiratory tract disease

Ears

Any tympanic membrane swelling to suggest abscessation?

SHELL

Scute quality–softness, pyramiding, ulceration, discharge, odour, wounds

LIMBS

Joint flexibility (compare limbs)
Swellings of joints or skin?
Reduced skin elasticity suggests dehydration
Nail overgrowth, sores on weight-bearing surfaces of feet
Mobility issues

SKIN

Swellings / masses?
Erythema?
Reduced elasticity suggests dehydration

RESPIRATORY SYSTEM

Limited due to shell and lack of access to skin. Damp cloth under stethoscope or electronic stethoscope has been recommended, but this author does not find auscultation very useful. Doppler blood flow monitor useful for evaluating heart sounds

COELOMIC CAVITY

Limited without further imaging. Pre-femoral digital palpation may find eggs or uroliths.

CLOACA

Discharge? Swelling? Odour? Prolapse?
Digital examination may allow identification of egg or urolith if stuck

OTHER

Microchipped?
Sex determination?

Figure 18.4 Checklist for clinical examination of Mediterranean tortoises.

18.4 Basic Techniques

18.4.1 Sample Collection

18.4.1.1 Blood Sampling

There are many potential venepuncture sites in chelonians, and choice can depend on species and clinician preference. Lymphodilution is a significant problem in chelonian blood sampling due to the anatomical proximity of lymph vessels to blood vessels, with least contamination occurring when sampling the jugular vein and most when using the dorsal coccygeal vein. Aseptic technique is important given that tortoises often have substantial debris on their skin. Sedation may be required for some more intractable tortoises.

3–6 ml/kg bodyweight can be safely taken from chelonians (Perpinan 2017), although this volume should be reduced for sick tortoises. Excessive negative pressure and the use of small needles can cause lysis of the large

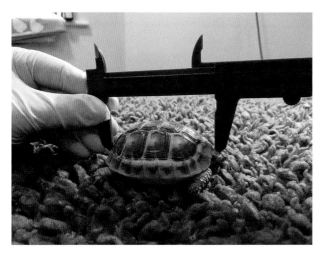

Figure 18.5 Measurement of straight carapace length (SCL) (*Source:* Courtesy of Sarah Brown).

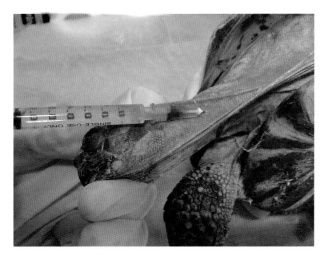

Figure 18.6 Jugular venepuncture (*Source:* Courtesy of Sarah Brown).

erythrocytes. EDTA may lyse chelonian blood cells, so samples should be collected in heparin for both haematological and biochemical analysis. Fresh smears should also be submitted as heparin may cause clumping of leucocytes and thrombocytes (Wilkinson 2004).

The main venipuncture sites used in Mediterranean tortoises are:

Jugular vein - Least likely to be lymph diluted. There are two branches – dorsal and ventral, which run along the length of the neck from the dorsal and ventral borders of the tympanic scale. The tortoise should be restrained by an assistant. The clinician extends the tortoise's neck and inserts the needle superficially in a caudal direction parallel to the neck, level to the dorsal or ventral aspect of the tympanic scale (Figure 18.6). Pressure should be applied after sampling as haematoma formation can be significant. The carotid artery may be sampled inadvertently

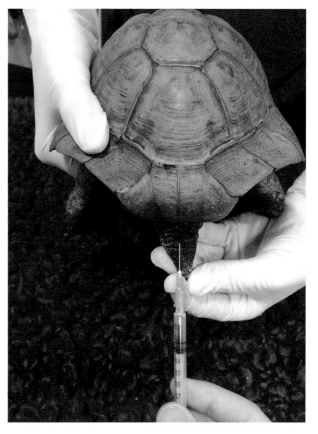

Figure 18.7 Site for accessing the dorsal coccygeal vein (*Source:* Courtesy of Sarah Brown).

in which case pressure should be applied for two to three minutes as large haematomas may form.

Dorsal coccygeal vein – lymphodilution can be an issue, and this site is often faecally contaminated and difficult to clean. Sample volume is less than for the jugular vein and females with shorter tails are more challenging. The needle is inserted into the dorsal midline of the tail at a 45° angle to the skin (Figure 18.7). If the needle touches the vertebral body it is gradually withdrawn until the more superficial vein is accessed.

Subcarapacial sinus (located in the dorsal midline, just ventral to the spine) – lymphodilution can be an issue and there is potential for damaging the spine. The needle is inserted into the dorsal midline of the skin above the neck, near the interface between the skin and carapace, and angled caudo-dorsally following the line of the carapace. If the underside of the carapace is touched, the needle should be withdrawn and repositioned. Bending the needle 30°, and using a 1–1½ inch needle are useful.

18.4.1.2 Faeces

Handling, or bathing the tortoise in warm water may encourage defaecation. Faecal samples may be examined by wet smear microscopy, sedimentation, flotation, and special staining for parasites. Faeces can contain 'parasite-like' plant elements, yeasts, and fungi which must be differentiated from true parasite infestations.

18.4.1.3 Urine

Urine samples may be obtained by free catch, and many tortoises will urinate on restraint. Urinalysis is not commonly performed in tortoises as urine is modified after renal clearance, but some valuable diagnostic information may still be obtained (Koelle 2000; Koelle and Hoffman 2002). Normal urine consists of clear fluid with some semi-solid white urates. Green urates (biliverdinuria) can be an indicator of hepatic dysfunction. The normal urine pH is alkaline in herbivorous tortoises such as the *Testudo* species (8.0–8.5). Acidic urine (<7) can be an indicator of prolonged anorexia (Wilkinson 2004). Due to contamination with faeces within the cloaca, urine is non-sterile. Urine specific gravity is less useful in tortoises as hyper-osmotic urine cannot be produced by the kidneys as reptiles lack the loop of Henle, and post-renal modification can occur by electrolyte and water exchange across the bladder wall. Normal values can be 1.003–1.014.

18.4.2 Fluid Therapy

Almost all hospitalised debilitated chelonia will benefit from fluid support. Dehydration is often only possible to assess when it has become well established. Severely dehydrated tortoises show sunken eyes and reduced skin elasticity. Measurement of serial urea and uric acid levels, along with packed cell volume (PCV) and weight will aid monitoring of response to fluid therapy. Overhydration is rare but vascular overload can result in individuals with renal dysfunction.

18.4.2.1 Choice of Fluid

Fluids should be warmed prior to administration. Maintenance requirements for chelonians are 10–30 ml/kg per 24 hours (Chitty and Raftery 2013), although there is little evidence-based information on fluid requirements for sick Mediterranean tortoises. Chelonians may withstand larger blood losses than mammals and birds as hypovolaemia can be compensated for by transferring from the large intracellular space (Chitty and Raftery 2013). Resorption of fluid from the bladder can also help to compensate for dehydration. Routes of fluid administration are given in Table 18.4.

Blood transfusions have rarely been reported in tortoises, and indeed would rarely be indicated as they can cope relatively well with low haematocrits.

18.4.3 Nutritional Support

Nutritional support is extremely important as many ill tortoises will not be eating voluntarily.

Crushing fragrant leaves or other foods and placing in front of the tortoise may encourage eating; smell is an important appetite stimulant for tortoises, especially if vision is compromised.

Where tortoises are anorexic, syringe feeding can be a viable option for home treatment by owners though risks aspiration pneumonia if large volumes are given too quickly or if the animal has a poor swallowing reflex. Oesophagostomy tube placement is often preferable.

Commercial diets exist for short and long-term support of nutrition. Simple or elemental nutritional supplements are preferred in the initial stages of assist feeding, but recovery diets with high fibre should be provided once gastrointestinal motility resumes.

The manufacturer's recommendations for quantity and dilution factors should be followed and ideally the food warmed before administration. Fluids and electrolytes should be replaced prior to giving food to avoid refeeding syndrome, an electrolyte imbalance caused by sudden reintroduction of food after prolonged anorexia. Small volumes of food should be given to start with and then gradually increased.

As the animal's condition improves, they will likely start to show interest in food and start eating voluntarily. Reduction or cessation of nutritional support should be based on an assessment of recovery and should ideally be tapered off within the reptile's own environment at home to avoid relapse when the animal is discharged.

18.4.4 Anaesthesia

A full clinical examination and diagnostic tests, based on the presenting signs and clinical condition of the patient should be completed prior to anaesthesia. If possible a pre-anaesthetic baseline blood sample should check levels of uric acid, urea, glucose, and electrolytes including ionised calcium plus a PCV and blood smear evaluation (Chitty and Raftery 2013). Pre and post-operative care should include planning fluid and nutritional care, heat provision, and an analgesia plan.

18.4.4.1 Induction

Induction should be via intravenous or intramuscular injection as tortoises will breath-hold for very long periods, making mask or chamber induction impossible. Intubation is achieved using small uncuffed tubes, or improvising tubes, such as cut-down dog urinary catheters or intravenous cannulas for very small patients. The glottis is located at the base of the tongue and access can be improved by placing a finger between the mandibles to push the tongue up and forwards. The tube should be placed approximately 2 cm down the trachea. Tortoises have a relatively short trachea before bifurcation, so it can be easy to intubate only one bronchus.

Table 18.4   Routes of fluid administration.

Fluid Therapy Routes	Administration	Comments
Bathing	Bathe twice daily in warm, shallow water	It is proposed that some chelonians will take up fluid well via the cloaca, although this has been disproved in aquatic chelonia (Peterson and Greenshields 2001). This technique also encourages drinking, urination, and defaecation. It may be a useful route for debilitated hospitalised tortoises.
Enteral Administration	1–5% body weight daily (10–50 ml/kg/24 hrs) in divided doses can be given. Water, electrolyte solutions, commercial liquid feeds, and liquidised food items can be used.	Preferred route for fluid therapy as long as the gastrointestinal tract is functioning.
● Stomach tubing (gavage)	Up to 15 ml/kg at a single dose	Excellent for short term nursing provided head can be easily accessed.
● Oesophagostomy tube placement	Up to 15 ml/kg per dose – monitor for regurgitation	Preferred for the administration of long-term medication, fluids and nutritional support. Patients tend to tolerate o-tubes well and will frequently eat around them.
Parenteral Administration	During initial stabilisation 1–3% body weight per 24 h can be administered safely (Kirchgessner and Mitchell 2009). Crystalloids such as glucose-saline or saline can be given as a continuous infusion intra-osseously or intravenously, or as boluses (e.g. epi-coelomically) of 5–10 ml/kg. Colloids are rarely used in practice.	May be required in more severe cases of dehydration. It has been suggested that lactated fluids (Hartmann's) should be avoided as lactic acidosis is common in stressed chelonians (Prezant and Jarchow 1997). Isotonic fluids are indicated for surgery, blood loss, and diarrhoea, whilst hypotonic solutions are indicated for chronic anorexia. There is little indication for hypertonic fluid administration.
● Epicoelomic	5–10 ml/kg given as boluses q 12–24 hours	Useful in practice.
● Intravenous	Continuous infusion preferred over infrequent off-the-needle boluses of 5–10 ml/kg.	Only suited to several debilitated chelonians requiring emergency treatment or anaesthetised animals. A jugular cut down is required for placement of an intravenous catheter which may then be sutured to the skin.
● Intracoelomic		Limited use due to poor absorption and risk of organ perforation (see therapeutics section)
● Subcutaneous	Limited to small volumes (1–2 ml/kg)	Absorption is likely to be slow.
● Intraosseous	10–30 ml/kg/day as a continuous infusion.	Rapid access to vascular system but may be painful and should be reserved for critical patients (see Therapeutics section).

18.4.4.2   Protocols

There are many injectable anaesthetic protocols described for tortoises. It is safest for the clinician to be familiar with one or two protocols (see Section 18.7.4). Doses may be adjusted based on the age and clinical condition of the patient. The author prefers intravenous induction with alfaxalone into the dorsal coccygeal vein. This gives approx- imately 15–20 minutes of surgical anaesthesia and can be topped up with repeat doses if needed, or the tortoise may be intubated and anaesthesia maintained with inhalant gas.

18.4.4.3   Maintenance

Inhalant gases such as isoflurane or sevoflurane are used. Intermittent positive pressure ventilation (IPPV) is important, particularly for longer procedures, due to profound respiratory depression during a surgical plane of anaesthesia with the absence of a diaphragm, and skeletal muscle relaxation. This may be done manually, but risks over-inflation of the lungs. A ventilator is recommended, with the peak airway pressure set at 12–15 cmH$_2$0 and a respiratory rate of 4–8 breaths a minute (Chitty and Raftery 2013).

18.4.4.4 Monitoring

Pedal and palpebral reflexes, plus jaw tone are useful to gauge the depth of anaesthesia.

Doppler flow monitoring over the carotid artery on the lateral neck is useful for monitoring heart rate audibly (Figure 18.8).

Temperature probes placed in the oesophagus or cloaca are useful to monitor trends. Hypothermia should be avoided by using heated operating tables, forced-air warming blankets, heat pads, and a high ambient temperature.

Pulse oximetry is less reliable in tortoises, although cloacal probes can be useful.

Electrocardiography (ECG) can help show arrhythmias, but is less useful in monitoring anaesthesia in tortoises as ECGs can be normal even if severe cardiopulmonary or brain compromise is present.

Capnography can be difficult to interpret in ventilated reptiles (Schumacher and Mans 2014) and needs further validation for reptilian patients.

18.4.4.5 Recovery

This may be slow, depending on the individual's clinical condition and the anaesthetic regime used. Core body temperature should be monitored and appropriate warming methods provided. Respiration is stimulated by high carbon dioxide and low oxygen levels, and so many clinicians will keep the tortoise intubated but provide IPPV using room air rather than oxygen to stimulate voluntary respiration.

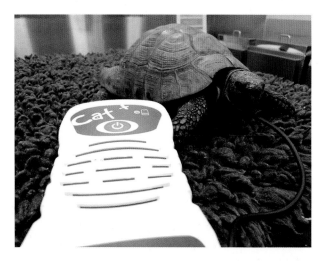

Figure 18.8 Placement of the Doppler probe over the lateral neck to monitor heart rate (*Source:* Courtesy of Sarah Brown).

18.4.4.6 Anaesthetic Emergencies

Tortoises can recover from prolonged periods of respiratory arrest, therefore every attempt should be made to aid resuscitation. In apparent respiratory arrest, the tortoise should be intubated and IPPV commenced. In cardiac arrest, adrenaline can be given intravenously, intraosseously, or via the endotracheal tube (Chitty and Raftery 2013), whilst continuing IPPV. Doxapram can be administered intravenously or intraosseously as a respiratory stimulant (Boyer 1998), whilst atropine can be used intravenously or intraosseously in severe bradycardia (Schumacher and Mans 2014).

18.4.5 Analgesia

The understanding of pain recognition and management in reptiles is still limited, and there appears to be much interspecies variation. It must be assumed that tortoises will feel pain and so a balanced analgesia plan starting prior to any potentially painful stimulus such as surgery should be implemented. Buprenorphine and butorphanol do not appear to have analgesic effects in reptiles so are not recommended (Sladky 2014). Tramadol, morphine, and methadone have been demonstrated to be effective in aquatic chelonia but no studies exist in Mediterranean tortoises to date (Sladky et al. 2007; Sladky and Johnson 2008; Baker et al. 2011). Local analgesia can be used to ameliorate analgesia during surgical intervention (Chitty and Raftery 2013; Chatigny et al. 2017).

Non-steroidal anti-inflammatory drugs (NSAIDs) such as meloxicam can be used together with opiates as part of a multimodal analgesic plan, or for management of chronic pain.

18.4.6 Euthanasia

Reptiles' slow metabolic rate and resistance to hypoxia can make euthanasia and death confirmation challenging (Baines and Rees Davies 2004; Leary et al. 2013). Euthanasia is generally performed by intravenous injection of 200 mg/kg pentobarbitone (McArthur 2004b). Prior sedation, for example with intramuscular ketamine, or intravenous or intramuscular alfaxalone is strongly recommended. Where intravenous access is not possible, for example in small juvenile tortoises, intracardiac injection through the plastron where the scutes intersect in the midline may be used after sedation, or alternatively using a longer needle introduced parallel to the neck and directed towards the midline. Intracoelomic injection is not recommended as uptake can be unpredictable and is likely to be painful (McArthur 2004b; Chitty and Raftery 2013).

Once the tortoise is unconscious, the brain should be pithed (mechanically disrupted), either through the roof of the mouth (more cosmetically palatable if the body is to be taken home by the owner) or through the foramen magnum. Freezing is not an acceptable method of euthanasia (Baines and Rees Davies 2004; Leary et al. 2013).

18.4.7 Death Confirmation

If not obviously in rigor mortis or showing signs of decomposition, this can be surprisingly difficult. Death may be confirmed by the lack of all withdrawal and ocular reflexes, no ECG trace (although ventricular pacing may give an ECG signal for up to 24 hours after death) and the use of Doppler or ultrasonography to show no cardiac motility (Baines and Rees Davies 2004; McArthur 2004b; Mader 2006; Chitty and Raftery 2013). It is recommended that owners be encouraged to collect their tortoise's body later the same day, or the next day, if there is any ambiguity over death confirmation.

18.4.8 Hospitalisation Requirements

It is imperative that suitable accommodation be available when admitting tortoise inpatients in practice. In particular, consideration should be given to heat provision, as keeping a reptile patient outside its POTZ will compromise recovery. Hospitalisation in a cat or dog kennel without appropriate heat provision is not acceptable.

Large plastic trays and aquaria can be quite simply adapted to provide appropriate short-term hospitalisation facilities (Figure 18.9). Conditions provided should approximate those described for captive husbandry, however modification such as replacing substrate with newspaper may be prudent for hygiene. Very debilitated individuals may not be able to move, and so temperatures should be monitored closely and kept within a smaller range to avoid hyper- or hypothermia.

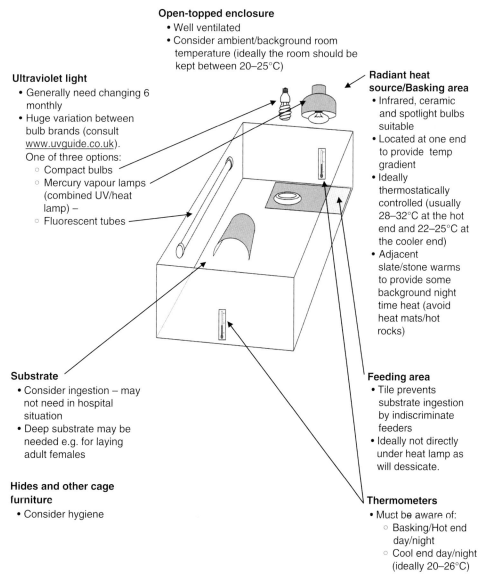

Open-topped enclosure
- Well ventilated
- Consider ambient/background room temperature (ideally the room should be kept between 20–25°C)

Ultraviolet light
- Generally need changing 6 monthly
- Huge variation between bulb brands (consult www.uvguide.co.uk). One of three options:
  - Compact bulbs
  - Mercury vapour lamps (combined UV/heat lamp) –
  - Fluorescent tubes

Radiant heat source/Basking area
- Infrared, ceramic and spotlight bulbs suitable
- Located at one end to provide temp gradient
- Ideally thermostatically controlled (usually 28–32°C at the hot end and 22–25°C at the cooler end)
- Adjacent slate/stone warms to provide some background night time heat (avoid heat mats/hot rocks)

Substrate
- Consider ingestion – may not need in hospital situation
- Deep substrate may be needed e.g. for laying adult females

Feeding area
- Tile prevents substrate ingestion by indiscriminate feeders
- Ideally not directly under heat lamp as will dessicate.

Hides and other cage furniture
- Consider hygiene

Thermometers
- Must be aware of:
  - Basking/Hot end day/night
  - Cool end day/night (ideally 20–26°C)

Figure 18.9 Generalised tortoise hospitalisation enclosure (*Source:* Illustration courtesy of Adam Naylor).

Gloves should be worn when handling patients, and changed between handling different individuals.

Hospitalisation sheets should be used to record any medications, fluid, and nutritional support given, and to record urination, defaecation, eating voluntarily, etc. The tortoise should be weighed daily and this recorded.

18.5 Common Medical and Surgical Conditions

18.5.1 Anorexia

It must be remembered that anorexia (lack of appetite) is not a disease, but a clinical sign (Goodman 2009) and so a thorough investigation is warranted. Common aetiologies for anorexia are shown in Table 18.5.

It can be difficult to differentiate between physiological anorexia, e.g. prior to egg-laying in females, and pathological anorexia. *T. horsfieldi* in the author's experience, will often show periods of poor or no appetite over the summer months when exposed to particularly high temperatures or prolonged photoperiod. This is consistent with their ability to aestivate in the wild. Careful history-taking may help with decision-making. Veterinary intervention is generally required if there is weight loss,

Table 18.5 Common factors in anorexia in Mediterranean tortoises.

Loss of energy reserves, e.g. post-hibernation. Termed 'depletion' (Chitty and Raftery 2013)
Poor husbandry (e.g. enclosure too cool, temperature fluctuation, lack of UVB lighting)
Inappropriate diet
Psychological stress (e.g. from overcrowding)
Systemic metabolic disease, e.g. renal failure, hepatic lipidosis
Systemic infectious disease, e.g. herpesvirus
Stomatitis/upper respiratory infection (often secondary to the cause of the anorexia)
Overgrown beak (relatively rare as a cause of anorexia)
Pain
Endoparasitism
Reproductive disease (e.g. egg binding or follicular stasis in females)
Gastrointestinal disease (e.g. foreign body)
Urinary tract disorders (chronic renal failure, urolithiasis)
Frost damage during hibernation – brain, digits, and eyes most commonly affected.
Blindness due to other causes

clinical evidence of disease, or persistent anorexia over a prolonged period of time.

Anorexia often occurs on waking from hibernation and the term Post-hibernation Anorexia (PHA) has been used as if this is a disease entity in itself. PHA has numerous causes and should be investigated and treated as for anorexia presenting at other times. Anorexia frequently occurs after hibernation as the tortoise is already in a vulnerable state. A recent survey of veterinary surgeons indicated that half the respondents had seen cases presenting with weight loss or anorexia following hibernation (BVA 2016). Cumulative effects of poor husbandry and diet, along with a poorly managed or excessively long hibernation period and concurrent disease compound this. The tortoise has insufficient metabolic resources to recover, leading to ongoing catabolism and further debilitation. The importance of correct hibernation preparation and management cannot be overstated.

The diagnostic approach will depend on the history and examination findings but as multiple factors are often present concurrently, a broad approach is needed. This often includes biochemistry, haematology, faecal analysis, and imaging (radiography, ultrasonography, endoscopy or CT). Culture and sensitivity, cytology, urinalysis, and specific pathogen detection may be utilised if indicated.

Treatment will vary and is dependent on achieving a diagnosis. In all cases failings in the husbandry must be addressed concurrently, both during hospitalisation and in the home environment. Fluid and nutritional therapy are crucial and oesophagostomy tubes are useful for long-term support and administration of medication. Reduction of stress and barrier nursing is important as many of these tortoises will be immunocompromised. Serial monitoring of blood values may be used to monitor response to therapy where applicable.

18.5.2 MBD and Accelerated Growth

MBD is a complex of conditions. The most common forms seen in Mediterranean tortoises are nutritional secondary hyperparathyroidism (NSHP) and renal secondary hyperparathyroidism (RSHP).

NSHP is most commonly seen in juvenile tortoises and can occur due to a dietary deficiency of calcium or vitamin D, excessive dietary phosphorus, lack of exposure to appropriate ultraviolet light, abnormally high growth rate (e.g. due to excess protein), or prolonged anorexia of any cause. The shell of a tortoise becomes rigid by 12 months of age, but affected tortoises will have progressively demineralised shells and bones, leading to issues with weight-bearing. Muscular weakness (and secondary organ prolapse), carapacial concavity over the pelvis, elongated beaks, overgrown claws, pyramiding of scutes, alterations in carapace conformation of juveniles, and egg retention in gravid females may be seen. Fractures are uncommon, but collapse of the humeral head may sometimes occur. Hypocalcaemic tetany is rarely seen in tortoises.

Radiography often shows poor bone density with decreased definition. Low ionised and total calcium, and elevated phosphate blood levels may be apparent, but affected individuals may be normocalcaemic due to sustained mineral release from bone. Reduced serum Vitamin D (as 25-hydroxycholecalciferol) levels support diagnosis (Eatwell 2008) but are not readily commercially available.

Treatment primarily involves correcting dietary and environmental issues, particularly diet and UVB light provision. Parenteral calcium therapy is rarely indicated and can be painful with potential side effects. Once normocalcaemic, calcitonin has been postulated to improve bone calcium deposition long term (McArthur 2004a), but there is minimal evidence for its efficacy and commercial availability is limited. Prognosis will vary according to the severity of signs. Most respond gradually over a period of weeks. The prognosis is poor if the shell is very soft or if renal dysfunction is concurrently present.

RSHP occurs due to either existing chronic renal disease or secondary to NSHP. These individuals can show the same signs as for NSHP but may be weak, anorectic, and dehydrated. Bloodwork may show hyperphosphataemia, hyperuricaemia, and a non-regenerative anaemia. Vitamin D levels can be low as its renal production will be affected. Radiography may show skeletal demineralisation, and also potentially renomegaly, urolithiasis, and gout-associated changes. Renal ultrasonography may be useful, and renal biopsy may allow a definitive diagnosis. However it is often difficult to justify invasive procedures in debilitated individuals with a guarded prognosis. Treatment involves fluid therapy, nutritional support, calcium supplementation, and allopurinol, but cases often have a guarded prognosis

Accelerated growth and shell-pyramiding are common in juvenile *Testudo* species and have been linked to excessive protein, excessive calorie intake, and low humidity. Accelerated growth also predisposes to NSHP and to reproductive issues such as dystocia in young females.

18.5.3 Renal Disease

Mediterranean tortoises are uricotelic, producing uric acid (and associated salts known as urates) as waste products. This is an evolutionary response to living in arid environments where energy and water are at a premium (McArthur et al. 2004) as urates precipitate out of solution without active concentration. Renal disease is common in tortoises and can have a variety of underlying causes.

These include:

Severe dehydration (e.g. after a poorly managed or excessively long hibernation);

Infection (bacterial, fungal, viral, e.g. picornavirus or protozoal, e.g. *Hexamita parva*); Pyelonephritis may arise from ascending urinary tract infection;

Toxins, e.g. iatrogenic aminoglycoside use;

Pelvic obstruction (post-renal disease) e.g. retained eggs, urolithiasis, gastrointestinal foreign body;

Diets high in purines (e.g. animal protein).

Clinical signs of renal disease are often non-specific, such as lethargy, anorexia, weight loss, dehydration, mucous membrane pallor, and weakness. There may be polydipsia and polyuria, but anuria is common. Oedema may occur secondary to protein-losing nephropathy or iatrogenic over-hydration in cases where the renal tubules are obstructed by urate deposits. Gout can occur due to the hyperuricaemia, leading to uric acid crystallisation in soft tissues (including kidneys, exacerbating pathology) and joints with associated lameness or swelling.

Definitive diagnosis of renal disease requires renal biopsy and histopathology (usually performed by pre-femoral endoscopy), but bloodwork showing elevated uric acid and normal, or elevated, urea levels plus hyperkalaemia is highly suggestive. Uric acid levels of greater than 1000 μmol/l carry a poor prognosis. Renal function tests are rarely performed in practice. Creatinine levels are considered a poor renal marker in tortoises (Wilkinson 2004). Fine needle aspiration of swollen joints or affected tissue will show uric acid crystals on cytology in cases of gout. Urine cytology and culture may be helpful, but due to cloacal anatomy, urine will be faecally contaminated. Urine specific gravity is not generally a useful marker of renal function, but changes in pH and urinary output can give an idea of response to treatment.

Treatment involves active fluid therapy, plus allopurinol treatment if uric acid levels are greater than 600 umol/l. This will only prevent further uric acid deposition. Recombinant urate oxidase (Rasburicase) therapy may be a promising treatment option, and can be given with allopurinol (Cope 2013). Oesophagostomy tube placement may facilitate fluid and nutritional support. Specific treatments such as antibiotics, anti-fungals, or anti-protozoals may be indicated, dependent on the primary cause. The tortoise's clinical condition, urine output and blood uric acid, urea and potassium levels should be regularly monitored. Euthanasia should be considered if the blood uric acid levels remain above 1000 umol/l as this is suggestive of intrinsic renal failure (Wilkinson 2004) or if the tortoise is not improving (e.g. starting to urinate actively) within 7–14 days of therapy (McArthur 2004b).

18.5.4 Urolithiasis

Bladder stones occur relatively commonly in Mediterranean tortoise species. The uroliths are usually composed of uric acid which forms solid aggregates during periods of dehydration. Other types of stones may form, e.g. struvite, but are rare. Tortoises can present with discomfort, secondary post-renal failure with urinary obstruction, or straining, or can be asymptomatic with uroliths found incidentally on radiography. Asymptomatic urolithiasis is suggestive of chronic dehydration or reduced urination.

Diagnosis is usually by radiography showing a solid opacity (Figure 18.10) though a very small proportion are radiolucent and require ultrasonography. Further work-up is required after diagnosis to assess the tortoise's hydration status and clinical condition – in particular renal parameters. If the tortoise is asymptomatic, and any husbandry or hydration issues are properly addressed, monitoring the size and location of the stone regularly by radiography alongside increasing fluid intake and bathing may be sufficient. In juvenile or very small tortoises, long-term treatment with allopurinol can help to prevent urolith enlargement so that, in time, the growing tortoise may be able to pass the urolith (Jepson 2016). For clinically affected cases, or those that do not pass the stone, surgical intervention is necessary. Uroliths lodged in the cloaca can be

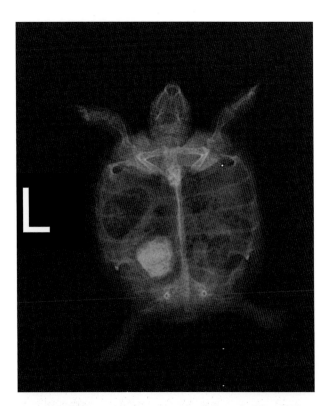

Figure 18.10 Dorsoventral radiograph of a juvenile *T. horsfieldi* showing a large radiopaque urolith (*Source:* Courtesy of Sarah Brown).

removed under anaesthesia either in entirety or piecemeal after breaking down in situ, with endoscopy and irrigation both helpful. If this is unsuccessful then cystotomy via a ventral plastral osteotomy is indicated (see Section 8.5.15). Lithotripsy under endoscopic guidance is an option, but rarely available to veterinary patients.

Prevention of urolithiasis is by correct feeding, good hydration, and good hibernation management.

18.5.5 Dystocia / Egg-Binding

This can be defined as a failure to deposit eggs within the time considered usual for the species concerned (McArthur 2004a) and is often a subjective assessment. The presence of calcified eggs on radiography is not necessarily a cause for concern or the explanation of any illness, but merely a sign of gravidity. However, chronic retention of eggs may occur and lead to clinical problems such as salpingitis, uterine or bladder rupture. There may be many reasons for egg retention including;

- Inadequate nesting site provision – tortoises may be very particular about nesting site location and substrate type;
- Competition for nesting sites;
- Intra/inter-species aggression;
- Inability to exhibit nesting behaviour due to stocking density;
- Inappropriate environmental provision, e.g. inappropriate substrate or temperature;
- Maternal or egg morphological and developmental abnormalities, e.g. over-sized eggs;
- Mechanical obstruction, e.g. urolith;
- Reproductive tract infection;
- Systemic illness (hypocalcaemia, dehydration etc.);
- Ectopic eggs (e.g. within the bladder).

The duration over which gravid females can carry eggs normally before oviposition is poorly defined so initially there may be no clinical signs. As the animal's health becomes compromised through systemic disease predisposing to dystocia, or dystocia itself, various signs are possible such as digging excessively, abnormal posture, hindlimb paresis, anorexia, lethargy, continuous or repetitive straining, and cloacal discharge. An egg may be visible at the cloaca.

Dystocia should be differentiated from normal gravidity as far as possible on the basis of clinical signs, history, radiography, ultrasonography, and general health assessment, but decision making can be complex as the point at which gravidity turns into dystocia is poorly defined. Chronically retained eggs are likely to have a thicker calcified shell on radiography, whilst eggs retained within the bladder may have irregular urate depositions around the shell. Ultrasonography can be useful to confirm the presence of eggs within the bladder.

If the tortoise is not systemically unwell and there is no obvious mechanical obstruction, then provision of appropriate environment with a nesting site may allow oviposition. These individuals should be regularly assessed to make sure that there is no progression to systemic illness. A nesting area should be at least four to five times larger than the carapace area of the female, contain substrate twice as deep as the carapace length and have a surface temperature of 30 °C (McArthur 2004a). As most chelonians lay eggs at night, excessive light should be avoided. If this does not induce egg-laying within 10–14 days then medical intervention may be required. Medical management should not be attempted if there are signs of mechanical obstruction, e.g. over-sized or conjoined eggs, prolapse, or ectopic eggs within the bladder. The tortoise is hospitalised and provided with a nesting area with appropriate heat, oral fluids and nutritional support provided prior to induction of oviposition (ideally after blood biochemistry to assess calcium levels and hydration status). If hypocalcaemic (ionised calcium <1 mmol/l), then calcium gluconate or borogluconate can be given, two to three hours prior to oxytocin. Beta-blockers such as atenolol may be given to help dilate the pseudocervix a few hours prior to oxytocin administration (McArthur 2004a). If egg expulsion does not occur after a single oxytocin injection, 50–100% of the original dose may be repeated after 4–12 hours. This may be continued in combination with fluid therapy whilst eggs continue to be produced at a rate greater than one every eight hours. If no eggs are produced and the tortoise is not systemically unwell, further attempts should be delayed for 10 days and then the protocol repeated.

If this is unsuccessful or the tortoise is becoming systemically unwell, surgical treatment should be performed after appropriate stabilisation. This is usually a salpingotomy or cystotomy via a plastronotomy to remove eggs. Bilateral ovariectomy is usually performed at the same time to prevent further reproductive problems. Rarely cloacal ovocentesis may be performed. This is a salvage procedure whereby the contents of one or more retained eggs may be aspirated via a needle and syringe per cloaca, e.g. if an over-sized egg is causing obstruction, but carries a risk of trauma or infection and eggs are rarely in a suitable position.

18.5.6 Follicular Stasis

Follicular stasis, or pre-ovulatory stasis, occurs when ovarian follicles are retained and do not either progress to ovulation or undergo atresia. Mediterranean tortoises have a reproductive cycle based on annual temperature variations (Chitty and Raftery 2013) but in captivity these temperature patterns are rarely achieved, leading to continued stimulation of follicle formation without ovulation in some individuals. Follicular stasis has also been proposed to be a failure of induced ovulation in long-term isolated females due to a lack of male pheromone or butting or biting behaviours (McArthur 2000).

Follicular stasis can lead to anorexia, hindlimb paresis, altered behaviour, and weight gain. Hepatic lipidosis, immunosuppression from hyperoestrogenism, a chronic catabolic state, and secondary bacterial oophoritis are common sequelae (McArthur 2004a).

This condition is a diagnosis of exclusion. Serial pre-femoral ultrasonography or coelioscopy to assess ovarian follicles showing non-progression of follicles over two to four weeks, and serial blood haematology and biochemistry showing leucopenia, hyperproteinaemia, hypercholesterolaemia, and hypercalcaemia can be suggestive. The presence of markedly different follicle sizes and co-existence of shelled eggs and mature follicles is also abnormal. If the tortoise is well, husbandry improvements and potentially introduction of a quarantined male at appropriate times may help. Bilateral ovariectomy via a coeliotomy after appropriate stabilisation is the treatment of choice (Figure 18.11). Medical management has so far proved unsuccessful. Prevention is by optimised husbandry and potentially the presence of a male at appropriate times of year, but much is still unclear regarding the underlying aetiology.

18.5.7 Cloacal Prolapse

Multiple tissues may protrude through the cloaca. To allow effective treatment, the tissue must be identified, its viability assessed, and the underlying cause investigated and addressed.

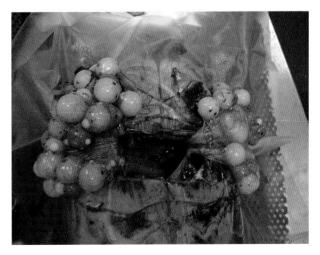

Figure 18.11 Plastronotomy in a tortoise with follicular stasis to carry out ovariectomy. Note the bevelled edge to plastronotomy site.

There is no single aetiology as many different organs may prolapse. Intermittent protrusion of the phallus in males, and occasionally the clitoris in females, is normal, especially on urination, defaecation, or handling, and should be distinguished from a persistent, abnormal prolapse (Figure 18.12).

Primary causes of cloacal prolapse include:

General weakness and debility;
Coelomic space-occupying lesion (e.g. urolithiasis, retained eggs, ectopic eggs, mass);

Localised trauma (excessive libido, mating injuries, substrate contamination);
Metabolic problems (e.g. hypocalcaemia);
Neurological issues;
Lower gastrointestinal or urogenital infection;
Endoparasitism;
Gastrointestinal foreign body.

Clinical signs show a structure protruding from the cloaca. There may be tenesmus and distress. The protruding tissue should be identified where possible.

18.5.7.1 Potential Tissues that May Prolapse

Cloaca – solid with no lumen. Shiny and pink. Urates may be seen coming from ureteral openings
Colon – smooth surface with a lumen. Shiny and pink. Faecal material may be present within the lumen
Oviduct – longitudinal striations on surface with a lumen. No faeces within lumen (Figure 18.13).
Bladder – thin walled with no lumen. May contain fluid.
Phallus – solid tissue with no lumen. Median groove may be visible.

Further investigations as to the underlying cause of the prolapse should be carried out, including history-taking, thorough clinical examination, bloodwork, radiography, faecal examination, and further imaging where indicated. Treatment will depend on the tissue prolapsed, its viability, and the underlying cause. Simply replacing the prolapse

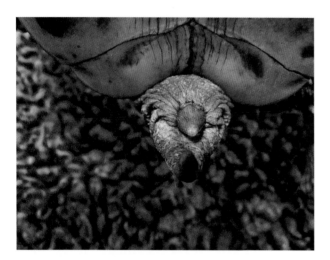

Figure 18.12 Normal transient prolapse of the phallus in a *T. hermanni* on handling (*Source:* Courtesy of Sarah Brown).

(a)

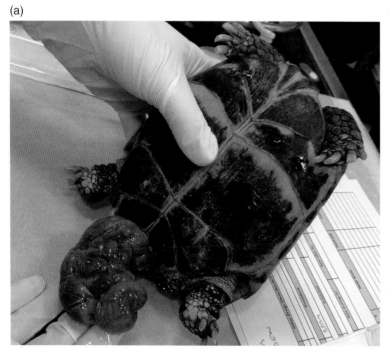

(b)

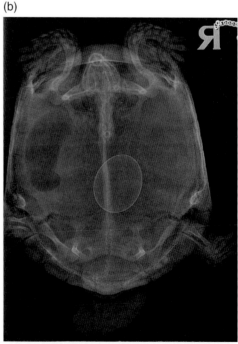

Figure 18.13 (a) Large oviductal prolapse in a young *T. horsfieldi*. This was due to straining to attempt to pass a single over-sized egg (*Source:* Courtesy of Sarah Brown). (b) Radiograph of same tortoise, note the large calcified egg and prolapsed soft tissues evident (*Source:* Courtesy of Sarah Brown).

with a purse-string suture without addressing and resolving the underlying cause will lead to recurrence.

Prolapses are emergency presentations and initial treatment will involve:

1) Gently lavaging prolapsed tissues with warmed sterile saline to remove contamination. Applying a 50% dextrose solution to the tissues will help to reduce oedema and allow easier reduction.
2) Applying lubricant gel to tissues to prevent desiccation.
3) Wrapping the tissues with a non-absorbent covering to stop further trauma or contamination.
4) Temporarily hospitalising animals in a substrate free enclosure. The enclosure should be warm but avoid intense heating that may desiccate prolapsed tissues.
5) Supportive care (analgesia, antibiotic cover, fluid and nutritional support).

Viable prolapsed tissues – should be cleaned, lubricated, and reduced under anaesthesia. Episiotomy to increase the cloacal orifice is sometimes necessary and should be repaired post-reduction. Once replaced, it should be ensured that the organ is completely inverted and not intussuscepted. Radiography and ultrasonongraphy can be useful to determine internal positioning post-reduction. Simple interrupted sutures can be placed on each side of the vent and removed after a few days to narrow the orifice and avoid repeated prolapse of tissue. Extensive colonic prolapses will require coeliotomy and colopexy.

Necrotic, traumatised, or infected prolapsed tissues – these tissues should be removed and the originating structure repaired. Underlying factors such as retained eggs or urolithiasis should also be addressed.

Amputation of oviductal tissue is possible, but a coeliotomy for bilateral ovariectomy and possibly salpingectomy is advised to prevent further pathology.

Removal of caudal intestinal tissue often requires coeliotomy for anastomosis of resected viable tissue and carries a more guarded prognosis.

Partial bladder resection will require a coeliotomy.

Amputation of the phallus is a more simple procedure and will not affect urination (but will affect fertility):

1) The tortoise is anaesthetised.
2) A haemostat is placed across the tissue close to the cloacal mucosa.
3) Monofilament polydioxanone transfixing ligatures are placed across the phallus base.
4) Distal tissues are removed. Over sewing the stump end is not necessary.
5) Analgesia and antibiotics should be given.

It is crucial that concurrent investigation of primary cause occurs after first aid measures and stabilisation are complete. Hedley and Eatwell (2014) evaluated recurrent prolapses and found that all involved underlying causes that had not been investigated or resolved on initial treatment.

18.5.8 Stomatitis and Pharyngitis

Stomatitis and pharyngitis are relatively common in tortoises. Affected individuals may show dysphagia or anorexia, hypersalivation, ventral neck swelling, diptheroid exudate on the tongue and oropharynx, oral inflammation, and petechiae of the oral mucous membranes. They can be associated with upper respiratory infections, otitis media and, less commonly, lower respiratory tract infections, oesophagitis, or gastritis.

Most cases have an underlying viral aetiology with secondary bacterial or fungal infection. Concurrent immunosuppression (e.g. recent hibernation, nutritional disease, or metabolic disease) or mixing of unquarantined tortoises will predispose individuals to stomatitis. Other more unusual causes include penetrating injury, ingestion of irritants, gout, and neoplasia. Investigation of stomatitis should include full clinical examination, history taking, and further investigations, such as bloodwork and radiography, to determine underlying causes.

Viral infection, in particular herpes, is a common cause of stomatitis, rhinitis, conjunctivitis, and glossitis. Currently four chelonian herpesviruses are recognised and exposure results in permanent infection with cycles of latency and recrudesence often associated with immune status. Pathogenicity is strain-dependent, and some individuals may be asymptomatic. Infections spread rapidly through colonies and consequently the virus is common in *Testudo* species farmed for the pet trade. Testudinid herpesvirus 1 and 3 commonly cause disease in Europe. TeHV1 is most commonly found in *T. horsfieldi* with low transmission and mortality. TeHV3 is more common in mainland Europe, usually in Hermann's tortoises, and has higher transmission and mortality rates (Marschang 2016). Spurthighed and marginated tortoises appear more resistant to disease, and may act as carriers, causing clinical disease in Hermann's and Horfield's tortoises if mixed with them (Marschang 2016). Acyclovir has been used with mixed results in confirmed herpes virus cases but side effects, including renal damage, are possible (McArthur 2004a; Gaio et al. 2007; Origgi 2012). Lysine has been suggested to help control herpes virus (Jepson 2016). Herpes-infected tortoises and their in-contacts should be kept in lifelong quarantine from others.

Iridoviruses (particularly ranaviruses) have recently emerged as a significant cause of mortality in wild chelonian populations (Johnson et al. 2008). Disease in pet species is usually associated with exposure to other infected reptiles or amphibians.

The field of chelonian virology is developing rapidly with further viral infections, e.g. picornaviruses implicated in stomatitis cases. Diagnosis of viral disease is by viral PCR testing of plain oropharyngeal swabs, viral isolation, or electron microscopy. Histopathology of tissues from deceased tortoises may be helpful. Serology is currently considered unreliable.

Bacterial or fungal stomatitis is usually secondary to immunosuppression or viral disease, and infections are often mixed. Oral samples should be taken for cytology and culture and sensitivity. Systemic or topical antibiotics or anti-fungal treatments based on sensitivity results should be given, alongside addressing the primary cause of immunosuppression. Fluid and nutritional support, usually with oesophagostomy tube placement, optimised husbandry, and barrier nursing are important. The oral discharge can be gently cleaned with cotton buds and dilute povidone iodine. Analgesia may be required in severe cases.

18.5.9 Upper Respiratory Disease (Runny Nose Syndrome – RNS)

Nasal discharge is common in Mediterranean tortoises and is often associated with various viral or bacterial infections. Mixed infections are often present. Many infections, such as herpes virus or *Mycoplasma agassizii* infection, will be latent and recrudesce when the individual is immunosuppressed (e.g. post-hibernation), whilst other bacterial and fungal infections will be opportunistic.

Affected tortoises show nasal discharge and some will also exhibit anorexia, lethargy, stomatitis, conjunctivitis, ocular discharge, increased respiratory noise, or dyspnoea. Necrosis of the external nares may occur, sometimes with oronasal fistulae developing.

A full clinical examination and husbandry review should be carried out. Blood biochemistry and haematology will screen for underlying disease. Culture and sensitivity testing may screen for opportunistic infections, but mycoplasmal culture is challenging. Cytology can indicate whether fungal organisms are present, indicating whether fungal culture is necessary. PCR testing for herpes viruses, *Mycoplasma* spp., iridovirus and *Chlamydia* are available for plain oropharyngeal swabs. Serology for *M. agassizii* and for chelonian herpes virus is available but may be difficult to interpret, as the presence of antibodies may indicate previous exposure rather than active disease. Repeated serological testing to demonstrate a rising titre, or concurrent use of serology and PCR techniques are more sensitive. Tests may not cover all viral serotypes and may not be

validated for every *Testudo* species. Imaging can help screen for lower respiratory disease – particularly Computed tomography (CT), or lateralateral and cranio-caudal horizontal beam radiographic views.

Treatment will depend on the causative agent. Concurrent diseases and husbandry insufficiencies should also be addressed. Appropriate systemic antimicrobial or anti-viral treatment can be useful. Even if a viral cause has been identified, antibiotics are usually necessary due to concurrent bacterial infection. Enrofloxacin or doxycycline are commonly used due to their anti-mycoplasmal properties. Nebulisation using saline or F10 has been used in some cases. Regular saline nasal flushing may help to clear the discharge and obtain diagnostic samples. Dilute iodine bathing of ulcerated areas is advised, along with barrier nursing and isolation of affected individuals. Those with herpes or *Mycoplasma* infections will be lifelong carriers. The main aim should be to improve the immune response by optimising husbandry and diet to minimise recrudescent episodes.

18.5.10 Lower Respiratory Disease

Tortoises with dyspnoea will often gape with their mouths and hold the neck extended. The forelimbs may 'pump' to help respiration (this should be differentiated with the normal 'pumping' sometimes seen when tortoises bask). There may be oral discharge and audible respiratory noise. Tortoises cannot cough so lower respiratory disease may not be evident until later in disease progression.

Differential diagnoses of dyspnoea include pneumonia, marked stomatitis or pharyngitis, tracheal or glottal obstruction, penetrating carapacial wounds, hyperthermia, or coelomic space-occupying masses. Potential causes of lung pathology include viral infection (herpes, iridovirus, and, picornavirus), bacterial infection (often opportunistic), parasitic infection (e.g. migrating ascarid larvae), inhaled toxins, neoplasia, aspiration pneumonia, and trauma.

Diagnosis will require full clinical examination, history-taking, and screening for concurrent disease. Radiographs should be taken to assess the lung fields with the cranio-caudal view most helpful to assess unilateral lung disease. Radiography is relatively insensitive in early pneumonia, so CT is preferred if available. Endoscopy of the trachea is possible on the larger Mediterranean tortoises but requires a small diameter endoscope. Focal lesions found on radiography may be assessed, sampled, and potentially treated endoscopically via a small carapacial osteotomy, whilst diffuse lung disease may be assessed endoscopically via a pre-femoral approach into the caudal lungs. Cytology and culture of samples taken via tracheal wash, tracheal swab, or endoscopy can be performed. Specific PCRs for viral and mycoplasmal causes can be performed.

Treatment involves supportive care with fluid and nutritional support and oxygen therapy, if needed, in the hospital environment. Depending on the cause, specific treatments such as targeted antimicrobials may be indicated. Viral treatment is generally supportive, as though anti-viral treatments for herpes infections have been used (e.g. acyclovir), efficacy is not proven. Nebulisation with F10 or antibacterial drugs is often used, although distribution of nebulised agents is undetermined. The prognosis may be guarded, depending on the underlying cause and severity of signs.

18.5.11 Drowning

Tortoises kept outside frequently fall into garden ponds. They often present as comatose with an absence of corneal, gag, or deep pain reflexes. Chelonia are very resilient to periods of anoxia and full but slow recovery is common, even after submersion of many hours. If non-responsive, the tortoise should be intubated and placed head down to drain fluid from lungs. Pumping of the limbs and head, IPPV and intravenous doxapram are useful. Fluid therapy, antibiotics, and NSAID therapy are advised. Frusemide has been suggested to encourage diuresis (Jepson 2016). Aspiration pneumonia is a possible sequel.

18.5.12 Trauma

Trauma presentations in tortoises occur usually due to bites from male conspecifics, dog bites, rodent bites (particularly during poorly managed hibernation), lawn mowers, and falling from a height. Burns can arise from inappropriate heat sources such as heat mats or radiators. Individuals may be clinically bright immediately post-trauma giving owners a false impression of the severity of injury.

Full clinical examination is required under opioid analgesia or sedation, depending on injuries and clinical status. Careful investigation of penetrating wounds and fractures should be carried out using radiography, endoscopy, or CT. The aim should be to establish whether there are communications with the coelomic cavity and what structures have been damaged. Healing may take months with intensive wound care and nursing, so owners must be informed and committed. Severe trauma may warrant euthanasia.

First aid should include haemostasis, analgesia, and sample collection for culture (if appropriate) prior to antibiotic therapy and flushing of wounds. If maggots are present, they should be removed. Permethrin-based products can be used, but ivermectin and other avermectins are contraindicated due to toxicity to chelonia. If coelomic communications are suspected, gentle lavage with sterile saline from below avoids flushing contaminants into the coelom. If coelomic communication is not likely then dilute iodine solutions can be used with more aggressive lavage. Any loose fragments of shell should be carefully removed. Wounds can be dressed with hydrocolloid gels and non-adhesive dressing to avoid further contamination.

Soft tissue wounds – uncontaminated fresh wounds can be debrided and closed under anaesthesia in an everting pattern and the sutures removed after 4–8 weeks. Contaminated wounds should be encouraged to heal by secondary intention. Surgical debridement may be necessary once tissue vitality is clear. Topical povidone-iodine cleaning and antibacterial ointments may be useful. Severe limb wounds may require partial or full limb amputation. A prop, e.g. toy wheel or solid hemisphere, can be placed under the plastron to improve balance post-amputation. Where wounds occur at the shell-skin interface, closure may be achieved by drilling small suture holes in the shell edge to allow suturing of the skin margin to the shell.

Shell wounds – daily lavage and dressing changes are appropriate even for full thickness penetrating wounds. Some wounds will require further debridement under general anaesthesia and the coelomic membrane may require repair if open. Unstable shell fissures or fractures require stabilisation. Screw and wire tension-band repair, plating, bridging, or other stabilisation techniques are carried out once infection is resolved. Patching of shell deficits is now not advised as the lack of visibility under the patch means that infection can go unnoticed. Osteomyelitis is a potential sequel to shell injuries.

Fluid and nutritional support is vital, along with systemic antibiotics (with a spectrum covering anaerobes) and analgesia. Fluid loss through wounds and burns is high, and placement of an oesophagostomy tube can greatly aid provisions as well as nutritional support and medication.

Limb fractures may be repaired by simple restriction of movement i.e. strapping the limb into the fossa, by external coaption, internal fixation, or a combination of methods. The choice will depend on the individual's age, size and bone quality, and the fracture site.

18.5.13 Ocular Disease

Ophthalmic examination is limited by the small eye and difficulty in inducing mydriasis as iridial muscles are under voluntary control. Anterior chamber examination is possible and fluoroscein staining can be used to assess for corneal ulcers. Corneal diseases include keratitis, cholesterol or lipid deposition (common in older tortoises), and ulceration. Hypopyon and hyphaema occur rarely. Cataracts are common in older individuals, and exposure to freezing during hibernation may induce ice crystallisation within the lens (the forebrain is likely to also be affected in these cases).

Palpebral and periocular swelling can be seen in tortoises with herpes virus, iridovirus, *Mycoplasma* spp., *Chlamydia* spp. and opportunistic bacterial infections (Figure 18.14). Hypovitaminosis A may play a role in susceptibility to such ocular clinical signs. Trauma, neoplasia, or photokeratitis caused by inappropriate UV lamps are less common causes.

Blindness in tortoises is not uncommon, but can be difficult to assess. Difficulty in finding food and navigating enclosures, or overt lesions such as corneal opacity may give rise to a suspicion of blindness. Tortoises often cope well without sight, relying on their well-developed sense of smell to find food.

Treatment will depend on the underlying cause, and in some cases, including lipid deposition or cataracts, no treatment is possible (Figure 18.15).

18.5.14 Septicaemia

Septicaemia is common in immunocompromised chelonians, such as those kept below the preferred temperature range or after a poorly managed hibernation period. Infections are usually gram-negative and entry occurs through wounds or dissemination from chronic lesions. Signs are non-specific but may include acute weakness, erythema of the plastron, mucous membranes petechiation, softening of the shell, and sudden death. The history often indicates poor husbandry, and there may be known previous infections. Diagnosis is often at post-mortem or presumptive. Blood culture would give definitive diagnosis

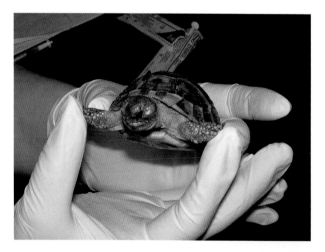

Figure 18.14 Severe blepharoedema and periocular abscessation in a juvenile tortoise (*Source:* Courtesy of Sarah Brown).

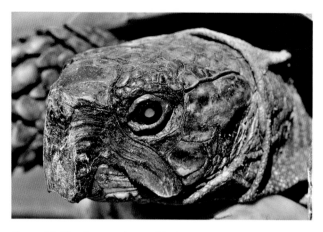

Figure 18.15 Cataract in an elderly *Testudo hermanni* (*Source:* Courtesy of T. Holtby).

but is rarely performed as contaminants are difficult to distinguish from infectious agents. Haematology may show toxic heterophils, sometimes with phagocytosed bacteria.

Treatment is antibiotics, ideally guided by culture and sensitivity, alongside fluid and nutritional support. Whilst awaiting results, broad spectrum antibiotic cover is started. The prognosis even with treatment can be guarded.

18.5.15 Surgery

Surgery in tortoises can be approached as for other companion animal species, with certain special considerations: having to perform an osteotomy for a coeliotomy (see later) and the need for IPPV during anaesthesia. When operating on extremities or the head, closure of the skin will require everting mattress sutures where possible, as reptilian skin has a strong tendency to invert, delaying healing (Mader et al. 2006). Aseptic site preparation is essential, with povidone-iodine based disinfectants generally preferred to chlorhexidine (McArthur and Hernandez-Divers 2004).

18.5.15.1 Coeliotomy

A plastronotomy will need to be performed to allow access to the coelomic cavity, e.g. for a cystotomy, ovariectomy, or salpingotomy. The anaesthetised tortoise is placed in dorsal recumbency and the incision site is marked as a square or rectangle, within the abdominal scutes, taking care not to include the pelvic and cardiac regions. The plastron is aseptically prepared and the incision made with a high speed saw or diamond cutting disc (Figure 18.16). Saline irrigation of the blade or disc will avoid localised thermal damage. The incision should be angled, with a larger external diameter, to give a bevelled edge and allow the plastral flap to fit securely back into position. The caudal incision can be partial to allow the plastral flap to be reflected caudally, or full thickness to remove the segment entirely.

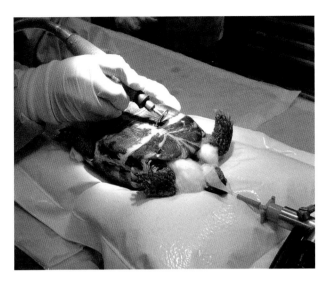

Figure 18.16   The plastron is incised using a diamond cutting disc after surgical preparation (*Source:* Courtesy of Sarah Brown).

The flap is lifted using a periosteal elevator to expose and detach the underlying musculature. The coelomic membrane is incised in the midline avoiding the paired ventral abdominal veins to access the coelomic viscera (Figure 18.11). The ventral abdominal veins can be ligated if disrupted.

Clear drapes, long-handled instruments and sterile cotton buds for tissue handling will help to ease the restrictions of operating within the coelomic cavity. Vascular clips, if available, can be invaluable.

After surgery, the coelomic membrane should be sutured and the plastral flap replaced. A mesh and expoxy resin can then be applied to give a waterproof covering. The tortoise should not be bathed for two to three weeks after a coeliotomy. The resin cover usually comes off after a few years, but may need to be removed and replaced sooner, e.g. in growing juveniles.

Systemic and local analgesia is vital along with appropriate hospitalisation with fluid and nutritional support. Oesophagostomy tubes may be placed at the same time as surgery to facilitate nursing care.

Coeliotomy may also be performed via a pre-femoral approach, but access is limited and endoscopy is usually needed for visualisation. This approach is not often used in Mediterranean tortoises due to their relatively small size and small pre-femoral fossae.

18.5.15.2   Oesophagostomy Tube Placement

The author usually places these with deep sedation via an intravenous alfaxalone bolus, but, in very debilitated animals, conscious placement with a local anaesthetic splash block and systemic analgesia may be preferable and appears minimally distressing for the patient.

1) Select a suitable tube (nasogastric Portex Feeding tubes, Infant 8F) and cut to approximately plastron length. A dog urinary catheter may be shortened and used in an emergency situation.
2) Mark tube at half the plastron length with a permanent pen to show the distance to advance into the oesophagus.
3) With the neck held in extension insert a long-handled curved haemostat into the oesophagus.
4) Push the tip laterally to protrude at the mid to distal third of the neck (the aim is to displace jugular and carotid arteries dorsally or ventrally)
5) Cut down over the tip of the instrument using a scalpel blade and push the tip through the oesophageal wall and skin. If bleeding occurs apply temporary pressure and place a mattress suture if necessary.
6) Grasp the end of the tube with the instrument tip and draw it through the incision and out of the mouth.
7) Reverse the tube and advance back down the oesophagus to the predetermined mark
8) Anchor tube to skin with a purse string suture then additional Chinese finger trap suture or surgical tape butterfly held in place with two mattress sutures.
9) Tape the tube to the nuchal scute and up over the carapace.

Tubes are generally well tolerated and can be left in place for months at a time. Placement allows home nursing and animals will frequently start eating with the tube still in place.

18.5.15.3   Microchipping

Microchipping provides a method of permanent identification of individual tortoises. This is useful for pet tortoises that may stray or be stolen, and is required for all CITES Annex A species – i.e. all *Testudo* species, other than *T. horsfieldi*, that are to be sold or exchanged, are on public display, or whose progeny are being sold or exchanged. Tortoises with carapace lengths of less than 60 mm may be temporarily exempted and a transaction certificate issued. When individuals reach sufficient size and the microchip is placed, the 'Article 10' certificate is applied for. The standard implantation site is the left hindlimb, and the preferred position is over the quadriceps muscle (WSAVA 2012). Hibernating tortoises should be implanted at least six weeks before the end of their active season in order to allow healing before hibernation.

The left hindlimb is extended and the site surgically scrubbed to try to reduce the risk of infection. The site can be infiltrated with local anaesthetic, taking care to use small volumes. There may be a functional lameness until the local anaesthetic clears. The chip should be implanted either subcutaneously or intramuscularly above the stifle in a proximal direction towards the hip. If there is any bleeding, pressure should be applied. Tissue glue or a mattress suture should be applied to the insertion site as there is increased risk of chip loss due to the inelasticity of reptilian skin. The tortoise should be kept in a clean environment and not bathed for a few days to reduce the risk of infection.

18.5.15.4 Beak Trimming

In some individuals the beak may become overgrown. This may be associated with MBD, accelerated growth, congenital abnormalities, infection, or trauma. Often the upper beak will grow to a rostral point, but in some cases the lower beak overgrows to protrude laterally. This can be trimmed carefully using a rotating sanding device, taking care to fully exteriorise the head and guard surrounding tissues (e.g. using a wooden tongue depressor as a gag and guard). Sedation may rarely be necessary. Regular correction is often required, and any underlying problems such as inappropriate diet or husbandry addressed.

18.6 Imaging

18.6.1 Radiography

Radiography is very useful in chelonians, although assessment of soft tissue structures is limited by the presence of the shell. High detail film screen systems are recommended. Sedation is rarely required. There are three standard views (Figure 18.17):

Dorso-ventral – the tortoise is placed in ventral recumbency with the head and limbs extended if possible.

Laterolateral – Ideally performed with a horizontal beam. The tortoise is placed on an object so that the limbs do not have traction with the floor. Alternatively, the tortoise can be taped to an object and rotated 90° to allow a lateral view from an overhead beam, although gravitational effects on internal organs may make interpretation more challenging.

Cranio-caudal – this provides a view of each lung (separated by a mid-line septum). Ideally a horizontal beam technique should be used, with the tortoise raised and legs extended. Otherwise the taping technique can be used, again with the potential interpretation issues.

Contrast studies using barium sulphate or iodinated non-ionic contrast media, e.g. iohexol, may be performed (Meyer 1998; Chitty and Raftery 2013). These can be useful for evaluating the gastrointestinal system. The contrast medium should be warmed to room temperature, given via stomach tube and serial radiographs taken. In reptiles, intestinal transit time will vary with temperature and agent

used, and can range from hours to days (Meyer 1998; Long et al. 2010; Mans 2013; Grosset et al. 2014). Meyer (1998) suggests using 7.5 ml/kg Gastrografin (amidotrizoate) in *T. hermanni*, giving a total transit time of 2.6 hours at 30.6 °C, 6.6 hours at 21.5 °C and 17.3 hours at 15.2 °C. Iodinated non-ionic contrast can also be used within the bladder to check whether an object visible on radiography is within the bladder or not (e.g. ectopic eggs, uroliths). Double contrast studies can be performed be introducing air into the bladder, reducing the positive contrast volume.

18.6.2 Ultrasonography

Ultrasonography can be a very useful non-invasive method for assessing soft tissue structures, such as the female reproductive system and the bladder, but is limited in tortoises to small acoustic windows. In Mediterranean tortoises a high frequency transducer (7.5 mHz) with a small footprint is deal. Sedation is rarely required. Usually the transducer is placed directly on the skin after application of acoustic gel, but a stand-off may be used in smaller individuals. The cervicobrachial window is used to assess the heart, major blood vessels, thyroid, liver, and gall bladder. The pre-femoral window can be used to visualise the reproductive tract (particularly ovarian follicles) and bladder. The liver and kidneys may be visible, depending on the individual's anatomy and the size of the pre-femoral window. The gastrointestinal tract may be imaged, but often the presence of gas impedes assessment.

18.6.3 Endoscopy

Rigid endoscopes are more commonly used, although flexible endoscopes can be useful when evaluating the gastrointestinal tract. Endoscopy can provide visual confirmation of diagnoses or abnormal findings, and provides an opportunity for biopsy and sampling. General anaesthesia, ventilation, and some form of insufflation are usually required.

Diagnostic endoscopic options include:

- Coelioscopy via the pre-femoral window;
- Evaluating the nares (often limited by the smaller size of these tortoises);
- Tracheoscopy via the glottis (often limited by the smaller size of these tortoises);
- Lower respiratory tract evaluation, e.g. investigation of focal lesion identified on radiography, via carapacial osteotomy;
- Lower respiratory tract evaluation via the pre-femoral window;
- Gastrointestinal tract via the mouth;
- Cystoscopy;
- Cloacoscopy.

(a)

(b)

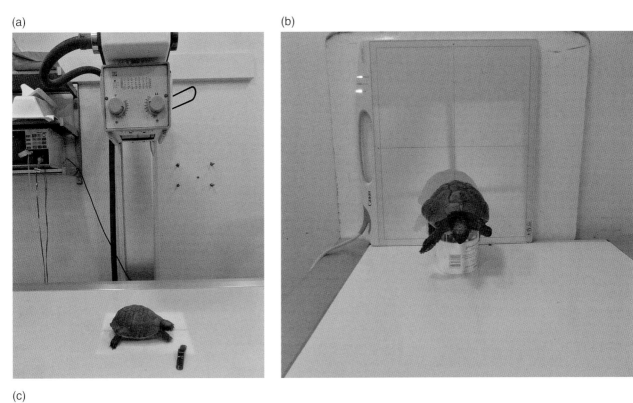

(c)

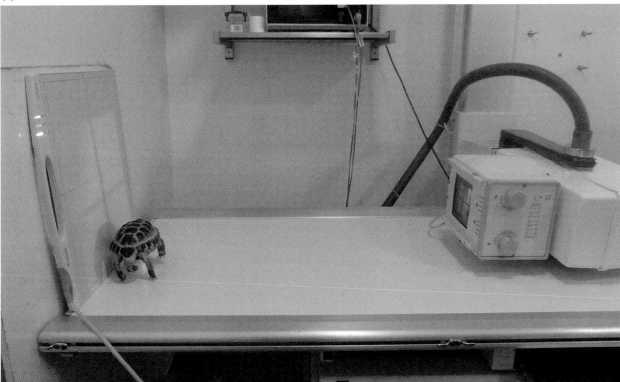

Figure 18.17 (a) Dorsoventral radiographic positioning. (b) Craniocaudal radiographic positioning. (c) Horizontal beam lateral radiographic positioning. (*Source:* Courtesy of Sarah Brown).

18.6.4 Advanced Imaging

CT and magnetic resonance imaging (MRI) are increasingly being used in chelonian patients. CT takes less time than MRI so can be performed without sedation or anaesthesia, although there is risk of movement artefact. Sedation will avoid this, or the limbs may be taped inside the shell to avoid movement. CT is useful for assessment of the skeletal system, spinal injury, internal organs, and gastrointestinal foreign bodies. A slice thickness of 1–2 mm should be used (Chitty and Raftery 2013). Contrast injection media may help visualise vasculature and organ systems (especially the hepatic, renal, and cardiopulmonary systems). There are no specified reptile doses for contrast media, although there are some suggested protocols (see Wyneken 2014).

MRI takes longer than CT so sedation or anaesthesia is usually required. It is useful for soft tissue detail, and indicated for space-occupying lesions, organomegaly, reproductive assessment, gastrointestinal foreign bodies, and respiratory disease. It is also a good choice for assessing neurological conditions. A slice thickness of 2–6 mm should be used with a field of view between 150–190 mm (Chitty and Raftery 2013).

18.7 Preventative Health Measures

There are no vaccinations or routine preventative health treatments recommended for Mediterranean tortoises. An annual or biannual veterinary check-up is recommended, including a faecal examination.

Endoparasites are common in pet Mediterranean tortoises, particularly oxyurids ('pinworms') and ascarid nematodes (Hedley et al. 2013). Other nematodes may occasionally be found, and protozoa are often found in elevated numbers secondary to other disease. The significance of low levels of endoparasitism can be questionable and indeed oxyurids may play a role in aiding digestion in wild tortoises. However, in captivity, a low burden can easily become significant due to the direct life cycle of parasites resulting in recurrent re-infection. Debility and enteric signs may be seen.

Routine deworming without faecal examination is not recommended due to the potential for development of resistance (especially given the limited range of 'safe' products available to use in chelonians), and the potential for adverse effects. Faecal examination (wet smears, or ideally flotation) should be carried out, and any significant parasites identified treated appropriately, whilst addressing environmental sources of infection. Tortoises can be bathed in a separate tray to encourage defaecation away from enclosure. Also, rotation of grazing areas outside helps to avoid an accumulation of parasites in one area.

Oxfendazole or fenbendazole have been historically used as anthelminthics in chelonia, and both seem effective against oxyurids (Gianetto et al. 2007). Aplastic anaemia and leucopaenia from bone marrow suppression, and gastrointestinal epithelial dysplasia may theoretically occur at high doses, as seen in other species (Howard et al. 2002; Graham et al. 2014). Clinical toxicosis has not been reported to date in *Testudo* species, though subclinical heteropaenia and transient biochemical parameter changes have been identified in Hermann's tortoises treated with fenbendazole (Neiffer et al. 2005). Careful assessment of risks and benefits should be considered when prescribing anthelmintics. To reduce the potential for toxicity, the tortoise should be weighed and a precise dose calculated. A faecal sample should be checked approximately two to four weeks after dosing to check efficacy.

Ivermectin or other avermectins should never be administered to tortoises due to the risk of severe toxic effects (Teare and Bush 1983).

Ectoparasitism is extremely rare in captive Mediteranean tortoises.

18.7.1 Annual vitamin injections

Often tortoise keepers present their tortoise for an annual multi-vitamin injection. If the environmental and nutritional provision is appropriate for the species, this is unnecessary, and an excess of vitamins may be detrimental. It is advised that such appointments be used to advise on correct husbandry and diet and to educate the keepers, and discuss other health monitoring options such as faecal examinations.

18.7.2 Claw Clipping

Claw clipping is rarely necessary. Overgrowth can sometimes be seen in younger individuals with generalised accelerated growth. Cat claw clippers or a rotating sanding nail trimmer can be used and silver nitrate pencils are suitable for cauterisation if there is any bleeding.

18.7.3 Neutering

Elective neutering is rarely performed in Mediterranean tortoises. Bilateral ovariectomy may be performed in cases of reproductive disease such as dystocia or follicular stasis in order to prevent further recurrence. This is usually performed via a midline plastron osteotomy (McArthur and Hernandez-Divers 2004), although endoscope-assisted pre-femoral ovariectomy may provide a viable alternative in larger individuals, avoiding osteotomy (Innis et al. 2007a). Attempts at medical manipulation of reproductive activtiy and behaviour have so far been minimally effective, although use of deslorelin implants has had a mixed response, with most effect seen in males showing signs of aggressive behaviour (Virbac, personal communication, 2017).

18.7.4 Formulary

There is very little pharmacokinetic data on the dosage and effectiveness of medications administered to Mediterranean

tortoises and doses are commonly extrapolated from other reptile species. Most medications given are unlicensed, and so the owner should sign an appropriate consent form. Common routes of medication administration are given in Table 18.6.

The formulary shows medications commonly given to Mediterranean tortoises which are available in general practice. Use is at the veterinary surgeon's discretion. It is not intended as a comprehensive list.

Table 18.6   Common routes of medication administration.

Route	Pros	Cons	Comments
Oral	In food medication simple for tortoises that are feeding	Medicated food should be hand-fed to ensure it is taken	
Gavage	Can be used to administer infrequent feeds/medication easily	Stressful for patient, consider placing oesophagostomy tube where repeated administration is expected	Gavage technique: 1) Select a suitable tube such as a crop tube, modified Jackson cat catheter, dog urethral catheters, or nasogastric feeding tube cut to approximately the length of the plastron (making sure the cut end is atraumatic). Use the widest possible bore to prevent tracheal intubation. 2) Mark tube at half the plastron length and lubricate. 3) A syringe containing the fluid to be given is attached to the tube and the tube is pre-filled (to prevent gavaging air). 4) Hold the tortoise in an upright position with the neck extended, and pass the tube dorsally along the roof of the mouth and pharynx. The tube should pass easily with no force. A gag (or a finger placed in the corner of the mouth) can be used to prevent the tortoise biting the tube.Fluids are administered slowly and the animal maintained in an upright position for a few minutes following administration to reduce regurgitation.
Subcutaneous	Small volumes can be given into skin folds in finely scaled areas.	Larger volumes cannot be injected due to the inelasticity of chelonian skin.	The skin should be cleaned with 10% povidone iodine or 4% chlorhexidine prior to any injection.
Intramuscular	Quadriceps muscles of hind legs or foreleg antebrachial muscles easily accessible	Small volumes possible, potential for iatrogenic radial nerve paralysis with antebrachial injections (Chitty and Raftery 2013)	The skin should be cleaned with 10% povidone iodine or 4% chlorhexidine prior to any injection. It is often suggested that drugs given to reptiles in the caudal part of the body may be cleared from the circulation by the kidneys due to the presence of a renal-portal shunt (Holz et al. 1997), or by the liver due to a first pass hepatic effect (Fink et al. 2018). There is no firm pharmacokinetic evidence at present to support this in Mediterranean tortoises, but where practical, cranial administration sites should be preferred.
Intravenous	Jugular and dorsal coccygeal veins accessible for injections	Repeated injection may be challenging, cut down technique necessary for jugular cannulation	See venepuncture notes

(Continued)

Table 18.6   (Continued)

Route	Pros	Cons	Comments
Epi-coelomic space	Useful for giving larger volumes of fluids to tortoises where oral or intravenous access is limited (e.g. smaller juveniles or larger intractable adults).		This is the potential space between the plastron and coelomic membrane. A needle is passed through the cranial plastronal inlet (parallel and just dorsal to the plastron between the head and forelimb). There should be no resistance to injection of fluid.
Intra-coelom	Possible in very small individuals where no other access is readily available	Absorption is very slow and there is a risk of organ perforation or injection into the lungs.	Access is via the pre-femoral fossa with the tortoise in lateral recumbency. The needle is directed to the ventral part of the fossa. Up to 3% bodyweight in fluids can be given via this route (Chitty and Raftery 2013).
Intra-osseous	Allows rapid access to the vascular system	Painful and reserved for critical patients	A spinal needle or hypodermic needle may be inserted into one of the following sites: plastron-carapacial bridge, gular plastron, distal ulna or proximal tibiotarsus. Use of a stylet avoids blockage of the catheter with a plug of bone during placement, but these sites remain prone to obstruction of fluid lines. Analgesia should be provided.
Topical	Useful for superficial dermal lesions or ocular therapy	Limited in tortoises due to the thickened nature of their skin	
Nebulisation	May be beneficial for respiratory tract disease	Dissemination of nebulised fluid unknown, particuarly for lower respiratory tract	Saline alone, or with antibiotics/disinfectants may be administered
In water		Not recommended as unreliable	

Formulary

Medication	Dose	Frequency	Comments
Anaesthetics			
Alfaxalone	5 mg/kg IV		15–20 minutes of surgical anaesthesia and can be topped up with repeat doses if needed. Otherwise, the tortoise may be intubated and anaesthesia maintained with inhalant gas under IPPV (Knotek 2014). Higher doses can be given IM but are less predictable
Propofol	4–10 mg/kg IV		Often little time for intubation before the tortoise wakes up. There are also reports of tissue necrosis occurring when propofol is injected into the subcarapacial sinus or coccygeal tail vein in other tortoise species (Chitty and Raftery 2013; Schumacher and Mans 2014).
Midazolam, Medetomidine, Ketamine	0.2 mg/kg (Mi), 0.1 mg/kg (Me), 2.5–5 mg/kg (K)		Can be reversed with atipamezole (0.5 mg/kg) IM +/− flumazenil (0.008 mg/kg IV)

(Continued)

Medication	Dose	Frequency	Comments

Antibiotics

Ideally these should be selected by culture and sensitivity. Antimicrobial combinations are popular where mixed infections are present or broad-spectrum cover required (e.g. enrofloxacin and ceftazidime). Topical cleaning with dilute iodine or chlorhexidine solutions is also useful.

Medication	Dose	Frequency	Comments
Amikacin	5 mg/kg IM	q 48 h	Potentially nephrotoxic (Caligiuri et al. 1990)
Ceftazidime	20 mg/kg IM	q72h	(Stamper et al. 1999)
Doxycycline	2.5–10 mg/kg PO	q 12–24 h	(Carpenter 2018)
Doxycycline	50 mg/kg IM initial dose, then 25 mg/kg	q 72 h	(Sporle et al. 1991)
Enrofloxacin	5–10 mg/kg IM, PO	q24–48h	Licensed in the UK, can be irritant when injected so use oral administration where possible (Sporle et al. 1991; Prezant et al. 1994; Raphael et al. 1994)
Marbofloxacin	10 mg/kg IM, 5 mg/kg IM	q 48 h q24h	(Coke et al. 2006)
Metronidazole	12.5–40 mg/kg PO	q 24 h	Use with caution due to effects on intestinal protozoal flora and adverse effects reported following administration at 20 mg/kg in red eared terrapins (Innis et al. 2007b)
Gentamicin (as Tiacil)	Topically on eyes	q8–12h	
Ofloxacin (as Exocin)	Topically on eyes	q8–12h	
Fusidic acid (as Isathal, Fucidin)	Topically on eyes and skin		Avoid steroid-containing preparations

Analgesia

Medication	Dose	Frequency	Comments
Lignocaine and bupivacaine	The dose should be kept below 2 mg/kg for each drug to avoid toxic doses		(Chitty and Raftery 2013)
Meloxicam	0.2 mg/kg IM, PO, IV	q24–48 h	(Divers et al. 2010; Uney et al. 2016)
Carprofen	1–4 mg/kg IM	q 24–72 h	(Lawton 1999)
Ketorolac	Topically on eyes		(Chitty and Raftery 2013)
Morphine	1–5 mg/kg SC, IM	q 24 h	(Sladky and Mans 2012)
Hydromorphone	0.5–1.0 mg/kg SC, IM	q 24 h	(Mans et al. 2012)
Methadone	3–5 mg/kg SC, IM	q 24 h	(Sladky et al. 2009)
Tramadol	5–10 mg/kg PO	q 48–72 h	(Baker et al. 2011; Norton et al. 2015; Spadola et al. 2015)

Antiviral

Medication	Dose	Frequency	Comments
Aciclovir	Topically to lesions (ointment)	q8–24h	(McArthur 2004b; Gaio et al. 2007; Origgi 2012)
	Systemic 80 mg/kg PO (syrup)	q8–24h	Efficacy not proven. Possible renal side effects.

Antiparasitics

Medication	Dose	Frequency	Comments
Fenbendazole	50–100 mg/kg PO	Repeat q14d for up to 4 treatments, or divide into three doses over three days	(Gianetto et al. 2007) Fenbendazole is metabolised to oxfendazole to take effect so tortoise must be in optimal condition for this conversion.
Oxfendazole	66 mg/kg PO	repeat after 14–28d	(Gianetto et al. 2007)

(Continued)

(Continued)

Medication	Dose	Frequency	Comments
Emodepsid/praziquantel (Profender, Bayer),	1.12 ml/kg topically		Shown to be effective against nematodes and cestodes (Mehlhorn et al. 2005; Schilliger et al. 2009)
Metronidazole	12.5–40 mg/kg PO		Use with caution due to effects on intestinal protozoal flora and adverse effects reported following administration at 20 mg/kg in red eared terrapins (Innis et al. 2007b)
Toltrazuril	15 mg/kg PO	q 48 h for three treatments	For coccidiosis (Gibbons and Steffes 2013)
Cypermethrin/piperonyl butoxide (F10 combined preparation)	Topical application		Used topically in myiasis treatment (avoid entering coelomic cavity or lungs) (Chitty and Raftery 2013)
Avermectins	Ivermectin and other avermectins should **not** be used in chelonians due to potential toxic effects (Teare and Bush 1983).		
Nebulisation agents			
F10 SC in saline	Dilute 1:250		(Chitty 2003)
Acetylcysteine	22 mg/ml sterile water		(Chitty and Raftery 2013)
Hypertonic saline			(Chitty and Raftery 2013)
Miscellaneous			
Adrenaline	0.1 mg/kg IV, IO or 0.2 mg/kg intra-tracheal		(Chitty and Raftery 2013)
Allopurinol	50 mg/kg PO	q24h for 30 days then q 72 h	For hyperuricaemia (Koelle 2001)
Allopurinol	10 mg/kg PO	q24h	for juveniles to prevent urolith enlargement (Jepson 2016)
Amidotrizoate (Gastrografin)	7.5 ml/kg PO		Radiographic contrast (Meyer 1998)
Atenolol	7 mg/kg PO	Single dose	can be given to help dilate a proposed pseudocervix 2–3 hours prior to oxytocin administration (McArthur 2004a)
Atropine	0.01–0.04 mg/kg IM, IV		(Schumacher and Mans 2014; Carpenter 2018)
Barium Sulphate	10 ml/kg PO		
Calcium borogluconate	100 mg/kg IV, IM, SC	q6–24h	Dilute 1:10 with water for injection or dextrose saline.
Calcium gluconate	50–100 mg/kg IM, SC	q6–24h	Dilute 1:10 with water for injection or dextrose saline.
Doxapram	5–10 mg/kg IM, IV, PO		(Boyer 1998)
Frusemide	5 mg/kg IM	q 12 h	(Jepson 2016)
Iohexol (Omnipaque)	10–20 ml/kg PO (reduce to 5 ml/kg for positive contrast cystography)		(Chitty and Raftery 2013)
Lactulose	0.5 ml/kg PO	q24h	(Jepson 2016)
Lysine	125 mg/kg PO	q 12 h	(Jepson 2016)
Oxytocin	1–5 IU/kg IM		If egg expulsion does not occur after a single injection, 50–100% of the original dose may be repeated after 4–12 hours (McArthur 2004a)
Rasburicase	0.2 mg/kg IM	q24h for 5 days	(Cope 2013)
Sibylin (milk thistle extract, medical grade. Samylin [VetPlus])	0.4 g/kg PO	q24h	(Chitty and Raftery 2013)
Silver sulphadiazine	Anti-bacterial skin barrier cream		(Hoppman and Wilson 2007)

References

Baines, F.M. and Rees Davies, R. (2004). The euthanasia of reptiles. *Veterinary Times* 34 (8): 89. and 34 (9): 12–14.

Baines, F., Chattell, J., Dale, J. et al. (2016). How much UV-B does my reptile need? The UV-tool, a guide to the selection of UV lighting for reptiles and amphibians in captivity. *Journal of Zoo and Aquarium Research* 4 (1): 42.

Baker, B.B., Sladky, K.K., and Johnson, S.M. (2011). Evaluation of the analgesic effects of oral and subcutaneous tramadol administration in red-eared slider turtles. *Journal of the American Veterinary Medical Association* 238 (2): 220–227.

Barrows, M., McArthur, S.J., and Wilkinson, R. (2004). Diagnosis. In: *Medicine and Surgery of Tortoises and Turtles* (eds. S.J. McArthur, R. Wilkinson, J. Meyer, et al.), 109–140. Oxford: Blackwell Publishing.

Boyer, T.H. (1998). Emergency care of Reptiles. *The Veterinary Clinics of North America. Exotic Animal Practice* 1 (1): 191–206.

BVA (2016). Don't leave your tortoise in a shoebox say vets. https://www.bva.co.uk/news-and-blog/news-article/don-t-leave-your-tortoise-in-a-shoebox-say-vets/ (accessed 20 September 2017).

Caligiuri, R., Kollias, G.V., Jacobsen, E. et al. (1990). The effects of ambient temperature on amikacin pharmacokinetics in gopher tortoises. *Journal of Veterinary Pharmacology and Therapeutics* 13: 287–291.

Carpenter, J.W. (2018). Reptiles. In: *Exotic Animal Formulary*, 5e (eds. J.W. Carpenter and C.J. Marion), 81–166. Amsterdam: Elsevier.

Chatigny, F., Kamunde, C., Creighton, C.M. et al. (2017). Uses and doses of local anesthetics in fish, amphibians, and reptiles. *Journal of the American Association for Laboratory Animal Science* 56 (3): 244–253.

Chitty, J.R. (2003). Use of a novel disinfectant agent in reptile respiratory disease. In: *Proceedings of the Association of Reptilian and Amphibian Veterinarians*, 65–67. Houston, TX: ARAV.

Chitty, J. and Raftery, A. (2013). *Essentials of Tortoise Medicine and Surgery*. Oxford: Wiley-Blackwell.

Coke, R.L., Isaza, R., Koch, D.E. et al. (2006). Preliminary single-dose pharmacokinetics of marbofloxacin in ball pythons (*python regius*). *Journal of Zoo and Wildlife Medicine* 37 (1): 6–11.

Cope, I. (2013). Fasturtec: A new treatment for renal disease in reptiles and birds? First International Conference on Avian, Herpetological & Exotic Mammal Medicine, Wiesbaden, Germany, 20–26 April 2013: 331.

Divers, S.J., Papich, M., McBride, M. et al. (2010). Pharmacokinetics of meloxicam following intravenous and oral administration in green iguanas (*Iguana iguana*). *American Journal of Veterinary Research* 71 (11): 1277–1283.

Eatwell, K. (2008). Plasma concentrations of 25-hydroxycholecalciferol in 22 captive tortoises (*Testudo* species). *Veterinary Record* 162 (11): 342–345.

Ernst, C.H. and Barbour, R.W. (1989). *Turtles of the World*. Washington, DC: Smithsonian Institution Press.

Fink, D.M., Doss, G.A., Sladky, K.K. et al. (2018). Effect of injection site on dexmedetomidine-ketamine induced sedation in leopard geckos (*Eublepharis macularius*). *Journal of the American Veterinary Medical Association* 253 (9): 1146–1150.

Gaio, C., Rossi, T., Villa, R. et al. (2007). Pharmacokinetics of acyclovir after a single oral administration in marginated Tortoises, *Testudo marginata*. *Journal of Herpetological Medicine and Surgery* 17 (1): 8–11.

Gianetto, S., Brianti, E., Poglayen, G. et al. (2007). Efficacy of oxfendazole and fenbendazole against tortoise (*Testudo hermanni*) oxyurids. *Parasitology Research* 100 (5): 1069–1073.

Gibbons, P.M. and Steffes, Z.J. (2013). Emerging infectious diseases of chelonians. *Veterinary Clinics: Exotic Animal Practice* 16 (2): 303–317.

Goodman, G. (2009). Clinical approach to the anorexic tortoise. *In Practice* 31: 156–163.

Gov.uk (2013). Endangered species: apply for a commercial use certificate. https://www.gov.uk/government/publications/endangered-species-application-for-commercial-use (accessed 24 September 2017).

Graham, J.E., Garner, M.M., and Reavill, R. (2014). Benzimidazole toxicosis in rabbits: 13 cases (2003-2011). *Journal of Exotic Pet Medicine* 23 (2): 188–195.

Grosset, C., Daniaux, L., Guzman, D.S. et al. (2014). Radiographic anatomy and barium sulfate contrast transit time of the gastrointestinal tract of bearded dragons (*Pogona vitticeps*). *Veterinary Radiology & Ultrasound* 55 (3): 241–250.

Hedley, J. and Eatwell, K. (2014). Cloacal prolapses in reptiles: a retrospective study of 56 cases. *Journal of Small Animal Practice* 55 (5): 265–268.

Hedley, J., Eatwell, K., and Shaw, D.J. (2013). Gastrointestinal parasitic burdens in UK tortoises: a survey of tortoise owners and potential risk factors. *Veterinary Record* 173: 525.

Highfield, A.C. (1994). *Tortoise Trust Guide to Tortoises and Turtles*. London: Carapace Press.

Highfield, A.C. (1996). *Practical Encyclopedia of Keeping and Breeding Tortoises and Freshwater Turtles*. London: Carapace Press.

Highfield, A.C. (2000). *The Tortoise and Turtle Feeding Manual.* London: Carapace Press.

Holz, P., Barker, I.K., Burger, J.P. et al. (1997). The effect of the renal portal system on pharmacokinetic parameters in the red-eared slider (*Trachemys scripta elegans*). *Journal of Zoo and Wildlife Medicine* 28 (4): 386–393.

Hoppman, E. and Wilson, H.W. (2007). Dermatology in reptiles. *Journal of Exotic Pet Medicine* 16 (4): 210–224.

Howard, L.L., Papendick, R., Stalis, I.H. et al. (2002). Fenbendazole and albendazole toxicity in pigeons and doves. *Journal of Avian Medicine and Surgery* 16 (3): 203–210.

Innis, C.J. (1994). Considerations in formulating captive tortoise diets. *Bulletin of the Association of Reptilian and Amphibian Veterinarians* 4 (1): 8–12.

Innis, C.J., Hernandez-Divers, S., and Martinez-Jimenez, D. (2007a). Coelioscopic-assisted prefemoral oophorectomy in chelonians. *Journal of the American Veterinary Medical Association* 230: 1049–1052.

Innis, C., Papich, M., and Young, D. (2007b). Pharmacokinetics of metronidazole in the red-eared slider turtle (*Trachemys scripta elegans*) after single intracoelomic injection. *Journal of Veterinary Pharmacology and Therapeutics* 30 (2): 168–171.

Jackson, O.F. (1980). Weight and measurement data on tortoises (*Testudo graeca* and *Testudo hermanni*) and their relationship to health. *Journal of Small Animal Practice* 21: 409.

Jepson, L. (2014). *Tortoise. Understanding and Caring for Your Pet.* London: Magnet & Steel.

Jepson, L. (2016). *Exotic Animal Medicine. A Quick Reference Guide*, 2e. St. Louis: Elsevier.

Jessop, M. (2009). Identification of tortoises. *In Practice* 31: 46–57.

Johnson, A.J., Pessier, A.P., Wellehan, J.F.X. et al. (2008). Ranavirus infection of free-ranging and captive box turtles and tortoises in the United States. *Journal of Wildlife Diseases* 44 (4): 851–863.

Kirchgessner, M. and Mitchell, M.A. (2009). Chelonians. In: *Manual of Exotic Pet Practice* (eds. M.A. Mitchell and T.N. Tully Jr.), 207–249. St. Louis, MO: Saunders/Elsevier.

Knotek, Z. (2014). Alfaxalone as an induction agent for anaesthesia in terrapins and tortoises. *Veterinary Record* 175: 327.

Koelle, P. (2000). Urinalysis in tortoises. In: *Proceedings of the Association of Reptilian and Amphibian Veterinarians*, 111–113. ARAV.

Koelle, P. (2001). Efficacy of allopurinol in European tortoises with hyperuricaemia. In: *Proceedings of the Association of Reptilian and Amphibian Veterinarians*, 185–186. ARAV.

Koelle, P. and Hoffman, R. (2002). Urinalysis in tortoises – Part II. In: *Proceedings of the Association of Reptilian and Amphibian Veterinarians*, 117. ARAV.

Lawton, M.P.C. (1999). Pain management after surgery. In: *Proceedings of the North American Veterinary Conference*, 782. ARAV.

Leary, S., Underwood, W., Anthony, R. et al. (2013). *AVMA Guidelines for the Euthanasia of Animals: 2013 Edition.* Schaumburg, IL: American Veterinary Medical Association.

Long, C.T., Page, R.B., Howard, A.M. et al. (2010). Comparison of Gastrografin to barium sulfate as a gastrointestinal contrast agent in red eared slider turtles (*Trachemys Scripta elegans*). *Veterinary Radiology & Ultrasound* 51 (1): 42–47.

Mader, D.R. (2006). Euthanasia. In: *Reptile Medicine and Surgery*, 2e (ed. D.R. Mader), 564–568. St. Louis: Saunders Elsevier.

Mader, D.R., Avery Bennett, R., Funk, R.S. et al. (2006). Surgery. In: *Reptile Medicine and Surgery*, 2e (ed. D.R. Mader), 581–630. St. Louis: Saunders Elsevier.

Mans, C. (2013). Clinical update on diagnosis and management of disorders of the digestive system of reptiles. *Journal of Exotic Pet Medicine* 22 (2): 141–162.

Mans, C., Lahner, L.L., Baker, B.B. et al. (2012). Antinociceptive efficacy of buprenorphine and hydromorphone in red-eared slider turtles (*trachemys scripta elegans*). *Journal of Zoo and Wildlife Medicine* 43 (3): 662–665.

Marschang, R.E. (2016). Viral diseases of reptiles. *In Practice* 38: 275–285.

McArthur, S.J. (2000). A review of 10 cases of follicular stasis in *Testudo* species. In: *Proceedings of the British Veterinary Zoological Society, Spring 2000*, 44–60. London: BVZS.

McArthur, S.J. (2004a). Problem solving approach to common diseases. In: *Medicine and Surgery of Tortoises and Turtles* (eds. S.J. McArthur, R. Wilkinson, J. Meyer, et al.), 309–377. Oxford: Blackwell Publishing.

McArthur, S.J. (2004b). Anaesthesia, analgesia and euthanasia. In: *Medicine and Surgery of Tortoises and Turtles* (eds. S.J. McArthur, R. Wilkinson, J. Meyer, et al.), 379–401. Oxford: Blackwell Publishing.

McArthur, S.J. and Barrows, M. (2004). General care of chelonians. In: *Medicine and Surgery of Tortoises and Turtles* (eds. S.J. McArthur, R. Wilkinson, J. Meyer, et al.), 87–107. Oxford: Blackwell Publishing.

McArthur, S.J. and Hernandez-Divers, S. (2004). Surgery. In: *Medicine and Surgery of Tortoises and Turtles* (eds. S.J. McArthur, R. Wilkinson, J. Meyer, et al.), 403–464. Oxford: Blackwell Publishing.

McArthur, S.J., Meyer, J., and Innis, C. (2004). Anatomy and physiology. In: *Medicine and Surgery of Tortoises and Turtles* (eds. S.J. McArthur, R. Wilkinson, J. Meyer, et al.), 35–72. Oxford: Blackwell Publishing.

Meek, R. (1984). Thermoregulatory behaviour in a population of Hermann's tortoise (Testudo hermanni) in southern Yugoslavia. *British Journal of Herpetology* 6: 387–391.

Mehlhorn, H., Schmahl, G., Frese, M. et al. (2005). Effects of a combinations of emodepside and praziquantel on parasites of reptiles and rodents. *Parasitology Research* 97 (1): 65–69.

Meyer, J. (1998). Gastrografin® as a gastrointestinal contrast agent in the Greek tortoise (*Testudo hermanni*). *Journal of Zoo and Wildlife Medicine* 29 (2): 183–189.

Neiffer, D.L., Lydick, D., Burks, K. et al. (2005). Hematologic and plasma biochemical changes associated with fenbendazole administration in Hermann's tortoises (*Testudo hermanni*). *Journal of Zoo and Wildlife Medicine* 36 (4): 661–672.

Norton, T.M., Cox, S., Nelson, S.E. Jr. et al. (2015). Pharmacokinetics of tramadol and *o*-desmethyltramadol in loggerhead sea turtles (*caretta caretta*). *Journal of Zoo and Wildlife Medicine* 46 (2): 262–265.

Origgi, F.C. (2012). Testudinid herpesviruses: a review. *Journal of Herpetological Medicine and Surgery* 22 (1–2): 42–54.

Perpinan, D. (2017). Chelonian haematology. 1. Collection and handling of samples. *In Practice* 39: 194–202.

Peterson, C.C. and Greenshields, D. (2001). Negative test for cloacal drinking in a semi-aquatic turtle (*Trachemys scripta*), with comments on the functions of cloacal bursae. *Journal of Experimental Zoology* 290 (3): 247–254.

Prezant, R.M. and Jarchow, J.L. (1997). Lactated fluid use in reptiles: Is there a better solution? In: *Proceedings of the Association of Reptilian and Amphibian Veterinarians*, 83–87. Houston, TX: ARAV.

Prezant, R.M., Isaza, R., and Jacobson, E.R. (1994). Plasma concentrations and disposition kinetics of Enrofloxacin in gopher tortoises (Gopherus polyphemus). *Journal of Zoo and Wildlife Medicine* 25 (1): 82–87.

Raphael, B.L., Papich, M., and Cook, R.A. (1994). Pharmacokinetics of Enrofloxacin after a single intramuscular injection in Indian star tortoises (Geochelone elegans). *Journal of Zoo and Wildlife Medicine* 25 (1): 88–94.

Schilliger, L., Betremieux, O., Rochet, J. et al. (2009). Absorption and efficacy of a spot-on combination containing emodepside plus praziquantel in reptiles. *Revista de Medicina Veterinaria* 160 (12): 557–561.

Schumacher, J. and Mans, C. (2014). Anesthesia. In: *Current Therapy in Reptile Medicine & Surgery* (eds. D.R. Mader and S.J. Divers), 134–153. St. Louis: Elsevier Saunders.

Scott, P.W. (1996). Nutritional Diseases in Reptile Medicine and Surgery. In: *Proceedings of the British Veterinary Zoological Society*. London: BVZS.

Sladky, K.K. (2014). Analgesia. In: *Current Therapy in Reptile Medicine & Surgery* (eds. D.R. Mader and S.J. Divers), 217–228. St. Louis: Elsevier Saunders.

Sladky, K.K. and Johnson, S.M. (2008). Current understanding of analgesic efficacy and associated side effects in reptiles. In: *Proceedings of the Annual Conference of the American Association of Zoo Veterinarians*, 116–117. Los Angeles, CA: AAZV.

Sladky, K.K. and Mans, C. (2012). Clinical anesthesia in reptiles. *Journal of Exotic Pet Medicine* 21 (1): 17–31.

Sladky, K.K., Miletic, V., Paul-Murphy, J. et al. (2007). Analgesic efficacy and respiratory effects of butorphanol and morphine in turtles. *Journal of the American Veterinary Medical Association* 230 (9): 1356–1362.

Sladky, K.K., Kinney, M.E., and Johnson, S.M. (2009). Effects of opioid receptor activation on thermal antinociception in red-eared slider turtles (*Trachemys scripta*). *American Journal of Veterinary Research* 70 (9): 1072–1078.

Spadola, F., Morici, M., and Knotek, Z. (2015). Combination of lidocaine/prilocaine with tramadol for short time anaesthesia-analgesia in chelonians: 18 cases. *Acta Veterinaria* 84: 71–75.

Sporle, H., Gobel, T., and Schildger, B. (1991). Blood levels of some anti-infectives in the Hermann's tortoise (*Testudo hermanni*). In: *Proceedings of the 4th International Colloquium on Pathology and Medicine of Reptiles and Amphibians*, 120–128. Giessen: Deutsche Veterinarmedizinische Gesellschaft.

Stamper, M.A., Papich, M.G., Lewbart, G.A. et al. (1999). Pharmacokinetics of ceftazidime in Loggerhead Sea turtles (Caretta caretta) after single intravenous and intramuscular injections. *Journal of Zoo and Wildlife Medicine* 30 (1): 32–35.

Teare, J.A. and Bush, M. (1983). Toxicity and efficacy of ivermectin in chelonians. *Journal of the American Veterinary Medical Association* 183 (11): 1195–1197.

The IUCN Red List of Threatened Species (2017). Version 2017–1. www.iucnredlist.org (accessed 21 May 2017).

Türkozan, O., Özdemir, A., and Kiremit, F. (2008). International testudo trade. *Chelonian Conservation and Biology* 7 (2): 269–274.

Uney, K., Altan, F., Aboubakr, M. et al. (2016). Pharmacokinetics of meloxicam in red-eared slider turtles (*Trachemys scripta elegans*) after single intravenous and intramuscular injections. *American Journal of Veterinary Research* 77 (5): 439–444.

Wilkinson, R. (2004). Clinical pathology. In: *Medicine and Surgery of Tortoises and Turtles* (eds. S.J. McArthur, R. Wilkinson, J. Meyer, et al.), 141–186. Oxford: Blackwell Publishing.

WSAVA (2012). Microchip identification guidelines. http://www.wsava.org/guidelines/microchip-identification-guidelines (accessed 30 May 2017).

Wyneken, J. (2014). Computed tomography and magnetic resonance imaging. In: *Current Therapy in Reptile Medicine & Surgery* (eds. D.R. Mader and S.J. Divers), 93–106. St. Louis: Elsevier Saunders.

19

African Tortoises

Marie Kubiak and Sarah Pellett

19.1   Introduction

African tortoises comprise a wide range of species with some overlap with Mediterranean species (see Chapter 18). This chapter will focus on those distinct species found only in Africa. It is important to be aware that, in contrast to Mediterranean tortoise species, the majority of African tortoise species do not hibernate, and prolonged cooling can be extremely detrimental.

African tortoises are all listed on CITES Appendices I and II, with the common captive species found on Appendix II, resulting in restrictions on exportation of wild individuals. The most severe restrictions affect Sulcata tortoises where no commercial exports are permitted (CITES 2019). Imports of terrestrial African tortoises into the USA are currently banned due to their potential for acting as vectors for *Ehrlichia,* or carriage of infected ticks (Baker et al. 2015). Captive breeding is well-established and provides a sustainable captive population for Leopard and Sulcata tortoises.

The basic environmental requirements and conservation status of selected African tortoise species are listed in Table 19.1.

19.2   Species

19.2.1   Spur-Thighed Tortoises

Testudo graeca and its subspecies are collectively known as 'Spur-thighed tortoises' and most likely comprise a complex of different species rather than a true single species (van Dijk et al. 2004). It has been postulated that European and Asian populations of *T. graeca* are genetically distinct from those from North Africa and that the Eurasian group should be redefined as *T. ibera* and the North African group as *T. graeca* but taxonomy of these animals remains

controversial (van der Kuyl et al. 2005). *T. graeca* subspecies typically have a hinged plastron (ventral aspect of shell), spurs on the caudal thigh, and the carapace (dorsal domed aspect of the shell) does not divide dorsal to the tail. Subspecies can be further differentiated visually by size and colouration (see Table 19.2), and this is important as subspecies that originate north of the Mediterranean Sea and those that have their origins in North Africa have some differing care requirements.

As warm climate adapted species, the ambient temperature is fundamental to the wellbeing of all African tortoises. For juveniles, temperatures can be controlled in an indoor enclosure such as a tortoise table or temperature controlled vivarium. Use of vivaria is reducing as these often result in restricted ventilation and reduced enclosure size in comparison to the open topped table enclosures. Outdoor access for grazing and sunlight exposure is of huge benefit to adult chelonians but requires a protected shelter such as a shed with supplementary heating and lighting for most of the year in temperate climes.

Full spectrum lighting including ultraviolet-A (UV-A) and UV-B wavelengths is essential to allow endogenous vitamin D3 activation for calcium absorption from the diet, maintain immunocompetence, stimulate normal reproductive activity, and support natural behaviours (Baines 2018). Natural unfiltered sunlight is ideal, but this may be limited in captivity in temperate climes. Artificial lights are available commercially and their output should be monitored to identify decreasing output, or routinely replaced every 6–12 months. A UV Index range of 1.0–2.6 is advised for this species (Baines et al. 2016).

The preferred substrate is a natural limestone soil mix and is provided at a depth to allow burrowing and create areas with variations in temperature and humidity within the enclosure. Woodchip or stone substrates may cause intestinal obstruction if ingested and do not allow for burrow formation.

Handbook of Exotic Pet Medicine, First Edition. Edited by Marie Kubiak.
© 2021 John Wiley & Sons Ltd. Published 2021 by John Wiley & Sons Ltd.
Companion website: www.wiley.com/go/kubiak/exotic_pet_medicine

Table 19.1 Basic environmental requirements and conservation status of selected African tortoise species.

	Typical enclosure	Ambient temperature (°C)	Basking temperature (°C)	Ultraviolet lighting	Diet	Hibernation	IUCN conservation status	CITES listing
North African *T. graeca* subspecies	Tortoise table, shed, and garden access	20–26	30–35	Yes	Weeds, grasses, flowers	Some subspecies	Vulnerable	Appendix II
African spurred or Sulcata tortoise (*Centrochelys sulcata*)	Insulated, heated large shed with reinforced walls and access to large garden/paddock	30	35–40	Yes	Grass, hay, leaves, cultivated cactus such as Opuntia, kiln dried grasses in winter	No	Vulnerable	Appendix II
Leopard tortoises (*Stigmochelys pardalis*)	Repurposed room, insulated shed and garden access	30	35–40	Yes	Grass, weeds, hay, leaves, cultivated cactus such as Opuntia, kiln dried grasses in winter	No	Least concern	Appendix II
Hingeback species (*Kinixys* spp.)	Repurposed room or large tropical vivarium	24–27	30	Yes, with shaded areas	Leaves, flowers, fruits, fungi, invertebrates, and carrion	No	Vulnerable/Data deficient	Appendix II
Aldabran tortoise (*Aldabrachelys gigantea*)	Insulated, heated large shed/barn with reinforced walls and access to large garden/paddock	24–26	30–34	Yes	Grass, hay, leaves, tree roots, root vegetables	No	Vulnerable	Appendix II
Pancake tortoise (*Malacochersus tornieri*)	Large vivarium with secured rock piles	20–25	35–40	Yes	Grasses, hay, weeds, flowers, and small quantities of fruit and vegetables	No	Vulnerable	Appendix II

Table 19.2 Characteristics of subspecies of *Testudo graeca*.

	Range	SCL	Weight	Appearance
Testudo g. graeca	North Africa and Southern Spain	Males up to 145 mm Females up to 180 mm	Males 550 g, females 1300 g	Highly domed carapace, Yellow/light brown with black centre to scutes, small caudal thigh spurs
Testudo g. ibera	Europe and Middle East predominantly, occasionally found in North Africa	Males up to 180 mm, females up to 210 mm	Males 1200 g, Females 2000 g	Broader, flatter carapace, light brown/green colour with dark brown centre to scutes, one or two well defined spurs
Testudo g. terrestris	Middle East	200–250 mm	Females up to 1300 g	Small and pale with a highly domed carapace and a yellow spot on each side of the head
Testudo. g. zarudnyi	Middle East	Females up to 280 mm	Females up to 3500 g	Small and pale with a narrow carapace that is wider caudally, dark brown colour with minimal patterning and translucent margins to carapace
Testudo g. flavominimaralis (not recognised subspecies)	Libya	Males 110–120 mm	unreported	Elongated carapace, bright yellow colour with dark dots, skin orange/yellow with a bright yellow scale on the top of the head
Testudo g. whitei (not recognised subspecies)	Algeria	Males up to 240 mm, females up to 280 mm	males 2400 g, females 2500 g	Broad, flat carapace, golden yellow with irregular lines of darker marking, yellow head, large laterally curved pale spurs
Testudo g. nabuelensis (not recognised subspecies)	Tunisia and Algeria (A visually similar population has been reported on Sardinia but taxonomy of these is undetermined)	Males up to 120 mm	Unreported	Bright yellow with black markings, head yellow with two bright yellow supranasal scales, hind feet have yellow scales caudally, spurs are small and may be paired

The wild diet for African *T. graeca* comprises a narrower variety of plants than is seen in its Mediterranean counterparts, but this likely reflects the more limited flora of the habitat (Andreu 1987; Rouag et al. 2008). Grasses made up 30% in one study, with the remainder as broad leaves and a negligible intake of invertebrates suggesting a generalist herbivorous approach (Rouag et al. 2008). *T. g. graeca* in contrast appears a specialist feeder, actively selecting more nutritious plants (including some considered toxic) (El Mouden et al. 2006). Captive diets should contain a variety of edible leaves, grasses, weeds, and flowers to provide a high calcium, high fibre, and a low sugar, fat, protein, and phosphorus diet. Commercial pelleted diets have vitamin, mineral, and protein values that vary widely, but are invariably low in fibre and water (Kik et al. 2003) and are not appropriate for herbivores.

Calcium supplementation is required to attempt to increase the calcium:phosphorus ratio of the captive diet closer to the natural diet (Highfield 2000). Calcium can be provided as a powder supplement for food, either as a calcium salt, or in combination with vitamins.

19.2.2 Sulcata Tortoise

Sulcata or African spurred tortoises (*Centrochelys sulcata*) originate in the sub-Saharan regions of Africa (Stearns 1989). These giant tortoises are often bought as juveniles and rehomed later in life when they approach adult size at 10–15 years of age and owners realise that the heating and space requirements to meet their needs are beyond their ability (Figures 19.1 and 19.2). Adults have been recorded to reach over 100 cm in length and weigh over 100 kg (Flower 1925). The sandy brown carapace has an irregular 'furrowed' or sulcate appearance, and the plastron is a pale brown. Both sexes have enlarged gular scutes for defence that are found projecting from the plastron and extend cranially from under the neck but these are larger in males (ARAV 2003). Sulcata tortoises also have prominent double caudal thigh spurs (Figure 19.3) but are easily differentiated from the much smaller *T. graeca* spur-thigh group.

Sulcata tortoises require heated accommodation year-round. As juveniles, housing can be indoors initially, with

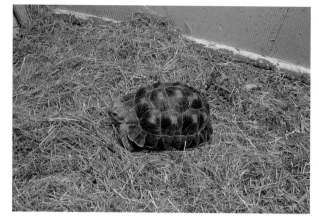

Figure 19.1 Subadult Sulcata at four years of age and 2.5 kg in weight.

deep soil substrate provided to enable burrowing to a depth of 30″ (ARAV 2003), with access to outdoor grazing during warmer periods. Adults, due to their size, cannot be maintained indoors. They require heated outdoor accommodation; often this is provided by a purpose built heated out-building with open access to grazing (Figure 19.4). This outdoor area should allow access to soil for digging and ideally a south-facing bank to facilitate basking. Sulcatas are large, strong tortoises able to demolish or dig under barriers, therefore enclosures must be robust with solid barriers extending under the soil. The social structure of a group is determined by the size and nature of the males and it is advisable to keep only one mature male per enclosure. If multiple animals are kept together, the space provided is often a limiting factor. Fighting can result if enclosure size is inadequate.

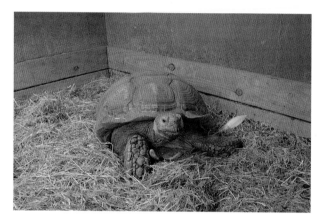

Figure 19.2 Mature male Sulcata tortoise at 60 kg bodyweight.

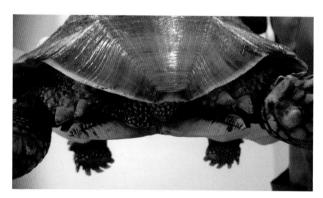

Figure 19.3 Appearance of double spurs in Sulcata tortoises.

(a)

(b)

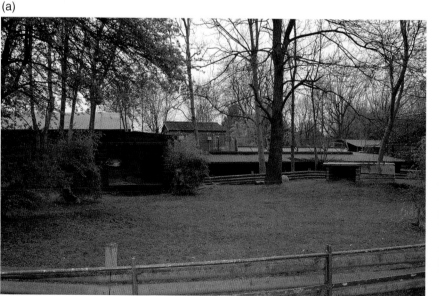
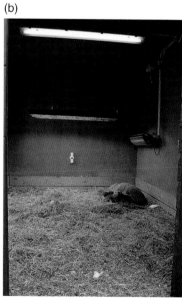

Figure 19.4 (a) Sulcata enclosure. (b) Interior of indoor shed shown in (a), note the heat and UVB provisions.

The indoor quarters should include heating and UV lighting. It is important that heat sources provide a wide area of heat to avoid focal overheating and thermal injury in basking animals. Multiple heat and UV lamps are often combined to provide a suitably large basking area.

Sulcatas originate from dry grasslands and feed on grasses, with opportunistic intake of succulent plants, flowers, and fruits (ARAV 2003). The captive diet is predominantly hay and grass, with supplemental leaves (e.g. Opuntia cactus, weeds, and salad leaves) when grazing is limited over winter. Adding limestone flour to soil can increase the calcium content of the grazing, or a calcium supplement can be administered daily. A large, shallow water vessel should be provided and water changed daily or more frequently if soiled.

19.2.3 Leopard Tortoise

Leopard tortoises (*Stigmochelys pardalis*) are a large tortoise species native to the arid areas of Eastern and Central Africa, with wild populations not currently under significant threat (Baker et al. 2015). They typically reach a weight of approximately 15 kg and a carapacial length of 35 cm. Leopard tortoises have a distinctive bright yellow carapace with melanistic patterning; this is an adaptation to provide camouflage in their native environment (Figure 19.5).

They can be a timid species in captivity, and may take a while to settle in and feed. Leopard tortoises require conditions and diet similar to those of Sulcatas, though enclosure size can be smaller to reflect the smaller individual size. Coarse grazing should be the mainstay of diet, supplemented by hay in winter, and calcium and vitamin supplementation of food is essential. Mixed sex groups have been maintained for this species but should be closely monitored for aggression or dominance of food sources.

19.2.4 African Hingeback Tortoises

African hingeback tortoises (*Kinixys* spp.) are small-to-medium sized tortoises with a distinctive hinged carapace. The caudal third of the carapace is able to move cranioventrally to close the caudal shell and protect the hindlimbs and tail.

This genus is difficult to maintain successfully in captivity (Innis 2000) and requires tropical conditions with constant day temperatures of 24–27 °C and 60–90% humidity. Deep moist substrate should be provided, and shaded or planted areas provided for cover. An enclosure should incorporate a shallow pond for constant access to water. Hingebacks are omnivorous, taking fruit, vegetation, fungi, invertebrates, and carrion opportunistically and the captive diet should reflect this (Luiselli 2003). Hingebacks are infrequently seen in captivity, with only Bell's hingeback (*Kinixys. belliana*) maintained with any frequency by private owners, though other species may be held within zoological collections.

19.2.5 Aldabran Tortoise

Aldabran tortoises (*Aldabrachelys gigantea*) originate from the islands of the Aldabra Atoll in the Seychelles and eclipse the Sulcata tortoise in terms of size with carapacial length of over 1 m and body weight of 240 kg in adults (Hatt 2008). Adults have an elongated neck for feeding from trees, slit-like nostrils and their size clearly differentiates them from other species (Figure 19.6). Their basic care is similar to that of Sulcata tortoises though basking temperatures are lower, space required is greater and diet is much broader, including roots and leaves. Mud wallows should also be considered for this species (Hatt 2008). Although captive breeding is increasing and these may be available to private owners, they are very challenging to maintain appropriately due to their large size.

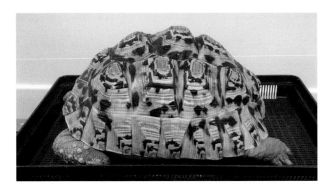

Figure 19.5 Leopard tortoises demonstrate distinctive shell patterning (*Source:* Courtesy of Sarah Pellett).

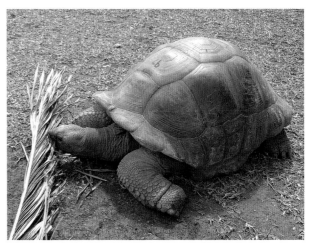

Figure 19.6 Aldabran tortoise (*Source:* Courtesy of Donna Stocking).

19.2.6 Pancake Tortoise
(Malacochersus tornieri)

The pancake tortoise is native to Tanzania and Kenya and is a specialist inhabitant of rocky outcrops (Malonza 2003). It has an unusual flexible, dorsoventrally flattened carapace with fenestrations in the bone, allowing for retreat into small crevices between rocks (Kabigumila 2002). It is found in zoological collections and captive bred specimens are occasionally held privately. These are small tortoises of 12–17 cm plastron length and weight of 200–600 g though some variation is seen with populations from different regions (Kabigumila 2002; Malonza 2003). Captive enclosures are predominantly indoor vivaria due to their small size and high temperature requirements. Providing a secure stack of rocks in the enclosure is ideal for simulating their rocky environment and allowing natural reclusive behaviours (Figure 19.7). Flat basking areas should be positioned under the heat and UV sources. They are able to climb so open topped enclosures should have high walls and rock features arranged to avoid escape. Although predominantly solitary, they will cohabit as pairs and larger groups of up to 11 animals have been observed (Loveridge and Williams 1957; Malonza 2003). Little information is available on natural diet, but captive populations are typically maintained on grass, leaves, and small amounts of fruit, with calcium and multivitamin supplementation.

A single egg is laid annually by wild breeding females during the dry season (Malonza 2003). In captivity, repeat clutches of one (or occasionally two eggs) may be laid every four to eight weeks.

19.2.7 Hibernation

Spur-thighed tortoises of North African origin, if hibernated at all, require a shorter hibernation period than their Mediterranean counterparts. It is recommended that they do not hibernate longer than 8–10 weeks, even in mature individuals, as opposed to the recommended 12 weeks with all other healthy Mediterranean species (Pellett et al. 2015). Other African tortoises should not be hibernated as they have not evolved to utilise this physiological mechanism. Periods of reduced activity in response to environmental conditions may be seen in many species in the wild, predominantly, aestivation (in hot conditions) and brumation (in cool conditions) but are physiologically distinct from hibernation.

19.3 Clinical Assessment

19.3.1 History Taking

As with other reptile species, captive management is a crucial factor in the health of animals and a full history must include a husbandry review. Low ambient or basking temperatures, lack of UV-B lighting, mixing different species, failure to quarantine new animals, and inappropriate diet are the most commonly deficient areas of care contributing to ill health. Particularly for larger species it is preferable to visit the facility where possible to assess husbandry in greater detail.

19.3.2 Handling

Handling of smaller species is straightforward with restraint of the animal by grasping the bridge of the shell on each side. Hingebacks are able to close the caudal plastron and carapace, so the hinge region and pre-femoral fossae should be avoided as fingers can be trapped. Large tortoises, such as adult Sulcatas, can cause serious damage to fingers if they retract the head or limbs during manual restraint and sedation should be considered for these animals if procedures are to be carried out or a complete examination is necessary.

19.3.3 Sex Determination

Sexual maturity is often size dependent, rather than age. For example, leopard tortoises may reach sexual maturity at 4 years of age in captivity, but their wild equivalents take 15 years to mature (Branch 1988; Innis and Boyer 2002). Sex determination is more challenging in juveniles as external differences may not become apparent until sexual maturity and there are individual variations.

Mature male tortoises have longer, thicker tails that curl around the caudal body and have a slit-like vent located distal to the margin of the shell (Figure 19.8) (Innis and Boyer 2002). The plastron may also be concave. Females have

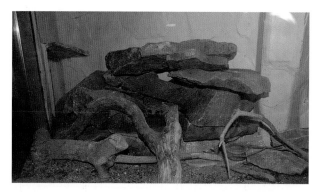

Figure 19.7 Pancake tortoise enclosure, incorporating secure rock pile to enable normal recluse behaviours (*Source:* Courtesy of Drayton Manor Park Zoo).

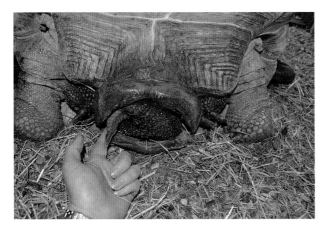

Figure 19.8 Male Sulcata, note the anal scute flaring and longer tail in comparison to the female in Figure 19.9.

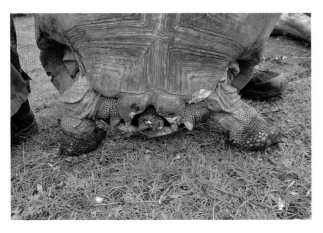

Figure 19.9 Female Sulcata tortoise with short tail and circular orifice at the level of the shell margin.

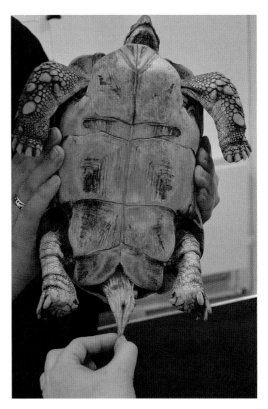

Figure 19.10 Male leopard tortoise, note the pronounced V-shaped notch in the plastron, and the slit-like vent located distal to the shell margin.

shorter tails with a more circular orifice (Figure 19.9). For the smaller species, females tend to be larger than males.

Male Leopard tortoises display a 'V' shaped notch for the tail opening, whereas in females the opening is typically 'U' shaped (Figure 19.10). Female leopard tortoises also have elongated hindleg nails (Innis and Boyer 2002). In Sulcata tortoises the gular scute projections are larger and the anal plastron scutes are more widely flared in males.

Plasma testosterone or follicle stimulating hormone stimulation test may also be potential options where external appearance is unclear but have yet to be validated in African species (Lance et al. 1992; Rostal et al. 1994). Laparoscopy may be used to directly assess the gonad and confirm sex (Innis and Boyer 2002) but is an invasive procedure and should not be considered a routine approach.

19.3.4 Clinical Examination

Before handling, observation of mobility, respiratory movements, and demeanour should be carried out. During clinical examination the shell is examined for injury or lesions and palpated to identify any areas of softening, though this is normal for Pancake tortoises. Limbs are palpated, joints flexed and extended, and skin, eyes, mouth, and nares observed for abnormalities. For oral examination, firm restraint of the head is needed and this is best achieved by allowing the tortoise to extend its neck and then placing a finger and thumb behind the head to prevent it withdrawing back into the shell. This can take a lot of time and patience and in some shy patients may not be possible (especially Leopard tortoises), or may risk handler injury in large individuals. Pushing the hindlegs into the shell or placing the tortoise in a warm water bath can encourage extension of the neck allowing the head to be grasped.

19.4 Basic Techniques

19.4.1 Sample Collection

Maximum sample volume is 0.6% bodyweight (i.e. 6 ml per kg) (Lloyd and Morris 1999) and in debilitated animals this should be reduced (Norton 2005).

Blood sample sites in small tortoises (and sedated large individuals) include the subcarapacial sinus, dorsal tail vein, and jugular veins. Lymph dilution can be a problem due to lymph vessels being in close association with veins, resulting in artefactual reduction of haematocrit, electrolyte, and tissue enzyme values (López-Olvera et al. 2003). As dilution is less commonly associated with jugular sample collection this is the preferred site (Gottdenker and Jacobson 1995). The jugular vein runs from the tympanum to the coelomic inlet and is accessed with the patient in lateral recumbency, with the head extended. Compression of the neck at the coelomic inlet may increase vessel size and visibility (Mans 2008). For large or uncooperative animals chemical sedation may be necessary.

The subcarapacial sinus is accessed by passing a pre-curved needle underneath the cranial lip of the carapace, dorsal to the neck to pass into the sinus on the underside of the cranial carapace (Hernandez-Divers et al. 2002). This site is harder to access in species with a high domed carapace but is often viable with both extended and retracted head positions.

The dorsal tail vein is relatively easy to collect samples from if the tail can be extended but lymph dilution is a common finding.

In intractable, conscious large individuals, the brachial vein may be the only accessible site, and this site also has the benefit of low lymph dilution potential (López-Olvera et al. 2003). A needle is inserted perpendicular to the humerus from the caudal aspect of the elbow, in a palpable groove adjacent to the bicipital tendon (Lloyd and Morris 1999; Mans 2008). The needle is advanced towards the elbow until blood is aspirated (Figure 19.11).

The occipital plexus has been described for blood-sampling of Pancake tortoises but this site results in lymph dilution and has potential for trauma to the brainstem so is best avoided (Raphael et al. 1994; Gottdenker and Jacobson 1995; Martínez-Silvestre et al. 2002).

Faecal samples can be collected as a freshly voided sample on handling or bathing, or warm saline can be instilled into the cloaca and colon using a soft rubber tube to stimulate defaecation or collect a dilute sample.

Bacteriology samples are collected directly from the lesion. Tracheal or pulmonary samples can also be collected under sedation by tracheal passage of a sterile catheter and direct aspiration of fluid and mucus, or by instilling sterile saline and re-aspirating fluid. In large species it is challenging to pass a catheter into the lungs and tracheal samples are more likely to be obtained.

19.4.2 Nutritional Support

Anorexia may be a consequence of chronic hypothermia and warming tortoises up to their correct thermal range

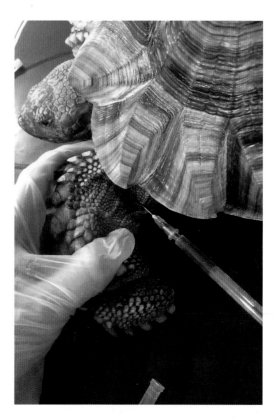

Figure 19.11 Blood sample collection from the brachial plexus in a Sulcata tortoise (*Source*: Courtesy of Sarah Pellett).

over one to two days can help restart self-feeding. Many tortoises use visual and olfactory stimuli to feed so brightly coloured or strong-smelling foods can encourage intake.

Nutritional support should be instigated when an animals loses 10% of body weight (Barten 2005). Nutritional requirements are calculated based on the Standard Metabolic Rate (SMR), with requirements of 1.1–2.5 SMR depending on individual animal status and activity. SMR is calculated in kcal, using a standard reptilian formula ($32[\text{bodyweight in kg}^{0.75}]$) (Pollock 2012). In chronically anorexic animals rehydration over a period of two to three days is necessary, followed by providing 40–75% of requirements initially to avoid refeeding syndrome (Barten 2005).

Herbivorous species can be assist fed using commercial liquid foods available for small hervbivorous mammals. Omnivores require addition of higher protein foods, available as omnivore liquid diets, or as a combination of herbivore and carnivore liquid foods. The stomach capacity of chelonians is approximately 2–5% of bodyweight and feeds should not exceed this volume (Pollock 2012).

Syringe feeding is poorly tolerated, time consuming, stressful for patients and risks aspiration of food material. Passing a gavage tube infrequently to administer a large volume into the stomach or distal oesophagus is possible in patients that can be readily restrained. A firm metal tube is typically used as rubber and plastic tubes may not withstand bites from tortoise patients. The tube should be of a wide enough diameter that it cannot pass inadvertently into the trachea, and have an atraumatic tip. The length should be pre-set to deliver food at the level of the distal oesophagus or stomach (generally coinciding with the junction of the humeral and pectoral scutes on the plastron: the second and third scutes in a cranio-caudal direction). The tortoise is restrained with the head and neck extended. The mouth is opened and the tube introduced into the mouth from one side, passed diagonally over the tongue and gently advanced down the oesophagus.

If enteral medication or feeding is likely to be needed repeatedly, or the patient is too large or strong to pass a gavage tube, then placement of a pharyngostomy tube under anaesthesia is recommended.

19.4.3   Fluid Therapy

Fluid absorption and regulation is compromised by cold temperatures, so patients should be maintained within their expected temperature gradient throughout treatment, and fluids should be warmed prior to administration.

A rough approximation of maintenance fluid requirements for tortoises is 10–20 ml/kg/day (Pollock and Arbona 2017), and deficits should be replaced, in addition to maintenance requirements, over 72–96 hours (Gibbons 2009). Isotonic fluids such as normal saline or Hartmann's solution are generally used, though hypotonic solutions, such as 0.45% saline, may be preferable for initial therapy of hyperkalaemic or severely dehydrated animals (Gibbons 2009).

Dehydration extent can be hard to evaluate in tortoises as evident skin folds are lacking but sunken eyes, absence of urination, hyperproteinaemia, and an elevated haematocrit value indicate dehydration (Divers and Cooper 2000). The epicoelomic (Figure 19.12) and enteric routes are commonly used for fluid therapy, see Table 18.4 for full details of options.

19.4.4   Anaesthesia

Anaesthesia or sedation may be challenging but is often essential for larger or stronger specimens to be able to complete a clinical examination and perform diagnostic tests, as well as for surgical procedures.

A pre-anaesthetic assessment to determine baseline respiratory rate, heart rate and rhythm is essential as these can be used as a comparison throughout anaesthesia and the recovery period. The chelonian must be warmed to its optimal temperature before administering any sedation or anaesthetic drug, and maintained at this temperature during and after the procedure.

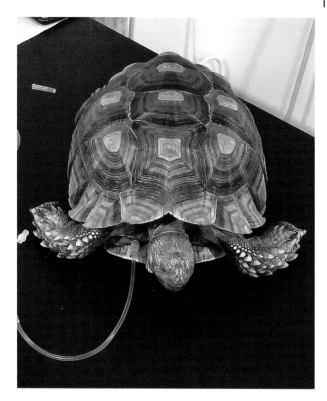

Figure 19.12   Epicoelomic fluid administration in a Sulcata tortoise (*Source:* Courtesy of Sarah Pellett).

Sedation should maintain spontaneous respiration, induce no significant cardiopulmonary depressive effect and maintain a response to stimuli. Drugs used are often short-acting or reversible. Minor surgical procedures such as skin abscess removal or hemipene amputation can be performed under sedation with the addition of local anaesthetic agents. Other minor procedures can be undertaken using sedation, such as oral examination, radiography, and blood sampling of larger chelonians or correction of beak overgrowth. Alfaxalone can be administered by intravenous or intramuscular (IM) injection, but the authors have seen highly variable responses when using the IM route. Anaesthetic options are listed in the formulary.

Induction with inhalational agents is not recommended due to prolonged or incomplete induction and health and safety implications for staff. Induction of anaesthesia is achieved with injectable agents, typically given intravenously using the same sites as for blood sample collection. Anaesthetics and analgesics may also be administered via the IM route, and this is believed to be quicker and have less variable onset times compared with subcutaneous (SC) injections. However SC routes are less painful, especially when large volumes are necessary, and resulting sedation depth is similar to that following IM injection (Mans 2015). Injection into the caudal body may result in increased clearance due to passage through the liver and renal portal system, so cranial sites are preferred (Holz et al. 1997).

Once induced, maintenance of anaesthesia can be achieved using volatile anaesthetics such as isoflurane or sevoflurane. A short, uncuffed endotracheal tube is used as the trachea bifurcates cranially and has complete cartilaginous rings (Sacchi et al. 2004). The glottis is visible at the base of the fleshy tongue and access can be improved using gentle external pressure on the underside of the cranial neck. Apnoea is common under anaesthesia (Bertelsen 2019) and intermittent positive-pressure ventilation (IPPV) using a mechanical small animal ventilator is advisable. If this is not available low pressure IPPV can be performed manually using an appropriate circuit such as the T-piece. The rate of IPPV is adjusted for individual requirements based upon the baseline data collected at the pre-anaesthetic assessment, the response of the patient, and the end-tidal carbon dioxide values during the procedure. As a general rule, to avoid over-inflation of the lungs, the inspiratory pressure should not exceed 12 cmH$_2$O.

Capnography values of end tidal CO$_2$ have been shown to have little or no correlation to pulmonary and arterial CO$_2$ concentration (Swenson et al. 2008). However, capnography remains useful in monitoring trends in the individual patient during an anaesthetic.

A Doppler probe can be used to assess heart rate and rhythm and is positioned over the carotid artery in larger chelonians, and the thoracic inlet in smaller individuals. An increase in heart rate during the procedure may indicate a response to pain or reducing plane of anaesthesia.

Head and limb withdrawal reflexes, palpebral and corneal reflexes, toe, tail, and cloacal pinch may be used as part of ongoing assessment but these reflexes are not always reliable.

As the procedure is nearing the end, the concentration of volatile anaesthetic should be tapered down with cessation at the end of the procedure. High oxygen concentrations in the lungs will significantly slow the return of spontaneous respiration, therefore the use of room air for ventilation during recovery is preferred to pure oxygen. Once spontaneous breathing occurs the chelonian is extubated and maintained within the appropriate ambient temperature range for the species. Once ambulatory, a basking spot can be reinstated.

19.4.5 Analgesia

Behavioural and physiological parameters associated with pain in chelonia may include an absence of normal behaviour, rubbing at an affected area, limb or head extension, changes in appetite, changes in activity levels, and changes to respiration and cardiac rate. Urination, defaecation, and thrusting of the head and limbs may be seen in response to an acute nociceptive stimulus (Wambugu et al. 2010). Baseline parameters and behavioural observations must be made before surgical or diagnostic interventions to allow comparisons after the procedure.

Morphine and pethidine have been shown to reduce response to a nociceptive stimulus at high doses in Speke's hingeback (*Kinixys spekii*), but flunixin, corticosteroids, and acetylsalicylic acid were ineffective (Wambugu et al. 2010). Clonidine has also been used experimentally in the same species, by intrathecal injection, to reduce response to a painful stimulus (Makau et al. 2017). Oral tramadol and local anaesthesia have been used together successfully for analgesia to enable penile amputation in a Leopard tortoise (Spadola et al. 2015).

19.4.6 Euthanasia

Euthanasia should be regarded as an act of humane killing with the minimum of pain, fear, and distress (Close et al. 1996). Pentobarbitone can be administered intravenously at 60–100 mg/kg (Fleming 2008). Sedation is advised if the chelonian cannot be restrained easily for access to the jugular vein or subcarapacial sinus. Once sedated, the occipital sinus is an alternative site but should be avoided in conscious animals. Maintaining the reptile at an appropriate temperature during the euthanasia process facilitates absorption and metabolism of the sedative and euthanasia agents (Music and Strunk 2016). The animal must be checked for cessation of a heart beat and then must be pithed to destroy the brain stem. Pithing involves insertion of a metal rod into the brainstem through the foramen magnum or roof of the mouth to physically disrupt tissues.

19.4.7 Hospitalisation Requirements

Tortoises hide signs of illness until later into the disease process, therefore stabilisation of the chronically debilitated reptile patient is often necessary before advanced diagnostics, treatment, or surgery can be performed and hospitalisation may be prolonged. As environmental conditions are crucial in patient health, appropriate heating, lighting, and nutrition must be available. Conditions for smaller species can be met temporarily using reptile vivaria with heat source and UV lighting as described under the husbandry section. Larger species may require an entire ward with appropriate heating and lighting. These large species can be difficult to manage longer-term without specialised facilities and may be better managed as out-patients with regular visits to the home facility if suitable.

19.5 Common Medical and Surgical Conditions

19.5.1 Infectious Disease

19.5.1.1 Upper Respiratory Tract Disease

Upper respiratory tract disease (URTD) is a common presentation of infectious disease seen in many tortoise species. Lesions may involve the nares, nasal cavity, mouth, and pharynx with nasal discharge, ocular discharge, and blepharitis common clinical presentations (Figure 19.13). Multifactorial causes are implicated involving various viruses, *Mycoplasma* species, other bacteria (usually as secondary opportunistic infections), and husbandry factors. Clinical disease can occur as an outbreak within a collection and is often seen when the animals are immunocompromised, with recrudescence of subclinical infection, or novel pathogen infection. If animals have been introduced into a group without adequate quarantine then pathogens may spread rapidly across a collection. Subclinical infections may be seen in some species due to co-evolution with pathogens, or acquired immunity in individuals, but these animals act as a source of infection for naïve animals within a collection (Wendland et al. 2006).

19.5.1.2 Viruses

Herpesvirus infections are commonly associated with URTD, with ocular and nasal discharge typically seen. Species variation in susceptibility and viral strain affects presentation. Leopard tortoises demonstrated URTD, intermittent paralysis, and 100% mortality (Drury et al. 1998) whereas the primary lesion seen in pancake tortoises was necrotic stomatitis, with hepatomegaly and gastritis less consistently seen (Une et al. 1999). Co-infection of a leopard tortoise with iridovirus and herpesvirus resulted in rhinitis, stomatitis, and pneumonia that resolved with supportive care (Benetka et al. 2007). Iridovirus alone has been reported to cause swelling of the head and neck and severe debilitation (McArthur 2004b). Tortoises with picornaviral infection may also develop necrotizing stomatitis, pharyngitis, conjunctivitis, rhinitis, pneumonia, ascites, and enteritis (Marschang and Ruemenapf 2002).

19.5.1.3 Bacteria

Mycoplasma agassizii and *M. testudineum* are common causes of URTD in North American and Mediterranean tortoise species, but reports in African tortoises are comparatively rare. Infection rates of 50% have been reported in Sulcata and Aldabran tortoises, and 68.6% of leopard tortoises tested however sample populations were small (Kolesnik et al. 2017). URTD associated with *M. agassizii* has been reported in the leopard tortoise and is widely reported in Spur-thighed tortoises (McArthur et al. 2002; Soares et al. 2004). Clinical picture is similar to other pathogens, with blepharitis, ocular and nasal discharge, and conjunctivitis (Jacobson et al. 1991). *Pasteurella testudinis* was isolated from multiple Leopard tortoises demonstrating dyspnoea, nasal discharge, pneumonia, and death (Henton 2003). No other pathogens were assessed and it is unknown whether the pasteurellosis was secondary to a viral or mycoplasmal primary infection.

19.5.1.4 Approach to URTD Cases

Presumptive diagnosis may be achieved by a thorough clinical examination, reviewing husbandry, nutrition, introduction of animals and biosecurity. Blood analysis and imaging are necessary to determine the overall health of the animal as co-morbidities are common. Specific pathogens can be identified by microbial culture and sensitivity (from oral or nasal secretions, or tracheal wash samples) and herpesvirus, picornavirus, ranavirus, and *Mycoplasma* PCR can be performed on tissue or dry swabs from affected regions. Significance of findings should be considered since many pathogens, such as picornaviruses, have been isolated from healthy individuals (Marschang and Ruemenapf 2002; The Pirbright Institute UK 2015).

Treatment is dependent on the causative agent but in all cases correction of environment and husbandry is essential, both during and after treatment. The tortoise should be kept at the high end of its temperature gradient, provided with a normal photoperiod incorporating UV-B light, and allowed warm daily baths to ensure good hydration. Minimising stressors is important, and this may include separating females from sexually active males, reducing population density, and minimising handling. Support feeding is often required and oesophagostomy tubes are generally

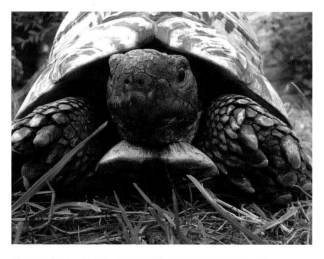

Figure 19.13 Nasal discharge in a leopard tortoise (*Source:* Courtesy of Donna Stocking).

well tolerated by most tortoises and are valuable for long-term administration of food and medication (McArthur 2004a).

Herpesvirus cannot be eliminated from infected chelonians and in this case optimal environmental conditions are essential to minimise recrudescence of infection. If *Mycoplasma* spp. are isolated then systemic antibiotics (typically oxytetracyclines or fluoroquinolones) can be administered but infection is rarely cleared and flare-ups require episodic treatment. Other treatments include nasal flushes and/or nebulization with medications such as F10 Antiseptic (Health and Hygiene [Pty] Ltd) diluted in saline to a concentration of 1 : 250. For hibernating species, hibernation must be avoided when clinically unwell, and length of hibernation for persisting carriers should be kept to no more than eight weeks.

19.5.1.5 Lower Respiratory Tract Disease

Lower respiratory tract disease may result from extension of upper respiratory tract infection, primary pathogens, or from opportunistic infections in immunocompromised individuals though published reports of common entities are lacking. Fungal pneumonia has been reported in Aldabran tortoises, with abscessation from *Paecilomyces fumosoroseus* and aspergillosis both described (Georg et al. 1963; Andersen and Eriksen 1968). Additionally, pneumonia and otitis media caused by intranuclear coccidian has been reported in a leopard tortoise (Jacobson 1997). A single case of suspected idiopathic pulmonary fibrosis has also been reported in a leopard tortoise with diffuse interstitial pattern on radiography, however concurrent presence of mycoplasma and a fungal granuloma in the lung complicate this diagnosis (Lim et al. 2013).

Radiography, or Computed tomography (CT) imaging, are valuable in identification of pulmonary lesions, and the craniocaudal view is preferred to assess the lung fields. A broncho-alveolar lavage is readily obtained in small species for diagnostic samples for cytology, culture, or PCR detection of specific pathogens. A sterile catheter is advanced down the trachea under sedation or anaesthesia, to allow warmed saline to be instilled into the lower respiratory tract and then a sample withdrawn. In large species access to the lung fields by this route is often not possible and an endoscopic approach to lesions may be necessary, with either a pre-femoral and trans-carapacial approach, dependent on target lesion location.

19.5.1.6 Miscellaneous Infections

A fatal *Helicobacter* septicaemia has been reported in a pancake tortoise (Stacy and Wellehan 2010). Weakness, lethargy, chronic anorexia, and oedema of the head and neck were identified prior to death. At necropsy, pericarditis with associated spiral bacteria and visceral bacteria presumed secondary to haematogenous dissemination were identified. PCR indicated that this was a novel species of *Helicobacter*. Concurrent intestinal cryptosporidiosis was identified in this animal.

SC abscessation can result from damage to the integument. The associated SC swelling tends to be firm due to fibrin content and a gradual increase in size may be noted in progressive lesions. Commonly affected sites are the forelimbs and neck. Surgical resection is necessary, with an incision made over the abscess. Where possible the associated capsule should be removed with the purulent core, and submitted for bacterial and fungal culture (Alworth et al. 2011). The abscess site is then flushed with a dilute disinfectant solution and may be left open for ongoing topical treatment, or sutured if abscess removal was complete (Alworth et al. 2011).

19.5.2 Parasites

19.5.2.1 Oxyurids

One study found 43.2% prevalence in a variety of tortoise species, with animals less than five years old more likely to be infected (Hallinger et al. 2018). Tortoises with confirmed infection included Sulcata, Leopard, Egyptian, Radiated, Aldabran, and Pancake tortoises. These 'pinworms' cover multiple genera of parasite that appear clinically indistinct, with apparent low pathogenicity however anorexia and death post-hibernation have been reported in a small number of cases with high levels of parasitism (Frank 1981; Martinez-Silvestre 2011). The lifecycle is direct so numbers can accumulate rapidly (Mitchell 2007). Diagnosis is by identification of asymmetrical pale brown ova, with one curved side and one flattened side. Infestation has been linked with ill health, poor hygiene, or inadequate husbandry. A review of management and health is indicated for animals with heavy burdens (Hallinger et al. 2018). Treatment with fenbendazole or oxfendazole is indicated for high burdens or in the presence of associated gastrointestinal signs (Giannetto et al. 2007). Benzimidazole-associated morbidity and mortality has been reported in Hermann's tortoises (*Testudo hermanni*) and so routine administration of anthelmintics is not advised (Neiffer et al. 2005).

19.5.2.2 Ascarids

Angusticaecum holopterum has been identified in Leopard and Sulcata tortoises with a prevalence of around 10%, though sample size for these species was small (Hallinger et al. 2018). In low numbers clinical disease is unlikely though visceral migration of larvae appears possible (Hedley et al. 2013). In higher burdens, gastrointestinal obstruction, intussusception, gastrointestinal ulceration, coelomitis, thromboembolism, and avascular necrosis have been reported (Keymer 1978; Frye 1991). Life cycle is direct and excreted eggs persist well under a range of environmental conditions, including exposure to many disinfectants making elimination difficult (Hallinger et al. 2018). Fenbendazole can be used for treatment of animals. Topical emodepside and praziquantel (Profender, Bayer) has also been used for endoparasite treatment (Mehlhorn et al. 2005; Brames 2008; Tang et al. 2017). Application to thin areas of skin, such as the axilla, may be a more practical, less stressful option than oral medication. In the giant species, the large volumes required may complicate application (Mans 2013).

19.5.2.3 Cryptosporidium

Cryptosporidiosis has been reported in the radiated tortoise (*Astrochelys radiata*), Egyptian tortoise (*Testudo kleinmanni*) and in a Pancake tortoise as a cause of enteritis (Graczyk et al. 1998; Griffin et al. 2010). Infection remains rare, with no positive samples identified in a population of 1054 tortoises assessed in one study (Hallinger et al. 2018). Acid-fast staining, immunofluorescent or PCR techniques are advisable to maximise sensitivity of testing (Hedley et al. 2013) but pathogenicity of detected cryptosporidia remains unclear and histology is needed to identify associated inflammation. No successful treatment has been identified in chelonia and euthanasia of confirmed clinical cases should be considered (Hedley 2012).

19.5.2.4 Other Protozoa

A range of motile protozoa are present in tortoise faeces and treatment is rarely necessary. If burdens are considered excessive, or are associated with clinical signs then metronidazole, iodoquinol, paromomycin, or chloroquine are treatment options (Hedley 2012)

19.5.2.5 Haemoparasites

A *Plasmodium* species (with concurrent flavivirus presence) has been suspected to be associated with a fatal haemorrhagic syndrome in a leopard tortoise (Drury et al. 2001). Affected tortoises demonstrated epistaxis, cloacal haemorrhage, biliverdinuria, and anaemia. Diagnosis was made based on identification of intracytoplasmic inclusions on blood smears but the aetiological agent was not confirmed. Successful treatment has not been reported in African tortoises, but chloroquine and primaquine were effective in Indian star tortoises (*Geochelone elegans*) (Redrobe 2000).

19.5.3 Non-infectious Disease

19.5.3.1 Metabolic Bone Disease

Metabolic bone disease is described as the most common medical disorder of captive chelonia, but this term encompasses multiple disease processes that result in disruption to calcium homeostasis and defective bone formation (Mautino and Page 1993). These include nutritional secondary hyperparathyroidism (NSHP), renal secondary hyperparathyroidism, osteoporosis, osteomalacia, and rickets (Heuser et al. 2014). In tortoises NSHP predominates, with resulting fibrous osteodystrophy (Mautino and Page 1993; Wright 1993). Juveniles are most frequently affected, followed by reproductively active females due to their greater physiological requirements for calcium (Jacobson 1994). To enable successful calcium homeostasis, calcium, vitamin D3, adequate temperatures, and normal organ function are required (see Table 19.3).

For non-breeding adults the recommended dietary calcium : phosphorus ratio is 2 : 1, however in growing leopard tortoise juveniles a ratio approximating 2 : 1 was inadequate and associated with development of NSHP (Fledelius et al. 2005). Vitamin D is required from the diet, or endogenous formation. Endogenous synthesis is initiated by exposure of dermal provitamin D to UVB light of wavelength 290–315 nm (Baines et al. 2016). Hydroxylation of the resulting cholecalciferol in the liver and kidney completes synthesis (Boyer 1995). Vitamin D3 enhances both calcium absorption from the intestinal tract and renal reabsorption of calcium to raise serum calcium levels (Innis 1994). Vitamin D3 doses for oral supplementation are still not clearly defined, with uptake appearing inferior compared with endogenous production (Oonincx et al. 2010).

Where calcium homeostasis is disrupted and serum ionised calcium levels reduce, parathyroid hormone (PTH) is secreted (Capen and Martin 1983). PTH raises serum calcium levels by increasing osteoclast activity to release calcium ions from bone, and increasing renal calcium reabsorption and phosphate excretion (Capen and Martin 1983). Without correction of the inciting cause PTH activity persists and progressive skeletal demineralisation occurs (Boyer 1995). Lethargy, softening of the shell, inability to walk, pathological fractures, shell abnormalities, flaccid paralysis, and dystocia are commonly seen (Figure 19.14) (Raiti and Haramati 1997; Eatwell 2008a). When the skeletal calcium supply becomes exhausted affected animals become lethargic, anorexic, and die (Boyer 1995).

Diagnosis is based upon assessment of diet, husbandry, serum biochemistry, and radiography (Boyer 1995). Plasma total calcium levels may be normal in the compensatory phase, but reduced later in the process when skeletal reserves of calcium are depleted (Boyer 1995; Raiti and Harmati 1997). Total calcium ranges can be broad, with 1.2–5.11 mmol/l reported in Hermann's tortoises, 2.39–3.67 mmol/l in Sulcata tortoises, and 2.22–6.21 mmol/l in Chinese three-striped turtles (*Cuora trifasciata*) (Andreani

Table 19.3 Factors commonly implicated in disruption to calcium homeostasis.

	Mechanism	Approach
Lack of dietary calcium	Inadequate available calcium for uptake. High oxalate foods can reduce available calcium content	Improve diet long-term, review supplementation, administer oral or injectable calcium preparations short-term
Excess dietary phosphorus	Dietary calcium is bound in insoluble calcium-phosphate salts preventing absorption, elevated serum phosphate levels induce parathyroid hormone release	Modify diet, consider administration of injectable calcium preparations short-term
Lack of UVB lighting (absence, incorrect wavelength of light, excessive distance from animal, failing output from old light)	Inability to form endogenous previtamin D3 (Raiti and Harmati 1997)	Improve husbandry with provision of appropriate lighting and monitoring of UVB output, administer oral Vitamin D3 short-term
Inadequate temperatures	Failure of conversion of previtamin D3 to cholecalciferol (Eatwell 2008b)	Provide appropriate heating and thermal monitoring using thermostats and maximum-minimum thermometers, administer oral Vitamin D3 short-term
Hepatic disease	Failure of conversion of cholecalciferol to 25-cholecalciferol in the liver, potential reductions in hepatic storage of 25-cholelcalciferol (Eatwell 2008b)	Supportive care and oral Vitamin D3 supplementation, consider endoscopy and liver biopsy for assessment of underlying pathology to enable targeted therapy of primary pathology
Renal disease	Failure of conversion of 25-cholecalciferol to 1,25-cholecalciferol in the kidney, impaired bone mineralisation due to uraemic/uricaemia acidosis, decreased phosphate elimination with precipitation of calcium and phosphorus in soft tissues and reduced serum calcium levels (Heuser et al. 2014)	Supportive care, fluid therapy and oral Vitamin D3 supplementation. Consider endoscopy and renal biopsy for assessment of underlying pathology to enable targeted therapy of primary pathology. In juvenile animals screen for picornavirus.

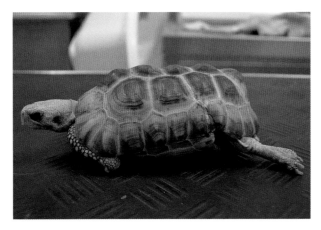

Figure 19.14 NSHP in a Bell's hingeback, note the inability to lift the body, pyramiding of shell and the degeneration of shell at the level of the hinge.

et al. 2014; Grioni et al. 2014; Eshar et al. 2016). The majority of this circulating calcium is bound to albumin and inactive. Interpretation of total calcium values should take albumin levels and physiological status into consideration as a serum calcium level within the reference range may be abnormal for a reproductively active or hyperalbuminaemic animal (Capen and Martin 1983). Ionised calcium accounts for 20% of circulating calcium and as the physiologically active fraction is considered more a more sensitive indicator (Eatwell 2007). Reported ionised calcium levels are 1.84–2.02 mmol/l for *Testudo* species (Eatwell 2008b). Phosphorus levels may be normal or increased depending on dietary levels, presence of folliculogenesis, and renal function (Capen and Martin 1983). Alkaline phosphatase may be elevated due to increased osteoclastic activity (Raiti and Harmati 1997). Vitamin D levels may be reduced. Reference values (as serum 25-hydroxycholecalciferol) in gopher tortoises (*Gopherus agassizii*) are 12.5–41.25 nmol/l, and in *Testudo* species are 24.41–32.42 nmol/l (Ullrey and Bernard 1999; Eatwell 2008b). Radiographs are valuable in advanced cases, demonstrating demineralisation and pathological fractures (Silverman 1993). Dual energy x-ray absorptiometry has been used to objectively assess more subtle alterations in bone mineral content but is not readily available (Fledelius et al. 2005).

Treatment comprises corrections of husbandry flaws, analgesia where bone changes are present, and exogenous provision of calcium and vitamin D until calcium regulation stabilises over weeks to months. Where significant deformities have been sustained that would hinder growth, egg laying, feeding, or mobility long-term, euthanasia should be considered. Malocclusion of the beak is a common consequence of mild–moderate NSHP and often requires corrective trimming long-term due to persistence of anatomical distortion even after bone mineralisation has normalised.

Renal secondary hyperparathyroidism has been described in juvenile tortoises with picornavirus nephropathy (Heuser et al. 2014). Reduced growth, plastron and carapacial softening, grey-black plastron discolouration, long bone deformities, hyperuricaemia, and high mortality were noted. Clinical signs were only seen in Indian star tortoises (*G. elegans*) and Spur-thighed tortoises (*T. graeca*) and typically started at four to six weeks of age with death by one year. All adults within the same group appeared unaffected (Heuser et al. 2014).

Toxicoses have been reported as a consequence of oversupplementation. An apparent excess of calcium (8 g/kg food, with a calcium : phosphorus ratio of 5 : 1) has been associated with mineralisation of soft tissues in leopard tortoises (Fledelius et al. 2005). Hypervitaminosis D has not been reported in chelonia to date but cases have been seen in other reptiles with excess of oral Vitamin D (Wallach and Hoessle 1966). Hypervitaminosis D is not a concern with endogenous synthesis as the conversion of provitamin D3 to previtamin d3 on exposure to UVB light is reversible and with exposure to excessive UVB light the products are degraded (Ferguson et al. 2003).

19.5.3.2 Shell Pyramiding

Shell pyramiding is the term applied to carapacial deformities associated with abnormally pronounced peaks and grooves (Figure 19.15). This should not be confused with the normal peaked appearance of some species from dry climes, notably the Sulcata tortoise. Pyramiding may result from metabolic bone disease, excess protein or calorie content of food, consistently high temperatures and abnormally low humidity (Wiesner and Iben 2003; Gerlach 2004; Heinrich and Heinrich 2016). Acquired shell deformities may lead to focal necrosis, weakening of peripheral margins, or an abnormally small shell compared to body size. Aldabran tortoises are reported to develop pronounced lesions under inappropriate conditions (Gerlach 2004). Prevention requires a multifactorial approach, which includes controlling food availability, ensuring an appropriate photoperiod, temperature, and humidity for the specific species and allowing a short hibernation period for the few African species that can hibernate (McArthur 2004c).

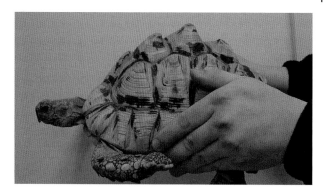

Figure 19.15 Pyramiding of the carapace in a leopard tortoise with a history of excessively rapid growth.

Changes cannot be reversed but will become less pronounced as shell growth normalises.

19.5.3.3 Calculi

Cloacal and bladder calculi comprising urate salts are reported as common in Sulcata tortoises (Che'Amat et al. 2012). Chronic dehydration, localised infection, excess dietary protein or oxalates and nutritional deficiencies have been postulated as causative factors (Mader 2006). One case series detailing three affected Sulcata tortoises described presentation with anorexia, straining, or failing to defaecate (Mans and Sladky 2012). All three cases had been maintained on a diet containing commercial dried pellets. Radiography demonstrates a radiopaque structure, or multiple structures, and cloacal endoscopy or cystoscopy can be used to visualise the calculi. Plastronotomy or pre-femoral coeliotomy can be used for surgical retrieval, or removal per cloaca can be attempted. Mans and Sladky (2012) report a successful approach for removal of cloacal calculi involving fragmentation using a guarded burr with endoscope-assisted fragment retrieval in Sulcata tortoises, with faster recovery than more invasive surgical techniques.

19.5.3.4 Shell Injuries

Traumatic injuries may be sustained from bites from dogs or foxes, animals being dropped, or conspecific trauma from aggression or mating attempts. Displacement or loss of over 30% of the shell, an inability to restore the shell integrity or concurrent damage to coelomic viscera, the head, or spine carry a grave prognosis and euthanasia should be considered (Fleming 2008). Where injuries are less severe, treatment can be attempted. Radiography provides valuable information as to whether the shell fractures affect only the superficial keratinised scutes, extend into the underlying bony scutes, or into the coelomic cavity. Primary closure of any fracture or cracks is not usually an option as most wounds are over six hours old by presentation and should be considered contaminated or infected (Crum 2013).

Management in these cases includes analgesia, lavage, topical and systemic antimicrobial therapy and regular dressing changes. Care must be taken when irrigating the wound not to introduce contamination deeper into the body. The chelonian must be positioned to direct the opening of the wound ventrally to allow for bone fragments, dirt, and foreign bodies to be flushed out from the wound and prevent fluid from pooling internally (Fleming 2008). Standard wet-to-dry dressings should then be applied to assist in the removal of debris (Fleming 2014).

Shell repair can be completed once infection has been addressed; a process that may take weeks. Displaced fractures can be reduced and aligned using wire or plates; metal bridges and/or fibreglass patches (Bennett 1989; Harwell 1989; Heard 1999; Richards 2001). Long-term fibreglass and epoxy repairs are no longer advised for traumatic and infected shell injuries as this may sustain infection if sequestra are trapped underneath, or hinder healing of the underlying tissues (Fleming 2014). Systemic antibiotics and analgesia must be continued until healing is well advanced, fractures are stable and clear of infection. External fixation is left in place for at least 6–12 months to enable full healing (Hernandez-Divers 2004).

Vacuum-assisted closure is a fairly novel technique used in shell trauma injuries that do not breach the coelomic cavity and has been used in Aldabran tortoises (Coke and Reyes-Fore 2006; Adkesson et al. 2007). Constant negative pressure of approximately 125 mmHg is applied over the wound aiding in the removal of fluid, bacteria, and other factors that inhibit granulation whilst stimulating the blood supply in the granulation bed (Fleming 2014; Marin et al. 2014). It is an excellent treatment choice for infected or large wounds giving a reduction in healing time (Adkesson et al. 2007) but the initial cost of equipment is comparatively high.

Shell necrosis as a consequence of thermal injury is occasionally seen, particularly in the larger species where chronic thermal damage of the dorsal carapace occurs due to an inappropriate heat source (Nevarez et al. 2008). A similar approach to treatment of traumatic injuries is taken once debridement of devitalised tissues, including any necrotic bone, has been carried out. Significant sequestrum presence or extensive under-running of superficial tissues can result in necessary exposure of large areas of underlying bone. These require protective dressings to prevent desiccation and allow a granulation bed to mature without ongoing trauma or exposure to potential pathogens.

19.5.3.5 Endocrine Disease

Hypothyroidism has been diagnosed in Aldabran tortoises (Frye and Dutra 1974). Clinical signs reported include oedema of the head and neck, goitre, and anorexia. Reference values are available for T4 in Aldabran tortoises (6–12 nmol/l) and Sulcata tortoises (2–9 nmol/l), (Teare 2002; Franco et al. 2009). Levothyroxine has been used successfully to elevate serum T4 in a Sulcata tortoise (Franco and Hoover 2009), however in this case the T4 was within the expected range for the species and the initial diagnosis of clinical hypothyroidism is uncertain.

19.5.3.6 Reproductive Disorders

Dystocia and pre-ovulatory stasis are common conditions, and approach is similar to that for Mediterranean tortoises, as described in Chapter 18. A pre-femoral approach may be a viable alternative to plastronotomy for surgical management of reproductive tract pathology in larger species, particularly ovariectomy. This technique results in shorter surgical time and faster healing than from a plastronotomy. The hind leg is retracted caudally and an incision is made in the centre of the pre-femoral fossa, followed by blunt dissection of the underlying soft tissue (Knafo et al. 2011). The aponeurosis of the ventral and oblique abdominal muscles is incised to permit access to the coelomic cavity. Use of an endoscope to identify and exteriorise the relevant section of the reproductive tract through the surgical incision is typically necessary but bilateral ovariosalpingectomy via a single pre-femoral incision has been carried out in Indian star tortoises without endoscopic guidance (Takami 2017). Bilateral incisions may be required for larger individuals. For small or juvenile individuals, a fully endoscopic intracoelomic approach may be necessary (Knafo et al. 2011). The coelomic membrane and muscle are closed with a simple continuous pattern and the skin is closed with horizontal mattress sutures, using polydioxanone (Knafo et al. 2011).

For pancake tortoises, the soft plastron can be incised with a scalpel for access to the coelomic cavity and plastronotomy closure using wire and wide gauge sutures overlain with acrylic is possible (Figure 19.16).

19.5.3.7 Neoplasia

Neoplasia is uncommon in tortoises with an overall prevalence of 1.4% (Garner et al. 2004) and scant reports in the literature. Of note is an apparent outbreak of lymphosarcoma in Sulcata tortoises that was suspected to have a viral origin, but no causative virus was identifiable (Duncan et al. 2002). Other published reports comprise a biliary duct adenoma in a pancake tortoise, and a soft tissue sarcoma in a Radiated tortoise that was successfully treated by forelimb amputation (Effron et al. 1977; Clabaugh et al. 2005).

(a)

(b)

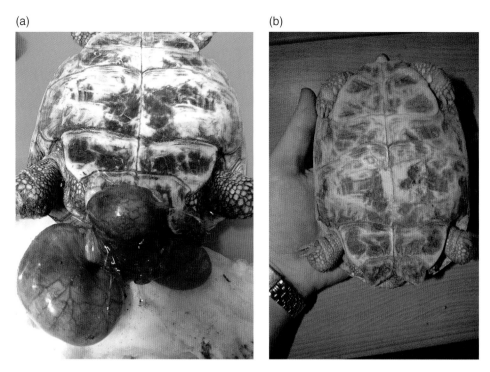

Figure 19.16   (a) Prolapse of both oviducts and one ovary with pathological accumulation of follicles in a pancake tortoise. (b) The same animal 18 months after plastronotomy to perform a bilateral ovariosalpingectomy, note the complete healing of the plastron.

19.6   Preventative Health Measures

Faecal examination can be an invaluable diagnostic tool used in practice to identify chelonian gastrointestinal parasites. Parasitology is advisable for all tortoises after purchase and then annually as part of a routine health check. Diagnosis can be made by demonstrating parasites or yeasts in faecal saline preparations and following flotation. Further diagnostics can be obtained by sending samples to specialist external exotics laboratories for culture and sensitivity, use of special staining techniques, and PCR analysis.

Direct faecal smears can be performed very easily in practice, requiring a microscope, slides, coverslips, and sterile saline. One drop of warmed saline is placed on to a slide with an equal amount of faecal material. The sample is then mixed to form a homogenous solution, a coverslip placed on top and the sample immediately examined under the microscope. Eggs and larvae can be visualised under the x10 objective and motile protozoa and cysts are examined under ×40. Lugol's iodine or a drop of new methylene blue may help to visualise parasites but will also kill them; movement of protozoans should therefore be assessed prior to staining.

Flotation techniques concentrate eggs and cysts and allow visualisation of these parasites. Saturated sodium chloride can be easily prepared by adding table salt to hot water until it no longer dissolves and commercial products, such as zinc sulphate, can also be purchased. 2–3 g of faeces are placed into a flotation chamber and the flotation solution is added and mixed and a coverslip is placed on top. This is then left undisturbed for 20–60 minutes, to allow the eggs to float to the surface. If using zinc sulphate it is better to examine after 20 minutes to avoid crystallisation (Wilkinson 2004). The coverslip is then lifted, placed on to a clean slide and examined under the microscope at ×10 and ×40 objectives.

19.6.1   Transponder Identification

Microchips have become the gold standard to identify individual animals. This is essential for paperwork such as for sale or movement of certain species subject to CITES restrictions. It is advised to microchip for identification purposes as the high value of tortoises means theft is not uncommon.

Microchip placement for chelonians is subcutaneously, in the proximal left hindlimb or in the quadriceps muscles of thin-skinned species. In giant species, the microchip is inserted subcutaneously in the tarsal area. Where limb restraint may not be possible due to the size and strength of the animal, sedation may be necessary.

19.7 Radiographic Imaging

Radiography is a useful diagnostic tool for chelonians presenting with lameness, suspected NSHP, gastrointestinal tract problems, respiratory tract disease, or urogenital system disorders. Conscious radiographs are often obtained during a consultation to assess bone density, the presence of retained eggs, bladder stones, radiodense foreign bodies, or obvious limb fractures.

Plain and contrast radiography can be performed depending on the individual case. Three views are required for the standard chelonian series; the dorsoventral, lateral, and cranio-caudal views using the horizontal beam. The cranio-caudal view allows the assessment of both lung fields which is important in respiratory disease.

19.7.1 Advanced Imaging

CT overcomes limitations of radiography such as superimposition of shell over viscera. It is useful in the giant species where other imaging modalities, such as ultrasonography, require sedation. CT provides excellent detail of bone allowing contrast showing cortical thickness and density. For chelonians, it provides assessment of structure and density of the shell, and in Mediterranean tortoises, densitometry values of 950–1300 HU have been suggested as normal in healthy specimens, whilst lower values (350–550 HU) have been seen in tortoises with NSHP (Wilkinson et al. 2004). CT may also be used to make a presumptive diagnosis of hepatic lipidosis. In male red-footed tortoises (*Geochelone carbonaria*) hepatic attenuation values lower than 20 HU were considered indicative of hepatic lipidosis (Marchiori et al. 2015). In Horsfield's tortoises values <50 HU were considered abnormal (Gumpenberger 2011) so there may be some species variation. Soft tissues do not emit high contrast signals, however, CT is useful to assess for ovarian follicles, lung fields, and to observe dystrophic calcification.

19.7.2 Ultrasonography

Ultrasonography is useful to examine soft tissue structures within the coelomic cavity and assess ocular tissues. It can be performed on conscious chelonians where tolerated but often requires sedation in larger species. The main indications are to assess for hepatic lipidosis, presence of free coelomic fluid and assessment of ovarian follicles. The acoustic windows in chelonians are the cervical windows and the pre-femoral fossa.

Formulary

	Dose	Interval	Comments
Chemical restraint/ anaesthetic agents			
Isoflurane	2–3%		Maintenance requirements for a surgical plane of anaesthesia (Schumacher and Yelen 2006).
Sevoflurane	3.5–4.5%		Maintenance requirements for a surgical plane of anaesthesia (Schumacher and Yelen 2006).
Alfaxalone	6–15 mg/kg IV to effect. Can be used IM at the higher dosages (up to 20 mg/kg)		Most reptile species (Schumacher and Yelen 2006) Variable effects have been described using this route.
Medetomidine + Ketamine	0.1 mg/kg (M) + 10 mg/kg (K) IV		Surgical anaesthesia in Galapagos tortoise (Knafo et al. 2011).
Medetomidine + midazolam + ketamine + morphine	0.15 mg/kg (M) + 2 mg/kg (Mi) + 2.5 mg/kg (K) + 1 mg/kg (Mo)		Light anaesthesia in Sulcata tortoise. Maintain with gaseous anaesthesia if necessary (Mans and Sladky 2012).
Propofol	IV 2–10 mg/kg, administered slowly to effect		Induction agent, for larger tortoises use the lower dose (Schumacher and Yelen 2006).

(Continued)

	Dose	Interval	Comments
Analgesia			
Bupivacaine	1–2 mg/kg local	Every 4–12 hours prn	(Schumacher and Yelen 2006)
	1 mg/kg intrathecal		Turtles/tortoises for regional anaesthesia and analgesia (Mans 2014)
Lidocaine	2–5 mg/kg local infiltration		Most species (Schumacher 1996).
	4 mg/kg intrathecal		Regional anaesthesia in chelonia (Mans 2014)
Lidocaine (L)/morphine (Mo)	2 mg/kg (L) + 0.1 mg/kg (Mo) intrathecal		Desert tortoises for analgesia for orchidectomy (Proença et al. 2014a)
Meloxicam	0.1–0.2 mg/kg PO, IM	Every 24 hours for 4–10 days	Chelonians – efficacy undetermined (Fleming 2008)
	0.2 mg/kg IM, IV, SC		Red-eared sliders plasma concentrations consistent with therapeutic efficacy for 48 hours administered IV and IM (Uney et al. 2016). Administered SC postsurgical in Mojave desert tortoises (Proença et al. 2014a, 2014b)
	0.5 mg/kg PO, IM		Red-eared sliders: absorption superior by IM route (Rojo-Solís et al. 2009)
Morphine	7.5 mg/kg SC, IM	Every 24 hours	Anti-nociceptive in Speke's hingeback (*Kinixys spekii*) (Wambugu et al. 2010)
Pethidine	20 mg/kg IM	Every 4 hours	Anti-nociceptive in Speke's hingeback (*Kinixys spekii*) (Wambugu et al. 2010)
Tramadol	5–10 mg/kg PO SC	Every 48–72 hours	Higher doses may affect ventilation (Baker et al. 2011)
	10 mg/kg PO		Chelonian analgesia (Spadola et al. 2015)
Antimicrobials			
Amikacin	5 mg/kg IM	Every 48 hours	Potentially nephrotoxic; use with caution in patients with renal insufficiency. Ensure adequate hydration (Caligiuri et al. 1990)
Ampicillin	50 mg/kg IM	Every 12 hours	Do not inject at the same site as aminoglycosides. Renally excreted (Spörle et al. 1991)
Ceftazidime	20–22 mg/kg IM IV	Every 72 hours	Extrapolated from other reptile species (Lawrence 1984; Stamper et al. 1999)
Doxycycline	5–10 mg/kg PO	Every 24 hours	Most reptile species for respiratory infection (Gibbons et al. 2013)
	50 mg/kg IM	Initial dose	(Spörle et al. 1991)
	25 mg/kg IM	Subsequently every 72 hours	
Enrofloxacin	10 mg/kg IM	Every 24 hours	(Spörle et al. 1991 – *Testudo hermanni*)
	5 mg/kg IM	Every 24–48 hours	Chelonians and most other reptiles. Hyperexcitation, incoordination, and diarrhoea reported in a Galapagos tortoise (Prezant et al. 1994; Casares and Enders 1996)
Gentamicin	6 mg/kg IM	Every 72–96 hours	(Raphael et al. 1985 – red-eared sliders at 24 °C)
			Potentially nephrotoxic
Metronidazole	20 mg/kg PO	Every 48 hours for 7 or more days	For most species of reptiles (Funk and Diethelm 2006)

(*Continued*)

(Continued)

	Dose	Interval	Comments
Oxytetracycline	5–10 mg/kg IM	Every 24 hours	(Gauvin 1993 – *Gopherus agassizii*)
Trimethoprim/ sulfadiazine or sulfamethoxazole	30 mg/kg IM	Every 24 hours for 2 doses, and then every 48 hours	Maintain hydration (Spörle et al. 1991)
Tylosin	5 mg/kg IM	Every 24 hours for 10–60 days	Most species of reptile for mycoplasmosis (Divers 1998)
Antiparasitics			
Chloroquine	50 mg/kg IM	Administer weekly for 3 doses	Effective against amoebic trophozoites but not cysts (McArthur 2004c)
	125 mg/kg PO	Administer every 48 hours for 3 doses	Haemoprotozoa in tortoises (Gibbons et al. 2013)
Emodepside (1.98%) + praziquantel (7.94%)	1.12 ml/kg topically		More research needed for efficacy data but appears safe (Mehlhorn et al. 2005; Schilliger et al. 2009)
Fenbendazole	50–100 mg/kg PO as a single dose, and then repeated as a single dose 14–28 days later	Administer as a single dose, and then repeat 14–28 days later	Holt (1982)
	50 mg/kg PO	Administer daily for three consecutive days	Wright (1997)
	100 mg/kg administered via intracolonic administration.	Given as a one-off dose	Innis (1995, 2008)
	100 mg/kg PO	Given as one-off dose	Giannetto et al. (2007)
Metronidazole	25 mg/kg PO	Given daily for 5 days	Amoebiasis in chelonians (Gibbons et al. 2013)
	20 mg/kg administered via intracoelomic injection	Administered every 48 hours	Not recommended, further safety trials required. Several deaths were reported in Red-eared sliders, a direct consequence of metronidazole administration was not confirmed (Innis et al. 2007)
Oxfendazole	66 mg/kg PO	Given as a single dose	(Giannetto et al. 2007)
Primaquine	0.75 mg/kg PO	Every 7 days for four treatments	For plasmodium treatment (Redrobe 2000)
Toltrazuril	15 mg/kg PO	Every 48 hours for 30 days	Tortoises for coccidiosis; further safety and efficacy trials needed (Gibbons and Steffes 2013)
Miscellaneous			
Calcium gluconate	50–100 mg/kg IM		1–2 hours prior to oxytocin therapy to induce oviposition (Innis and Boyer 2002)
Levothyroxine	0.25 mg/kg PO	Every 24 hours	For hypothyroidism, monitor T4 levels (Franco and Hoover 2009)
Oxytocin	1–10 IU/kg IM	Up to three treatments at 90 minute intervals	Preferably administered after calcium for optimal effects on inducing oviposition (Innis and Boyer 2002)

References

Adkesson, M.J., Travis, E.K., Weber, M.A. et al. (2007). Vacuum-assisted closure for treatment of a deep shell abscess and osteomyelitis in a tortoise. *Journal of the American Veterinary Medical Association* 231 (8): 1249–1254.

Alworth, L.C., Hernandez, S.M., and Divers, S.J. (2011). Laboratory reptile surgery: principles and techniques. *Journal of the American Association for Laboratory Animal Science* 50 (1): 11–26.

Andersen, S. and Eriksen, E. (1968). Aspergillose bei einer Elephantenschildkrote (*Testudo gigantea elephantina*). In: *X Internationalen Symposiums uber die Erkrankungen der Zootiere*. Berlin: Akademie der Wissenschaften der DDR.

Andreani, G., Carpene, E., Cannavacciuolo, A. et al. (2014). Reference values for hematology and plasma biochemistry variables, and protein electrophoresis of healthy Hermann's tortoises (Testudo hermanni ssp.). *Veterinary Clinical Pathology* 43 (4): 573–583.

Andreu, A.C. (1987). Ecologia dinamica poblacional de la tortuga mora, Testudo graeca, en Donana. Doctoral dissertation. University of Seville, Spain.

ARAV (2003). African spurred tortoise, *Geochelone sulcate*, client handout. *Journal of Herpetological Medicine and Surgery* 13 (4): 45–46.

Baines, F. (2018). True full spectrum lighting for zoo animals. In: *Proceedings of the British Veterinary Zoological Society*, 20. BVZS.

Baines, F., Chattell, J., Dale, J. et al. (2016). How much UV-B does my reptile need? The UV-tool, a guide to the selection of UV lighting for reptiles and amphibians in captivity. *Journal of Zoo and Aquarium Research* 4 (1): 42–63.

Baker, B.B., Sladky, K.K., and Johnson, S.M. (2011). Evaluation of the analgesic effects of oral and subcutaneous tramadol administration in red-eared slider turtles. *Journal of the American Veterinary Medical Association* 238: 220–227.

Baker, P.J., Kabigumila, J., Leuteritz, T. et al. (2015). Stigmochelys pardalis. The IUCN Red List of Threatened Species. https://dx.doi.org/10.2305/IUCN.UK.2015-4. RLTS.T163449A1009442.en.

Barten, S.L. (2005). Thinking inside the box: anorexia in box turtles and small tortoises. In: *Proceeding of the North American Veterinary Conference, Orlando, Florida, Jan 8–12*, 1266–1268. Gainesville, FL: North American Veterinary Conference.

Benetka, V., Grabensteiner, E., Gumpenberger, M. et al. (2007). First report of an iridovirus (genus Ranavirus) infection in a leopard tortoise (*Geochelone pardalis pardalis*). *Wiener Tierärztliche Monatsschrift* 94 (9/10): 243.

Bennett, R.A. (1989). Reptilian surgery part II: management of surgical diseases. *Compendium on Continuing Education for the Practising Veterinarian* 11: 111–112.

Bertelsen, M.F. (2019). Anaesthesia and analgesia. In: *BSAVA Manual of Reptiles* (eds. S. Girling, P. Raiti and BSAVA), 200–209. Gloucester, UK: BSAVA Library.

Boyer, T.H. (1995). Metabolic bone disease in reptiles. In: *Proceedings of North American Veterinary Conference*, 638. Gainesville, FL: North American Veterinary Conference.

Brames, H. (2008). Efficacy and tolerability of Profender in reptiles: spot on treatment against nematodes. *Exotic DVM* 10 (3): 29–34.

Branch, B. (1988). *Field Guide to the Snakes and Other Reptiles of Southern Africa*. Cape Town, South Africa: Struik.

Caligiuri, R.L., Kollias, G.V., Jacobson, E.R. et al. (1990). The effects of ambient temperature on amikacin pharmacokinetics in gopher tortoises. *Journal of Veterinary Pharmacology and Therapeutics* 13: 287–291.

Capen, C.C. and Martin, S.L. (1983). Calcium-regulatory hormones and diseases of the parathyroid glands. In: *Textbook of Veterinary Internal Medicine* (eds. S.J. Ettinger and E.C. Feldman), 1581–1584. Philadelphia: WB Saunders.

Casares, M. and Enders, F. (1996). Enrofloxacin side effects in a Galapagos tortoise (Geochelone elephantopus nigra). In: *Proceedings of Annual conference, American Association of Zoo Veterinarians*, 446–448. American Association of Zoo Veterinarians.

Che'Amat, A., Gabriel, B., and Chee, N.W. (2012). Cystic calculi removal in African spurred tortoise (*Geochelone sulcata*) using transplastron coeliotomy. *Veterinary World* 5 (8): 489–492.

CITES (2019). Appendices. https://www.cites.org/eng/app/appendices.php (accessed 11 March 2019).

Clabaugh, K., Haag, K.M., Hanley, C.S. et al. (2005). Undifferentiated sarcoma resolved by forelimb amputation and prosthesis in a radiated tortoise (*Geochelone radiata*). *Journal of Zoo and Wildlife Medicine* 36 (1): 117–121.

Close, B., Banister, K., Baumans, V. et al. (1996). Recommendations for euthanasia of experimental animals: part 1. *Laboratory Animals* 30 (4): 293–316.

Coke, R.L. and Reyes-Fore, P.A. (2006). Treatment of a carapace infection in an Aldabra tortoise, *Geochelone gigantea*, with negative pressure wound therapy. *Journal of Herpetological Medicine and Surgery* 16 (3): 102–106.

Coke, R.L., Hunter, R.P., Isaza, R. et al. (2003). Pharmacokinetics and tissue concentrations of azithromycin in ball pythons (*Python regius*). *American Journal of Veterinary Research* 64: 225–228.

Crum, D.A. (2013). Orthopaedics and fracture repair. In: *Clinical Veterinary Advisor Birds and Exotic Pets* (eds. J. Mayer and T.M. Donnelly), 125–127. St Louis: Elsevier.

van Dijk, P.P., Corti, C., Mellado, V.P. et al. (2004). Testudo graeca. The IUCN Red List of Threatened Species 2004. https://www.iucnredlist.org/species/21646/9305693 (accessed 2 September 2017).

Divers, S.J. (1998). Empirical doses of antimicrobial drugs commonly used in reptiles. *Exotic DVM* 1: 23.

Divers, S.J. and Cooper, J.E. (2000). Reptile hepatic lipidosis. *Seminars in Avian and Exotic Pet Medicine* 9 (3): 153–164.

Drury, S.E.N., Gough, R.E., McArthur, S. et al. (1998). Detection of herpesvirus-like and papillomavirus-like particles associated with diseases of tortoises. *The Veterinary Record* 143 (23): 639.

Drury, S.E.N., Gough, R.E., and McArthur, S.D.J. (2001). Detection and isolation of a flavivirus-like agent from a leopard tortoise (*Geochelone paradalis*) in the United Kingdom. *Veterinary Record* 148 (14): 462.

Duncan, M., Christopher, J.D., and Randall, E.J. (2002). Lymphosarcoma in African Spurred Tortoises (*Geochelone sulcata*). In: *Annual Proceedings-American Association of Zoo Veterinarians*, 71. Knoxville, TN: American Association of Zoo Veterinarians.

Eatwell, K. (2007). Effects of storage and sample type on ionized calcium, sodium and potassium levels in captive tortoises, *Testudo* spp. *Journal of Herpetological Medicine and Surgery* 17: 84–91.

Eatwell, K. (2008a). Hypocalcemia in a Tunisian tortoise (*Furculachelys nabeulensis*). *Journal of Herpetological Medicine and Surgery* 18 (3): 117–122.

Eatwell, K. (2008b). Plasma concentrations of 25-hydroxycholecalciferol in 22 captive tortoises (*Testudo* species). *Veterinary Record* 162 (11): 342–345.

Effron, M., Griner, L., and Benirschke, K. (1977). Nature and rate of neoplasia found in captive wild mammals, birds, and reptiles at necropsy. *Journal of the National Cancer Institute* 59 (1): 185–198.

El Mouden, E.H., Slimani, T., Kaddour, K.B. et al. (2006). *Testudo graeca graeca* feeding ecology in an arid and overgrazed zone in Morocco. *Journal of Arid Environments* 64 (3): 422–435.

Eshar, D., Gancz, A.Y., Avni-Magen, N. et al. (2016). Selected plasma biochemistry analytes of healthy captive sulcata (African spurred) tortoises (*Centrochelys sulcata*). *Journal of Zoo and Wildlife Medicine* 47 (4): 993–999.

Ferguson, G.W., Gehrmann, W.H., Karsten, K.B. et al. (2003). Do panther chameleons bask to regulate endogenous vitamin D3 production? *Physiological and Biochemical Zoology* 76 (1): 52–59.

Fledelius, B., Jørgensen, G.W., Jensen, H.E. et al. (2005). Influence of the calcium content of the diet offered to leopard tortoises (*Geochelone pardalis*). *Veterinary Record* 156 (26): 831–835.

Fleming, G. (2008). Clinical technique: chelonian shell repair. *Journal of Exotic Pet Medicine* 17: 246–258.

Fleming, G.J. (2014). New techniques in chelonian shell repair. In: *Current Therapy in Reptile Medicine and Surgery* (eds. D.R. Mader and S.J. Divers), 205–212. St. Louis, MO: Elsevier Saunders.

Flower, M.S.S. (1925). Contributions to our knowledge of the duration of life in vertebrate animals. III. Reptiles. *Proceedings, Zoological Society of London* 60 (3): 911–925.

Franco, K.H. and Hoover, J.P. (2009). Levothyroxine as a treatment for presumed hypothyroidism in an adult male African spurred tortoise (*Centrochelys* [formerly *Geochelone*] *sulcata*). *Journal of Herpetological Medicine and Surgery* 19 (2): 42–44.

Franco, K.H., Famini, D.J., Hoover, J.P. et al. (2009). Serum thyroid hormone values for African spurred tortoises (*Centrochelys* [formerly *Geochelone*] *sulcata*). *Journal of Herpetological Medicine and Surgery* 19 (2): 47–49.

Frank, W. (1981). Endoparasites. In: *Diseases of the Reptilia*, vol. 1 (eds. J.E. Cooper and O.F. Jackson), 291–358. London: Academic Press.

Frye, F.L. (1991). Applied clinical nonhemic parasitology of reptiles. In: *Biomedical and Surgical Aspects of Captive Reptile Husbandry*, 2e, vol. 1 (ed. F.L. Frye), 281–325. Malabar, FL: Krieger.

Frye, F.L. and Dutra, F.R. (1974). Hypothyroidism in turtles and tortoises. *Veterinary Medicine, Small Animal Clinician* 69 (8): 990.

Funk, R.S. and Diethelm, G. (2006). Reptile formulary. In: *Reptile Medicine and Surgery*, 2e (ed. D.R. Mader), 1119–1139. St. Louis: Sanders/Elsevier.

Garner, M.M., Hernandez-Divers, S.M., and Raymond, J.T. (2004). Reptile neoplasia: a retrospective study of case submissions to a specialty diagnostic service. *The Veterinary Clinics of North America. Exotic Animal Practice* 7 (3): 653–671.

Gauvin, J. (1993). Drug therapy in reptiles. *Seminars in Avian and Exotic Pet Medicine* 2 (1): 48–59.

Georg, L.K., Williamson, W.M., Tilden, E.B. et al. (1963). Mycotic pulmonary disease of captive giant tortoises due to *Beauvaria bassiana* and *Paecilomyces fumoso-roseus*. *Sabouraudia* 2 (2): 80–86.

Gerlach, J. (2004). Effects of diet on the systematic utility of the tortoise carapace. *African Journal of Herpetology* 53 (1): 77–85.

Giannetto, S., Brianti, E., Poglayen, G. et al. (2007). Efficacy of oxfendazole and fenbendazole against tortoise (*Testudo hermanni*) oxyurids. *Parasitology Research* 100 (5): 1069–1073.

Gibbons, P.M. (2009). Critical care nutrition and fluid therapy in reptiles. Proceedings of the 15th Annual International Veterinary Emergency and Critical Care Symposium, Sept 9–13, Chicago, IL: 91–94.

Gibbons, P.M. and Steffes, Z.J. (2013). Emerging infectious diseases in chelonians. *The Veterinary Clinics of North America. Exotic Animal Practice* 16: 303–317.

Gibbons, P.M., Klaphake, E., and Carpenter, J.W. (2013). Reptiles. In: *Exotic Animal Formulary*, 4e (ed. J.W. Carpenter), 83–182. St. Louis: Elsevier.

Gottdenker, N.L. and Jacobson, E.R. (1995). Effect of venipuncture sites on hematologic and clinical biochemical values in desert tortoises (*Gopherus agassizii*). *American Journal of Veterinary Research* 56 (1): 19–21.

Graczyk, T.K., Cranfield, M.R., Mann, J. et al. (1998). Intestinal cryptosporidium sp. infection in the Egyptian tortoise, *Testudo kleinmanni*. *International Journal for Parasitology* 28 (12): 1885–1888.

Griffin, C., Reavill, D.R., Stacy, B.A. et al. (2010). Cryptosporidiosis caused by two distinct species in Russian tortoises and a pancake tortoise. *Veterinary Parasitology* 170 (1–2): 14–19.

Grioni, A., Ho, K.K., Karraker, N.E. et al. (2014). Blood clinical biochemistry and packed cell volume of the Chinese three-striped box turtle, *Cuora trifasciata* (Reptilia: Geoemydidae). *Journal of Zoo and Wildlife Medicine* 45 (2): 228–238.

Gumpenberger, M. (2011). Chelonians. In: *Veterinary Computed Tomography* (eds. T. Schwarz and J. Saunders), 533–544. Oxford, UK: Wiley-Blackwell/Blackwell Publishing Ltd.

Hallinger, M.J., Taubert, A., Hermosilla, C. et al. (2018). Occurrence of health-compromising protozoan and helminth infections in tortoises kept as pet animals in Germany. *Parasites & Vectors* 11 (1): 352.

Harwell, G. (1989). Repair of injuries to the chelonian plastron and carapace. In: *Current Vet Therapy 10: Small Animal Practice* (ed. R.W. Kirk), 789–791. Philadelphia, PA: WB Saunders.

Hatt, J.M. (2008). Raising giant tortoises. In: *Zoo and Wild Animal Medicine: Current Therapy*, vol. 6 (eds. M.E. Fowler and R.E. Miller), 144–153. St. Louis, MO: Saunders / Elsevier.

Heard, D.J. (1999). Shell repair in turtles and tortoises: a heretical approach. In: *Proceedings of the North America Veterinary Conference*. Gainesville, FL: North American Veterinary Conference.

Hedley, J. (2012). Survey of gastrointestinal parasites in the United Kingdom. RCVS Diploma thesis, RCVS library. http://knowledge.rcvs.org.uk/document-library/diplomas-dzm-12-1 (accessed 11 March 2019).

Hedley, J., Eatwell, K., and Shaw, D.J. (2013). Gastrointestinal parasitic burdens in UK tortoises: a survey of tortoise owners and potential risk factors. *Veterinary Record* 173 (21): 525.

Heinrich, M.L. and Heinrich, K.K. (2016). Effect of supplemental heat in captive African leopard tortoises (*Stigmochelys pardalis*) and spurred tortoises (*Centrochelys sulcata*) on growth rate and carapacial scute pyramiding. *Journal of Exotic Pet Medicine* 25 (1): 18–25.

Henton, M.M. (2003). *Pasteurella testudinis* associated with respiratory disease and septicaemia in leopard (Geochelone pardalis) and other tortoises in South Africa. *Journal of the South African Veterinary Association* 74 (4): 135–136.

Hernandez-Divers, S.J. (2004). Surgery: principles and techniques. In: *BSAVA Manual of Reptiles*, 2e (eds. S. Girling and P. Raiti), 147–167. Gloucester: BSAVA.

Hernandez-Divers, S.M., Hernandez-Divers, S.J., and Wyneken, J. (2002). Angiographic, anatomic and clinical technique descriptions of a subcarapacial venipuncture site for chelonians. *Journal of Herpetological Medicine and Surgery* 12 (2): 32–37.

Heuser, W., Pendl, H., Knowles, N.J. et al. (2014). Soft plastron, soft carapace with skeletal abnormality in juvenile tortoises. *Tierärztliche Praxis. Ausgabe K, Kleintiere/Heimtiere* 42 (05): 310–320.

Highfield, A.C. (2000). *The Tortoise and Turtle Feeding Manual*. London: Carapace Press.

Holt, P.E. (1982). Efficacy of fenbendazole against nematodes of reptiles. *Veterinary Record* 110: 302–304.

Holz, P., Barker, I.K., Burger, J.P. et al. (1997). The effect of the renal portal system on pharmacokinetic parameters in the red-eared slider (*Trachemys scripta elegans*). *Journal of Zoo and Wildlife Medicine* 28 (4): 386–393.

Innis, C. (1994). Considerations in formulating captive tortoise diets. *Bulletin of the Association of Reptilian and Amphibian Veterinarians* 4 (1): 8–12.

Innis, C. (1995). Per-cloaca worming of tortoises. *Bulletin of the Association of Reptilian and Amphibian Veterinarians* 5: 4.

Innis, C.J. (2000). Captive care of Bell's hingeback tortoise, *Kinixys belliana*. *Journal of Herpetological Medicine and Surgery* 10 (1): 26–28.

Innis, C. (2008). Clinical parasitology of the chelonian. In: *Proceedings of the North American Veterinary Conference, Orlando*, 1783–1785. Gainesville, FL: North American Veterinary Conference.

Innis, C.J. and Boyer, T.H. (2002). Chelonian reproductive disorders. *Veterinary Clinics: Exotic Animal Practice* 5 (3): 555–578.

Innis, C., Papich, M., and Young, D. (2007). Pharmacokinetics of metronidazole in the red-eared slider turtle (*Trachemys scripta elegans*) after single intracoelomic injection. *Journal of Veterinary Pharmacology and Therapeutics* 30: 168–171.

Jacobson, E.R. (1994). Causes of mortality and diseases in tortoises: a review. *Journal of Zoo and Wildlife Medicine* 25 (1): 2–17.

Jacobson, E.R. (1997). Diseases of the respiratory tract of chelonians. *Verh Ber Erkrg Zootiere* 38: 1–5.

Jacobson, E.R., Gaskin, J.M., Brown, M.B. et al. (1991). Chronic upper respiratory tract disease of free-ranging desert tortoises (Xerobates agassizii). *Journal of Wildlife Diseases* 27 (2): 296–316.

Kabigumila, J. (2002). Morphometrics of the pancake tortoise (*Malacochersus tornieri*) in Tanzania. *Tanzania Journal of Science* 28 (2): 33–46.

Keymer, I.F. (1978). Diseases of chelonians: (1) Necroscopy survey of tortoises. *Veterinary Record* 103: 548–552.

Kik, M.J.L., Dorrestein, G.M., and Beynen, A.C. (2003). Evaluation of 15 commercial diets and their possible relation to metabolic diseases in different species of reptiles. *Verh ber Erkrg Zootiere* 41: 1–5.

Knafo, S.E., Divers, S.J., Rivera, S. et al. (2011). Sterilisation of hybrid Galapagos tortoises (*Geochelone nigra*) for island restoration. Part 1: endoscopic oophorectomy of females under ketamine-medetomidine anaesthesia. *Veterinary Record* 168 (2): 47.

Kolesnik, E., Obiegala, A., and Marschang, R.E. (2017). Detection of mycoplasma spp., herpesviruses, topiviruses, and ferlaviruses in samples from chelonians in Europe. *Journal of Veterinary Diagnostic Investigation* 29 (6): 820–832.

van der Kuyl, A.C., Ballasina, D.L., and Zorgdrager, F. (2005). Mitochondrial haplotype diversity in the tortoise species *Testudo graeca* from North Africa and the Middle East. *BMC Evolutionary Biology* 5 (1): 29.

Lance, V.A., Valenzuela, N., and Von Hildebrand, P. (1992). A hormonal method to determine sex of hatchling giant river turtles, *Podocnemis expansa*: application to endangered species. *Journal of Experimental Zoology* 270: 16A.

Lawrence, K. (1984). Preliminary study on the use of ceftazidime, a broad-spectrum cephalosporin antibiotic, in snakes. *Research in Veterinary Science* 36: 16.

Lim, C.K., Kirberger, R.M., Lane, E.P. et al. (2013). Computed tomography imaging of a leopard tortoise (*Geochelone pardalis pardalis*) with confirmed pulmonary fibrosis: a case report. *Acta Veterinaria Scandinavica* 55 (1): 35.

Lloyd, M. and Morris, P. (1999). Chelonian venipuncture techniques. *Bulletin of the Association of Reptilian and Amphibian Veterinarians* 9 (1): 26–29.

López-Olvera, J.R., Montané, J., Marco, I. et al. (2003). Effect of venipuncture site on hematologic and serum biochemical parameters in marginated tortoise (*Testudo marginata*). *Journal of Wildlife Diseases* 39 (4): 830–836.

Loveridge, A. and Williams, E.E. (1957). *Revision of the African Tortoises and Turtles of the Suborder Cryptodira*. Cambridge, MA: The Museum of Comparative Zoology.

Luiselli, L. (2003). Afrotropical tortoise species (genus *Kinixys*). *Contributions to Zoology* 72 (4): 211–220.

Mader, D.R. (2006). Calculi: urinary. In: *Reptile Medicine and Surgery* (ed. D.R. Mader), 763–771. Philadelphia: WB Saunders.

Makau, C.M., Towett, P.K., Abelson, K.S.P. et al. (2017). Modulation of formalin-induced pain-related behaviour by clonidine and yohimbine in the Speke's hinged tortoise (*Kiniskys spekii*). *Journal of Veterinary Pharmacology and Therapeutics* 40 (5): 439–446.

Malonza, P.K. (2003). Ecology and distribution of the pancake tortoise, *Malacochersus tornieri* in Kenya. *Journal of East African Natural History* 92 (1): 81–97.

Mans, C. (2008). Venipuncture techniques in chelonian species. *Lab Animal* 37 (7): 303–305.

Mans, C. (2013). Clinical update on diagnosis and management of disorders of the digestive system of reptiles. *Journal of Exotic Pet Medicine* 22: 141–162.

Mans, C. (2014). Clinical technique: intrathecal drug administration in turtles and tortoises. *Journal of Exotic Pet Medicine* 23: 67–70.

Mans, C. (2015). Reptile sedation, anesthesia and analgesia. In: Proceedings 2nd International Conference on Avian, Herpetological and Exotic Mammal Medicine. CD-ROM: 69–72

Mans, C. and Sladky, K.K. (2012). Endoscopically guided cloacal calculi removal in three African spurred tortoises (*Geochelone sulcata*). *Journal of the American Veterinary Medical Association* 240: 869–875.

Marchiori, A., da Silva, I.C.C., de Albuquerque Bonelli, M. et al. (2015). Use of computed tomography for investigation of hepatic lipidosis in captive *Chelonoidis carbonaria* (Spix, 1824). *Journal of Zoo and Wildlife Medicine* 46 (2): 320–324.

Marin, M.L., Norton, T.M., and Mettee, N.S. (2014). Vacuum-assisted wound closure in chelonians. In: *Current Therapy in Reptile Medicine and Surgery* (eds. D.R. Mader and S.J. Divers), 197–204. St. Louis, MO: Elsevier Saunders.

Marschang, R.E. and Ruemenapf, T.H. (2002). Virus "X": characterizing a new viral pathogen in tortoises. In: *Proceedings of the Conference of the Association of Reptilian and Amphibian Veterinarians. Reno*, 101–102. ARAV.

Martinez-Silvestre, A. (2011). Massive *Tachygonetria* (Oxyuridae) infection in a Hermann's tortoise (*Testudo hermanni*). *Consulta Journal Special Edition* 2011: 409–412.

Martínez-Silvestre, A., Perpinan, D., Marco, I. et al. (2002). Venipuncture technique of the occipital venous sinus in freshwater aquatic turtles. *Journal of Herpetological Medicine and Surgery* 12 (4): 31–32.

Mautino, M. and Page, C.D. (1993). Biology and medicine of turtles and tortoises. *The Veterinary Clinics of North America. Small Animal Practice* 23 (6): 1251–1270.

McArthur, S. (2004a). Feeding techniques and fluids. In: *Medicine and Surgery of Tortoises and Turtles* (eds. S. McArthur, R. Wilkinson and J. Meyer), 257–271. Oxford: Blackwell Publishing.

McArthur, S. (2004b). Interpretation of presenting signs. In: *Medicine and Surgery of Tortoises and Turtles* (eds. S. McArthur, R. Wilkinson and J. Meyer), 273–300. Oxford: Blackwell Publishing.

McArthur, S. (2004c). Problem-solving approach to common diseases of terrestrial and semi-aquatic chelonians. In: *Medicine and Surgery of Tortoises and Turtles* (eds. S. McArthur, R. Wilkinson and J. Meyer), 347–349. Oxford: Blackwell Publishing.

McArthur, S., Windsor, H., Bradbury, J.M. et al. (2002). Isolation of Mycoplasma agassizii from UK captive Chelonians (Testudo horsfieldii and Geochelone pardalis) with upper respiratory tract disease. In: 14th International Congress of the International Organisation for Mycoplasmology, Vienna. Bethesda, MD: International Organisation for Mycoplasmology.

Mehlhorn, H., Schmahl, G., Frese, M. et al. (2005). Effects of a combination of emodepside and praziquantel on parasites of reptiles and rodents. *Parasitology Research* 97: S64–S69.

Mitchell, M.A. (2007). Parasites of reptiles. In: *Flynn's Parasites of Laboratory Animals*, 2e (ed. D.G. Baker), 177–216. Iowa: Blackwell Publishing.

Music, M.K. and Strunk, A. (2016). Reptile critical care and common emergencies. *Veterinary Clinics: Exotic Animal Practice* 19: 591–612.

Neiffer, D.L., Lydick, D., Burks, K. et al. (2005). Hematologic and plasma biochemical changes associated with fenbendazole administration in Hermann's tortoises (*Testudo hermanni*). *Journal of Zoo and Wildlife Medicine* 36 (4): 661–673.

Nevarez, J.G., Rademacher, N., and Shaw, S. (2008). Carapace Sequestrum in an African spurred tortoise, *Geochelone sulcata*. *Journal of Herpetological Medicine and Surgery* 18 (2): 45–51.

Norton, T.M. (2005). Chelonian emergency and critical care. *Seminars in Avian and Exotic Pet Medicine* 14 (2): 106–130.

Oonincx, D.G.A.B., Stevens, Y., Van den Borne, J.J.G.C. et al. (2010). Effects of vitamin D3 supplementation and UVB exposure on the growth and plasma concentration of vitamin D3 metabolites in juvenile bearded dragons (*Pogona vitticeps*). *Comparative Biochemistry and Physiology Part B: Biochemistry and Molecular Biology* 156 (2): 122–128.

Pellett, S., Wissink-Argilaga, N., and Stocking, D. (2015). Species specific identification and husbandry requirements for chelonia in UK collections. *VetCPD* 2 (1): 8.

Pollock, C. (2012). Feeding the hospitalized tortoise or turtle. Lafeber Website. https://lafeber.com/vet/feeding-the-hospitalized-turtle-or-tortoise (accessed 2 January 2019).

Pollock, C. and Arbona, N.(2017). Fluid administration in reptiles. Lafeber Website. https://lafeber.com/vet/fluid-administration-in-reptiles (accessed 30 March 2018).

Prezant, R.M., Isaza, R., and Jacobson, E.R. (1994). Plasma concentrations and disposition kinetics of enrofloxacin in gopher tortoises (*Gopherus polyphemus*). *Journal of Zoo and Wildlife Medicine* 25 (1): 82–87.

Proença, L.M., Fowler, S., Kleine, S. et al. (2014a). Single surgeon coelioscopic orchiectomy of desert tortoises (*Gopherus agassizii*) for population management. *Veterinary Record* 175: 404.

Proença, L.M., Fowler, S., Kleine, S. et al. (2014b). Coelioscopic-assisted sterilization of female Mojave Desert tortoises (*Gopherus agassizii*). *Journal of Herpetological Medicine and Surgery* 24 (3): 95–100.

Raiti, P. and Haramati, N. (1997). Magnetic resonance imaging and computerized tomography of a gravid leopard tortoise (*Geochelone pardalis pardalis*) with metabolic bone disease. *Journal of Zoo and Wildlife Medicine* 28 (2): 189–197.

Raphael, B., Clark, C.H., and Hudson, R. (1985). Plasma concentration of gentamicin in turtles. *The Journal of Zoo Animal Medicine* 16 (4): 136–139.

Raphael, B.L., Klemens, M.W., Moehlman, P. et al. (1994). Blood values in free-ranging pancake tortoises (*Malacochersus tornieri*). *Journal of Zoo and Wildlife Medicine* 25: 63–67.

Redrobe, S.P.(2000). Treatment of suspected plasmodium infection in star tortoises (Geochelone elegans). IAAAM Proceedings. https://www.vin.com/apputil/content/defaultadv1.aspx?id=3864479&pid=11257& (accessed 13 June 2019).

Richards, J. (2001). Metal bridges – a new technique of turtle shell repair. *Journal of Herpetological Medicine and Surgery* 11: 31.

Rojo-Solís, C., Ros-Rodriguez, J.M., Valls, M. et al. (2009). Pharmacokinetics of meloxicam (Metacam) after intravenous, intramuscular, and oral administration in red-eared slider turtles (*Trachemys scripta elegans*). In: *Proceedings of the American Association of Zoo Veterinarians*, 228. Knoxville, TN: The American Association of Zoo Veterinarians.

Rostal, D.C., Grumbles, J.S., Lance, V.A. et al. (1994). Non-lethal sexing techniques for hatchling and immature desert tortoises (*Gopherus agassizii*). *Herpetological Monographs* 8: 83–87.

Rouag, R., Ferrah, C., Luiselli, L. et al. (2008). Food choice of an Algerian population of the spur-thighed tortoise, *Testudo graeca*. *African Journal of Herpetology* 57 (2): 103–113.

Sacchi, R., Galeotti, P., Fasola, M. et al. (2004). Larynx morphology and sound production in three species of Testudinidae. *Journal of Morphology* 261 (2): 175–183.

Schilliger, L., Betremieux, O., Rochet, J. et al. (2009). Absorption and efficacy of a spot-on combination containing emodepside plus praziquantel in reptiles. *Revue de Médecine Vétérinaire* 160 (12): 557–561.

Schumacher, J. (1996). Reptiles and amphibians. In: *Lumb and Jones' Veterinary Anesthesia*, 3e (eds. J.C. Thurman, W.J. Tranquilli and G.J. Benson), 670–685. Baltimore, MD: Williams and Wilkins.

Schumacher, J. and Yelen, T. (2006). Anaesthesia and analgesia. In: *Reptile Medicine and Surgery* (ed. D.R. Mader), 442–452. St. Louis, MO: Elsevier.

Silverman, S. (1993). Diagnostic imaging of exotic pets. *The Veterinary Clinics of North America. Small Animal Practice* 23 (6): 1287–1299.

Soares, J.F., Chalker, V.J., Erles, K. et al. (2004). Prevalence of mycoplasma agassizii and chelonian herpesvirus in captive tortoises (Testudo sp.) in the United Kingdom. *Journal of Zoo and Wildlife Medicine* 35 (1): 25–34.

Spadola, F., Morici, M., and Knotek, Z. (2015). Combination of lidocaine/prilocaine with tramadol for short time anaesthesia-analgesia in chelonians: 18 cases. *Acta Veterinaria Brno* 84 (1): 71–75.

Spörle, H., Gobel, T., and Schildger, B. (1991). Blood levels of some anti-infectives in the spur-thighed tortoise (Testudo hermanni). Proceedings of the 4th International Colloquium on the Pathology of Reptiles and Amphibians, Bad Nauheim, Germany: 120–128

Stacy, B.A. and Wellehan, J.F. Jr. (2010). Fatal septicemia caused by helicobacter infection in a pancake tortoise (*Malacochersus tornieri*). *Journal of Veterinary Diagnostic Investigation* 22 (4): 660–662.

Stamper, M.A., Papich, M.G., Lewbart, G.A. et al. (1999). Pharmacokinetics of ceftazidime in loggerhead sea turtles (*Caretta caretta*) after single intravenous and intramuscular injections. *Journal of Zoo and Wildlife Medicine* 30 (1): 32–35.

Stearns, B.C. (1989). The captive status of the African spurred tortoise *Geochelone sulcata*: recent developments. *International Zoo Yearbook* 28 (1): 87–98.

Swenson, J., Henao-Guerrero, P.N., and Carpenter, J.W. (2008). Clinical technique: use of capnography in small mammal anesthesia. *Journal of Exotic Pet Medicine* 17 (3): 175–180.

Takami, Y. (2017). Single-incision, prefemoral bilateral oophorosalpingectomy without coelioscopy in an Indian star tortoise (*Geochelone elegans*) with follicular stasis. *Journal of Veterinary Medical Science* 79 (10): 1675–1677.

Tang, P.K., Pellett, S., Blake, D. et al. (2017). Efficacy of a topical formulation containing Emodepside and Praziquantel (Profender® Bayer) against nematodes in captive tortoises. *Journal of Herpetological Medicine and Surgery* 27 (3–4): 116–122.

Teare, J.A. (2002). Reference ranges for physiological values of captive wildlife. International Species Inventory System, 2 Apple Valley, MN.

The Pirbright Institute UK (2015). Torchvirus A. https://www.picornaviridae.com/torchivirus/torchivirus_a/torchivirus_a.htm (accessed 05 May 2015).

Ullrey, D.E. and Bernard, J.B. (1999). Vitamin D: metabolism, sources, unique problems in zoo animals, meeting needs. In: *Zoo and Wild Animal Medicine*, 4e (eds. M.E. Fowler and R.E. Miller), 63–78. Philadelphia, PA: WB Saunders.

Une, Y., Uemura, K., Nakano, Y. et al. (1999). Herpesvirus infection in tortoises (*Malacochersus tornieri* and *Testudo horsfieldii*). *Veterinary Pathology* 36 (6): 624–627.

Uney, K., Altan, F., Aboubakr, M. et al. (2016). Pharmacokinetics of meloxicam in red-eared slider turtles (*Trachemys scripta elegans*) after single intravenous and intramuscular injections. *American Journal of Veterinary Research* 77 (5): 439–444.

Wallach, J.D. and Hoessle, C. (1966). Hypervitaminosis D in green iguanas. *Journal of the American Veterinary Medical Association* 149 (7): 912–914.

Wambugu, S.N., Towett, P.K., Kiama, S.G. et al. (2010). Effects of opioids in the formalin test in the Speke's hinged tortoise (*Kinixy's spekii*). *Journal of Veterinary Pharmacology and Therapeutics* 33 (4): 347–351.

Wendland, L.D., Brown, D.R., Klein, P.A. et al. (2006). Upper respiratory tract disease (Mycoplasmosis) in tortoises. In: *Reptile Medicine and Surgery*, 2e (ed. D. Mader), 931–938. St. Louis: Elsevier-Saunders.

Wiesner, C.S. and Iben, C. (2003). Influence of environmental humidity and dietary protein on pyrimidial growth of carapaces in African spurred tortoises (*Geochelone sulcata*). *Journal of Animal Physiology and Animal Nutrition* 87: 66–74.

Wilkinson, R. (2004). Clinical pathology. In: *Medicine and Surgery of Tortoises and Turtles* (eds. S. McArthur, R. Wilkinson and J. Meyer), 141–186. Oxford: Blackwell.

Wilkinson, R., Hernandez-Divers, S., Lafortune, M. et al. (2004). Diagnostic imaging techniques. In: *Medicine and Surgery of Tortoises and Turtles* (eds. S. McArthur, R. Wilkinson and J. Meyer), 187–238. Oxford: Blackwell.

Wright, K.M. (1993). Metabolic bone disease in reptiles. *Reptile and Amphibian Magazine* 2: 60–68.

Wright, K.M. (1997). Common medical problems of tortoises. In: *Proceedings of North American Veterinary Conference*, 769–771. Gainesville, FL: North American Veterinary Conference.

20

Terrapins
Ian Sayers and Marie Kubiak

There is much variation in common terms used to describe the different sub-classifications of chelonia. For the purposes of this chapter, the term terrapin is used to refer to semi-aquatic fresh water chelonia; with terrestrial tortoises and marine turtles not included. Due to their popularity as pets and the heavy bias towards this genus in the published literature, *Trachemys* species will be the primary focus. Other less frequently kept genera may be referenced where pertinent information is available, e.g. *Chrysemys* (Painted Turtles); *Emys* (Pond Turtles); *Graptemys* (Map Turtles) and *Terrapene* (Box Turtles).

Trachemys scripta subspecies are specifically listed in EU Regulation (1143/2014) on invasive alien (non-native) species. Since the introduction of the Invasive Alien Species legislation, it has become an offence to breed, trade, or move *T. scripta* subspecies and hence captive numbers should reduce over the coming years as no new animals are available. Owners are permitted to maintain owned animals for their natural lifespan. Rescue centres are permitted to take in surrendered individuals and can elect to maintain them as non-breeding animals for their natural lifespan or euthanase individuals. Transfer to an alternative rescue facility may also become a possibility. Maintenance of an oviparous species as non-breeding is simple as eggs can be removed and destroyed, or animals kept as single sex groups. Within the United Kingdom (UK) it is also illegal to release non-native species, including all chelonia, under the Wildlife and Countryside Act, 1985. Some states in the USA prohibit ownership and breeding of red-bellied sliders (*T. s. elegans*), and a nationwide ban on sales of individuals under 4 inches in carapacial length is in place.

20.1 Husbandry

Poor husbandry remains a significant contributory factor to disease in reptiles and it is essential to reproduce the parameters found in a reptile's natural environment when keeping them in captivity. Basic requirements for common species are included in Table 20.1.

20.1.1 Enclosure Size

Enclosures should be large enough to provide an adequate temperature gradient and have sufficient space to allow expression of natural fight/flight behaviour when threatened. The minimum size for a higher standard temporary enclosure (for animals in commercial establishments in the UK) would be approximately 2 m × 1.2 m × 0.9 m, with a water depth of 25 cm for an adult *Trachemys* species, with a land to water ratio of 25:75 (DEFRA 2018). However, these recommendations apply to temporary holding facilities which would be smaller than those intended for long term husbandry. Permanent enclosures for pet animals would be expected to significantly exceed to these minimum standards. Reported minimum home ranges for Painted turtles (*Chrysemys picta*) and red-bellied sliders are 89 and 327 ha respectively, which clearly highlights the limitations of a small scale captive facility (Jaeger and Cobb 2012).

20.1.2 Temperature

Reptiles are poikilothermic, regulating their body temperature by behavioural means and that temperature can vary between species, and for individuals at differing times. For a given physiological status (e.g. post-prandial, vitellogenesis) there is a preferred body temperature (PBT) to optimise the specific function. As status and PBT will vary over time, a range of temperatures that allow animals to attain the expected range of PBT should be provided and is known as the Preferred Optimum Temperature Zone (POTZ) (Norton 2005). The temperature range should be provided by use of both a primary and secondary heat source.

Handbook of Exotic Pet Medicine, First Edition. Edited by Marie Kubiak.
© 2021 John Wiley & Sons Ltd. Published 2021 by John Wiley & Sons Ltd.
Companion website: www.wiley.com/go/kubiak/exotic_pet_medicine

Table 20.1 Biological parameters of selected semi-aquatic turtles.

	Yellow-bellied slider (Trachemys scripta scripta)	Red-eared slider (Trachemys scripta elegans)	False map turtle (Graptemys pseudogeographica)	Eastern box turtle (Terrapene carolina carolina)
Lifespan	30–40 years	30–40 years	25–35 years	40 years (up to 100 years reported) (Carr 1952; Ernst et al. 1994)
Adult size	Females up to 29 cm, males up to 23 cm	Females up to 33 cm, males up to 23 cm	Females up to 26 cm, males up to 16 cm	Approximately 15×10 cm, males tend to be slightly larger than females (Ernst et al. 1994)
Age at sexual maturity	8 years in females, 5 years in males (Mitchell and Pague 1990)	5–7 years for females, 2–5 years for males	8–14 years for females, 4–6 years for males (Ernst et al. 1984; Vogt 1993)	By 5 years of age
Incubation length	69–95 days	59–110 days	58–85 days (Ernst et al. 1984; Vogt 1993)	50–70 days
Incubation conditions	20–27 °C produces all males and 29.4–35 °C produces all females with mixed sex groups in intermediate temperatures (Ewert and Nelson 1991; Crews 1996)	20–27 °C produces all males and 29.4–35 °C produces all females with mixed sex groups in intermediate temperatures (Ewert and Nelson 1991; Crews 1996)	Eggs incubated at 25 °C produce all males, eggs incubated at 30 °C produce all females (Ewert and Nelson 1991)	22–27 °C produce males, above 28 °C produces females (Ernst et al. 1994)
Heart rate	30 bpm at 22 °C (Akers and Damm 1963)	15–30 bpm at 20–24 °C (as low as 1 bpm in hibernation, up to 50 bpm at 30 °C)	20–21 bpm at 20 °C, 5–6 bpm in torpor at 5 °C (Akers and Damm 1963; Semple et al. 1970)	39 bpm at 22 °C (Akers and Damm 1963)
Respiratory rate	1–2/min at 30 °C (Jackson 1971)	1–2/min at 30 °C (Jackson 1971) (absent in hibernation)	No data	4–5/min (Altland and Parker 1955)
Ambient temperature	20–24 °C (McArthur and Barrows 2004)	20–24 °C (McArthur and Barrows 2004)	22–26 °C	22–26 °C
Basking temperature	32–35 °C	29–34 °C	31–35	29–34 °C
Water temperature	24–27 (Johnson 2004b)	24–27 °C (Johnson 2004b)	21–24	Primarily terrestrial though mud and shallow pools should be available
UV index (Baines et al., 2016)	1.0–3.5	1.0–3.5	1.0–3.5	0.7–1.0
Diet	Omnivores with greater tendency towards herbivory with age	Omnivores with greater tendency towards herbivory with age	Omnivores with tendency towards insectivory	Broad omnivorous diet, young more carnivorous, adults feed more on fruit, flowers, roots, and fungi
Physical appearance	Dorsoventrally flattened appearance to ovoid carapace, olive to dark brown colouration to shell and skin with yellow highlights. Broad yellow band on lateral head and bright yellow plastron.	Distinctive bilateral red stripe on lateral face. Carapace predominantly green in juveniles maturing to brown in adults. Plastron yellow with variable darker markings. Fine lines cover the skin and carapace and are thought to aid camouflage.	The carapace has low spines along the dorsal midline and a serrated appearance to the caudal margin. A complex series of pale lines is present over the predominantly brown carapace but is most pronounced in juveniles	Hinged plastron to allow almost complete closure of the shell, yellow/orange markings to predominantly brown carapace and skin

The primary heat source provides ambient heat at the lowest appropriate temperature in the POTZ. A secondary heat source should provide a focal basking area at the higher end of the POTZ during the day, creating a gradient of temperatures encompassing the POTZ across the enclosure. Ceramic heat emitters, infra-red bulbs, or mercury vapour lamps may be considered as a secondary heat source. It is important not to rely on incandescent bulbs as an ambient primary heat source as they would need to remain on overnight but 24 hours light exposure is a significant stressor.

All heat sources should be positioned and protected to prevent direct contact with the animal and should be thermostatically controlled. Temperatures should be monitored daily by use of data-logging thermometers, measuring the maximum and minimum temperatures at the extremes of the temperature gradient. An overnight temperature drop by reliance on the primary ambient heat source alone is advisable to maintain circadian rhythms.

A water heater, as commonly used for aquaculture, is required to maintain a suitable temperature of the aquatic section of the enclosure. If water temperature is too high then the stimulus to bask may be lost, resulting in shell deterioration. If water temperature is too low this may impact adversely upon the metabolism, reducing appetite and immunocompetence. Whilst adults may be able to survive colder water temperatures by entering a brumation period, this is a temporary survival strategy and prolonged cooling will result in debilitation.

20.1.3 Lighting

Reptiles visualise ultraviolet (UV) wavelength light as well as that within the human visible spectrum, and also rely on UV light for reproductive and behavioural cues (Baines et al. 2016). UV-B light is necessary for endogenous Vitamin D3 synthesis and should be considered an essential requirement (Acierno et al. 2006). Ordinary glass prevents transmission of UV-B and so exposure to natural sunlight through a window is not sufficient. A full spectrum light source should be placed overhead and in close association with the basking heat source to replicate exposure to natural sunlight, but not in a position where water splashes are likely. Areas of shade should also be provided in the enclosure, both on land and in water. Lamps should be replaced as output diminishes over time to maintain an appropriate UV index. If monitoring is not possible, lamps should be regularly replaced according to manufacturer recommendations. If the UV index is excessive, or wavelength is incorrect, ophthalmic and dermatological problems can result (Gardiner et al. 2009). A photoperiod of 13–14 hours light and 10–11 hours dark will replicate that which occurs in the terrapin's natural environment for most species (Baines et al. 2016).

20.1.4 Humidity

Evaporation from the water source will generally maintain adequate humidity levels, but it is important that a lower relative humidity is achieved at the basking site. Together with good ventilation and heat, this will allow the shell to dry out during basking, and help avoid proliferation of bacteria and fungi.

20.1.5 Water Quality

Water hygiene can deteriorate rapidly as *Trachemys* species feed in water, and remnants of food, urination, and defaecation contaminate the water. It may be suitable to move smaller specimens into a separate smaller container for feeding (Johnson 2004b) that is more easily cleaned, but it is still likely a water filtration device will be required for faecal material and organic debris from plants and the microbiome. Enclosure size and design, number of animals and plant growth will guide filter type required (see Chapter 22), and canister filters are most commonly used for small scale enclosures. Water quality should be monitored weekly using commercial aquatic kits to assess ammonia, nitrate, and nitrite levels.

20.1.6 Diet

Trachemys species are considered to be omnivorous with juveniles and gravid females tending to be more carnivorous than adults. (Clark and Whitfield 1969; Johnson 2004b). It is thought that the higher protein intake is beneficial for growth in small terrapins, and for egg production for large females (Bouchard and Bjorndal 2006; Works and Olson 2018).

For maintenance of adult *Trachemys* species, a diet of 60–70% plant matter and 30% invertebrate or vertebrate material should be provided to reflect the natural diet (Parmenter and Avery 1990). Diet can be supplemented by growing aquatic plants within the enclosure as these should make up a substantial part of the diet for adults (Calvert 2004). Food should be offered two or three times weekly for a period of 30–40 minutes (Calvert 2004). Commercial terrapin pelleted diets can be used as part of the diet but should not be fed in excess of the manufacturer's recommendations. Over-feeding results in obesity which may be seen as soft tissue protruding from the fossae around the limbs (Zwart 2000).

20.1.7 Handling

Commonly presented patients are usually easily handled by using one or both hands, depending on size. Most terrapins can be lifted using a bilateral grip caudal to the

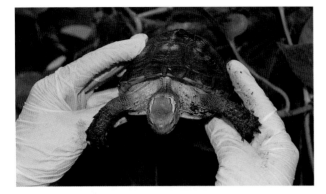

Figure 20.1 Restraint of a docile species with bilateral grip at the plastrocarapacial bridges (*Source:* Photo courtesy of Drayton Manor Park Zoo).

forelimbs, at the plastrocarapacial bridge (Figure 20.1). Whilst most individuals are amenable, be aware that some individuals can be more aggressive and may bite. Attempts to bite can be quite active and painful minor soft tissue injuries can result. For aggressive individuals the hands can be placed at the level of the prefemoral fossae (shell apertures around the hindlimbs), taking care not to place fingers within the fossae as limb retraction may cause compression. This grip is less secure.

Good hygiene is required as *Salmonella* carriage is common in aquatic and semi-aquatic chelonia, and over 200 000 cases of human salmonellosis have been associated with *Trachemys* species (Johnson 2004b; Gaertner et al. 2008). The routine wearing of disposable gloves is recommended, alongside washing hands with warm running water and soap between patients.

20.1.8 Sex Determination

The most reliable characteristic for sex determination is the pre-cloacal tail length. The male has a longer, thicker tail with a distally placed cloacal orifice (the vent) (Figure 20.2). The position of the vent in females is closer to the tail base, usually proximal to the carapacial margin (Figure 20.3). In individuals over 10 cm carapace length, species-specific secondary sexual characteristics can also be used. The forelimb nails of *Trachemys* species males are longer than in females and may be used for courtship (Moll and Legler 1971; Thomas 2002). The hind claws of *Trachemys* females are longer than those of the male and may be associated with nest construction (Warner et al. 2006). Male Eastern box turtles (*Terrapene c. carolina*) have a red iris, females have a brown iris.

The use of ultrasound may also be useful in visualising ovarian follicle development in females using probes of appropriate frequency and footprint, via the pre-femoral fossa.

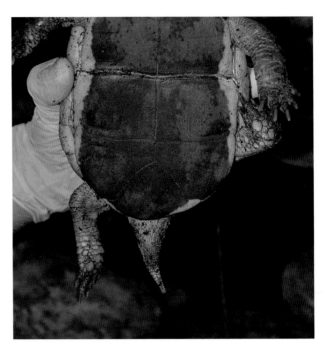

Figure 20.2 Male *Cuora flavimarginata*, note the long tail and distally located vent (*Source:* Photo courtesy of Drayton Manor Park Zoo).

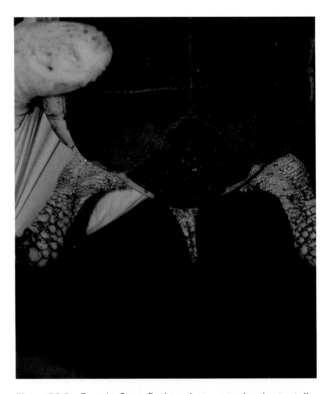

Figure 20.3 Female *Cuora flavimarginata*, note the shorter tail and vent located under the carapacial margin (*Source:* Photo courtesy of Drayton Manor Park Zoo).

Endoscopy may be considered as another tool for sex determination. Cloacoscopy, to visually inspect the phallus/clitoris, has been reported to only be 57% accurate in red-bellied sliders, whilst coelioscopy, to examine the gonads, was found to be 100% accurate (Perpinan et al. 2016). Whilst coelioscopy is of value for sexing juveniles of all species, it is an invasive procedure requiring general anaesthesia and surgical access. Other methods should be utilised where possible.

20.2 Clinical Examination

A thorough history collection and husbandry review should be part of any patient's clinical examination (see Figure 20.4).

The patient should be visually assessed prior to examination. Activity, response to stimuli, resting respiratory rate, and respiratory pattern are all valuable information that may alter following handling. Individuals should be able to support their bodies and walk without the plastron (lower shell) dragging on the ground, and when placed in water should be able to submerge and float in a level, symmetrical manner and make purposeful movements to alter level. Alterations in buoyancy may indicate abnormal mass or foreign body presence, or asymmetrical reductions in air filling in the lower respiratory tract.

Generally, systematic examinations start at the head and work towards the tail and follow similar protocols as for other species. However, opening of the mouth is often resented and is usually performed later in the examination. Erythema of the mucous membranes and apigmented areas of shell may be indicative of a generalised inflammatory process. Oral examination may also reveal petechial haemorrhages. Externally visible tympanic membranes should be flat and symmetrical, a raised tympanum is highly suggestive of aural abscessation. The shell and skin surfaces should be assessed for any ulceration, thickening, and excessive or retained shedding. Limbs and head should be withdrawn rapidly on handling and demonstrate no asymmetry or masses. Information gained by palpation may be limited due to the presence of the shell but masses or eggs may be palpated via the pre-femoral fossa.

Clinical examination is limited by the presence of the shell and, together with the common presentation of animals with non-specific signs such as lethargy and anorexia, means that broad diagnostic procedures may be necessary at initial presentation to narrow the differential diagnoses. Initial investigation of clinically unwell animals with no clear cause will usually include radiography, haematology, and serum biochemistry. Faecal analysis is indicated if gastrointestinal clinical signs are present.

20.2.1 Blood Sample Collection

Circulating blood volume is approximately 5–8% of body weight and up to 10% of circulating volume can be taken from a healthy animal (Murray 2000; Eatwell et al. 2014). A maximum of 0.5–0.8 ml/100 g can be collected though volume taken may need to be reduced for debilitated

HISTORY	TERRESTRIAL ENVIRONMENT	REPRODUCTIVE DATA
• Species (common and scientific names)	• Method of ambient and basking heat provision?	• Social structure
• Sex and age		• Reproductively active?
• Reason for presentation	• Max, min and average daytime/night time temps?	• Last contact with opposite sex?
KEEPER/COLLECTION DETAILS	• How is humidity varied and monitored?	• Breeding history
• Captive-bred or wild-caught?	• What type of ultra-violet lighting is provided?	• Prevention of breeding used (if a controlled species)
• Appropriate licence available (if indicated)?	• What is the photoperiod?	**DISEASE CONTROL**
• Duration of ownership?	• Substrate used?	• Quarantine programme? How long?
• Previous ownership details?		• What disinfectants are used?
• Disease history and any previous veterinary treatment?	**AQUATIC ENVIRONMENT**	
• Contact with other animals (and their health status)	• Water temperature and heating method	
OBSERVATIONS	• Water quality checked regularly?	
• Appetite?	• Filter system?	
• Activity and mobility?	• How often is water changed?	
• Faecal output?	**NUTRITION**	
HOUSING	• Diet offered/frequency of feeding	
• Indoors, outdoors or both?	• Diet eaten	
• Diagram / photo / description	• Plants within enclosure	
• Size of enclosure (land and water)	• Supplementation	
	• Any changes in appetite/food selection?	

Figure 20.4 Common factors to assess on patient history and husbandry review.

animals. Complete haematology and biochemistry is possible on low sample volumes but may not be possible in very small individuals. In these cases total protein (TP), glucose, and a blood smear can be assessed with minimal samples and even this limited information can be very useful.

Venepuncture can be a little more challenging than in domestic species as the vessels are not readily visible. Additionally, lymphoid vessels run close to veins at a number of sites (Murray 2000; Eatwell et al. 2014) and concurrent lymph sampling can alter results, however careful technique can help minimise negative impacts (Waters et al. 2001). Dependent upon the size of the animal, 22–27 G needles will be required, with 1.0–2.5 ml syringes.

Asepsis during sampling is important. Cutaneous bacterial load in terrapins will reflect water populations and poor environmental hygiene will result in increased skin contamination. Removal of any gross contamination and topical disinfection is advisable prior to venipuncture.

The preferred site is the external jugular vein as there is minimal chance of lymphodilution (Redrobe and MacDonald 1999; Eatwell et al. 2014). The patient should be restrained with the neck extended and forelimbs restrained caudally. The vein is more dorsal and superficial than in mammals and may be seen as linear bulge, running from the level of the tympanum to the base of the neck. Pressure at the 'thoracic' inlet can aid visualisation but blind sampling may be necessary. After sampling ensure haemostasis by applying suitable pressure, or significant haematoma formation may occur.

The subcarapacial sinus is situated below the cranial aspect of the carapace in the midline, at the level of the caudal cervical vertebrae. The needle is inserted at the junction of the skin and shell and advanced caudo-dorsally until blood is aspirated. A 1–2 inch needle is required in adult *Trachemys* terrapins and there is potential for lymphodilution from nearby lymph vessels. If clear fluid is noted flowing into the hub of the needle then the sample should be discarded and a fresh attempt made.

The dorsal coccygeal vein is situated in the dorsal midline of the tail immediately above the vertebrae. The area is frequently contaminated with faecal material so pre-sample cleansing must be thorough. A 1 ml syringe and 25 G needle, or insulin syringe, is preferred for this site.

Once the sample is collected, fresh blood should be used to make smears and the remainder of the sample placed in a lithium heparin blood tube. Manual haematology is necessary due to nucleation of red cells, thus good quality fresh smears are preferred to those made from heparinised samples where cell clumping is often seen.

20.2.2 Nutritional Support

Physiological anorexia is commonly seen in terrapins relating to reproductive activity or a reduction in environmental temperatures. As terrapins generally feed in water, any alteration to time spent in the water may interfere with feeding behaviour. It can be difficult to differentiate physiological or environmental effects from the pathological anorexia that is a non-specific sign seen with a wide range of disease processes (Norton 2005). In an otherwise clinically well animal that is maintaining body condition it is often prudent to thoroughly review husbandry and correct any concerns to assess whether feeding normalises without further intervention. Loss of condition, reduction in bodyweight, or prolonged anorexia of two weeks or more without a discernible environmental cause does merit nutritional support in many cases. Additionally, where clinical signs of disease are present nutritional support may improve the response to therapy (Bonner 2000). However, feeding should not be initiated until the patient has been hydrated and factors that may be impacting on gastrointestinal motility (e.g. hypocalcaemia) have been addressed (Norton 2005).

Nutritional support for some sick reptiles may be as simple as provision of oral fluids and electrolytes to ensure the gastrointestinal tract is suitably hydrated. For others, tempting with/hand feeding favourite food items may encourage feeding. For others, where neither of these approaches is successful assisted feeding, i.e. placement of food items directly into the mouth, or syringe feeding may be required. Syringe feeding carries a potential for aspiration and gavage administration of food is preferred. If repeated gavage is likely to be required in the longer term, placement of oesophagostomy tubes in the first instance may reduce overall stress.

20.2.3 Gavage Feeding

Gavage tubes may be metal, as are frequently used in avian patients, or made of other softer materials - typically silicone or rubber. A silicone or rubber tube may be less likely to cause trauma but is more likely to be bitten through by larger patients. Use of oral gags may protect these tubes.

The gavage tube should be pre-measured to the level of the stomach which is positioned at 33–50% of the plastron length (Norton 2005). The patients head and neck should be extended, and the tube can be aligned on the underside of the patient with the tip at the level of the stomach and the proximal portion of the tube near the mouth, where it can then be marked as an indicator to prevent excess advancement of the tube. With the patients head restrained, the lubricated tube is introduced via the oral commissure.

Some patients may need the mouth to be manually opened and kept open via digital pressure on the mandible but many terrapins will open the mouth as a defensive response to stimulation. The gavage tube is then advanced across the mouth (avoiding the visible glottis), down the oesophagus and into the stomach. Once in the stomach the liquid feed can be gradually introduced. Foodstuff should be warmed to an appropriate temperature and instilled slowly to avoid damage to the gastric mucosa or inducing regurgitation.

20.2.3.1 Oesophagostomy Tube Placement

Placement of an oesophagostomy tube is advisable when long-term nutritional support or medication is anticipated, or for cases with disease processes, surgical intervention, or traumatic injury affecting the head or oral cavity.

A flexible, soft tube approximately 30–50% of the oesophageal diameter should be selected (Norton 2005; McCormack 2015). The stomach is located at the level of 33–50% of the plastron length, and the distance from tube insertion point on the neck to the stomach should be measured and pre-marked on the tube to be used (Norton 2005). The patient is anaesthetised and held in lateral recumbency with the head and neck extended (Figure 20.5). The left side of the neck is most commonly used to avoid the larger right jugular vein. The skin is aseptically prepared and curved haemostatic forceps passed through the mouth to tent up the skin on the lateral neck and displace vessels (Figure 20.6) (Divers 2001). A scalpel is used to incise the skin and oesophagus over the forceps to expose the tips. The tube is then grasped by the forceps and pulled through the incision and out of the mouth (Figure 20.7). The tube is redirected and gently advanced down the oesophagus using straight forceps, feeding the remaining tube in from the side of the neck until the pre-marked length is reached. The glottis should be visualised and confirmed clear, and radiography can be used to confirm gastric positioning of the tube tip. A purse-string

suture around the incision site is used to secure the tube, with secondary security provided by either a Chinese finger trap suture (Figure 20.8) or creation of a tab of waterproof tape around the insertion of the tube and suturing of this to the skin (Divers 2001). The external portion of the tube is then secured to the dorsal carapace with acrylic or waterproof tape to prevent patient interference and allow easy access for feeding or medication. The tube can be retained in place for months with minimal potential for adverse effects (McCormack 2015). Flushing the tube with water after feeds is necessary to prevent clogging of the tube. Any blockages can usually be alleviated by alternating aspiration and flushing with warm water.

It is often necessary to keep animals out of water whilst initial incisions heal which may disrupt resumption of

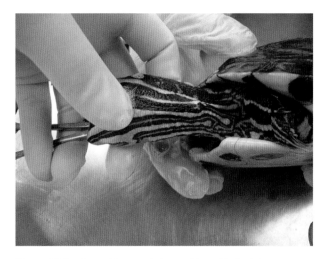

Figure 20.6 Curved haemostats used to guide incision placement for oesophagostomy tube insertion.

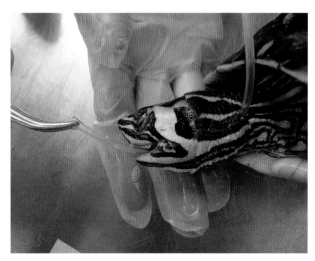

Figure 20.7 Withdrawal of oesophagostomy tube via the mouth following insertion.

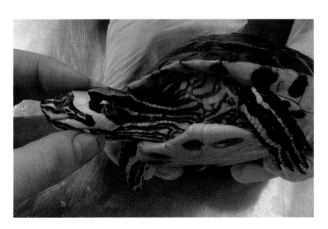

Figure 20.5 Yellow bellied slider anaesthetised and positioned for oesophagostomy tube placement.

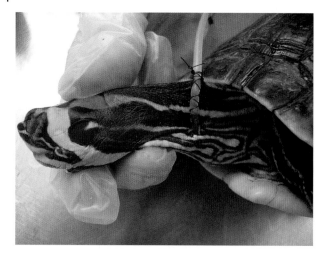

Figure 20.8 Oesophagostomy tube secured in place using a Chinese finger trap suture.

normal behaviours such as feeding or defaecation (DeSouza et al. 2005). Presence of the oesophogostomy tube for assist feeding means this is unlikely to be detrimental but access to water is also important to maintain skin health and muscle tone and patients should be returned to water as soon as is reasonable.

Self-feeding is possible with an appropriately sized tube and once this resumes then feeding via the tube can be withdrawn. Maintenance of weight in a self-feeding animal for four days indicates that the tube can be removed (Divers 2001). The securing sutures can be removed conscious in many animals, the tube withdrawn and the placement site allowed to heal by secondary intention. However, it is often preferable to remove the tube under anaesthesia and suture the oesophagus and skin, or skin alone, to hasten healing and allow rapid return to the water.

20.2.3.2 Dietary Choice

For initial nutritional support, following prolonged periods of anorexia, simple electrolyte solutions are preferred to support fluid therapy and avoid re-feeding syndrome and associated electrolyte aberrations (Mans and Braun 2014). After rehydration, confirmed by clinical assessment of hydration, weight gain, and passage of urine, liquid foods can be introduced. Suggested daily volumes to administer anorexic animals are dependent on the diet used but are typically in the region of 5–7 ml/kg bodyweight (Rees Davies and Klingenberg 2004; Norton 2005). Starting with these smaller volumes is advised, gradually increasing over several days to 10–20 ml/kg. The gastric volume is estimated to be 20 ml/kg bodyweight so no single feed should ever exceed this volume (Bonner 2000). The exact quantity fed will depend on the manufacturer guidelines of the preparation used. Proprietary elemental complete diets for omnivores

are available, though combinations of herbivore and carnivore or insectivore diets can be suitable alternatives.

20.2.4 Fluid Therapy

Maintenance requirements are 15–25 ml/kg/day for chelonia, with smaller patients requiring the higher end of the range (Norton 2005). Crystalloids are most frequently used as dehydration is the most common reason for fluid therapy in reptiles (Lawton 2005; Pees and Girling 2019). Lactic acidosis is common in chelonia and lactated solutions are not considered to carry additional advantages (Prezant and Jarchow 1997; Pees and Girling 2019). Where available, serum electrolyte measurement should be considered to aid fluid preparation choice. A full discussion of fluid therapy routes is detailed in Table 18.4.

For mild dehydration, the oral and subcutaneous routes may be used but uptake can be slow and inconsistent. The epicoelomic route is also appropriate and is more reliable. Although absorption of fluid via the cloaca has been postulated for terrestrial chelonia, it does not appear a valid route in *Trachemys* species (Peterson and Greenshields 2001).

Where dehydration is moderate–severe, the epicoelomic route is favoured. This site is readily accessible and fluid appears to be rapidly absorbed (McArthur 2004a). The epicoelomic potential space is located dorsal to the plastron and ventral to the pectoral muscles (Norton 2005). A needle is placed into skin overlying the plastron and is advanced, maintaining a horizontal aspect in relation to the plastron towards the opposite hindleg. Volumes of 10 ml/kg appear to be well tolerated at this site.

For animals with marked dehydration, continuous infusion via an intravenous or intraosseous cannula is preferred. Rates of 1 ml/kg/h are used, but up to 5 ml/kg/h may be administered for short-term rehydration over 1–2 hours (Maclean and Raiti 2004). Overhydration is possible due to the slow elimination of excess fluids (Norton 2005), and is of greater concern in animals with renal compromise. Jugular cannula placement requires a cutdown technique under anaesthesia, and maintenance can be difficult (Bonner 2000). Intraosseous cannula sites include the distal humerus, distal tibia, or caudal aspect of the plastrocarapacial bridge (Lawton 2005). Spinal needles or hypodermic needles with a stylet are used, and anaesthesia is required for placement (Norton 2005). Once placed, positive pressure infusion devices are required to maintain fluid flow through an intraosseous catheter, though during surgical procedures bolus administration may be sufficient. In animals with Nutritional Secondary Hyperparathyroidism (NSHP), the intraosseous route is not appropriate.

20.2.5 Anaesthesia

Intravenous administration of induction agents is preferred for a quick and predictable induction, see the formulary for anaesthesia protocols and doses. Alfaxalone given intravenously into the subcarapacial sinus results in rapid induction of anaesthesia (Knotek 2014). Alfaxalone given by the intramuscular route requires higher doses and may not produce surgical anaesthesia but is useful for sedation (Kischinovsky et al. 2013). Propofol is an alternative intravenous induction agent with similar induction times and a dose-dependent duration of action (Divers 1996).

Intramuscular administration of ketamine alone requires high doses to achieve a surgical plane of anaesthesia and sufficient muscle relaxation, with resulting protracted recovery periods of several days (Boyer 1992a). Combination of ketamine with other sedatives has given more reliable sedation and recovery. Subcutaneous administration of medetomidine and ketamine combinations have been demonstrated to be as effective as intramuscular administration, with potential to give larger volumes than the intramuscular route (Mans 2015). Injections are typically given in the front half of the body to reduce theoretical concerns regarding renal clearance and first pass effects due to the renal and hepatic portal veins.

Intranasal administration of ketamine and dexmedetomidine have been reported and resulted in safe sedation for intubation and minor procedures though volume required is a limiting factor (Schnellbacher et al. 2012; Cermakova et al. 2017). Atipamezole antagonism via the intranasal route resulted in reversal of the sedation associated with dexmedetomidine (Schnellbacher et al. 2012).

Skeletal muscle movement is required for effective respiration in chelonia due to the lack of diaphragmatic and costal movements. Spontaneous respiration may continue to occur slowly, or intermittently, during anaesthesia but it is not adequate to maintain oxygenation, or depth of anaesthesia when using volatile agents. Endotracheal intubation and intermittent positive pressure ventilation (IPPV) is required for anaesthesia. Intubation is usually straightforward as the glottis is rostrally positioned at the base of the tongue (Figure 20.9). Care should be taken to choose endotracheal tubes that give a snug fit, but do not traumatise the respiratory epithelium. Silicone endotracheal tubes are now available as small as 1.0 mm with a rigid introducer, and for small patients intravenous cannulae can also be used but narrow diameter tubes are prone to obstruction by respiratory secretions. The use of low dead space circuits and connectors is recommended. The trachea of chelonia bifurcates quite cranially, so care should be taken not to advance tubes excessively and inadvertently ventilate a

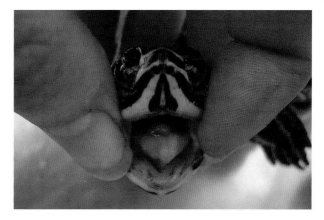

Figure 20.9 The glottis is readily identifiable as a fleshy mass at the base of the tongue.

single lung (McArthur 2004b; Scheelings 2019). Inflation at both axillary fossae should be confirmed on IPPV prior to securing the ET tube.

IPPV can be performed by trained personnel, but a small animal ventilator is preferred. The level and depth of respiration for each individual should be monitored prior to anaesthesia, this should then be matched by the ventilator when the patient is anaesthetised. These ventilation parameters are then reliably maintained throughout anaesthesia, reducing the potential for overinflation and possible rupture of the delicate lung, or underinflation. For surgical coeliotomy however, ventilator parameters will need reviewing once the coelomic membrane is breached as resistance to ventilation will markedly decrease.

Maintaining patient temperature is crucial in reptiles as metabolic rate (and hence metabolism of drugs) is temperature dependent and deep cloacal or oesophageal temperature measurement is valuable for monitoring trends (Norton 2005). A Doppler probe can be secured over the carotid artery for the entirety of the procedure to enable assessment of cardiac rate and rhythm. Side-stream capnography connectors are preferred to reduce dead space, and capnography can be useful to monitor trends in expired CO_2 however end tidal CO_2 values may not directly reflect circulating levels (Swenson et al. 2008).

It is important to be aware that the respiratory stimulus in reptiles is low partial pressure of oxygen in the blood (Redrobe 2004; Scheelings 2019). The main impact of this is usually observed at the end of anaesthesia where volatile anaesthetic agents have been delivered in 100% oxygen carrier, when recovery times and return to spontaneous breathing can be protracted. Using room air for IPPV at the end of anaesthesia is to be recommended.

20.2.6 Analgesia

Signs of pain in terrapins are subtle, but neural pathways of pain perception in reptiles appear equivalent to mammals (Terashima and Liang 1994; Sneddon et al. 2014) and it should be assumed that terrapins experience pain even if it is not readily recognised by an observer.

Previously butorphanol was a preferred opioid but more recent work indicates that it has no benefit above placebo and causes respiratory depression (Sladky et al. 2007; Kinney et al. 2011). Analgesia in *Trachemys* species appears effected by mu-receptors, and so mu-receptor agonists such as morphine, hydromorphone, or methadone are considered the most appropriate choices for analgesia (Sladky et al. 2007; Sladky et al. 2009; Baker et al. 2011; Mans et al. 2012). Tramadol has also been shown to have anti-nociceptive effects in *T. s. scripta* (Giorgi et al. 2015).

Even less information is available on the efficacy of non-steroidal anti–inflammatory drugs, though meloxicam has been assessed in *Trachemys* species and is used commonly for analgesia. Intramuscular and intravenous doses of 0.2 mg/kg result in plasma concentrations that would be provide analgesia in other species, however oral administration was reported to result in poor uptake and low plasma concentrations (Di Salvo et al. 2016; Uney et al. 2016). Pharmacodynamic data is lacking to confirm the analgesic effects of this class of therapeutics in terrapins.

20.2.7 Euthanasia

Reptiles can endure hypoxia for considerable periods (Johlin and Moreland 1933) and evidence suggests the central nervous system of decapitated reptiles may continue to perceive painful stimuli (Cooper et al. 1984). Historically hypothermia and freezing have been used for euthanasia but this is not appropriate, unless for specimens under 4 g undergoing rapid whole body freezing by submersion in liquid nitrogen (Cooper 2004).

The preferred method of euthanasia is by overdose of pentobarbital, ideally administered intravenously (McArthur 2004b). Venous access may be difficult in the debilitated patient but can be facilitated by sedation. Pentobarbital administered into tissue or the coelomic cavity can cause irritation and a slow response, particularly if body temperature is not maintained (Leary et al. 2013).

The use of a Doppler probe, or echocardiography, can be used to confirm cessation of cardiac activity. Agonal movements can be protracted but purposeful movement and reflex responses should be absent. Pithing should then be carried out to arrest brainstem activity and prevent recovery (Cooper et al. 1984). This is achieved by inserting a rod into the brainstem via the roof of the mouth or the foramen magnum. The use of suitable sized needles or dental hand tools can be useful alternatives.

20.2.8 Hospitalisation Requirements

Hospitalisation requires provision of the same basic husbandry essentials previously detailed i.e. suitable temperature gradient, lighting, and water quality. For short-term hospitalisation, enclosure size requirements may be reduced, small enclosures may also be preferable to reduce activity levels and facilitate regular capture.

It may also be necessary to withhold access to water temporarily whilst surgical sites or wounds are in an early stage of healing. However these aspects need to be considered in a 'cost benefit' assessment with overall animal welfare paramount and full facilities should be available to transition patients into during recuperation.

20.3 Common Medical and Surgical Conditions

20.3.1 Infectious Disease

20.3.1.1 Respiratory Tract Disease and Stomatitis

Ranaviruses are emerging pathogens of reptiles and have been described in red eared sliders (RES), Eastern painted turtles (*Chrysemys picta picta),* Eastern box turtles (*Terrapene c. carolina*), Chinese softshell turtles (*Trionyx sinensis*), and Florida box turtles (*Terrapene carolina bauri*) (Mao et al. 1997; Chen et al. 1999; Johnson et al. 2008; Goodman et al. 2013). Reported cases are predominantly from North America but have also been described in Europe and Asia. Clinical signs include lethargy, anorexia, stomatitis, conjunctivitis, nasal discharge, and subcutaneous oedema, and mortality is high (Marschang 2011). Experimental transmission of an isolated ranavirus to box turtles (*Terrapene ornata ornata*) and RES resulted in the same clinical presentation, confirming viral pathogenicity (Johnson et al. 2007). Hypoproteinaemia and hypoalbuminaemia have been demonstrated to develop in infected RES (Moore et al. 2014). Both ELISA and PCR techniques have been used to confirm infection. Co-infection of ranavirus, *Mycoplasma,* and a herpes virus has been reported in Eastern box turtles, associated with a mortality rate of 48% (n = 27) (Sim et al. 2016). Attempted treatment of cases comprises supportive care, fluid therapy, assisted feeding, antiviral therapy, and management of secondary infections (Sim et al. 2016).

Terrapene herpesvirus 1 (TerHV1) has been reported in Eastern box turtles. One case in a juvenile was associated with dyspnoea, lethargy, and dehydration on emergence from brumation, and subsequent death despite supportive therapy (Sim et al. 2015). Post-mortem examination showed a severe necroulcerative rhinitis, stomatitis, oesophagitis, and pneumonia. Co-infection with ranavirus and TerHV1 resulted in lethargy, stomatitis, cloacitis, conjunctivitis, and blepharitis in a group of 27 Eastern box turtles. Post-mortem examination showed similar necroulcerative stomatitis, oesophagitis, gastritis, enterocolitis, hepatitis, nephritis, and pulmonary oedema but the role of the herpesvirus is unclear (Sim et al. 2015). Antiviral therapy is unvalidated but has been reported in some cases and would be considered prudent given limited treatment options (Sim et al. 2015).

Mycoplasma has been associated with blepharitis, conjunctivitis, mucopurulent ocular and nasal discharge, and weight loss in Eastern box turtles and three toed box turtles (*Terrapene carolina triunguis*) (Feldman et al. 2006; Palmer et al. 2016). The bacterium detected on PCR of oronasal discharge samples appears distinct to *Mycoplasma agassizii*, which is responsible for mycoplasmosis in terrestrial chelonia, and is proposed as a novel species (Feldman et al. 2006). Asymptomatic prescence of a mycoplasma species has also been reported in bog turtles (*Glyptemys muhlenbergii*), eastern box turtles, and spotted turtles (*Glyptemys insculpta*) so pathogenicity remains unclear (Ossiboff et al. 2015a). *M. agassizii* has been identified by PCR in RES with pneumonia (Jacobson et al. 2014). The prevalence of *Mycoplasma* species in captive RES is undetermined but has been assessed in free-living individuals in California, USA. A range in prevalence of 0–14.3% was reported, varying with geographic region, and no herpes or ranaviruses were detected in the 33 red-eared sliders assessed (Silbernagel et al. 2013). Culture of *Mycoplasma* species is often unsuccessful and PCR remains the mainstay of diagnosis. Treatment of clinically affected animals includes use of macrolides, tetracyclines, and fluoroquinolones (Berry et al. 2002; Feldman et al. 2006). Mycoplasmosis is recognised as a lifelong, often recurrent, infection in terrestrial chelonia (Berry et al. 2002) and would be expected to be similar in terrapins.

20.3.1.2 Viral Hepatitis

Fatal herpesvirus infection associated with lethargy, anorexia, pulmonary, and subcutaneous oedema has been reported in Pacific pond turtles (*Actinemys marmorata*), painted turtles (*C. picta*), Eastern river cooters (*Pseudemys concinna concinna*), and three species of map turtle (*Graptemys geographica, Graptemys pseudogeographica* and *Graptemys barbouri*) (Frye et al. 1977; Cox et al. 1980; Jacobson et al. 1982; Jungwirth et al. 2014; Ossiboff et al. 2015b). Diagnosis is typically made on post-mortem histopathology of the liver, with marked hepatic necrosis and large eosinophilic intranuclear inclusions to hepatocytes

noted, but biopsy could be considered for ante-mortem testing of suspect cases. Molecular analysis in two reports identified a herpesvirus, termed Emydid herpesvirus 1 (Jungwirth et al. 2014; Ossiboff et al. 2015b). Subclinical carriage of virus has been demonstrated, and individual species susceptibility may affect pathogenicity (Jacobson et al. 1982; Ossiboff et al. 2015b). Treatment of suspected cases comprises supportive care, fluid therapy, assisted feeding, antiviral therapy, and symptomatic therapy but prognosis is guarded where clinical signs are present.

A presumptive circovirus has been identified by electron microscopy in a painted turtle (*Chrysemys* sp.) with splenic and hepatic necrosis (Jacobson 2007).

20.3.1.3 Aural Abscessation

Aural abscesses are common in aquatic chelonia, particularly *Trachemys* and *Terrapene* species (Joyner et al. 2006; Yardimci et al. 2010; Mader 2015). Presentation is typified by swelling of the tympanic scales, which can be pronounced (Figure 20.10). This may extend medially resulting in the presence of exudate at the opening of the eustachian tube on the lateral walls of the pharynx (Divers 2015). Abscessation can be unilateral or bilateral (Yardimci et al. 2010; Tatli et al. 2016). The true aetiopathogenesis of the problem is unknown, but sub-optimal husbandry as a result of inadequate temperature, water quality, and nutrition are all contributory factors resulting in immune suppression, squamous metaplasia, and secondary bacterial infection (Murray 2006; Yardimci et al. 2010; Tatli et al. 2016). It is essential to assess and correct underlying factors, as well as the abscess itself.

The reptilian response to bacterial infection differs from mammals, with fibrin deposition and formation of solid, fibrin-rich purulent material (Norton 2005). The fibrous nature of the abscess means that drainage is ineffective (Fraser and Girling 2004) and antibiotic penetration into the abscess is usually limited (McArthur 2004c; Tatli et al.

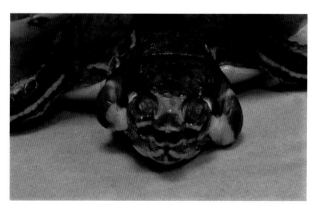

Figure 20.10 Bilateral aural abscessation in a yellow-bellied slider.

2016). Surgical treatment is necessary for treatment (Fraser and Girling 2004). A 3–4 mm incision is made through the full thickness of the tympanum, to enable *en bloc* removal of the caseated material (Açık et al. 2018). The deep portions of the tympanic cavity should then be examined and any remaining material removed, followed by flushing of the eustachian tube. During flushing, endotracheal intubation with the pharynx packed is advisable to prevent aspiration (Murray 2006). Swabs may be collected to guide antibiotic therapy. Bacteria present vary, with gram negative commensals and opportunistic invaders most frequently identified (Joyner et al. 2006). Earlier authors advise removal of half of the tympanum and to maintain the site as an open wound post-operatively (McArthur 2004c; Murray 2006). More recent reports advise suturing of the incision in a simple interrupted pattern, alongside antibiotic use, with no associated complications (Yardimci et al. 2010; Tatli et al. 2016) and this would seem more appropriate for species requiring access to water.

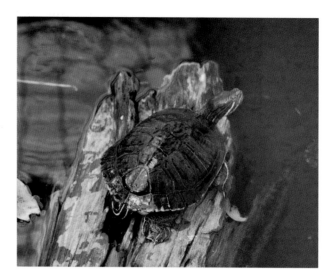

Figure 20.11 This wild red-eared slider is using a natural platform to enable basking, facilitating thermoregulation and maintaining integumental health (*Source:* Photo courtesy of Sarah Pellett).

20.3.1.4 Septicaemic Cutaneous Ulcerative Disease (SCUD)

SCUD appear to be a consequence of poor hygiene and immunosuppression resulting from inappropriate husbandry factors (Köbölkuti et al. 2008; Feldman and Feldman 2011). Abrasions and trauma to the shell or skin allow bacterial penetration and localised infection, followed by systemic spread of bacteria. Affected animals often demonstrate discolouration or sloughing of shell scutes, skin ulceration, lethargy, anorexia, and emaciation, progressing to septicaemia and death (Jesús et al. 2013). On examination affected areas of shell may also feel soft on compression or have a foetid smell (Feldman and Feldman 2011). Shell lesions greater than $2\,cm^2$ or that involve a bone area greater than $1\,cm^2$ carry a poor prognosis (Feldman and Feldman 2011).

Treatment is antibiotic therapy based on culture and sensitivity of samples collected from lesions, or blood culture, and improvement of husbandry (Köbölkuti et al. 2008). *Citrobacter freundii* is commonly isolated and is considered to be the primary cause of SCUD but this bacterium is also commonly isolated from asymptomatic terrapins (Hossain et al. 2017a). Antibacterial resistance, in particular resistance to fluoroquinolones, is common in *C. freundii* and empirical therapy may result in treatment failure (Hossain et al. 2017b,c). *C. freundii* is often identified in combination with other opportunistic bacterial and fungal pathogens, including *Serratia* spp. which result in localised lysis and may potentiate progression of *Citrobacter* spp. infection (Soccini and Ferri 2004; Köbölkuti et al. 2008). Complete debridement of necrotic areas of shell has been reported to be effective at halting lesions (Feldman and Feldman 2011).

Prevention involves optimising husbandry and hygiene, with particular focus on using non-abrasive materials within the enclosure, designing enclosures to avoid sharp drops into water that can result in collisions with the tank base, and provision of adequate basking opportunities to allow the shell to fully dry (Figure 20.11) (Feldman and Feldman 2011).

20.3.2 Non-infectious Disease

20.3.2.1 Metabolic Bone Disease (MBD)

MBD is a term used to describe a number of disease entities affecting bone health across species. NSHP is the commonest cause in reptiles (Calvert 2004). The aetiopathogenesis is similar to other reptiles, with lack of UV-B lighting, inadequate temperatures and inappropriate diet, frequently implicated. A more comprehensive review of NSHP is included in Chapter 19. Clinical signs in terrapins include softening of the shell and facial bones with secondary deformity of the carapace and beak, compromised swimming or ambulation, anorexia, lethargy, and muscular tremors (Zwart 2000; Calvert 2004). Radiography is valuable in advanced cases to allow full assessment of long bones and shell, and to subjectively assess bone density. As with other reptiles, treatment is aimed at improving husbandry to rectify deficits in temperature, UV exposure, and nutrition allowing gradual improvement of bone mineralisation. Frequently deformities are permanent. The impact these deformities have depends upon the severity and site, and thus affect prognosis.

Pseudogout is the deposition of crystals other than monosodium urate around joints, and typically involves crystals of calcium salts (Jones and Fitzgerald 2009). Postulated causes include excess dietary calcium, phosphorus, or vitamin D, and chronic renal compromise (Jones and Fitzgerald 2009). This condition has been reported in a painted turtle with a 1 cm mass over the stifle in this case, which affected joint mobility (Chambers et al. 2009). Limb amputation was carried out and articular calcium pyrophosphate crystal deposition were confirmed on histopathology. Initial recovery was unremarkable, however the animal died two months later and no necropsy was possible.

20.3.2.2 Follicular Stasis

Follicular or pre-ovulatory stasis may be a consequence of poor husbandry or concurrent medical conditions resulting in failure of developed follicles to be ovulated (Johnson 2004a). It should be a differential diagnosis for any female terrapin presenting with vague signs of anorexia or lethargy (Johnson 2004). Secondary bacterial infection of follicles can cause a more acute presentation with weakness, debilitation, and erythema of the plastron. Ultrasound is preferred for assessment of follicles (Cheng et al. 2010). Pre-ovulatory follicles in red-eared sliders can exceed 21 mm (Perez-Santigosa et al. 2008) but these should be ovulated with shelled eggs evident within the oviduct subsequently. If normal development and ovulation of follicles does not occur over several weeks, or if clinical signs in the presence of enlarged follicles support pathological ovarian activity, ovariectomy, or ovariosalpingectomy is indicated. Salpingectomy alone is contra-indicated as it has no impact upon ovarian pathology and can result in subsequent issues including coelomitis (Mader et al. 2006). Elective ovariectomy may also be a consideration to prevent ovarian pathology or to prevent breeding, particularly in species such as *T. scripta* where breeding is not permitted in many regions. A transplastron approach has been used widely (see Chapter 18), but a pre-femoral approach, with or without the use of endoscopic equipment, reduces healing times and potential post-operative complications (Bel et al. 2014). The ovary is exteriorized through a pre-femoral incision, the multiple contributing vessels ligated and the ovary sharply dissected. Bilateral incisions may be necessary to access both ovaries in larger individuals if endoscopic assistance is not available.

20.3.2.3 Post-Ovulatory Stasis

Dystocia and retained or ectopic eggs have all been reported in red-eared sliders (Bel et al. 2014). Typically eggs are held within the vagina in chelonia until they are laid (Mans and Sladky 2012). Oviposition in free-ranging terrapins occurs between April and June, with most breeding females laying a single clutch (Perez-Santigosa et al. 2008; Rose 2011). The presence of eggs is often an incidental finding on radiographs and it is frequently not clear how long the eggs have been present as physiological retention of eggs has been reported for up to six months (Innis and Boyer 2002; McArthur 2004c; Mans and Sladky 2012).

Dystocia is the failure to deposit eggs within the expected time for the species, and this can be difficult to accurately determine in chronic cases without knowledge of the duration of egg presence (McArthur 2004c). In acute cases where oviposition has started but is not completed within 48–72 hours, a diagnosis of dystocia is more confidently made (Johnson 2004a). Radiography is indicated to assess the number, shape and size of eggs present, and enables assessment of whether or not the eggs can physically pass through the pelvis. Non-obstructive dystocia in a clinically well terrapin may be an indicator that an appropriate nest site has not been made available, or that oviductal contractions have been limited by calcium availability. Provision of nesting sites with various substrates is recommended, alongside correction of any other husbandry deficiencies and management of concurrent health concerns. If egg retention persists then use of oxytocin may be indicated (Tucker et al. 2007). The action of oxytocin is dependent upon availability of calcium and disruption to calcium homeostasis is common in captive reptiles. Supplementation of calcium prior to oxytocin use is recommended (Norton 2005). The use of injectable calcium supplementation requires thorough pre-treatment assessment of hydration status, electrolytes, and other blood parameters (McArthur 2004c) and oral preparations may be preferred. Oxytocin use should be avoided if there is any concern that eggs have become adherent to the oviduct wall, as there is the potential for oviductal rupture (Johnson 2004a) and owners should be made aware of the potential complications prior to use. Concurrent use of beta-blockers may also be beneficial (McArthur 2004c).

If medical attempts to remedy retained eggs or dystocia are unsuccessful then a surgical approach is indicated. Potentially a pre-femoral approach similar to that for ovariectomy may be considered, but size disparity between egg and fossa may require collapse of the eggs (Raiti 2013; Bel et al. 2014). Egg collapse is associated with concerns for coelomic contamination thus a transplastron approach may be the preferred technique despite concerns for longer healing times and post-operative complications (Raiti 2013; Bel et al. 2014).

20.3.2.4 Hypovitaminosis A

Hypovitaminosis A is most common in omnivorous terrapins (Zwart 2000) and causes epithelial squamous cell metaplasia and hyperkeratosis. Typically it is seen as bulging and swelling of the eyelids (Zwart 2000) but any epithelium can be affected, and consequences can include aural abscessation, respiratory infections, and renal dysfunction. Treatment is based on improved husbandry, with particular focus on providing a balanced diet with vitamin A supplementation. Injectable preparations may be used but carry a potential for hypervitaminosis A, or excess of other constituents if a multivitamin preparation is used. The prognosis can be poor for some individuals if left untreated, with mortality observed as a result of the effects of squamous metaplasia in other organs (Millichamp 2004; Zwart 2000).

20.3.2.5　Penile Prolapse

The male terrapin has a single phallus situated on the ventral floor of the proctodeum. The normal phallus is exteriorised during sexual behaviour, or a small portion may be seen normally when droppings are passed. If it fails to be retracted then engorgement can occur with varying degrees of desiccation and or trauma and eventually necrosis results. Penile prolapse is rarely seen in *Trachemys* species (Korkmaz et al. 2013). The underlying aetiology can be varied and include straining to pass faeces, a coelomic space occupying mass, obesity, NSHP, localised trauma, or infection (McArthur and Hernandez-Divers 2004; Korkmaz et al. 2013). Underlying causes must be identified where possible otherwise resolution is unlikely (Hedley and Eatwell 2014).

If the prolapse is persistent then the phallus should be cleaned and the prolapse gently reduced. Placement of retaining sutures can help to maintain the reduction, and both lateral vent sutures and a single purse-string suture to reduce vent aperture can be used (Norton 2005). Sutures can be removed after 14 days if treatment has been successful (Barten 2006a). Systemic antibiosis is indicated where necrosis or trauma has occurred.

If the phallus is non-viable then amputation should be carried out. This is achieved by placement of transfixing ligatures across the base of the phallus in the anaesthetised patient (Nisbet et al. 2011; Korkmaz et al. 2013). Although amputation may affect fertility, the phallus has no involvement in urination.

20.3.2.6　Trauma

The most common trauma presentations include shell fractures as a result of falls or drops, or bite injuries from dogs and wildlife (Barten 2006b).

Soft tissue injuries alone are uncommon due to the ability of terrapins to withdraw soft tissues fully into the shell. Haemostasis may be achieved by application of pressure, ligation of vessels, or electrosurgery as appropriate. Analgesia, flushing with sterile saline or dilute disinfect-

ants and primary closure is appropriate for fresh, uncontaminated wounds. Wounds over six hours old should be considered contaminated and closure delayed pending initiation of antibiotic therapy and assessment of tissue viability. Limb amputation may be necessary for severe injuries but long-term outcomes are not reported for captive animals. In the partially aquatic wood turtle (*G. insculpta*), single limb amputation in wild animals did not appear to overtly impact on mobility or feeding ability but a high incidence of further traumatic injuries may suggest that mobility was suboptimal (Walde et al. 2003; Saumure et al. 2007).

Where shell injuries are present, radiography is necessary to fully assess fractures, taking care to assess potential involvement of the fused vertebrae and spinal cord as some injuries may not be externally evident. Fresh wounds can be considered contaminated but not infected and shell fractures less than six hours old may be suitable for primary closure (Mitchell 2002; Barten 2006b). Fracture sites should be lavaged to remove contaminants and described disinfectants include dilute povidone-iodine and dilute chlorhexidine, with povidone iodine preferred, then rinsed with isotonic saline (McArthur and Hernandez-Divers 2004; Penn-Barwell et al. 2012; Pothiappen et al. 2014). For injuries older than six hours, or when the interval is unclear, wounds should be considered to be infected (McArthur and Hernandez-Divers 2004). Control of any infection is necessary before any closure to prevent abscess or persistent sequestrum formation (McArthur and Hernandez-Divers 2004). Wet-to-dry dressings can be applied and changed every 24 hours, with flushing of defects or application of topical antibacterial treatments at each dressing change. Local and systemic antibiotic therapy is often prudent for contaminated wounds (Alworth et al. 2011). Trauma that exposes the coelomic cavity and infected wounds are associated with poorer prognosis (Alworth et al. 2011).

Fixation of shell fractures will depend on fracture type and location (see Table 20.2). Anaesthesia is needed for this as manipulation of shell fragments is painful (Vella 2009). Any nonvital or questionable tissue should be debrided, and the wound and surrounding area flushed with warmed saline and cleaned with 0.05% chlorhexidine or 0.1% povidone iodine (Strachan 1996; Watt 2005). Displaced fragments should be aligned. Resection of an overlapped segment instead of realignment is likely to result in significant haemorrhage and potential alteration of anatomy, and should be avoided if possible. Close apposition of shell fragments is ideal and results in healing with 12–18 weeks in uncomplicated cases, though fixation implants are typically left in place for 6–12 months (Alworth et al. 2011). Even where apposition of fragments is not fully achievable

Table 20.2 Shell fracture repair options (Vella 2009; Alworth et al. 2011; Joshi and Darji 2017).

	Technique	Pros	Cons
Bandaging	External coaption of the shell is suitable for carapacial fractures with minimal displacement	Non-invasive, simple	Not waterproof requiring dry docking during healing, immobilisation effects may be minimal
Cast	Moulded or printed cast applied round fracture	Useful for plastrocarapacial bridge fractures	Casts are large and may impede movement, fracture site not easily accessed to assess for complications
Adhesive tape	Waterproof, fibrous tape (e.g. 3 M Filament tape) applied to manually reduced fractures	Non-invasive, simple, can be a useful first-aid measure to stabilise fractures until a more permanent alternative is possible	Not suitable for fractures under tension
Sealant cover	Epoxy resin or acrylic applied over fracture site.	Waterproof, simple technique for non-displaced fractures. Valuable option for fractures repaired by other techniques to provide waterproofing of the site for rapid return to water.	Not suitable as a sole technique for fractures under tension. Exothermic materials can cause localised necrosis, cover allows infections to progress without detection, shell growth may be affected and shell integrity compromised.
Cable ties	Cable ties and their fastenings are attached using acrylic on either side of the fracture. The tie is threaded through the fastening and tightened to hold the fracture in reduction	No disruption to underlying bone layers, technically simple and resist moderate tension. Waterproof and do not extend dry docking phase	Less resilient than metal implants
Bone plates	Plates are applied across fractures and screws applied to secure position	Secure, rigid fixation	May require multiple plates for larger fractures, screws breach the shell barrier and creation of insertion points may extend the dry-docked period, potential for implant failure
Wiring	Screws are inserted either side of the fracture and wire looped round repeatedly in a figure of 8, tightened and secured	Simple technique	Not as stable as plate fixation, screws breach the shell barrier, potential for implant failure

most defects will eventually granulate and mineralise to allow healing over 6–30 months (Roffey and Miles 2018).

It may be necessary to keep the patient out of water in the initial treatment and recovery period but prolonged periods away from water can contribute to stress and dehydration (Barten 2006b). Fracture repair with a temporary resin or acrylic seal over defects may allow for return to water within 24 hours (Alworth et al. 2011). Alternatively waterproof dressing materials can be applied to allow short periods in water daily. Plastic screw-top containers have been attached with waterproof resin over shell defects in *Trachemys scripta elegans* to provide a watertight seal for continuous access to water but still permit dressing changes (Sypniewski et al. 2016). For dorsal carapacial injuries, access to a shallow water bath may be a suitable short-term measure.

20.3.2.7 Neoplasia

Published cases of neoplasia in freshwater turtles are listed in Table 20.3.

20.4 Imaging

20.4.1 Radiography

Terrestrial tortoises can undergo radiography using physical immobilisation (e.g. within a box or elevated on a radiolucent block) but terrapins restrained in this way will typically attempt escape or withdraw into the shell (Mans et al. 2013). Image quality of chelonia within their shells is reduced due to superimposition of bony structures over viscera and reduced pulmonary inflation (Mans et al.

Table 20.3 Published cases of neoplasia in freshwater turtles.

Common name	Scientific name	Neoplasm	Site	Comments	Reference
Red eared slider	*Trachemys scripta elegans*	Malignant ovarian teratoma	Ovary	Presented with egg retention, exploratory laparotomy demonstrated large ovarian mass and the terrapin died during surgery	Newman et al. (2003)
Red eared slider	*Trachemys scripta elegans*	Teratoma	Ovary	Euthanased to control invasive species, incidental finding	Hidalgo-Vila et al. (2006)
Red eared slider	*Trachemys scripta elegans*	Papillary carcinoma	Thyroid	Found post-mortem	Gál et al. (2010a)
Red eared slider	*Trachemys scripta elegans*	Dysgerminoma (2)	Ovary	Symptoms included anorexia, altered swimming and buoyancy, and extension of the head and neck	Frye et al. (1988)
Red eared slider	*Trachemys scripta elegans*	Haemangioma	Oesophagus	Presented for dysphagia, mass identified on radiography and endoscopy and terrapin euthanased	Gál et al. (2009a)
Red eared slider	*Trachemys scripta elegans*	Squamous cell carcinoma	Lateral head	Initially suspected to be aural abscess, debrided but animal died after 1 month	Ardente et al. (2011)
Yellow bellied slider	*Trachemys scripta scripta*	Squamous cell carcinoma	Cervical skin	Presented with ulcerated mass, surgical excision and electrochemotherapy used successfully	Lanza et al. (2015)
European pond turtle	*Emys orbicularis*	Chondroma	Tarsus	Examined as part of wildlife survey	Aleksić-Kovačević et al. (2013)
European pond turtle	*Emys orbicularis*	Adenoma	Lacrimal gland	Examined as part of wildlife survey	Aleksić-Kovačević et al. (2013)
European pond turtle	*Emys orbicularis*	Squamous cell carcinoma	Mouth	Metastasis to liver	Billups and Harshbarger (1976)
Eastern box turtle	*Terrapene carolina carolina*	Carcinoma	Skin	Wildlife casualty presented with concurrent traumatic injury	Schrader et al. (2010)
Common box turtle	*Terapene carolina*	Adenocarcinoma	Kidney	Metastases to liver	Ippen (1972)
Florida red-bellied turtle	*Pseudemys nelsoni*	Adenocarcinoma	Harderian gland	Rapidly growing periocular mass, euthanased	Gál et al. (2009b)
Bog turtle	*Glyptemys muhlenbergii*	Soft tissue sarcoma	Forelimb	Managed by amputation, no recurrence 2yrs post-operatively	Latney et al. (2017)
Mata mata	*Chelus fimbriatus*	Adenocarcinoma	Oesophagus	Found at post-mortem examination after sudden death. Concurrent hepatocellular adenoma identified	Lombardini et al. (2013)
Northern red-bellied cooter	*Pseudemys rubriventris*	Mucinous melanophoroma	Forelimb	Brown-black fluid with spindle cell population on fine needle aspirate	Bielli et al. (2015)

Common name	Species	Tumour type	Location	Notes	Reference
Soft-shelled turtle	*Pelodiscus sinensis*	Soft tissue sarcoma	Skin	Laboratory animal euthanased on diagnosis of a mass	Syasina et al. (2006)
Williams' mud turtle	*Pelusios williamsi*	Papilloma	Skin	Autogenous vaccine created to suspected herpesviral cause but died before response could be assessed	Široky et al. (2018)
West African black mud turtle	*Pelusios subniger*	Carcinoma	Stomach	Metastases to kidney	Cowan (1968)
Asian leaf turtle	*Cyclemys dentata*	Adenocarcinoma	Hindlimb	Euthanased on presentation for a fast-growing mass	Gál et al. (2010b)
Indian black turtle	*Geoemyda trijuga*	Carcinoma	Thyroid	Metastases to mediastinum	Cowan (1968)
Chinese box turtle	*Cuora flavimarginata*	Lymphoid leukaemia	Multifocal	Presented with anorexia, dyspnoea, and lethargy. Marked leukocytosis and atypical lymphoblasts. Euthanased	Bezjian et al. (2013)
Common snapping turtle	*Chelydra serpentina*	Fibroma	Skin of forelimb		Gonzales-Viera et al. (2012)
Common snapping turtle	*Chelydra serpentina*	Fibroma	Skin of forelimb	Surgical excision reported to have good outcome	Thomeeran et al. (2018)
Common snapping turtle	*Chelydra serpentina*	Dysgerminoma	Ovary	Concurrent carapacial necrosis and poor body condition, euthanased	Machotka et al. (1992)
Alligator snapping turtle	*Macrochelys temminckii*	Fibroma	Skin		Gonzales-Viera et al. (2012)

2013). Sedation may be preferable to improve positioning and radiograph quality.

As with other species, orthogonal views are usually required but in chelonia a third orthogonal view is advisable for full assessment i.e. dorsoventral, laterolateral, and craniocaudal views. The laterolateral and craniocaudal views are best achieved with a horizontal beam to avoid distortion of anatomy, in particular reduction of lung field size and associated reduction of sensitivity of radiography for pulmonary lesions (Mans et al. 2013). Interpretation of images is challenging due to the dorsoventrally flattened shape of most species and superimposition of the shell (DeShaw et al. 1996).

Common findings on radiographs include traumatic injuries to the shell, pulmonary opacities associated with lower respiratory tract infections, intestinal foreign bodies and presence of eggs. The craniocaudal view is most valuable for pulmonary assessment as there is no superimposition of other viscera over the field of interest (Mans et al. 2013). Eggs are radiographically visible on the dorsoventral view six to seven days after ovulation in yellow pond turtles (*Mauremys mutica*), with increasing mineralisation of the egg shell during gestation (Cheng et al. 2010). It is common to find small stones in low numbers within the gastrointestinal tract of terrapins and these are typically an incidental finding. Gastrointestinal obstruction associated with a large quantity of stones has been reported in red-eared and D'Orbigny's sliders (*Trachemys dorbigni*) and clinical signs included anorexia, lethargy, and failure to pass faeces (Rahal et al. 1998; de Oliveira et al. 2009). In both cases plastronotomy and enterotomy to remove the stones were successful in resolving clinical signs.

20.4.2 Ultrasonography

Manual restraint of animals with a limb held extended to expose either the cervicobrachial or pre-femoral fossa is usually adequate for ultrasonographic examination (Figures 20.12 and 20.13), but sedation may be required for aggressive individuals. A 7.5–10 MHz probe is suitable for most species (Martorell et al. 2004), but patient size can be a limiting factor due to probe footprint being greater than the available acoustic window. The use of stand-off pads may help but the surrounding bone can still compromise images obtained (Redrobe 1997). The right cervicobrachial window is preferred for echocardiographic assessment and objective assessment of cardiac size has been described in red-eared sliders using this approach (Poser et al. 2011). The pre-femoral fossae are used for evaluation of the lower intestinal tract, liver, gall bladder, kidneys, urinary bladder, and gonads (Martorell et al. 2004; Cheng et al. 2010).

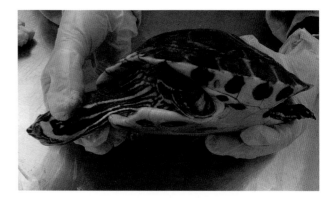

Figure 20.12 Yellow bellied slider restrained conscious for access to the cervicobrachial fossa in front of the forelimb. Retracting the forelimb caudally during scanning reduces patient movement.

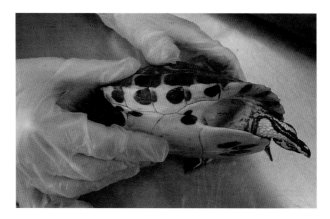

Figure 20.13 Yellow bellied slider restrained conscious for access to the pre-femoral fossa in front of the hindlimb. Retracting the hindlimb caudally during scanning reduces patient movement.

20.4.3 Advanced Imaging

Computed tomography (CT) and magnetic resonance imaging (MRI) are both valuable imaging modalities for chelonia as the complications of shell superimposition seen in radiography are overcome. CT is particularly valuable for pulmonary assessment. Whilst CT is a rapid technique, it is still advised to consider the use of sedation or short-term anaesthesia to minimise movement or positioning artefacts (Mans et al. 2013) particularly if contrast studies are to be performed.

MRI may be superior for soft tissue assessment but requires a slice thickness of less than 5 mm to be of value in these small patients (Głodek et al. 2016) and 1–2 mm slice thickness is preferred. Data acquisition is longer than for CT, typically 60 minutes (Raiti 2019) and so sedation or anaesthesia is indicated to prevent movement blur. MRI topography of red-eared and yellow-bellied sliders, as well as river cooters (*Pseudemys concinna*), has been reported (Summa et al. 2012; Mathes et al. 2017).

Formulary of selected drugs

Medication	Dose	Interval	Comments
Anaesthesia			
Alfaxalone	5 mg/kg IV		15–40s for induction, 20–35 mins anaesthesia in red-eared sliders (Knotek 2014). This dose was not effective when given intranasally (Cermakova et al. 2017).
Alfaxalone	10–20 mg/kg IM		Assessed in red-eared sliders. Sedation adequate to permit intubation in majority of cases at lower dose, and in all animals at higher dose (at 20 °C). At higher temperatures efficacy is reduced (Kischinovsky et al. 2013)
Propofol	10–15 mg/kg IV		15-25 mins of surgical anaesthesia (Divers 1996) Loss of deep pain sensation only occurred in 20% of patients at 10 mg/kg highlighting the requirement of additional analgesia (Ziolo and Bertelsen 2009). Higher dose of 20 mg/kg result in 58–122 mins of anaesthesia (Ziolo and Bertelsen 2009).
Dexmedetomidine and ketamine	0.2 mg/kg (D) and 10 mg/kg (K) intracloacal or intranasal		Assessed in red-bellied sliders. Unpredictable results by the intracloacal route, may be suitable for sedation for short procedures (Morici et al. 2017). Intranasal route provided moderate to deep sedation for minor procedures, reversible with atipamezole intranasally (Schnellbacher et al. 2012).
Dexmedetomidine, midazolam, and ketamine	0.1 mg/kg (D), 1 mg/kg (M) and 2 mg/kg (K) SC		Sedation of red-eared sliders for imaging, partially reversible using atipamezole (1 mg/kg) and flumazenil (0.05 mg/kg) (Mans et al. 2013)
Isoflurane	0.5–2% for maintenance		For maintenance of anaesthesia (Mans and Sladky 2012). Has been used for induction at 4–5% (Reyes et al. 2015) but this tends to be prolonged and incomplete
Analgesia			
Hydromorphone	0.5 mg/kg SC	q24h	Anti-nociceptive response seen in red-eared sliders (Mans et al. 2012)
Morphine	2 mg/kg SC, IM	q24–48h	Demonstrated anti-nociceptive effects for 42 hrs in red-eared sliders (Kinney et al. 2011)
Tramadol	10 mg/kg IM	q48h	Anti-nociceptive response demonstrated in yellow-bellied sliders (Giorgi et al. 2015)
Meloxicam	0.2 mg/kg IM, IV	q48h	Pharmacokinetic study in red-eared sliders (Uney et al. 2016). Oral bioavailability appears poor (Di Salvo et al. 2016)
Ketorolac	0.25 mg/kg IM	q24h	Pharmacokinetic study in common box turtles (Cerreta et al. 2019)
Lidocaine	2 mg/kg SC		Local anaesthetic block for coeliotomy, can be combined with bupivacaine (Raiti 2013)
Bupivacaine	2 mg/kg SC		Local anaesthetic block for coeliotomy, can be combined with lidocaine (Raiti 2013)
Antibiotics			
Gentamicin	2.5 mg/kg IM	q72h	Injection site appears not to affect pharmacokinetics in red-eared sliders (Holz et al. 1997)
Carbenicillin	115 mg/kg IM	q24h	Marginally greater bioavailability if injected in the forelimb compared to hindlimb in red-eared sliders (Holz et al. 1997)
Enrofloxacin	5 mg/kg IM	q48h	In red-eared sliders (James et al. 2003) Pharmacokinetics based on intracoelomic injection in yellow-bellied sliders indicated less frequent dosing was required (q8d) but this route was associated with a pain response (Giorgi et al. 2013)
Enrofloxacin	10 mg/kg PO	q 48h	In red-eared sliders (James et al. 2003)
Oxytetracycline	41 mg/kg for first dose then 21 mg/kg IM	q72h	Extrapolated from loggerhead turtle dose (Harms et al. 2004)

(Continued)

(Continued)

Medication	Dose	Interval	Comments
Cefovecin	10 mg/kg SC	q12–24h	In red-eared sliders (Sypniewski et al. 2017)
Ceftazidime	20 mg/kg IM	q5d	In common box turtles, yellow-bellied sliders and river cooters, injectable solution can be frozen for 25 days to preserve 90% efficacy (Cerreta et al. 2018)
Voriconazole	10 mg/kg SC	q12h	In red-eared sliders. Dose was not sufficient to maintain effective concentrations continuously but was potentially associated with adverse effects of paraplegia in two animals and voriconazole should be used with caution (Innis et al. 2014)
Acyclovir	80–200 mg/kg PO	q12–24h	Extrapolated from tortoise doses (McArthur et al. 2002). Serum concentrations attained in *Terrapene* spp. using 80 mg/kg were subtherapeutic (Allender et al. 2013)
Valacyclovir	40 mg/kg PO	q24h	Results in serum concentrations in *Terrapene* spp. that would be considered suitable for herpesvirus therapy in humans (Allender et al. 2013)
Antiparasitics			
Levamisole	10 mg/kg SC, IM	q 14–28d	In red-eared sliders (Corum et al. 2019)
Fenbendazole	100 mg/kg PO or by gavage	q 48h for 3 treatments, repeat course after 3 weeks	For intestinal nematode infections in *Terrapene* spp. (Boyer 1992b)

Ivermectin is toxic in chelonia and should not be used (Teare and Bush 1983)

Miscellaneous			
10% calcium gluconate	50 mg/kg IM	once	For induction of oviposition or treatment of hypocalcaemia in *Terrapene* spp. (Barten 1990)
Oxytocin	10–20 IU/kg IM		For induction of oviposition, preferably after calcium administration. Effects seen after 30-60 mins in *Terrapene* spp., can be repeated if unsuccessful (Boyer 1992b)

References

Acierno, M.J., Mitchell, M.A., Roundtree, M.K. et al. (2006). Effects of ultraviolet radiation on 25-hydroxyvitamin D3 synthesis in red-eared slider turtles (*Trachemys scripta elegans*). *American Journal of Veterinary Research* 67 (12): 2046–2049.

Açık, M.N., Ünsaldı, S., Melek, Ş. et al. (2018). First isolation of *Pseudomonas aeruginosa* from ear abscess of a red-eared slider (*Trachemys scripta elegans*). *Kafkas Üniversitesi Veteriner Fakültesi Dergisi* 24 (4): 623–625.

Akers, T.K. and Damm, M.G. (1963). The effect of temperature on the electrocardiograms of two species of turtles. *Copeia* 1963 (4): 629–634.

Aleksić-Kovačević, S., Özvegy, J., Krstić, N. et al. (2013). Skin and skeletal system lesions of European pond turtles (*Emys orbicularis*) from natural habitats. *Acta Veterinaria Hungarica* 62 (2): 180–193.

Allender, M.C., Mitchell, M., Yarborough, J. et al. (2013). Pharmacokinetics of a single oral dose of acyclovir and valacyclovir in north American box turtles (*Terrapene sp.*). *Journal of Veterinary Pharmacology and Therapeutics* 36 (2): 205–208.

Altland, P.D. and Parker, M. (1955). Effects of hypoxia upon the box turtle. *American Journal of Physiology-Legacy Content* 180 (2): 421–427.

Alworth, L.C., Hernandez, S.M., and Divers, S.J. (2011). Laboratory reptile surgery: principles and techniques. *Journal of the American Association for Laboratory Animal Science* 50 (1): 11–26.

Ardente, A.J., Christian, L.S., Borst, L.B. et al. (2011). Clinical challenge. *Journal of Zoo and Wildlife Medicine* 42 (4): 770–773.

Baines, F., Chattell, J., Dale, J. et al. (2016). How much UV-B does my reptile need? The UV-tool, a guide to the selection of UV lighting for reptiles and amphibians in captivity. *Journal of Zoo and Aquarium Research* 4 (1): 42–63.

Baker, B.B., Sladky, K.K., and Johnson, S.M. (2011). Evaluation of the analgesic effects of oral and subcutaneous tramadol administration in red-eared slider turtles. *Journal of the American Veterinary Medical Association* 238 (2): 220–227.

Barten, S.L. (1990). Clinical problems of iguanas and box turtles. In: *Proceedings of the Eastern States Veterinary Conference*, 269–270. The Eastern States Veterinary Association.

Barten, S.L. (2006a). Penile prolapse. In: *Reptile Medicine and Surgery*, 2e (ed. D.R. Mader), 862–864. St. Louis, MO: WB Saunders.

Barten, S.L. (2006b). Shell damage. In: *Reptile Medicine and Surgery*, 2e (ed. D.R. Mader), 893–899. St. Louis, MO: Elsevier.

Bel, L., Kiss, A., Pestean, C. et al. (2014). Prefemoral oophorectomy in red eared terrapins (*Trachemys scripta elegans*). *Lucrari Stiintifice Medicina Veterinara* 47 (4): 5–9.

Berry, K.H., Brown, D.R., Brown, M. et al. (2002). Reptilian mycoplasmal infections. *Journal of Herpetological Medicine and Surgery* 12 (3): 8–20.

Bezjian, M., Diep, A.N., de Matos, R. et al. (2013). Chinese box turtle (*Cuora flavomarginata*) with lymphoid leukemia characterized by immunohistochemical and cytochemical phenotyping. *Veterinary Clinical Pathology* 42 (3): 368–376.

Bielli, M., Forlani, A., Nardini, G. et al. (2015). Mucinous melanophoroma in a northern red-bellied Cooter (*Pseudemys rubriventris*). *Journal of Exotic Pet Medicine* 24 (1): 71–75.

Billups, L.H. and Harshbarger, J.C. (1976). Naturally occuring neoplastic diseases. XI. Reptiles. In: *Handbook of Laboratory Animal Science* (eds. E.C. Melby and N.H. Altman), 343–356. Cleveland OH: CRC Press.

Bonner, B.B. (2000). Chelonian therapeutics. *The Veterinary Clinics of North America. Exotic Animal Practice* 3: 257–332.

Bouchard, S.S. and Bjorndal, K.A. (2006). Ontonogenetic diet shifts and digestive constraints in the omnivorous freshwater turtle *Trachemys scripta*. *Physiological and Biochemical Zoology: Ecological and Evolutionary Approaches* 79: 150–158.

Boyer, T.H. (1992a). Clinical anesthesia of reptiles. *Bulletin of the Association of Reptilian and Amphibian Veterinarians* 2 (2): 10–13.

Boyer, T.H. (1992b). Common problems of box turtles (*Terrapene* spp) in captivity. *Bulletin of the Association of Reptilian and Amphibian Veterinarians* 2 (1): 9–14.

Calvert, I. (2004). Nutrition. In: *BSAVA Manual of Reptiles*, 2e (eds. S.J. Girling and P. Raiti), 18–39. Gloucester, UK: BSAVA.

Carr, A. (1952). *Handbook of Turtles*. Ithaca, NY: Cornell University Press.

Cermakova, E., Ceplecha, V., and Znotek, Z. (2017). Efficacy of two methods of intranasal administration of anesthetic

drugs in red-eared terrapins (*Trachemys scripta elegans*). *Veterinarni Medicina* 62 (02): 87–93.

Cerreta, A.J., Lewbart, G.A., Dise, D.R. et al. (2018). Population pharmacokinetics of ceftazidime after a single intramuscular injection in wild turtles. *Journal of Veterinary Pharmacology and Therapeutics* 41 (4): 495–501.

Cerreta, A.J., Masterson, C.A., Lewbart, G.A. et al. (2019). Pharmacokinetics of ketorolac in wild eastern box turtles (*Terrapene carolina carolina*) after single intramuscular administration. *Journal of Veterinary Pharmacology and Therapeutics* 42 (2): 154–159.

Chambers, J.K., Suzuki, T., and Une, Y. (2009). Tophaceous pseudogout of the femorotibial joint in a painted turtle (*Chrysemys picta*). *Journal of Veterinary Medical Science* 71 (5): 693–695.

Chen, Z.X., Zheng, J.C., and Jiang, Y.L. (1999). A new iridovirus isolated from soft-shelled turtle. *Virus Research* 63 (1–2): 147–151.

Cheng, Y., Chen, T., Pin-Huan, Y. et al. (2010). Observations on the female reproductive cycles of captive Asian yellow pond turtles (*Mauremys mutica*) with radiography and ultrasonography. *Zoo Biology* 29: 50–58.

Clark, D.B. and Whitfield, J. (1969). Dietary shift in the turtle *Pseudemys scripta* (Schoept) from youth to maturity. *Copeia* 969 (4): 704–706.

Cooper, J. (2004). Humane euthanasia and post-mortem examination. In: *BSAVA Manual of Reptiles*, 2e (eds. S.J. Girling and P. Raiti), 168–183. Gloucester, UK: BSAVA.

Cooper, J.E., Ewbank, R., and Rosenberg, M.E. (1984). Euthanasia of tortoises. *Veterinary Record* 114: 635.

Corum, O., Durna Corum, D., Atik, O. et al. (2019). Pharmacokinetics of levamisole in the red-eared slider turtles (*Trachemys scripta elegans*). *Journal of Veterinary Pharmacology and Therapeutics* 42 (6): 654–659.

Cowan, D.F. (1968). Diseases of captive reptiles. *Journal of the American Veterinary Medical Association* 153: 848–859.

Cox, W.R., Rapley, W.A., and Barker, I.K. (1980). Herpesvirus-like infection in a painted turtle (*Chrysemys picta*). *Journal of Wildlife Diseases* 16 (3): 445–449.

Crews, D. (1996). Temperature-dependent sex determination: the interplay of steroid hormones and temperature. *Zoological Science* 13: 1–13.

DEFRA (2018). The Animal Welfare (Licensing of Activities Involving Animals) (England) Regulations 2018. In: *Guidance Notes for Conditions for Selling Animals as Pets*, 70–73. London: DEFRA.

DeShaw, B., Schoenfeld, A., Cook, R.A. et al. (1996). Imaging of reptiles: a comparison study of various radiographic techniques. *Journal of Zoo and Wildlife Medicine* 27 (3): 364–370.

DeSouza, R.A.M., Deconto, I., Lange, R.R. et al. (2005). Comparison of therapeutic protocols used for chelonian Shell wound repair in red-eared sliders. *Exotic DVM* 7 (3): 53.

Di Salvo, A., Giorgi, M., Catanzaro, A. et al. (2016). Pharmacokinetic profiles of meloxicam in turtles (*Trachemys scripta scripta*) after single oral, intracoelomic and intramuscular administrations. *Journal of Veterinary Pharmacology and Therapeutics* 39 (1): 102–105.

Divers, S.J. (1996). The use of propofol in reptile anesthesia. *Proceedings of the Association of Reptile and Amphibian Veterinarians*: 57–59.

Divers, S.J. (2001). Esophagostomy tube placement in chelonians. *Exotic DVM* 2 (6): 27–30.

Divers, S.J. (2015). Clinical approach to tortoises and turtles. In *Building Exotics Excellence: One City, One Conference, ExoticsCon Main Conference Proceedings*. 541–551.

Eatwell, K., Hedley, J., and Barron, R. (2014). Reptile haematology and biochemistry. *In Practice* 36: 34–42.

Ernst, C., Barbour, R., and Lovich, J. (1984). *Turtles of the United States and Canada*. Washington and London: Smithsonian Institution Press.

Ernst, C., Barbour, R., and Lovich, J. (1994). *Turtles of the United States and Canada*, 2e. Washington, DC: Smithsonian Institution Press.

Ewert, M.A. and Nelson, C.E. (1991). Sex determination in turtles: diverse patterns and some possible adaptive values. *Copeia* 1999 (1): 50–69.

Feldman, M.L. and Feldman, M.B. (2011). A tale of two shell diseases: observations of two shell diseases present in breeding operations of the red-eared slider turtle (*Trachemys scripta elegans*). *Turtle and Tortoise Newsletter* 15: 25–29.

Feldman, S.H., Wimsatt, J., Marchang, R.E. et al. (2006). A novel mycoplasma detected in association with upper respiratory disease syndrome in free-ranging eastern box turtles (*Terrapene carolina carolina*) in Virginia. *Journal of Wildlife Diseases* 42 (2): 279–289.

Fraser, M.A. and Girling, S.J. (2004). Dermatology. In: *BSAVA Manual of Reptiles*, 2e (eds. S.J. Girling and P. Raiti), 184–198. Gloucester, UK: BSAVA.

Frye, F.L., Oshiro, L.S., Dutra, F.R. et al. (1977). Herpesvirus-like infection in two Pacific pond turtles. *Journal of the American Veterinary Medical Association* 171 (9): 882–884.

Frye, F.L., Eichelberger, S.A., Harshbarger, J.C. et al. (1988). Dysgerminomas in two red-eared slider turtles (*Trachemys scripta elegans*) from the same household. *The Journal of Zoo Animal Medicine* 19 (3): 149–151.

Gaertner, J.P., Hahn, D., Jackson, J. et al. (2008). Detection of salmonellae in captive and free-ranging turtles using enrichment culture and polymerase chain reaction. *Journal of Herpetology* 42 (2): 223–232.

Gál, J., Jakab, C., Szabó, Z. et al. (2009a). Haemangioma in the oesophagus of a red-eared slider (*Trachemys scripta elegans*). *Acta Veterinaria Hungarica* 57 (4): 477–484.

Gál, J., Demeter, Z., Palade, E. et al. (2009b). Harderian gland adenocarcinoma in a Florida red-bellied turtle (Pseudemys Nelsoni) – case report. *Acta Veterinaria Hungarica* 57 (2): 275–281.

Gál, J., Csikó, G., Pásztor, I. et al. (2010a). First description of papillary carcinoma in the thyroid gland of a red-eared slider (*Trachemys scripta elegans*). *Acta Veterinaria Hungarica* 58 (1): 69–73.

Gál, J., Mándoki, M., Sátorhelyi, T. et al. (2010b). In situ complex adenocarcinoma on the femoral part of the hindlimb in an Asian leaf turtle (*Cyclemys dentata*). *Acta Veterinaria Hungarica* 58 (4): 431–440.

Gardiner, D.W., Baines, F.M., and Pandher, K. (2009). Photodermatitis and photokeratoconjunctivitis in a ball python (*Python regius*) and a blue-tongue skink (*Tiliqua* species). *Journal of Zoo and Wildlife Medicine* 40 (4): 757–766.

Giorgi, M., Rota, S., Giorgi, T. et al. (2013). Blood concentrations of enrofloxacin and the metabolite ciprofloxacin in yellow-bellied slider turtles (*Trachemys scripta scripta*) after a single intracoelomic injection of enrofloxacin. *Journal of Exotic Pet Medicine* 22 (2): 192–199.

Giorgi, M., Salvadori, M., De Vito, V. et al. (2015). Pharmacokinetic/pharmacodynamic assessments of 10 mg/kg tramadol intramuscular injection in yellow-bellied slider turtles (*Trachemys scripta scripta*). *Journal of Veterinary Pharmacology and Therapeutics* 38 (5): 488–496.

Głodek, J., Adamiak, Z., and Przeworski, A. (2016). Magnetic resonance imaging of reptiles, rodents, and lagomorphs for clinical diagnosis and animal research. *Comparative Medicine* 66 (3): 216–219.

Gonzales-Viera, O., Bauer, G., Bauer, A. et al. (2012). Cutaneous fibroma in a captive common snapping turtle (*Chelydra serpentina*). *Journal of Comparative Pathology* 147 (4): 574–576.

Goodman, R.M., Miller, D.L., and Ararso, Y.T. (2013). Prevalence of ranavirus in Virginia turtles as detected by tail-clip sampling versus oral-cloacal swabbing. *Northeastern Naturalist* 20 (2): 325–333.

Harms, C.A., Papich, M.G., Stamper, M.A. et al. (2004). Pharmacokinetics of oxytetracycline in loggerhead sea turtles (*Caretta caretta*) after single intravenous and intramuscular injections. *Journal of Zoo and Wildlife Medicine* 35 (4): 477–488.

Hedley, J. and Eatwell, K. (2014). Cloacal prolapses in reptiles: a retrospective study of 56 cases. *Journal of Small Animal Practice* 55 (5): 265–268.

Hidalgo-Vila, J., Martinez-Silvestre, A., and Díaz-Paniagua, C. (2006). Benign ovarian teratoma in a red-eared slider turtle (*Trachemys scripta elegans*). *Veterinary Record* 159 (4): 122.

Holz, P., Barker, I.K., Burger, J.P. et al. (1997). The effect of the renal portal system on pharmacokinetic parameters in the red-eared slider (*Trachemys scripta elegans*). *Journal of Zoo and Wildlife Medicine* 28 (4): 386–393.

Hossain, S., Wimalasena, S.H.M.P., De Zoysa, M. et al. (2017a). Prevalence of *Citrobacter* spp. from pet turtles and their environment. *Journal of Exotic Pet Medicine* 26 (1): 7–12.

Hossain, S., Wimalasena, S.H.M.P., and Heo, G.J. (2017b). Virulence factors and antimicrobial resistance pattern of *Citrobacter freundii* isolated from healthy pet turtles and their environment. *Asian Journal of Animal and Veterinary Advances* 12: 10–16.

Hossain, S., De Silva, B.C.J., Wimalasena, S.H.M.P. et al. (2017c). High prevalence of quinolone resistance genes in *Citrobacter freundii* isolated from pet turtles. *Asian Journal of Animal and Veterinary Advances* 12: 212–217.

Innis, C.J. and Boyer, T.H. (2002). Chelonian reproductive disorders. *Veterinary Clinics: Exotic Animal Practice* 5 (3): 555–578.

Innis, C.J., Young, D., Wetzlich, S. et al. (2014). Plasma concentrations and safety assessment of voriconazole in red-eared slider turtles (*Trachemys scripta elegans*) after single and multiple subcutaneous injections. *Journal of Herpetological Medicine and Surgery* 24 (1): 28–35.

Ippen, R. (1972). Ein Beitrag zu den Spontantumoren bei Reptilien. In: *XIV. Internationales Symposium über die Erkrankungen der Zootiere*. Berlin: Akademie der Wissenschaften der DDR.

Jackson, D.C. (1971). The effect of temperature on ventilation in the turtle, *Pseudemys scripta elegans*. *Respiration Physiology* 12 (2): 131.

Jacobson, E.R. (2007). Viruses and viral diseases of reptiles. In: *Infectious Diseases and Pathology of Reptiles*, 395–460. Boca Raton, FL: Taylor & Francis.

Jacobson, E.R., Gaskin, J.M., and Wahlquist, H. (1982). Herpesvirus-like infection in map turtles. *Journal of the American Veterinary Medical Association* 181 (11): 1322–1324.

Jacobson, E.R., Brown, M.B., Wendland, L.D. et al. (2014). Mycoplasmosis and upper respiratory tract disease of tortoises: a review and update. *The Veterinary Journal* 201 (3): 257–264.

Jaeger, C.P. and Cobb, V.A. (2012). Comparative spatial ecologies of female painted turtles (*Chrysemys picta*) and red-eared sliders (*Trachemys scripta*) at Reelfoot Lake,Tennessee. *Chelonian Conservation and Biology* 11 (1): 59–67.

James, S.B., Calle, P.P., Raphael, B.L. et al. (2003). Comparison of injectable versus oral enrofloxacin

pharmacokinetics in red-eared slider turtles, *Trachemys scripta elegans*. *Journal of Herpetological Medicine and Surgery* 13 (1): 5–10.

Jesús, L.G., Miryam, Q.U., and Víctor, F.A. (2013). Septicemic cutaneous ulcerative disease in a multi-species collection of semi-aquatic turtles. *Revista de Investigaciones Veterinarias del Perú (RIVEP)* 24 (4): 561–564.

Johlin, J.M. and Moreland, F.B. (1933). Studies on the blood of the turtle after complete anoxia. *The Journal of Biological Chemistry* 103: 107–114.

Johnson, J.D. (2004a). Urogenital system. In: *BSAVA Manual of Reptiles*, 2e (eds. S.J. Girling and P. Raiti), 261–272. Gloucester, UK: BSAVA.

Johnson, J.H. (2004b). Husbandry and medicine of aquatic reptiles. *Seminars in Avian and Exotic Pet Medicine* 13 (4): 223–228.

Johnson, A.J., Pessier, A.P., and Jacobson, E.R. (2007). Experimental transmission and induction of ranaviral disease in western ornate box turtles (*Terrapene ornata ornata*) and red-eared sliders (*Trachemys scripta elegans*). *Veterinary Pathology* 44 (3): 285–297.

Johnson, A.J., Pessier, A.P., Wellehan, J.F. et al. (2008). Ranavirus infection of free-ranging and captive box turtles and tortoises in the United States. *Journal of Wildlife Diseases* 44 (4): 851–863.

Jones, Y.L. and Fitzgerald, S.D. (2009). Articular gout and suspected pseudogout in a basilisk lizard (*Basilicus plumifrons*). *Journal of Zoo and Wildlife Medicine* 40 (3): 576–578.

Joshi, M.M. and Darji, P.P. (2017). Shell fracture repair in red eared slider (Trachemys scripta elegans) using k-wire and cortical screws: a case report. http://www.veterinarypaper.com/pdf/2017/vol2issue5/PartA/2-4-1-127.pdf (accessed 15 July 2019).

Joyner, P.H., Brown, J.D., Holladay, S. et al. (2006). Characterization of the bacterial microflora of the tympanic cavity of eastern box turtles with and without aural abscesses. *Journal of Wildlife Diseases* 42 (4): 859–864.

Jungwirth, N., Bodewes, R., Osterhaus, A.D. et al. (2014). First report of a new alphaherpesvirus in a freshwater turtle (*Pseudemys concinna concinna*) kept in Germany. *Veterinary Microbiology* 170 (3–4): 403–407.

Kinney, M.E., Johnson, S.M., and Sladky, K.K. (2011). Behavioral evaluation of red-eared slider turtles (*Trachemys scripta elegans*) administered either morphine or butorphanol following unilateral gonadectomy. *Journal of Herpetological Medicine and Surgery* 21 (2): 54–62.

Kischinovsky, M., Duse, A., Wang, T. et al. (2013). Intramuscular administration of alfaxalone in red-eared sliders (*Trachemys scripta elegans*) – effects of dose and body temperature. *Veterinary Anaesthesia and Analgesia* 40 (1): 13–20.

Knotek, Z. (2014). Alfaxalone as an induction agent for anaesthesia in terrapins and tortoises. *The Veterinary Record* 175 (13): 327.

Köbölkuti, L.B., Czirják, G.Á., Cadar, D. et al. (2008). Septicemic/systemic cutaneous ulcerative diseases (SCUD) in captive red eared slider (*Trachemys scripta elegans*) – first report in Romania. *Bulletin of University of Agricultural Sciences and Veterinary Medicine Cluj-Napoca* 65 (2): 362.

Korkmaz, M., Saritas, K.Z., and Demirkan, I. (2013). Surgical treatment of penile prolapse in a red eared slider (*Trachemys scripta elegans*). *Research Journal for Veterinary Practitioners* 2 (1): 17–18.

Lanza, A., Baldi, A., and Spugnini, E.P. (2015). Surgery and electrochemotherapy for the treatment of cutaneous squamous cell carcinoma in a yellow-bellied slider (*Trachemys scripta scripta*). *Journal of the American Veterinary Medical Association* 246 (4): 455–457.

Latney, L.T.V., Beguesse, K., Newton, A.L. et al. (2017). Management of a Soft Tissue Sarcoma in a bog turtle (*Glyptemys muhlenbergii*). *Journal of Herpetological Medicine and Surgery* 27 (1–2): 12–17.

Lawton, M. (2005). Intraosseus fluid therapy in chelonia. In: *Proceedings of the North American Veterinary Conference*, 1297. Gainesville, FL: Eastern States Veterinary Association.

Leary, S., Underwood, W., Anthony, R. et al. (2013). *AVMA Guidelines for the Euthanasia of Animals: 2013 Edition*. Schaumburg, IL: American Veterinary Medical Association.

Lombardini, E.D., Desoutter, A.V., Montali, R.J. et al. (2013). Esophageal adenocarcinoma in a 53-year-old Mata Mata turtle (*Chelus fimbriatus*). *Journal of Zoo and Wildlife Medicine* 44 (3): 773–776.

Machotka, S.V., Wisser, J., Ippen, R. et al. (1992). Report of dysgerminoma in the ovaries of a snapping turtle (*Chelydra serpentina*) with discussion of ovarian neoplasms reported in reptilians and women. *In vivo (Athens, Greece)* 6 (4): 349–354.

Maclean, B. and Raiti, P. (2004). Emergency care. In: *BSAVA Manual of Reptiles*, 2e (eds. S.J. Girling and P. Raiti), 63–70. Gloucester, UK: BSAVA.

Mader, D. (2015). Clinical conditions affecting the head of reptiles. In: *Proceedings of the Association of Reptile and Amphibian Veterinarians*, 563–570. ARAV.

Mader, D., Avery Bennet, R., Funk, R.S. et al. (2006). Surgery. In: *Reptile Medicine and Surgery*, 2e (ed. D.R. Mader), 581–630. St. Louis, MO: Saunders Elsevier.

Mans, C. (2015). Reptile sedation, anesthesia and analgesia. Proceedings 2nd International Conference on Avian, Herpetological and Exotic Mammal Medicine (CD-ROM), 69–72.

Mans, C. and Braun, J. (2014). Update on common nutritional disorders of captive reptiles. *Veterinary Clinics: Exotic Animal Practice* 17 (3): 369–395.

Mans, C. and Sladky, K.K. (2012). Diagnosis and management of oviductal disease in three red-eared slider turtles (*Trachemys scripta elegans*). *The Japan Society of Applied Physics* 53: 234–239.

Mans, C., Lahner, L.L., Baker, B.B. et al. (2012). Antinociceptive efficacy of buprenorphine and hydromorphone in red-eared slider turtles (*Trachemys scripta elegans*). *Journal of Zoo and Wildlife Medicine* 43 (3): 662–665.

Mans, C., Drees, R., Sladky, K.K. et al. (2013). Effects of body position and extension of the neck and extremities on lung volume measured via computed tomography in red-eared slider turtles (*Trachemys scripta elegans*). *Journal of the American Veterinary Medical Association* 243 (8): 1190–1196.

Mao, J., Hedrick, R.P., and Chinchar, V.G. (1997). Molecular characterization, sequence analysis, and taxonomic position of newly isolated fish iridoviruses. *Virology* 229 (1): 212–220.

Marschang, R.E. (2011). Viruses infecting reptiles. *Viruses* 3 (11): 2087–2126.

Martorell, J., Espada, Y., and de Gopegui, R.R. (2004). Normal echoanatomy of the red-eared slider terrapin (*Trachemys scripta elegans*). *Veterinary Record* 155 (14): 417–420.

Mathes, K.A., Schnack, M., Rohn, K. et al. (2017). Magnetic resonance imaging measurements of organs within the coelomic cavity of red-eared sliders (*Trachemys scripta elegans*), yellow-bellied sliders (*Trachemys scripta scripta*), coastal plain cooters (*Pseudemys concinna floridana*), and hieroglyphic river cooters (*Pseudemys concinna hieroglyphica*). *American Journal of Veterinary Research* 78 (12): 1387–1399.

McArthur, S. (2004a). Feeding techniques and fluids. In: *Medicine and Surgery of Tortoises and Turtles* (eds. R. Wilkinson, S. McArthur and J. Meyer), 257–272. Oxford, UK: Wiley-Blackwell.

McArthur, S. (2004b). Anaesthesia, analgesia and euthanasia. In: *Medicine and Surgery of Tortoises and Turtles* (eds. R. Wilkinson, S. McArthur and J. Meyer), 379–401. Oxford, UK: Wiley-Blackwell.

McArthur, S. (2004c). Problem-solving approach to common diseases of terrestrial and semi-aquatic chelonians. In: *Medicine and Surgery of Tortoises and Turtles* (eds. R. Wilkinson, S. McArthur and J. Meyer), 309–377. Oxford, UK: Wiley-Blackwell.

McArthur, S. and Barrows, M. (2004). General care of chelonians. In: *Medicine and Surgery of Tortoises and Turtles* (eds. R. Wilkinson, S. McArthur and J. Meyer), 87–107. Oxford, UK: Wiley-Blackwell.

McArthur, S. and Hernandez-Divers, S. (2004). Surgery. In: *Medicine and Surgery of Tortoises and Turtles* (eds. R. Wilkinson, S. McArthur and J. Meyer), 403–464. Oxford, UK: Wiley-Blackwell.

McArthur, S., Blahak, S., Köelle, P. et al. (2002). Chelonian herpesvirus. *Journal of Herpetological Medicine and Surgery* 12 (2): 14–31.

McCormack, S. (2015). A guide to esophagostomy tube placement in chelonians. http://lafeber.com/vet/a-guide-to-esophagostomy-tube-placement-in-chelonians (accessed 15 July 2019).

Millichamp, N.J. (2004). Ophthalmology. In: *BSAVA Manual of Reptiles*, 2e (eds. S.J. Girling and P. Raiti), 199–209. Gloucester, UK: BSAVA.

Mitchell, M.A. (2002). Diagnosis management of reptile orthopaedic injuriesand. *Veterinary Clinics of North America* 5 (1): 97–114.

Mitchell, J.C. and Pague, C.A. (1990). Body size, reproductive variation, and growth in the slider turtle at the northeastern edge of its range. In: *Life History and Ecology of the Slider Turtle* (eds. W. Gibbons and H.W. Avery), 146–151. Washington, DC: Smithsonian Institution Press.

Moll, E. and Legler, J.M. (1971). The life history of a neotropical slider turtle, *Pseudemys scripta* (Schoepff). Panama. *Bulletin of the Los Angeles County Museum of Natural History: Science* 11: 102.

Moore, A.R., Allender, M.C., and MacNeill, A.L. (2014). Effects of Ranavirus infection of red-eared sliders (*Trachemys scripta elegans*) on plasma proteins. *Journal of Zoo and Wildlife Medicine* 45 (2): 298–305.

Morici, M., Interlandi, C., Costa, G.L. et al. (2017). Sedation with intracloacal administration of dexmedetomidine and ketamine in yellow-bellied sliders (*Trachemys scripta scripta*). *Journal of Exotic Pet Medicine* 26 (3): 188–191.

Murray, M.J. (2000). Reptilian laboratory medicine. In: *Laboratory Medicine Avian and Exotic Pets* (ed. A.M. Fudge), 185–197. Philadelphia, PA: WB Saunders.

Murray, M.J. (2006). Aural abscesses. In: *Reptile Medicine and Surgery*, 2e (ed. D.R. Mader), 742–750. St. Louis, MO: Saunders Elsevier.

Newman, S.J., Brown, C.J., and Patnaik, A.K. (2003). Malignant ovarian teratoma in a red-eared slider (*Trachemys scripta elegans*). *Journal of Veterinary Diagnostic Investigation* 15 (1): 77–81.

Nisbet, H.O., Yardimci, C., Ozak, A. et al. (2011). Penile prolapse in a red eared slider (*Trachemys scripta elegans*). *Kafkas Üniversitesi Veteriner Fakültesi Dergisi* 17 (1): 151–153.

Norton, T.M. (2005). Chelonian emergency and critical care. *Seminars in Avian and Exotic Pet Medicine* 14 (2): 106–130.

de Oliveira, F.S., Delfini, A., Martins, L. et al. (2009). Obstrução intestinal e enterotomia em tigre d'água (*Trachemys dorbignyi*). *Acta Scientiae Veterinariae* 37: 307–310.

Ossiboff, R.J., Raphael, B.L., Ammazzalorso, A.D. et al. (2015a). A *Mycoplasma* species of Emydidae turtles in the northeastern USA. *Journal of Wildlife Diseases* 51 (2): 466–470.

Ossiboff, R.J., Newton, A.L., Seimon, T.A. et al. (2015b). Emydid herpesvirus 1 infection in northern map turtles (*Graptemys geographica*) and painted turtles (*Chrysemys picta*). *Journal of Veterinary Diagnostic Investigation* 27 (3): 392–395.

Palmer, J.L., Blake, S., Wellehan, J.F. Jr. et al. (2016). Clinical *Mycoplasma* sp. infections in free-living three-toed box turtles (*Terrapene carolina triunguis*) in Missouri, USA. *Journal of Wildlife Diseases* 52 (2): 378–382.

Parmenter, R.R. and Avery, H.W. (1990). The feeding ecology of the slider turtle. In: *Life History and Ecology of the Slider Turtle* (eds. W. Gibbons and H.W. Avery), 257–265. Wasington, DC: Smithsonian Institution Press.

Pees, M. and Girling, S.J. (2019). Emergency care. In: *BSAVA Manual of Reptiles*, 3e (eds. S.J. Girling and P. Raiti), 101–114. Gloucester, UK: BSAVA.

Penn-Barwell, J.G., Murray, C.K., and Wenke, J.C. (2012). Comparison of the antimicrobial effect of chlorhexidine and saline for irrigating a contaminated open fracture model. *Journal of Orthopaedic Trauma* 26 (12): 728–732.

Perez-Santigosa, N., Diaz-Paniagua, C., and Hidalgo-Vila, J. (2008). The reproductive ecology of exotic *Trachemys scripta elegans* in an invaded area of southern Europe. *Aquatic Conservation: Marine and Freshwater Ecosystems* 18: 1302–1310.

Perpinan, D., Martinez-Silvestre, A., Bargallo, F. et al. (2016). Correlation between endoscopic sex determination and gonad histology in pond slider *Trachemys scripta* (Reptilia: Testudines: Emydidae). *Acta Herpetologica* 11 (1): 91–94.

Peterson, C.C. and Greenshields, D. (2001). Negative test for cloacal drinking in a semi-aquatic turtle (*Trachemys scripta*), with comments on the functions of cloacal bursae. *Journal of Experimental Zoology* 290 (3): 247–254.

Poser, H., Russllo, G., Zanella, A. et al. (2011). Two-dimensional and Doppler echocardiographic findings in healthy non-sedated red-eared slider terrapins (*Trachemys scripta elegans*). *Veterinary Research Communications* 35: 511–520.

Pothiappen, P., Palanivelrajan, M., Thangapandiyan, M. et al. (2014). Carapace fracture and its management in a red-eared slider turtle (*Trachemys scripta*). *The Indian Veterinary Journal* 91 (9): 86–87.

Prezant, R.M. and Jarchow, J.L. (1997). Lactated fluid use in reptiles: is there a better solution. In: *Annual Conference of the Association of Reptile and Amphibian Veterinarians. Houston, TX*, 83–87. Association of Reptile and Amphibian Veterinarians.

Rahal, S.C., Teixeira, C.R., Castro, G.B. et al. (1998). Intestinal obstruction by stones in a turtle. *The Canadian Veterinary Journal* 39 (6): 375.

Raiti, P. (2013). Prefemoral salpingotomy and salpingoscopy in a red-eared slider (*Trachemys scripta elegans*) with pathologic egg retention. *Journal of Herpetological Medicine and Surgery* 23 (3–4): 60–63.

Raiti, P. (2019). Non-invasive imaging. In: *BSAVA Manual of Reptiles*, 3e (eds. S.J. Girling and P. Raiti), 134–159. Gloucester, UK: BSAVA.

Redrobe, S. (1997). An introduction to chelonian radiography and ultrasonography. *British Chelonia Group, Testudo* 4 (4): 34–41.

Redrobe, S. (2004). Anaesthesia and analgesia. In: *BSAVA Manual of Reptiles*, 2e (eds. S.J. Girling and P. Raiti), 131–146. Gloucester, UK: BSAVA.

Redrobe, S. and MacDonald, J. (1999). Sample collection and clinical pathology of reptiles. *The Veterinary Clinics of North America: Exotic Animal Practice* 2 (3): 709–730.

Rees Davies, R. and Klingenberg, R.J. (2004). Therapeutics and medication. In: *BSAVA Manual of Reptiles*, 2e (eds. S.J. Girling and P. Raiti), 115–130. Gloucester, UK: BSAVA.

Reyes, C., Fong, A.Y., and Milsom, W.K. (2015). Distribution and innervation of putative peripheral arterial chemoreceptors in the red-eared slider (*Trachemys scripta elegans*). *Journal of Comparative Neurology* 523 (9): 1399–1418.

Roffey, J. and Miles, S. (2018). Turtle shell repair. In: *Reptile Medicine and Surgery in Clinical Practice* (eds. B. Doneley, D. Monks, R. Johnson, et al.), 397–408. Hoboken, NJ: Wiley Blackwell.

Rose, F.L. (2011). Annual frequency of clutches of *Pseudemys texans* and *Trachemys scripta* at the headwaters of the San Marcos river in Texas. *The Southwestern Naturalist* 56 (1): 61–65.

Saumure, R.A., Herman, T.B., and Titman, R.D. (2007). Effects of haying and agricultural practices on a declining species: the north American wood turtle, *Glyptemys insculpta*. *Biological Conservation* 135 (4): 565–575.

Scheelings, T.F. (2019). Anatomy and physiology. In: *BSAVA Manual of Reptiles*, 3e (eds. S.J. Girling and P. Raiti), 1–25. Gloucester, UK: BSAVA.

Schnellbacher, R.W., Hernandez, S.M., Tuberville, T.D. et al. (2012). The efficacy of intranasal administration of dexmedetomidine and ketamine to yellow-bellied sliders (*Trachemys scripta scripta*). *Journal of Herpetological Medicine and Surgery* 22 (3): 91–98.

Schrader, G.M., Allender, M.C., and Odoi, A. (2010). Diagnosis, treatment, and outcome of Eastern box turtles (*Terrapene carolina carolina*) presented to a wildlife clinic in Tennessee, USA, 1995–2007. *Journal of Wildlife Diseases* 46 (4): 1079–1085.

Semple, R.E., Sigsworth, D., and Stitt, J.T. (1970). Seasonal observations on the plasma, red cell, and blood volumes of two turtle species native to Ontario. *Canadian Journal of Physiology and Pharmacology* 48 (5): 282–290.

Silbernagel, C., Clifford, D.L., Bettaso, J. et al. (2013). Prevalence of selected pathogens in Western pond turtles and sympatric introduced red-eared sliders in California, USA. *Diseases of Aquatic Organisms* 107 (1): 37–47.

Sim, R.R., Norton, T.M., Bronson, E. et al. (2015). Identification of a novel herpesvirus in captive Eastern box turtles (*Terrapene carolina carolina*). *Veterinary Microbiology* 175 (2–4): 218–223.

Sim, R.R., Allender, M.C., Crawford, L.K. et al. (2016). Ranavirus epizootic in captive Eastern box turtles (*Terrapene carolina carolina*) with concurrent herpesvirus and *Mycoplasma* infection: management and monitoring. *Journal of Zoo and Wildlife Medicine* 47 (1): 256–270.

Široky, P., Frye, F.L., Dvorakova, N. et al. (2018). Herpesvirus associated dermal papillomatosis in Williams' mud turtle *Pelusios williamsi* with effects of autogenous vaccine therapy. *Journal of Veterinary Medical Science* 80 (8): 1248–1254.

Sladky, K.K., Miletic, V., Paul-Murphy, J. et al. (2007). Analgesic efficacy and respiratory effects of butorphanol and morphine in turtles. *Journal of the American Veterinary Medical Association* 230 (9): 1356–1362.

Sladky, K.K., Kinney, M.E., and Johnson, S.M. (2009). Effects of opioid receptor activation on thermal antinociception in red-eared slider turtles (*Trachemys scripta*). *American Journal of Veterinary Research* 70 (9): 1072–1078.

Sneddon, L.U., Elwood, R.W., Adamo, S.A. et al. (2014). Defining and assessing animal pain. *Animal Behaviour* 97: 201–212.

Soccini, C. and Ferri, V. (2004). Bacteriological screening of *Trachemys scripta elegans* and *Emys orbicularis* in the Po plain (Italy). *Biologia* 14: 201–207.

Strachan, D.B. (1996). Topical therapy of wounds. *Australian Veterinary Practitioner* 26 (1): 34.

Summa, N.M., Risi, E.E., Fusellier, M. et al. (2012). Magnetic resonance imaging and cross-sectional anatomy of the coelomic cavity in a red-eared slider (*Trachemys scripta elegans*) and yellow-bellied sliders (*Trachemys scripta scripta*). *Journal of Herpetological Medicine and Surgery* 22 (3–4): 107–116.

Swenson, J., Henao-Guerrero, P.N., and Carpenter, J.W. (2008). Clinical technique: use of capnography in small mammal anesthesia. *Journal of Exotic Pet Medicine* 17 (3): 175–180.

Syasina, I.G., Hur, J.W., Kim, E.M. et al. (2006). Histopathological and DNA content analysis of a dermal sarcoma in the soft-shelled turtle *Pelodiscus sinensis*. *Fisheries and Aquatic Sciences* 9 (3): 107–114.

Sypniewski, L.A., Hahn, A., Murray, J.K. et al. (2016). Novel shell wound care in the aquatic turtle. *Journal of Exotic Pet Medicine* 25 (2): 110–114.

Sypniewski, L.A., Maxwell, L.K., Murray, J.K. et al. (2017). Cefovecin pharmacokinetics in the red-eared slider. *Journal of Exotic Pet Medicine* 26 (2): 108–113.

Tatli, Z.B., Sen, Z.B., and Gulaydin, A. (2016). Aural abscess in a red-eared slider turtle (*Trachemys scripta elegans*). *Harran Üniversitesi Veteriner Fakültesi Dergisi* 5 (2): 170–172.

Teare, J.A. and Bush, M. (1983). Toxicity and efficacy of ivermectin in chelonians. *Journal of the American Veterinary Medical Association* 183 (11): 1195–1197.

Terashima, S.I. and Liang, Y.F. (1994). C mechanical nociceptive neurons in the crotaline trigeminal ganglia. *Neuroscience Letters* 179 (1–2): 33–36.

Thomas, R.B. (2002). Conditional mating strategy in a long-lived vertebrate: ontogenetic shifts in the mating tactics of male slider turtles (*Trachemys scripta*). *Copeia* 2002 (2): 456–461.

Thomeeran, H., Selvarajah, G.T., Mazlan, M. et al. (2018). Cutaneous fibroma in a common snapping turtle (*Chelydra serpentina*). *Jurnal Veterinar Malaysia* 30 (2): 19–22.

Tucker, J.K., Thomas, D.L., and Rose, J. (2007). Oxytocin dosage in turtles. *Chelonian Conservation and Biology* 6 (2): 321–324.

Uney, K., Altan, F., Aboubakr, M. et al. (2016). Pharmacokinetics of meloxicam in red-eared slider turtles (*Trachemys scripta elegans*) after single intravenous and intramuscular injections. *American Journal of Veterinary Research* 77 (5): 439–444.

Vella, D. (2009). Effective modern shell repair techniques for turtles. In: *Effective Modern Shell Repair Techniques for Turtles*. South Turramurra, New South Wales, Australia: The Veterinarian, Sydney Magazine Publishers.

Vogt, R. (1993). *Systematics and Ecology of the False Map Turtle Complex Graptemys pseudogeographica*. Ann Arbor, MI: A Bell & Howell Company.

Walde, A.D., Bider, J.R., Daigle, C. et al. (2003). Ecological aspects of a wood turtle, *Glyptemys insculpta*, population at the northern limit of its range in Quebec. *The Canadian Field-Naturalist* 117 (3): 377–388.

Warner, D.A., Tucker, J.K., Filoramo, N.I. et al. (2006). Claw function of hatchling and adult red-eared slider turtles (*Trachemys scripta elegans*). *Chelonian Conservation and Biology* 5 (2): 317–320.

Waters, M., Lopez, J., Brewer, B. et al. (2001). Subcarapacial sampling in tortoises. In: *Proceedings of the British Veterinary Zoological Society Meeting, RVC, UK; 10–11 November*, 45. London: British Veterinary Zoological Society.

Watt, P. (2005). Wound care: urgency in emergency. Emergency medicine and critical care. *Post Graduate Foundation in Veterinary Science, Proceedings* 358: 321–339.

Works, A.J. and Olson, D.H. (2018). Diets of two nonnative freshwater turtle species (*Trachemys scripta* and *Pelodiscus sinensis*) in Kawai Nui march, Hawaii. *Journal of Herpetology* 52 (4): 444–452.

Yardimci, B., Yardimci, C., Ural, K. et al. (2010). Auricular abscessation in red-eared sliders (*Trachemys scripta elegans*). *Kafkas Üniversitesi Veteriner Fakültesi Dergisi* 16 (5): 879–881.

Ziolo, M.S. and Bertelsen, M.F. (2009). Effects of propofol administered via the supravertebral sinus in red-eared sliders. *Journal of the American Veterinary Medical Association* 234 (3): 390–393.

Zwart, P. (2000). Nutrition of chelonians. In: *Zoo Animal Nutrition* (eds. J. Nijboer, J.M. Hatt, et al.), 33–44. Fürth: Filander Verlag.

21

Amphibians

Stephanie Jayson

21.1 Introduction

The Class Amphibia consists of three extant orders: Anura (frogs and toads), Caudata (salamanders) and Gymnophiona (caecilians). Although amphibians may not be common patients, they are kept by private keepers in significant numbers. The UK amphibian pet trade was evaluated in 1992–1993 and 2004–2005 and trends showed that both numbers and costs of amphibians in the pet trade are increasing (Tapley et al. 2011). In 2018, it was estimated that there were 100 000 pet frogs and toads in the UK (PFMA 2019). Commonly kept species include the White's tree frog (*Ranoidea caerulea*), African clawed frog (*Xenopus laevis*) and Argentine horned frog (*Ceratophrys ornata*). Salamanders, such as the fire salamander (*Salamandra salamandra*) and axolotl (*Ambystoma mexicanum*) are less common pets. The axolotl is unusual amongst amphibians in that it exhibits neotony, meaning that it reaches sexual maturity without metamorphosis and retains its juvenile aquatic form throughout adulthood.

The amphibian pet trade has been implicated in the global spread of amphibian infectious disease and has contributed to amphibian population declines. Therefore, a call has been made for improved legislation and enforcement (Auliya et al. 2016).

Biological parameters of commonly kept species are given in Table 21.1.

21.2 Husbandry

21.2.1 Enclosure

The anuran or salamander enclosure should be built from non-abrasive materials that do not warp or leach chemicals (e.g. glass is preferred over plastic) (Barnett et al. 2001). The enclosure should be easily serviced with minimal disturbance, escape-proof, permit ventilation and allow provision of temperature, humidity, precipitation, and light gradients that mimic the amphibian's wild microhabitat, including consideration of seasonal variation (Barnett et al. 2001). A typical pet terrestrial anuran or salamander enclosure is a glass-walled terrarium with a mesh roof which permits ventilation and partial penetration of ultraviolet-B (UV-B) radiation, waterproof base, front ventilation, and lockable single or double front doors. For pet aquatic amphibians, a glass-walled aquarium with a secure mesh lid which permits ventilation is frequently used.

Daily enclosure maintenance should involve checking lighting, temperature, water quality, and humidity levels, removal of any faecal material, uneaten food items, shed skin, and dead or overgrown plants, checking water features, and cleaning and refilling any unfiltered water bodies (Lentini 2013).

21.2.2 Substrate

The substrate choice is species-dependent. Depth, humidity, particle size, and chemical properties need to be considered (Barnett et al. 2001). Humidity gradients are essential for terrestrial amphibians to allow osmoregulation and both water-logged substrates and exceptionally dry substrates can cause disease (Barnett et al. 2001).

As a general example for terrestrial amphibians, a base layer of clean gravel or lightweight expanded clay aggregate from a reliable source may be used, with a depression in one corner for a small pool (Poole and Grow 2012). The gravel should be covered, for example by at least a 2 cm layer of sphagnum or sheet moss which has been soaked and then rinsed prior to use in the enclosure, or by coconut fibre covered with a layer of sphagnum moss (Poole and Grow 2012). Coconut fibre is friable so if it is used, a substrate divider such as fibreglass window screen or shade-cloth should be used to separate the coconut fibre

Handbook of Exotic Pet Medicine, First Edition. Edited by Marie Kubiak.
© 2021 John Wiley & Sons Ltd. Published 2021 by John Wiley & Sons Ltd.
Companion website: www.wiley.com/go/kubiak/exotic_pet_medicine

Table 21.1 Biological parameters of commonly kept species.

Species	White's tree frog (*Ranoidea caerulea*)	African clawed frog (*Xenopus laevis*)	Argentine horned frog (*Ceratophrys ornata*)	Axolotl (*Ambystoma mexicanum*)
Lifespan	Average 16 years (up to 20+ years)	Typically 10–15 years (up to 25+ years)	Typically 6–7 years (up to 16+ years)	Typically 5–6 years (up to 30+ years)
Adult bodyweight	50–90 g	Average 60 g (males), 145 g (females)	Large females up to 480 g	60–110 g
Adult snout-vent length	5–11 cm	10–15 cm	8–15 cm	15–45 cm (average 20 cm)
Temperature gradient	Day: 25–30 °C (with basking spot of 35 °C). Use lower day temperature in Winter. Night: 18–21 °C	18–24 °C (water temperature)	Day: 24–28 °C Night: 18 °C Use lower temperatures to induce brumation period	16–18 °C (water temperature)
UV-B radiation	UVI range 0.7–1.6. 12 hour photoperiod	Low level UV-B radiation. 12–14 hour photoperiod	Low level UV-B radiation. 9–12 hour photoperiod	No UV-B radiation.
Humidity	60–70% Lower humidity in Winter in conjunction with reduced daytime temperature	N/A (fully aquatic)	80% Allow to become dry in conjunction with lower temperatures to induce brumation period	N/A (fully aquatic)
Microhabitat	Terrestrial, arboreal, rocks, foliage, grasslands, wetlands	Aquatic, muddy freshwater ponds (use fine sand substrate or bare glass base, not a rocky substrate)	Terrestrial, fossorial, leaf litter, forest floor, grasslands, croplands	Aquatic, freshwater lakes

UVI = UV Index.

from the gravel or clay aggregate (Poole and Grow 2012). Alternatively, the gravel may be covered by a safe, clean, organic soil manufactured for amphibians; this is particularly useful as a substrate if developing a naturalistic, bioactive enclosure with live plants and invertebrates (Courteney-Smith 2016).

21.2.3 Refugia

All anurans and salamanders should be provided with refugia as they provide both hiding areas and microclimates (Poole and Grow 2012). Examples include cork bark, wood, dried leaves, halved coconut shells and inverted plastic tubs with an opening in one side (Poole and Grow 2012). Refugia should be opaque to provide privacy, not contaminated with chemicals and placed in a stable position to avoid movement which could potentially traumatise the amphibian. Terraces may be considered for territorial species to partition the space (Poole and Grow 2012).

21.2.4 Visible Light, Ultraviolet Light, and Temperature Gradients

Lighting should provide a gradient of heat, visible light, and ultraviolet lighting of wavelength 290–315 nm (UV-B) in tandem (i.e. the area of the enclosure with the highest temperature should have the highest UV-B radiation and visible light to mimic sunlight) and these parameters should reflect those of the species' wild microhabitat (Baines et al. 2016).

Typically, temperate species are kept within a temperature range of 18–24 °C, with consideration of lower temperatures or a brumation period in the Autumn and Winter, tropical lowland species are kept at 24–30 °C and tropical montane species are kept at 18–24 °C. Eggs and larvae of most Neotropical hylid and dendrobatid frogs are kept at 25–27 °C (Poole and Grow 2012). Heat can be provided by fitting heat pads and lamps outside the enclosure, guarded heat pads and lamps within the enclosure or by heating the entire room where the enclosure is kept, the latter being preferable as lamps and pads can affect humidity unpredictably, overheat animals, cause thermal burns, and dry out the enclosure

(Poole and Grow 2012). If heat pads and lamps are used, a thermostat should be fitted to allow temperature control. Air conditioning units may be used to control room temperature (Poole and Grow 2012); however, the enclosure should not be positioned directly under the unit as it may dry the enclosure. Water bodies may be cooled or heated to the appropriate temperature using water heaters or chillers within the enclosure (Poole and Grow 2012). Alternatively, an external reservoir of water may be heated or cooled to the correct temperature before adding it to the enclosure (Poole and Grow 2012). Maximum and minimum temperatures within the enclosure should be recorded daily.

UV-B radiation is important as it enables the conversion of provitamin D3 in the skin to pre-vitamin D3, which undergoes temperature-dependent isomerisation to form vitamin D3. Vitamin D3 plays an important role in calcium metabolism and, in mammal species, has been shown to have autocrine and paracrine functions (Baines et al. 2016). UV radiation also has direct effects on the skin's immune system, barrier function, and pigment formation (Baines et al. 2016). The UV-Tool (BIAZA RAWG 2018) is an online document that can be used to choose a gradient of UV-B levels for a species based on their Ferguson zone, which describes thermoregulatory behaviour and microhabitat preferences (Baines et al. 2016). An appropriate UV-B lamp can then be chosen based on the animal's Ferguson zone and enclosure size (Baines et al. 2016). Use of a UV Index meter is recommended to determine the optimal positioning of the UV-B lamp and to regularly check if the desired UV-B gradient is being maintained over time (Baines et al. 2016). All species should have access to refugia with no UV-B exposure regardless of their Ferguson Zone (Baines et al. 2016). Lamps should be inaccessible to amphibians to prevent burns (e.g. by using wide wire mesh) and placed above the animal such that the eyes are shaded from direct exposure (Baines et al. 2016). Ordinary glass, plastics, or other materials which may prevent UV-B transmission should not be placed between the light and the animal (Baines et al. 2016).

21.2.5 Humidity and Water Quality

Humidity and water quality are very important as amphibians osmoregulate and absorb oxygen through their skin, which must be kept moist to maintain the ability for gas exchange (Poole and Grow 2012). Humidity should reflect the microhabitat of the species in the wild, be routinely monitored using a hygrometer, and may be maintained in an amphibian enclosure using automatic misting systems or hand spraying (Poole and Grow 2012).

There are several different water sources which may be used in enclosures for anurans and salamanders. Municipal water is most frequently used; however, it typically contains chlorine or chloramines as a disinfectant, both of which are toxic to amphibians (Odum and Zippel 2008). Municipal water should be tested for chlorine and chloramines and allowed to aerate for 24 hours before use to eliminate free chlorine (Odum and Zippel 2008). If chloramines are present, a filter specifically designed for chloramine removal or chemical treatment (e.g. with a sodium thiosulphate conditioner) is required (Odum and Zippel 2008). Alternative outdoor supplies include well water, rainwater, water that collects in ponds, streams, and lakes, and bottled spring water (Odum and Zippel 2008). However, well water may be hard with a high pH if pumped through limestone bedrock, high in phosphates and nitrates from fertilisers in agricultural areas, supersaturated with nitrogen and carbon dioxide, high in hydrogen sulphide and low in oxygen; rainwater may be acidic in places with high air pollution, too soft for some species, and may be contaminated with chemicals; water from ponds, streams, and lakes may be contaminated with chemicals; and bottled spring water may be contaminated with chemicals and hard with a high pH if pumped through limestone bedrock (Odum and Zippel 2008). All outdoor water sources could also contain pathogens from free-living wildlife, *Batrachochytrium dendrobatidis* being an important risk, therefore natural water sources are not suitable for biosecure populations of amphibians (Odum and Zippel 2008). Reverse osmosis (RO) water is an alternative water source; however, it is too pure to use on its own therefore salts and trace elements or a known quantity of municipal water is typically added to avoid osmotic imbalance in anurans and salamanders (Odum and Zippel 2008).

Open and semi-closed systems are the two main water systems used for amphibian enclosures. In an open system, a fresh source of water is continually or intermittently (e.g. using a timer) added to the enclosure, remains within the enclosure for a short period of time and is then fully discharged; whereas in a semi-closed system, partial water changes are intermittently performed and biological, chemical, and mechanical filters used continuously to maintain water quality (Odum and Zippel 2008).

In a semi-closed system, partial water changes typically involve removal of 10–20% of the total water volume every one to two weeks and replacement with a similar volume of fresh water; however, the frequency and volume of water changes required depends on the results of regular water quality testing and will vary with the number and size of animals in the enclosure, the volume of water, feeding frequency, filter efficiency, and plants in the enclosure (Odum and Zippel 2008; Poole and Grow 2012). Temperature, pH, ammonia (NH_3/NH_4^+), nitrite (NO_2^-), nitrate (NO_3^-), hardness, alkalinity and trace elements including potentially toxic metals (e.g. copper) should be tested in all water sources and temperature, pH, ammonia, nitrite, and nitrate monitored weekly in an established enclosure or daily when an enclosure is first set up (Odum and Zippel 2008; Poole and Grow 2012).

Mechanical filters may be wad-type, cannister, or slow or rapid sand filters and their function is to remove particulate matter prior to chemical and biological filtration (Odum and Zippel 2008). Mechanical filters should be cleaned regularly (at least weekly) to remove particulate matter (Odum and Zippel 2008; Poole and Grow 2012).

Chemical filters remove dissolved substances from water and should be replaced regularly to avoid saturation and release of toxic substances back into the water, typically every two to four weeks although this depends on the amount of filter media and the chemical load (Odum and Zippel 2008). Activated carbon is a useful chemical filter for amphibian enclosures as it removes organic compounds, free chlorine, and some ions (e.g. copper), whilst microparticulate matter (e.g. some bacteria) is caught in the porous matrix (Odum and Zippel 2008).

Biological filters contain nitrifying bacteria that convert toxic nitrogenous compounds (ammonia and nitrites) to a less toxic form (nitrates). Ammonia is present in the enclosure as it is the main nitrogenous waste product of aquatic amphibians and it is produced by decomposing bacteria and uneaten food (Odum and Zippel 2008; Poole and Grow 2012). It exists in its more toxic non-ionic form (NH_3) at higher temperatures and pH levels (Odum and Zippel 2008). Nitrifying bacteria within the biological filter require a suitable substrate on which to grow (e.g. ceramics or aquarium gravel), a source of food (ammonia and nitrites) and an oxygen supply, achieved by circulating oxygenated water through the biofilter at an appropriate rate fast enough to produce an aerobic environment but slow enough to allow bacteria time to absorb nitrogenous waste (Odum and Zippel 2008; Poole and Grow 2012). The biological filter can take several weeks to months to establish and it should only be cleaned as and when needed by rinsing gently with dechlorinated water (Odum and Zippel 2008; Poole and Grow 2012). Plants also play a useful role in biological filtration by removing organic and inorganic wastes from the water system (Odum and Zippel 2008). Appropriate plants for amphibian enclosures have been reviewed and examples include pothos species, ferns, tropical and temperate ivys, club mosses, moisture-tolerant bromeliads and submerged aquatic plants for salamanders, whilst plants that are high in oxalates should be avoided (Poole and Grow 2012).

21.2.6 Diet

The nutrient requirements and nutrient absorptive efficiency of anuran and salamander species are largely unknown, therefore provision of an appropriate captive diet can be a difficult task (Ferrie et al. 2014; Livingston et al. 2014). Most larval anurans are herbivorous or detritivorous, whilst a smaller number are oophagous (being fed infertile ova by their mother), omnivorous, or carnivorous (Wright 2001b). Herbivorous tadpoles may be fed a diet of flaked fish food for herbivorous fish supplemented with spirulina tablets; aquatic vegetation and algae should also be present (Wright 2001b). Detritivorous tadpoles may be reared on a combination of algae, diatoms, and artificial food such as that designed for filter-feeding invertebrates and fish fry (Wright 2001b). Carnivorous tadpoles and larval salamanders may be offered various whole and chopped invertebrates and vertebrates such as earthworms, bloodworms, tubifex worms, and freshwater fish, whilst some larvae may take a pelleted or flaked food for carnivorous fish or reptiles (Wright 2001b). Smaller carnivorous tadpoles and larval salamanders may initially need to be fed smaller food items such as small crustaceans (Wright 2001b). Omnivorous tadpoles can be provided with flaked or pelleted food for omnivorous fish, occasionally offered those items fed to carnivorous tadpoles, and aquatic vegetation and algae should also be present (Wright 2001b). Flaked foods should be offered in such a way that they will be consumed immediately (e.g. floating food for surface-feeding tadpoles) as loss of B vitamins from flaked food may occur rapidly and has been associated with disease (Wright 2001b).

Post-metamorphic anurans and salamanders are predominantly insectivores and should be fed live invertebrates of an appropriate size and movement to stimulate feeding as they rely predominantly on visual cues to detect prey items (Duellman and Trueb 1994b). For arboreal species, invertebrates should also be chosen that will attach to cage furniture or vegetation where the amphibians are located (Ferrie et al. 2014). Most wild post-metamorphic anurans and salamanders feed on a wide variety of invertebrates which in turn feed on a wide variety of food sources. In contrast, most captive amphibians are fed a small number of invertebrate species due to the limited availability of commercially raised invertebrates, difficulty in rearing certain invertebrate species in-house in sufficient quantities to feed anurans and unsuitability of certain invertebrate species to elicit a feeding response (Ferrie et al. 2014). It is therefore likely that the nutritional composition of captive diets are suboptimal and nutritional disorders have been well documented (Wright and Whitaker 2001a). As a general rule, invertebrates fed to captive amphibians are low in calcium, with an inverse calcium: phosphorus ratio, and low in vitamin A (Ferrie et al. 2014). Therefore, supplementation of captive invertebrates by dusting (coating invertebrates in a powdered specific nutrient supplement) and gut loading (providing invertebrates a specific nutrient-rich diet in order to fill their gastrointestinal tract with the supplement) is recommended to increase calcium and vitamin A levels, in particular to aim for a dietary calcium:phosphorus ratio of 2:1 (Ferrie et al. 2014). Gut loading invertebrates with a diet of 5–8% calcium for two to three days prior to offering the invertebrates to anurans is recommended and provision of fresh water rather than using produce as a water source for invertebrates is advised to increase intake of the gut-loading diet (Livingston et al. 2014). For dusting, a high calcium supplement is recommended as this has been shown to increase the calcium: phosphorus ratio of certain cricket species for up to 5.5 hours (Michaels et al. 2014b). Amphibians should be fed at times to coincide with their peak activity periods to encourage intake and ensure that food is eaten as soon as possible after being offered so that supplements are still coating the invertebrates and the gut loading diet is retained in the invertebrate gastrointestinal tract at the time of ingestion (Michaels et al. 2014b; Wright 2001b).

Most anurans and salamanders do not drink water; instead water intake occurs by cutaneous uptake and some water intake derives from ingested food (Ferrie et al. 2014). Terrestrial anurans particularly absorb water via the 'drink patch', a highly permeable area of skin in the ventral pelvic region, which they press against standing water for extended periods of time to increase water uptake (Ferrie et al. 2014). An appropriate water body for the species should be provided to enable water uptake.

21.2.7 History-Taking

In preparation for the consultation, information should be gathered on the natural history and captive husbandry of the species, particularly relating to habitat requirement, behaviour, breeding, and diet so that appropriate questions may be asked during history-taking (Barnett et al. 2001). However, this information is not available for all species and may be difficult to source (Michaels et al. 2014a). Information on wild environmental parameters and diet may also be identified on review of the scientific literature and general amphibian husbandry documents are available through organisations such as Amphibian Ark (Amphibian Ark 2017). Specifically, the enclosure design should be reviewed (photographs of the enclosure brought in by the owner can be useful) and information gathered on sources of heating and lighting and how these are monitored and recorded, substrate, refugia, water quality management, cleaning regime and quarantine procedures (Clayton and Gore 2007). Information on prior disease screening of the owner's collection, the source from which they derived and any other amphibians that they may have come into contact with should be obtained. The composition and source of the diet, including any supplements, should also be reviewed (Clayton and Gore 2007). Prior administration of any medication and potential toxin exposure should also be covered

(Clayton and Gore 2007). A thorough history of the problem in question and any other affected animals in the collection should be obtained.

21.2.8 Handling

Safe handling requires different techniques for larval and post-metamorphic anurans and salamanders. Direct handling of larval anurans and salamanders should be avoided; instead nets or scoops may be used to transfer larvae to a clear plastic bag containing their usual tank water for visual examination (Green 2001). Adult anurans and salamanders may be handled with moistened powder-free gloves (Chai 2015a). Nitrile gloves are preferred as exposure to latex and vinyl gloves has been associated with mortality in certain species (Gutleb et al. 2001). Gloves not only reduce the risk of trauma to delicate amphibian skin but also reduce the risk of zoonotic pathogen transfer and exposure to potentially toxic compounds in amphibian skin secretions (Wright 2001a). Medium-large adult anurans may be safely restrained around the waist just cranial to the hindlimbs (Figure 21.1) (Wright 2001a). Species that tend to have a calm temperament such as the White's tree frog (*R. caerulea*) may be held in the palms of the handler's gloved hands (Figure 21.2). To restrain small adult anurans, the hindlimbs may be held near the base between the handler's thumb and forefinger and the anuran's body supported by a second hand (Figure 21.3). Medium-large salamanders may be grasped immediately behind the forelimbs initially then the grip secured in front of the hindlimbs, taking care to avoid grasping the tail as this can result in tail autotomy, whilst small adult salamanders are best restrained with a loose grip encircling the whole body (Wright 2001a). Chemical restraint may provide a safer alternative than conscious handling in species that are particularly sensitive to handling. Defensive behavioural displays may be observed when anurans and salamanders are restrained, such as inflation, micturition, or biting (Figure 21.1) (Wright 2001a).

21.2.9 Sex Determination

Sexual dimorphism exists in many anuran species. Typically, the female is larger than the male; however, in some species both sexes are of equal size or the male can be slightly larger (Duellman and Trueb 1994a). Spines may be present in males which can be prepollical (just before the first digit) or projecting from the proximal humerus (Duellman and Trueb 1994a). Nuptial excrescences can develop on the prepollices of males during the breeding season; these are typically conical protuberances in the dermis that have a cornified covering due to thickening of the stratum germinativum layer of the

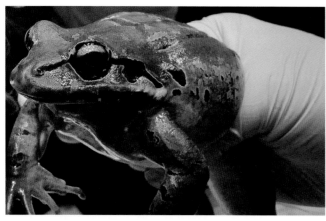

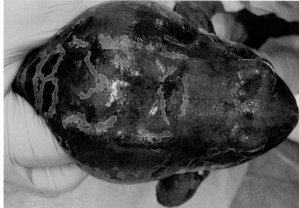

Figure 21.1 Restraint of adult mountain chicken frogs (*Leptodactylus fallax*) around the waist just cranial to the hindlimbs. Note that the body of these frogs appears inflated, a common defensive behavioural display observed in anurans when handled (*Source:* Images courtesy of ZSL Veterinary Department).

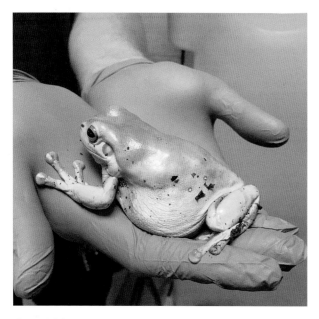

Figure 21.2 Adult White's tree frogs (*Ranoidea caerulea*) may be held in the palm of the hands, as shown with this gravid female (*Source:* Image courtesy of ZSL Veterinary Department).

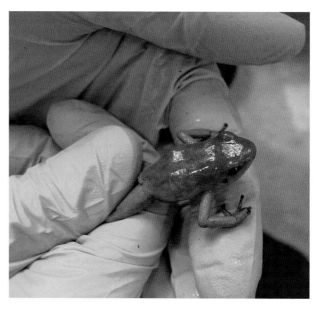

Figure 21.3 Restraint of an adult bicolored poison dart frog (*Phyllobates bicolor*). The hindlimbs are held near the base between the handler's thumb and forefinger and the anuran's body is supported by a second hand (*Source:* Image courtesy of ZSL Veterinary Department).

epidermis, which is often pigmented with melanin (Figure 21.4). These excrescences are present in nearly all anurans which breed in water and tend to either be absent or minimally developed in land-breeding anurans (Duellman and Trueb 1994a). Hypertrophied forelimbs may develop in males alongside nuptial excrescences and many other secondary sexual characteristics of the phalanges exist in anurans (Duellman and Trueb 1994a). Other secondary sexual characteristics in males of certain anuran species include larger sharp odontoids or tusks, cornified labial spines, glands on the ventrum, more numerous and cornified tubercles on the dorsum, hairlike projections on the flanks and

thighs, a cloacal extension or 'tail', a protruding spiny vent, a pigmented vocal sac, a larger tympanum, protrusion of the columella through the tympanum and the *linea masculinea*, bands of fibrous connective tissue which extend along the dorsal and ventral edge of the *M. obliquus* (Duellman and Trueb 1994a). There may also be an overall difference in colouration between males and females (Duellman and Trueb 1994a).

Like anurans, female salamanders are typically slightly larger than males, but they can be the same size in many species and in a small number of species males are larger than females (Duellman and Trueb 1994a). Other sexually

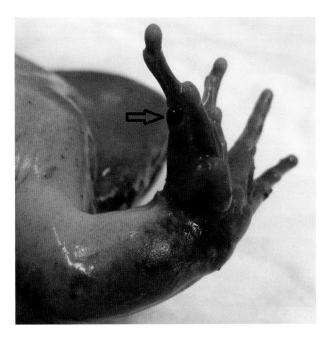

Figure 21.4 Pigmented nuptial excrescence on the prepollex of an anaesthetised male mountain chicken frog (*Leptodactylus fallax*) during the breeding season (*Source:* Image courtesy of ZSL Veterinary Department).

dimorphic characters in males of salamander species during the breeding season include a swollen vent due to enlargement of cloacal glands, more extensive caudal fins (and dorsal fins in newts), development of bright colouration, courtship glands, enlarged cirri (the lip margin encompassing the end of the nasolabial grooves), elongate monocuspid premaxillary teeth, nuptial excrescences, and hypertrophied limb musculature (Duellman and Trueb 1994a).

21.2.10 Clinical Examination

Visual examination is recommended prior to handling, preferably in the animal's transport carrier to minimise disturbance. Information can be gathered on respiratory rate, body condition, skin condition including colouration and any lesions, posture, ambulation, and behaviour (Clayton and Gore 2007).

The anuran or salamander may then be restrained for physical examination. Ocular examination with an ophthalmoscope and slit lamp is recommended as corneal and lenticular lesions are common (Whitaker and Wright 2001; Williams 2012). Aquatic and larval frogs lack eyelids whereas terrestrial adults have short eyelids and a translucent conjunctival fold, and most salamanders have well-developed eyelids (Whitaker and Wright 2001). A blink reflex may be elicited by gentle palpation of the cornea, whilst the pupillary light reflex may be elicited using a bright focal light source (Whitaker and Wright 2001);

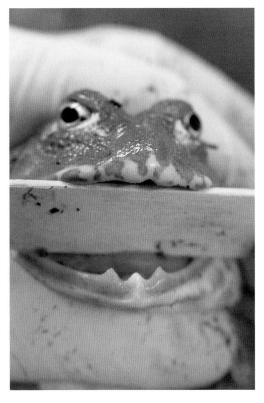

Figure 21.5 Oral examination of an African bullfrog (*Pyxicephalus adspersus*) using a wooden tongue depressor (*Source:* Image courtesy of ZSL Veterinary Department).

however, the amphibian pupil may constrict in response to light even in an enucleated eye due to autonomous activity therefore the presence of this reflex should be interpreted with caution (Williams 2012). Other neurological reflexes include the limb withdrawal reflex, elicited by grasping the limb distally and extending it, and the righting reflex, elicited by placing the anuran in dorsal recumbency (Whitaker and Wright 2001). The nares should be inspected for excessive mucous or bubbles which may suggest underlying respiratory disease (Whitaker and Wright 2001). Oral examination may be performed by gently opening the mouth with a small flat piece of plastic card, waterproof paper, an oral speculum, or tongue depressor (Figure 21.5), taking care not to cause trauma to the mandible (Whitaker and Wright 2001). Heart rate and rhythm may be determined using a Doppler probe placed on the cranioventral coelom in the region of the sternum (Whitaker and Wright 2001). Coelomic palpation can be useful, particularly to assess for coelomic masses; however, palpation should be performed early on during the clinical examination as anurans often inflate with air after handling which limits examination (Figure 21.1) (Whitaker and Wright 2001). Hydration status should be assessed as dehydration is common, as indicated by tacky skin, skin tenting, sunken eyes, lack of urination when handled, and reduced prominence of the lingual or ventral abdominal vein (Clayton and Gore 2007). Bodyweight measurement may be performed with the amphibian restrained in a plastic bag or carrier and is important to allow accurate calculation of medication doses (Whitaker and Wright 2001).

21.3 Diagnostic Tests

21.3.1 Blood Sampling

Blood sampling is most often performed for haematology, biochemistry, blood culture, and virology. The venepuncture site should be cleaned with sterile saline or dilute chlorhexidine first (1 : 40 dilution) (Whitaker and Wright 2001). The volume of blood (ml) that can safely be withdrawn is 1% of bodyweight (g) in healthy individuals or 0.5% of bodyweight in ill anurans or salamanders (Chai 2015a). A 25–27 gauge needle and heparinised 1 ml syringe is suitable for most species (Chai 2015a). The preferred venepuncture site in most anurans is the ventral abdominal vein (Figure 21.6); however, cardiocentesis under sedation or anaesthesia may be required for smaller anurans, in which blood is withdrawn from the ventricle via a needle inserted into the heart apex (Chai 2015a). The preferred venepuncture site in medium to large salamanders is the ventral tail vein in the proximal third of the tail via a lateral approach (Baitchman and Herman 2015). The ventral abdominal vein is an alternative option. Cardiocentesis under sedation or anaesthesia may be necessary for smaller salamanders weighing less than 10 g; the heart is located just cranial to the thoracic girdle (Baitchman and Herman 2015). Lithium heparin is

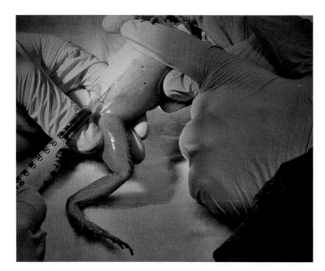

Figure 21.6 Blood collection from the ventral abdominal vein of an anaesthetised juvenile mountain chicken frog (*Leptodactylus fallax*) (*Source:* Image courtesy of ZSL Veterinary Department).

the recommended anticoagulant as EDTA may lyse amphibian red blood cells. Haematology reference intervals are published for commonly kept species (Whitaker and McDermott 2018). For less commonly kept species, comparison may be made to field data or values in the zoological database Species360® for the same or closely related species, although care should be taken to ensure that these reference intervals include only healthy animals.

21.3.2 Faecal Analysis

Faecal samples should be examined fresh as some protozoa will encyst in the environment or when refrigerated (Whitaker and Wright 2001). Fresh faeces can be obtained by target feeding an individual and placing them on moist paper towel in a clean container. This method will also help to avoid sampling free-ranging organisms (Whitaker and Wright 2001). Routine parasitology is recommended with a wet mount (0.9% saline) and flotation (e.g. saturated salt solution) (Whitaker and Wright 2001). Many metazoa and protozoa are considered normal in moderate numbers and bacteriology is of little significance except if there is pure growth of a single isolate (Whitaker and Wright 2001). If it is not possible to obtain a fresh faecal sample, a cloacal wash may be performed by inserting a lubricated urinary or intravenous catheter of appropriate size into the cloaca and gently instilling up to 1 ml of saline then aspirating the material and examining it immediately (Whitaker and Wright 2001).

21.3.3 Skin Swabs, Scrapes, and Smears

Skin swabs for bacteriology, mycology, Gram and Ziehl-Neelsen staining are useful in the investigation of skin disease. If chytridiomycosis is suspected or being screened for in adult anurans or salamanders, a plain swab should be used to swab each foot, the ventral thighs and the ventral coelomic surface, particularly the drink patch, with three to five sweeps at each site and submitted for *B. dendrobatidis* (Bd) and *B. salamandrivorans* (Bsal) polymerase chain reaction (PCR) (Pessier et al. 2017). For tadpoles, the swab should instead be inserted into the mouth and rotated several times (Pessier et al. 2017). It is important to check with the laboratory which swabs are most appropriate and how they should be stored, for example a fine-tipped rayon swab with a plastic handle should be used and the sample air-dried and kept at or below 23 °C for testing by real time Taqman PCR (Pessier et al. 2017).

Skin scrapes are useful to assess for the presence of parasites, bacteria, and fungal elements (e.g. *Saprolegnia*). The edge of a cover slip or blunted scalpel blade is gently pulled over the skin lesion, material smeared onto a glass slide with a drop of tank water or saline and a cover slip added prior to microscopy (Whitaker and Wright 2001). Fungal elements may be more easily visualised with Lugol's iodine or lactophenol blue stain. For lesions such as rostral abrasions and cloacal prolapses which may be damaged by a skin scrape, an impression smear may be made and stained using Gram and Ziehl-Neelsen stains (Whitaker and Wright 2001).

21.3.4 Nutritional Support

Assist feeding may be required in anorexic debilitated anurans and salamanders. Some anurans and salamanders may open the mouth if a food item is lightly touched against the mouth; otherwise an oral speculum such as a flat plastic card or waterproof paper may be used to gently open the mouth by inserting it at the philtrum (Wright and Whitaker 2001a). Food items such as killed invertebrates can then be placed in the caudal oral cavity and the speculum removed to allow the amphibian to swallow or a gavage tube may be inserted into the gastrointestinal tract to administer a liquid formula (Wright and Whitaker 2001a). The gavage tube should be pre-measured and no longer than a third to a half of the animal's body length to avoid trauma to the stomach and a powdered critical care formula suitable for carnivores may be used (Wright and Whitaker 2001a).

The daily caloric needs (kcal/day) of an amphibian can be calculated by multiplying the resting oxygen consumption by the standard conversion of 0.0048 (kcal/ml of oxygen) and by 24 (hours/day). Oxygen consumption is temperature and species dependent. For example, the daily caloric needs of a 50 g frog kept at 25 °C would be:

$$0.174(50)^{0.84} \times 0.0048 \times 24 = 0.54 \, \text{kcal} / \text{day}.$$

For an ill anuran or salamander, at least 50% more than the daily caloric needs should be provided and bodyweight regularly monitored to help guide nutritional support (Wright and Whitaker 2001a).

21.3.5 Fluid Therapy

Provision of fluid therapy is highly important in terrestrial amphibians as the rate of evaporative water loss via the skin is greater in amphibians than in other vertebrates, dehydration is common in ill amphibians, and the skin is involved in osmoregulation and respiration in some species (Clayton and Gore 2007).

Transdermal fluid therapy is appropriate in all cases and is often sufficient for rehydration (Clayton and Gore 2007). Fluid that is hypotonic (e.g. 0.6% saline) or isotonic (e.g. amphibian Ringer's solution) to amphibian plasma should be used (Clayton and Gore 2007). Amphibian Ringer's solu-

tion can be made by mixing the appropriate amounts of various salts (6.6 g NaCl, 0.15 g KCl, 0.15 g $CaCl_2$ and 0.2 g $NaHCO_3$) in 1 l of RO, carbon-filtered, or distilled water (Clayton and Gore 2007). The base chemicals can be purchased from chemical supply companies. If Amphibian Ringer's solution is not available, an alternative isotonic solution that may be used is four parts Hartmann's (lactated Ringer's) solution with 1 part dextrose 5% (Clayton and Gore 2007; Chai 2015a). Bolus soaking (e.g. for one hour once to twice daily) or continuous soaking in a shallow bath may be used depending on the degree of dehydration (Clayton and Gore 2007). The nares and mouth should be positioned above the water to avoid aspiration of fluid. The transdermal method of fluid therapy is also appropriate for aquatic anurans and salamanders. As aquatic amphibians live in fluid which is hypotonic to amphibian plasma, fluid diffuses across the permeable skin and excess fluid must be excreted, predominantly via the kidneys, and electrolytes conserved (Clayton and Gore 2007). Diseased aquatic anurans and salamanders tend to retain excessive fluid and lose electrolytes, therefore bathing in isotonic rather than hypotonic fluid is preferred (Clayton and Gore 2007).

Injectable routes of fluid therapy may be considered for more severely dehydrated anuran and salamander patients. Typically, reptile Ringer's solution is used (equal parts of 2.5% dextrose, 0.45% sodium chloride, and lactated Ringer's solution) (Clayton and Gore 2007). Delivery routes include: (i) subcutaneous injection into the dorsal lymph sacs, along the lateral body wall or thigh in anurans; (ii) intracoelomic injection approached via the caudoventral lateral body wall to avoid coelomic organs and the ventral abdominal vein in anurans and salamanders; (iii) intravenous injection into the midline abdominal vein in anurans or ventral tail vein in salamanders; and (iv) intraosseous injection via an intravenous catheter placed normograde into the tibiofibula or retrograde into the femur in anurans and salamanders (Clayton and Gore 2007). Typically, boluses of 10 ml/kg are administered and repeated as needed.

21.3.6 Anaesthesia and Analgesia

Anaesthetic options are listed in Table 21.2. The most frequently used anaesthetic agent in anurans and salamanders is MS-222 (tricaine methanesulfonate). It has a wide safety margin and can be used to anaesthetise all life stages (Baitchman and Stetter 2014). MS-222 powder is dissolved in distilled water or amphibian Ringer's solution to the required concentration and, as it is acidic, must be buffered to the optimal pH for the species with sodium bicarbonate (Baitchman and Stetter 2014). The animal should be placed in an induction chamber (e.g. plastic bag or box) which contains an induction dose of the anaesthetic solution; this should cover approximately half of the body of adult anurans and salamanders (Baitchman and Stetter 2014). Once induced, the anuran or salamander should be removed from the induction chamber and rinsed regularly with oxygenated clean distilled water or amphibian Ringer's solution to maintain hydration (Figure 21.7) (Baitchman and Stetter 2014). A dilution of the MS-222 solution, typically half the induction concentration, may be used as a bath or syringed over the patient to maintain anaesthesia (Baitchman and Stetter 2014).

Isoflurane may be used as an alternative anaesthetic agent in adult anurans and salamanders. Induction may be slow and recovery rapid if chamber induction is used; whilst topical application and bath immersion provide more effective and longer lasting anaesthesia (Baitchman and Stetter 2014). If applied topically, the isoflurane mixture should be rinsed from the patient's skin following induction and anaesthesia typically lasts 45–80 minutes (Baitchman and Stetter 2014). For longer surgical procedures or if the plane of anaesthesia becomes too light, a 50% concentration of the induction solution may be applied or 1–2% isoflurane may be delivered in oxygen via a short endotracheal tube with the cuff inflated, placed just inside the glottis in large adult anurans and salamanders (Baitchman and Stetter 2014). Sevoflurane has also been used as a topical gel for anaesthetic induction and has a 4.5 times more rapid recovery than isoflurane (Whitaker and McDermott 2018).

Benzocaine is an effective anaesthetic agent in most anurans and salamanders (Whitaker and McDermott 2018). Benzocaine is available as a powder which is not easily soluble in water and must be dissolved in ethanol first, with no more than 1% ethanol in the final anaesthetic solution, or as a topical anaesthetic gel marketed for toothache in humans (Orajel®) which can be dissolved in water to the appropriate concentration (e.g. 1 g of 20% Orajel per litre of water, equivalent to a 200 mg/l bath, may be used; although unexpected mortality was reported in *Bufo fowleri* at this concentration) (Baitchman and Stetter 2014).

Alfaxalone may be administered intramuscularly resulting in muscle relaxation and immobility (West 2017). Immersion in a bath of alfaxalone solution resulted in 10–30 minutes of light anaesthesia in oriental fire bellied toads (*Bombina orientalis*) and may be considered for anurans weighing less than 100 g for which it would be difficult to accurately measure the volume required for intramuscular administration (West 2017). Anaesthesia has also successfully been induced in axolotls (*A. mexicanum*) by immersion in alfaxalone for induction, followed by irrigation of the gills and skin with 10 mg/ml alfaxalone as needed to deepen the plane of anaesthesia (West 2017).

Monitoring should involve assessment of reflexes, respiration, and heart rate. The righting reflex is lost at a light anaesthetic depth and the withdrawal reflex reduces during anaesthetic induction and is lost at a surgical anaesthetic depth (Baitchman and Stetter 2014). Respiration may be monitored by observation of gular movement. Gular movement decreases as the patient becomes anaesthetised and typically ceases altogether during anaesthesia (Baitchman and Stetter 2014). Cutaneous respiration will still occur, and the skin should be kept moist to enable this; however, during longer procedures supplemental oxygen should also be provided (e.g. by bubbling oxygen into a shallow water bath containing the patient or by intubation) (Baitchman and Stetter 2014). Heart rate may be monitored by direct visualisation in most anurans when they are positioned in dorsal recumbency or by using a Doppler probe (Figure 21.8) and a significant decrease from baseline

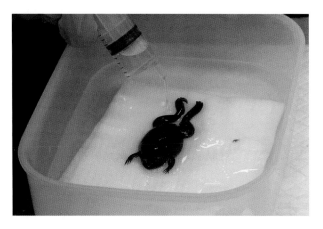

Figure 21.7 Amphibian Ringer's solution is regularly applied to the skin of this anaesthetised Lake Oku clawed frog (*Xenopus longipes*) (*Source:* Image courtesy of ZSL Veterinary Department).

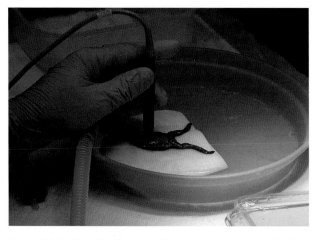

Figure 21.8 Use of a Doppler ultrasound probe to monitor the heart rate of an anaesthetised Lake Oku clawed frog (*Xenopus longipes*) (*Source:* Image courtesy of ZSL Veterinary Department).

values suggests that the anaesthetic plane is too deep (Baitchman and Stetter 2014).

There is little published information regarding analgesia in amphibians. NSAIDs are most often used (Whitaker and McDermott 2018). Opioids have not been well studied but may be considered peri-operatively for surgical procedures. The relative analgesic potency of opioid receptors is similar to that in mammals, with μ-receptors greater than δ-receptors which are greater than κ-receptors therefore full or partial μ-agonists may be considered most useful (Baitchman and Stetter 2014; Whitaker and McDermott 2018). Local anaesthetic agents may be used topically on skin or for local infiltration but with caution to avoid toxicity (Chai 2016; Whitaker and McDermott 2018).

21.3.7 Euthanasia

Prolonged immersion in a high concentration of tricaine methanesulfonate (e.g. 10 g/l), buffered to a neutral pH with sodium bicarbonate, is one of the most frequently used and least stressful methods of euthanasia for both larval and adult anurans and salamanders (Wright 2001a; Leary et al. 2013; Whitaker and McDermott 2018). However, immersion in 5 g/l tricaine methanesulfonate for as long as one hour was required to ensure death of all *X. laevis* in one study (Torreilles et al. 2009), therefore if a shorter time frame than one hour is allowed then a secondary euthanasia technique is recommended for this species once loss of consciousness has been achieved. Application of topical benzocaine hydrochloride gel to the ventrum (20% concentration, 20 mm × 1 mm application) is an effective alternative in some species (Leary et al. 2013). Administration of barbiturates, such as pentobarbital sodium 60 mg/kg by intravenous or intracoelomic injection (or in the lymph sacs in anurans) is also acceptable (Whitaker and McDermott 2018). Rapid freezing may be acceptable if it results in immediate death, for example, this is likely to be achieved if anurans or salamanders which have a body weight of less than 4 g and do not have freeze-tolerance strategies are placed into liquid nitrogen (Leary et al. 2013). Other methods of freezing are not considered acceptable (Leary et al. 2013). A Doppler probe can be used to confirmation cessation of the heart beat following euthanasia. However, the amphibian heart can continue to beat after brain function has ceased therefore confirmation of death by pithing is recommended (Leary et al. 2013). The pithing site in anurans is the foramen magnum, which can be found as a slight midline skin depression caudal to the skull with the neck flexed (Leary et al. 2013). Although pithing is used as a secondary method of euthanasia in an unconscious anuran or salamander, it is not considered acceptable as a primary method of euthanasia (Leary et al. 2013).

21.4 Common Medical and Surgical Conditions

21.4.1 Infectious Diseases

21.4.1.1 Bacterial Disease

Bacterial diseases occur commonly in anurans and salamanders secondary to trauma, viral infection, and mycotic skin infections (Baitchman and Herman 2015; Chai 2015a). The most well described bacterial infections in anurans and salamanders are bacterial dermatosepticaemia, flavobacteriosis, mycobacteriosis, and chlamydiosis (Densmore and Green 2007). Clinical signs of bacterial dermatosepticaemia may include erythema of the ventrum and extremities (hence the historical name 'red leg syndrome'), anorexia, swelling, oedema, coelomic effusion, skin erosion, ulceration, sloughing, and necrosis, and sudden death (Densmore and Green 2007). Previously attributed to *Aeromonas hydrophila* infection, it is now recognised that infection with a wide variety of other Gram-negative bacilli and some Gram-positive bacteria (*Staphylococcus* and *Streptococcus*) may produce similar signs. Treatment involves parenteral antibiotics based on culture and sensitivity testing and supportive care (Densmore and Green 2007).

Flavobacteriosis due to infection with bacteria from the genus *Flavobacterium* has been reported in anurans and salamanders and may cause similar clinical signs to dermatosepticaemia, with effusions in the lymphatic sacs, hydrocoelom, lingual or corneal oedema, panophthalmitis, petechiation, and visceral congestion, and mortality may be high (Densmore and Green 2007). Diagnosis is based upon culture and PCR testing and treatment should be based on bacterial culture and antibiotic sensitivity testing.

Atypical mycobacteriosis has been described in anurans and salamanders due to infection with various environmental mycobacteria (including *Mycobacteria marinum, M. chelonei,* and *M. liflandii*) and it can present subclinically or with non-specific signs such as weight loss, lethargy, anorexia, bloating, ulcerative or nodular dermatitis, localised ocular disease, subcutaneous oedema, coelomic effusion, abnormal buoyancy in aquatic species, or sudden death (Martinho and Heatley 2012). Diagnosis may be made ante mortem by demonstration of pink-red filamentous rods on Ziehl-Neelsen stained impression smears from lesions or coelomic aspirates (Martinho and Heatley 2012). Swab samples may also be collected for mycobacterial culture or PCR-based techniques to identify the type of mycobacteria involved. However, no effective treatments have been described in amphibians, the risk of systemic disease or recurrence following treatment is high, and there is a risk of zoonosis therefore euthanasia is recommended (Martinho and Heatley 2012). At post mortem examination, granulomatous lesions of the skin and any internal organ, particularly the liver, may be identified.

Chlamydia infection can cause a disease in anurans very similar to that of bacterial dermatosepticaemia and ranaviral infection (Densmore and Green 2007). Clinical signs may include skin petechiation and sloughing, coelomic distension due to hydrocoelom, fluid accumulation in lymphatic sacs, lethargy, cutaneous depigmentation, and interstitial pneumonia (Densmore and Green 2007). Diagnosis may be based on histopathology, in which granulomatous inflammation may be identified in the liver, spleen, heart, lungs, and kidneys with intracytoplasmic basophilic inclusions in hepatocytes, and liver tissue may be submitted for cell culture, immunofluorescence, immunohistochemistry, transmission electron microscopy, and PCR testing (Reed et al. 2000; Densmore and Green 2007). Treatment with oral tetracycline antibiotics is recommended (Densmore and Green 2007). Disease associated with a novel genus within the family Chlamydiaceae has also been described in captive salamanders and was characterised by anorexia, lethargy, oedema, abnormal gait, and 100% mortality rate (Martel et al. 2012). Hepatitis was identified on histological examination of some of the affected individuals and chlamydial infection was identified based on a combination of immunohistochemical staining, transmission electron microscopy, and PCR performed on liver tissue samples (Martel et al. 2012).

21.4.1.2 Viral Disease

Ranaviruses, large double-stranded DNA viruses from the genus *Ranavirus* and family Iridioviridae, are the most significant pathogenic amphibian viruses (Densmore and Green 2007; Chai 2015a). Ranavirus infection in anurans and salamanders may be subclinical, although the mechanisms for this are poorly understood, or it may result in clinical disease with mass morbidity and mortality within a population (Lesbarrères et al. 2012). Clinical signs typically observed in affected anurans and salamanders in the USA include erratic swimming, haemorrhages, and swelling in larvae, whilst in Europe either a chronic disease characterised by skin ulceration or a peracute disease characterised by systemic haemorrhages is typically seen in adults (Lesbarrères et al. 2012). Histological changes include foci of necrosis in the skin and viscera, especially the liver and haematopoietic tissue of the kidney and spleen, and basophilic intracytoplasmic inclusions may be present, particularly in hepatocytes (Densmore and Green 2007). Diagnosis of ranavirus infection can be confirmed ante mortem by conventional PCR testing of toe clip or tail clip samples and post mortem by electron microscopy, immunohistochemistry, conventional or quantitative-PCR (qPCR) testing of liver or kidney samples (Gray et al. 2017; Leung et al. 2017;

Allender 2018). There are no specific treatments for ranaviruses and vaccines are in the early stages of development (Gray et al. 2017). Ranaviruses are likely to be able to persist in aquatic systems for one to three weeks depending on temperature and microbiota (Gray et al. 2017). Various disinfectants (Virkon®, Nolvasan®, bleach, and ethanol) are known to inactivate ranaviruses and may be used following an outbreak in isolated aquatic systems (Gray et al. 2017).

21.4.1.3 Fungal Disease

Chytridiomycosis, caused by the fungal pathogen *B. dendrobatidis* (Bd), is the most significant fungal disease of anurans and has been associated with amphibian population declines globally (Densmore and Green 2007). Chytrid fungi are ubiquitous in moist and aquatic environments and infection with Bd occurs in the keratinizing stratified squamous epithelium of the skin of postmetamorphic anurans and the mouthparts of larval anurans (Baitchman and Pessier 2013). Whilst larval anurans are typically subclinically infected, postmetamorphic anurans may show clinical signs of lethargy, dehydration, dysecdysis, skin hyperaemia, abnormal posture, loss of the righting reflex, abnormal behaviour such as lack of a flight response when captured, and mortality rates may be high (Densmore and Green 2007). Death occurs due to electrolyte depletion due to disruption of electrolyte transport across affected skin (Baitchman and Pessier 2013).

Salamanders appear to be relatively resistant to disease caused by Bd; however, in 2010 a novel species of chytrid fungus emerged, *B. salamandrivorans* (Bsal), which can cause ulcerative skin disease and a short period of anorexia followed by mortality in salamanders (Martel et al. 2013). Bsal spread from Asia to Europe and thus far it has affected wild European salamanders in Belgium, Germany, and the Netherlands, as well as captive salamanders in Germany and the United Kingdom (Martel et al. 2013; Cunningham et al. 2015; Sabino-Pinto et al. 2015; Spitzen-van der Sluijs et al. 2016).

Diagnosis of chytrid fungus infection may be made post mortem by histopathology of affected skin samples, particularly those obtained from the ventral pelvis, hindlegs, and feet (Baitchman and Pessier 2013). Typical findings of chytridiomycosis due to Bd infection are epidermal hyperplasia and hyperkeratosis with Bd thalli (fungal bodies) within the stratum corneum (Baitchman and Pessier 2013); whereas typical findings of chytridiomycosis due to Bsal infection are epidermal ulceration with keratinocytes containing one centrally located Bsal thallus at the periphery of these erosions (Martel et al. 2013). Ante mortem testing for both Bd and Bsal may be performed by PCR testing of skin swab samples obtained using the technique outlined in *Skin swabs, scrapes, and smears* (Blooi et al. 2013).

Various treatments for chytridiomycosis exist (Table 21.2) and there is no single treatment protocol that is suitable for all species and life stages, therefore safety and effectiveness should always be researched prior to use. Itraconzaole baths are most widely used to treat Bd infection in post-metamorphic anurans (Baitchman and Pessier 2013). The bath solution should be a depth to reach approximately midway along the animal's dorsum when in a sitting position, should be agitated frequently to evenly distribute the medication and to ensure all skin surfaces are covered, and the animal should be rinsed at the end of each treatment (Baitchman and Pessier 2013). Use of itraconazole baths in salamanders to successfully clear asymptomatic Bd infection has also been described and no side-effects were reported when the granulated preparation of itraconazole was used (Sporanox®) (Michaels et al. 2018). As Bd organisms can persist for a long time in moist environments, animals should be placed in a clean disinfected enclosure after each treatment, ideally a sparse, easily-cleaned enclosure, and strict biosecurity should be adhered to prevent Bd re-infection and spread to other amphibians (Baitchman and Pessier 2013). The effectiveness of treatment should be checked by performing post-treatment Bd PCR, ideally with three PCR tests over a 14-day post-treatment period (Baitchman and Pessier 2013). The permanent enclosure of affected animals should be broken down and all contents disinfected prior to the return of successfully-treated animals to their enclosure (Baitchman and Pessier 2013). Clinically ill animals should also be provided with supportive care including fluid therapy, antibiotics to prevent secondary bacterial infections, and assisted feeding if anorexic (Baitchman and Pessier 2013).

Chytridiomycosis due to Bsal infection has been successfully treated using high temperature treatment (>25°C for at least 10 days) (Blooi et al. 2015a) or using a combination of polymyxin E submersion baths (2000 IU/ml for 10 minutes) followed by spraying with voriconazole (12.5 µg/ml) twice a day for 10 days with the animals kept at 20°C (Blooi et al. 2015b).

Saprolegniasis is another common fungal disease which affects aquatic anurans and salamanders (Chai 2015a). Infection with *Saprolegnia* spp. presents as erythematous or ulcerated skin lesions with a cotton wool-like fungal growth on the surface (Chai 2015a). Treatment is usually initiated based on observation of typical cotton wool-like lesions alone; however, confirmation of the diagnosis may be made by collecting and examining these lesions as described in *Skin swabs, scrapes and smears*. Treatment options include methylene blue, potassium permanganate, and benzalkonium chloride (Table 21.2).

21.4.1.4 Parasitic Disease

Many parasites have been documented in captive anurans and salamanders and the decision to treat depends on the type of organisms, parasite load, and associated clinical signs (Chai 2015a). Some of the most commonly identified nematodes in anurans are:

1) *Rhabdia* sp., lungworms which may also encyst in other organs causing granuloma formation.
2) filarial nematodes (e.g. *Dracunculus*, *Foleyella*) which are found in the subcutis, as well as the coelomic cavity and tissues in the case of *Foleyella*.
3) *Pseudocapillaroides xenopi*, a capillarioid nematode found in the epidermis of *Xenopus* sp. (Chai 2015a).

Lungworms (*Rhabdia* sp.) and intestinal nematodes (*Strongyloides* sp.) are amongst the most common nematodes in salamanders (Baitchman and Herman 2015).

Treatment of nematode infection is recommended if there are any unthrifty animals, mortalities, or if there is diarrhoea, blood (>5–10 RBCs/hpf), or evidence of inflammation (> 1–5 WBCs/hpf) on a Romanowsky-stained faecal smear, mucus, or a high parasite burden (>5 strongyle larvae/hpf) identified on direct or flotation faecal examination (Whitaker and McDermott 2018). Several different anti-parasitic medications have been used successfully to treat nematode infections in amphibians (Table 21.2) and filarial nematodes may be directly removed via a skin incision (Chai 2015a).

Trematodes and cestodes are typically present as larval forms in anurans and salamanders as they represent an intermediate host (Klaphake 2009). Clinical signs are usually minimal but focal pathology may be observed due to encysted larvae or more significant pathology may occur due to migration of the parasites through tissues (Klaphake 2009; Chai 2015a). The acanthocephalan *Acanthocephalus ranae* may infect the stomach and intestine of anurans and can cause gastrointestinal perforation, coelomitis, and death; however, the life cycle involves an arthropod intermediate host therefore infection in captivity is usually self-limiting (Klaphake 2009; Chai 2015a).

Anurans and salamanders have many commensal protozoa in the gastrointestinal tract (Klaphake 2009). Potentially pathogenic protozoa in anurans include:

1) *Entamoeba ranarum*, which has trophozoites that mature to the cyst form in the colon, and typically causes anorexia, weight loss, gastrointestinal signs, oedema, and coelomic fluid accumulation and can also affect the kidneys and cause hepatic abscessation.
2) *Microsporidium* sp. (e.g. *Pleistophora myotrophica*) which affect the striated muscles and cause wasting and poor body condition.

3) Myxozoa including *Chloromyxum* sp., which affects the kidneys, *Myxidium immersum*, which is found free-floating in the gall bladder, and *Myxobolus hylae*, which affects the reproductive organs.

4) Coccidia, including *Eimeria* and *Isospora*, which can affect the gastrointestinal tract and kidneys, causing weight loss, diarrhoea, dehydration, and nephritis.

5) Trypanosomes, haemoprotozoa that can cause haemorrhage, anaemia, swollen lymph glands, and death, and are typically introduced to captive amphibians via feeder fish or other live food. Therefore, placing food items in a hypertonic bath for five minutes then rinsing prior to feeding is recommended as a preventative measure (Chai 2015a; Klaphake 2009).

Metronidazole is the treatment of choice for amoebiasis in anurans (Table 21.2); treatment is recommended if large numbers of amoeba are present on faecal examination or an amphibian appears unwell in the presence of amoeba (Klaphake 2009).

Pathogenic protozoa in salamanders include two protozoal organisms of the Mesomycetozoea class: *Ichthyophonus* spp., which cause myositis with ulceration and secondary infection, and *Amphibiocystidium* spp. which cause subcutaneous and hepatic cysts and can also affect anurans (Baitchman and Herman 2015). No treatment has been described for these protozoal species (Baitchman and Herman 2015).

Trombiculid mites are the most commonly described external parasites of anurans and salamanders, especially plethodontid salamanders (Baitchman and Herman 2015; Chai 2015a). Trombiculid mite larvae burrow through the skin into the dermis where they feed on tissue and induce an inflammatory reaction (Baitchman and Herman 2015). The feet are most frequently affected and ivermectin is the treatment of choice for larvae (Table 21.2). All other life stages of the mite live in the environment and soil can be oven-heated to kill the mites (Klaphake 2009). External leeches and copepods may be observed in anurans and salamanders and can be treated with saline baths (Klaphake 2009).

21.5 Non-infectious Diseases

21.5.1 Rostral Abrasions

Rostral abrasions (Figure 21.9) are very common in captive anurans and are typically caused by trauma to the rostrum in stressed or nervous animals, especially during and post-transport (Chai 2015a). Disturbance to the animal and its enclosure should be minimised and husbandry reviewed to assess for any environmental sources of stress such as lack

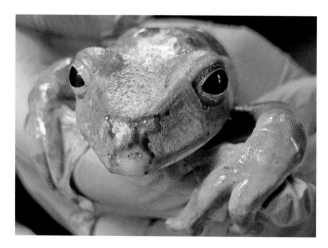

Figure 21.9 Rostral abrasion in a Fea's tree frog (*Rhacophorus feae*) under treatment. Note the hyperpigmentation at the healing wound margin (*Source:* Image courtesy of ZSL Veterinary Department).

of refugia (Chai 2015a). Impression smears and swabs of rostral abrasions may be collected for Ziehl-Neelsen staining and culture and sensitivity to rule out secondary mycobacterial or other bacterial infection, particularly for deep or non-healing ulcers which might require topical or systemic antibiotic treatment based on culture and sensitivity results (Chai 2015a). Orabase® Protective Paste (ConvaTec Inc.) may also be applied to deep or non-healing rostral abrasions (Mylniczenko 2008). This semi-solid paste adheres to moist lesions, assisting healing by providing a temporary protective cover and barrier against osmotic losses (Mylniczenko 2008).

21.5.2 Oedema Syndrome

Oedema syndrome, or accumulation of fluid in the coelomic cavity and tissues, is common in both anurans and salamanders and may be caused by a variety of underlying disease processes. Differential diagnoses include cardiac failure, lymph heart failure, renal disease, hepatic disease, hypocalcaemia (as this may reduce the frequency and force of lymph heart contractions), osmotic imbalances (e.g. due to skin disease or exposure to water with low dissolved solutes), retained ova, or bacterial and viral infections (Wright 2001c; Chai 2015a; Clancy et al. 2015). Aspiration of fluid for cytology and culture was the most useful diagnostic test to identify an infectious aetiology in one study of dendrobatid frogs with oedema syndrome (Clancy et al. 2015). Ultrasound examination may be useful to evaluate the heart, liver, and kidneys in larger anurans and salamanders and blood sampling may be performed for haematology and biochemistry, particularly to evaluate renal and hepatic parameters. The prognosis for generalised oedema syndrome is guarded given the poor prognosis associated with many of the underlying disease processes. Supportive care is recommended, including bathing the affected animal in hypertonic amphibians Ringer's solution (7.3 g NaCl, 0.17 g KCl, 0.17 g CaCl₂ and 0.22 g NaHCO₃ dissolved in 1l of RO, carbon-filtered, or distilled water) or 10% Whitaker-Wright solution, i.e. 10 ml of 100% Whitaker-Wright solution (113 g NaCl, 8.6 g MgSO4, 4.2 g CaCl2, 1.7 g KCl in 1l distilled water) to 90 ml distilled water, with reassessment at least every four hours and subsequent maintenance in an isotonic solution when oedema has significantly reduced in volume (Wright 2001c; Wright and Whitaker 2001b; Clayton and Gore 2007). The underlying cause should also be treated if known. Initiation of antibiotic therapy (enrofloxacin 10 mg/kg PO q 24 h) was the only treatment positively associated with case success in a study of dendrobatid frogs with oedema syndrome (Clancy et al. 2015).

21.5.3 Nutritional Disease

Metabolic bone disease occurs relatively commonly in anurans and salamanders in captivity, either due to nutritional secondary hyperparathyroidism (NSHP) or renal secondary hyperparathyroidism (RSHP) (Klaphake 2010). NSHP is more common and typically affects juvenile amphibians due to inadequate oral calcium, low dietary calcium:phosphorus ratio, inadequate oral cholecalciferol, inadequate UV-B radiation, inappropriate heating, or a combination of these factors, whilst RSHP tends to occur in older individuals with declining renal function (Klaphake 2010). High phosphorus or fluoride levels in the water supply may also be a contributory factor to metabolic bone disease in anurans (Shaw et al. 2012). Clinical signs may include skeletal deformities, pathologic fractures, tetany, oedema, intestinal and cloacal prolapse, generalised weakness, gas accumulation in the gastrointestinal tract, and death (Hadfield and Whitaker 2005). Diagnosis is made based on poor bone density, misshapen bones, thin bone cortices, and pathologic fractures on radiographs (Hadfield and Whitaker 2005). If presenting with tetany and gastrointestinal disease, calcium gluconate (100–200 mg/kg SC) should be administered (Hadfield and Whitaker 2005; Whitaker and McDermott 2018). Following resolution of tetany or in cases presenting without tetany or gastrointestinal disease, oral calcium gluconate or calcium glubionate, as well as oral vitamin D3 (e.g. 1 ml/kg of Zolcal-D®, Vetark Professional), should be administered and improvement in bone density monitored with repeat radiographs (Hadfield and Whitaker 2005). To address the underlying cause, the diet, water source, heating, and UV-B lighting provision should be reviewed and corrected.

Obesity has been described in captive anurans, most commonly White's tree frogs (*Ranoidea caerulea*), horned frogs (*Certaophrys* spp.), and the African bullfrog (*Pyxicephalus adspersus*), and captive salamanders, typically the axolotl (*A. mexicanum*) and tiger salamander (*Ambystoma tigrinum*), due to the high fat content of most captive amphibian diets and inactivity (Wright and Whitaker 2001a). Obese individuals typically present with an enlarged coelom due to fat deposition in the coelomic fat bodies and *R. caerulea* may also deposit fat in crests over the eyes which obscure vision if they become sufficiently enlarged (Wright and Whitaker 2001a). Active foraging species may be encouraged to lose condition by increasing activity levels, e.g. by providing a larger enclosure or adding new cage furniture, whilst the amount of food offered per week may be reduced for sit-and-wait foragers (Wright and Whitaker 2001a). Lipid keratopathy is another common disease of captive anurans which is thought to be nutritional in origin, presenting as a white corneal opacity which usually protrudes from the cornea (Wright and Whitaker 2001a; Williams 2012). High cholesterol levels in captive diets or other compositional differences between the fatty acid content of captive and wild diets of amphibians have been suggested as likely contributory factors (Wright and Whitaker 2001a; Williams 2012). High-cholesterol items should be limited and total caloric intake reduced to prevent further progression of corneal lesions; however, no treatment is known and the condition may be painful so analgesia should be considered (Chai 2015a).

Hypovitaminosis A has been described in several anuran families and occurs due to low vitamin A levels in most captive invertebrate food items (Ferrie et al. 2014). Clinical signs may include a shortened tongue which prevents prehension of food (short tongue syndrome) and was described in Wyoming toads (*Anaxyrus baxteri*) due to squamous metaplasia of the tongue epithelium, poor reproductive success, reduced larval survival, and poor function of the immune system (Ferrie et al. 2014). A diagnosis may be made based on clinical signs, histopathological evidence of squamous metaplasia, and response to treatment; liver and blood vitamin A levels may also be tested but normal values have not been established (Ferrie et al. 2014). Treatment involves vitamin A supplementation which is most consistently achieved by the oral route, e.g. by dusting or gut loading invertebrates with a vitamin A supplement (Ferrie et al. 2014).

21.5.4 Surgery

Surgeries performed in anurans and salamanders include wound repair, mass removal, prolapse repair and replacement, coeliotomy (for exploratory laparotomy, gastrotomy, enterotomy, cystotomy or reproductive surgery), digit and limb amputation, enucleation, and lens surgery (Chai 2016). The patient should be adequately hydrated prior to surgery; it is recommended to soak the anuran or salamander for one hour pre-operatively in a shallow water bath (Chai 2016). Amphibian Ringer's solution at the preferred temperature for the species is used by the author. Pre-operative fasting is not typically required, although large anurans may be fasted for 24–48 hours prior to coelomic surgery to aid visualisation and reduce the risk of anaesthetic-associated ileus (Chai 2016). Adequate analgesia should be provided as described in *Anaesthesia and analgesia* (Chai 2016). Dilute chlorhexidine (e.g. a sterile gauze soaked with 0.75% chlorhexidine solution applied to the skin for 10 minutes), povidone–iodine solution (diluted 1 : 10 in sterile saline) or sterile saline alone may be used to prepare the surgical site and clear plastic drapes are preferred to isolate the surgical site and reduce cutaneous evaporative water loss (Chai 2016). Size 11 or 15 scalpel blades, microsurgical instruments, or surgical kits designed for small exotic animals, sterile cotton-tipped applicators for haemostasis and some form of magnification are recommended for amphibian surgery (Chai 2016).

When performing coeliotomy, the coelomic membrane should be elevated and incised following the initial skin incision, taking care to avoid the midline ventral abdominal vein, lungs, gastrointestinal tract and bladder (Chai 2016). Single layer closures are adequate for the gastrointestinal tract and urinary bladder when gastrotomy, enterotomy, or cystotomy are performed (Chai 2016). Absorbable suture material such as polyglactin (VICRYL®, Ethicon) or polydioxanone (PDS®, Ethicon) is suitable for coelomic organs and muscle (Chai 2016). The coeliotomy incision should be closed in two layers with a simple continuous pattern in the coelomic membrane and muscle and

interrupted everting sutures in the skin (Chai 2016). Monofilament nylon, plus cyanoacrylate tissue adhesives if needed, is suitable for use in skin closure (Chai 2016). Prior to proceeding with limb amputation, it is particularly important in anurans to consider that some species require both forelimbs to maintain posture, ambulation or food manipulation and both hindlimbs for reproduction (Chai 2016). Limb amputation in salamanders may result in limb regeneration therefore the amputation site should be left open and kept clean as surgical closure of the skin at the amputation site prevents limb regeneration (Baitchman and Herman 2015). If enucleation is performed, care must be taken to avoid traumatising the membrane separating the eye and oral cavity and the surgical site is typically left to heal by second intention (Chai 2016). It is possible that some species could have difficulty swallowing following enucleation; however, many animals do well after surgery (Mylniczenko 2008).

21.6 Diagnostic Imaging

Radiography is most frequently used for diagnosis of metabolic bone disease, radiodense choleliths, osteoarthritis, fractures, and the presence of foreign bodies (Figure 21.10) (Chai 2015a). This can be performed conscious in most amphibians with the animal in a closed plastic box or shallow water bath (Chai 2015a). Use of mammography film or digital radiography with processing algorithms designed for amphibians are useful to show fine detail in smaller species.

Ultrasonography is most often used to assess cardiac, hepatic and renal architecture, coelomic masses, and for fluid aspiration for culture and cytology in cases of coelomic effusion. High frequency probes such as a high

(a)   (b)

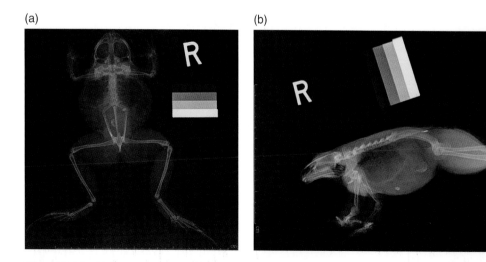

Figure 21.10   (a) Dorsoventral and (b) Lateral radiographs of an adult mountain chicken frog (*Leptodactylus fallax*). This individual has a radiodense cholelith, granular radiodense material in the gastrointestinal tract and osteoarthritis of the right stifle (*Source:* Images courtesy of ZSL Veterinary Department).

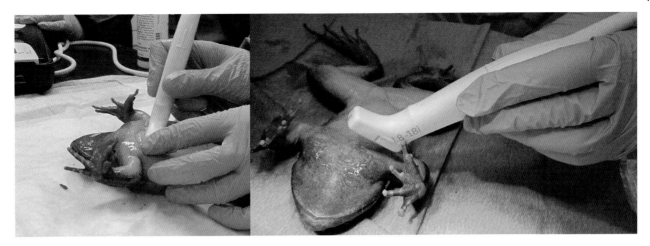

Figure 21.11 Use of a high frequency hockey stick linear probe for ultrasound examination of anaesthetised mountain chicken frogs (*Leptodactylus fallax*) (*Source:* Images courtesy of ZSL Veterinary Department).

frequency hockey stick linear probe (Figure 21.11) are useful for anurans to provide fine detail. To reduce skin irritation, direct probe contact can be avoided by using a water-filled plastic bag or container or by using water-based ultrasonography gel (Chai 2015a).

Endoscopy may be performed in the anaesthetised anuran or caudate to retrieve foreign bodies from the upper gastrointestinal tract, directly visualise coelomic organs, and collect tissue samples (Chai 2015b). Given the small size of anurans and caudates, typically a 1.9 mm diameter integrated telescope or 2.7 mm diameter oblique rigid telescope with a 4.8 mm diameter protection sheath and 1 or 1.7 mm diameter endoscopic grasping forceps are used (Chai 2015b). For coelioscopy, the anuran or caudate is placed in dorsal recumbency, the skin aseptically prepared as for other surgical procedures, the telescope introduced into the coelom via a 3 mm paramedian incision through the skin and coelomic membrane and carbon dioxide used to insufflate the pleuroperitoneal cavity (Chai 2015b). Following coelioscopy, the coelomic membrane and skin should be closed in a single layer with simple interrupted sutures and the sutures removed after four to eight weeks (Chai 2015b).

Use of computed tomography (CT) for diagnostics in amphibians is in its infancy. CT has been used to compare bone mineralisation between wild European spadefoot toads (*Pelobates fuscus*) and captive individuals of the species which were housed with different levels of UV-B radiation and dietary supplements (van Zijll Langhout et al. 2017). The bone mineralisation of the femur and thickest part of the skull parietal bone was measured in Hounsfield units (HUs) and HUs compared between the groups (van Zijll Langhout et al. 2017). The HUs in the femurs of captive adult animals which were fed a calcium and vitamin D3 supplemented diet but never had exposure to UV-B radiation were significantly higher than the HUs in the femurs of captive adult animals which were exposed to natural UV-B

light but received no calcium or vitamin D3 supplementation, suggesting that this species may reply more heavily on dietary vitamin D3 than vitamin D3 formed through UV-B exposure (van Zijll Langhout et al. 2017).

21.7 Preventative Health Measures

To prevent introduction of disease to the amphibian collection, owners should be advised on appropriate quarantine measures for newly acquired amphibians. The length of the quarantine period, infectious disease screening and treatment required during quarantine depends on a risk assessment for each new animal or group of animals entering the collection (Pessier et al. 2017). Animals that have an overall low risk are those from a source that is known to have good biosecurity practices, can provide complete health history information, and is a single species facility or a population which has been isolated long-term at a mixed species facility (Pessier et al. 2017). Animals with a high risk are those from a source with unknown or poor biosecurity practices, unknown health history or a history of unexplained mortality or morbidity, recent identification of pathogens that can be population-limiting (e.g. Bd, Bsal, or ranaviruses) or cause significant clinical disease (e.g. mycobacteriosis or pathogenic parasites) and that mixes amphibian species from different sources and geographic locations in a single room or water system (Pessier et al. 2017). Low risk animals require shorter quarantine periods and less diagnostic testing (e.g. 30 day period; test animals at least once for Bd and Bsal), whereas high risk animals require a longer quarantine period and more extensive diagnostic testing (e.g. 60–90 day period; test animals 2–3 times for Bd and Bsal) (Pessier et al. 2017). Necropsy and histopathology is recommended for any animals that die within the quarantine period and faecal parasite examination is recommended in the first week and one week before the expected end of the quarantine period (Pessier et al. 2017). The quarantine period should be lengthened if there are unexplained mortalities, significant pathogens identified, ongoing health problems or treatment for an infectious disease is not yet complete (Pessier et al. 2017).

The quarantine enclosure should ideally be in a dedicated room or building away from other amphibians and dedicated footwear, protective clothing, tools and equipment used for servicing the quarantine animals (Pessier et al. 2017). Specific work-flow patterns should be used to reduce the risk of transferring potential pathogens from amphibians in quarantine to amphibians in the main collection (Pessier et al. 2017). Hands should be washed between servicing different enclosures or a new set of disposable gloves used for each enclosure and tools should be cleaned and disinfected between enclosures (Pessier et al. 2017).

21.8   Medications and Formulary

The semipermeable nature of amphibian skin allows use of topical formulations and medicated baths. Care should be taken to avoid drugs containing irritants or whose pH causes skin irritation (Whitaker and Wright 2001). Short-term baths in a container separate to the main tank are preferred to avoid effects on the filtration system (Whitaker and Wright 2001). If in-tank medication is used, the carbon and biological filters should be removed to avoid deactivation of the drug and destruction of nitrifying bacteria (Whitaker and Wright 2001). Oral medication may be administered by opening the mouth with an atraumatic speculum (e.g. plastic card) and inserting a blunted flexible tube (e.g. urinary catheter) or microliter syringe (Whitaker and Wright 2001). Subcutaneous injections may be performed in anurans but are difficult to perform in salamanders due to adherence of the skin to the underlying musculature (Whitaker and Wright 2001). Intramuscular injections are given in the foreleg musculature if they are excreted or metabolised by the kidneys or liver due to the presence of renal and hepatic portal systems (Whitaker and Wright 2001). Intravenous injections are rarely performed due to the small size of amphibian patients, however injection into the ventral abdominal vein, lingual vein, or heart may be possible in larger patients (Whitaker and Wright 2001). Intracoelomic injections are injected just off midline with the amphibian in dorsal recumbency with the head tipped slightly down (Whitaker and Wright 2001). Injection into a lymph sac (e.g. dorsal lymph sac in anurans just craniolateral to the urostyle) allows rapid drug uptake (Whitaker and Wright 2001). Doses for commonly used medications in amphibians are presented in Table 21.2.

Acknowledgements

The author would like to thank Dr. Christopher Michaels PhD FLS, Herpetology Section Team Leader at ZSL London Zoo, for helpfully reviewing and providing some of the husbandry information.

Table 21.2   Selected commonly used drugs in amphibians. Adapted from Baitchman and Stetter (2014), Chai (2016), and Whitaker and McDermott (2018).

Drug	Dose	Main use
Anaesthetics		
MS-222	1 g/l	Anaesthetic induction (adults)
	0.2–0.5 g/l	Anaesthetic induction (larvae and neotenous species)
Isoflurane	3–5% isoflurane in oxygen in an induction chamber	Anaesthetic induction (adults)
	0.025–0.035 ml/g BW topically using a mixture of isoflurane 3 ml, K-Y® Jelly 3.5 ml, water 1.5 ml	
	2–3 ml/l in an induction bath or bubbled into water to effect	
Sevoflurane	3 ml sevoflurane, 3.5 ml K-Y Jelly, 1.5 ml water combined and used topically as a gel	Anaesthetic induction (adults)
Benzocaine	200–300 mg/l bath to effect	Anaesthetic induction (adults)
	50 mg/l bath to effect	Anaesthetic induction (larvae)
Alfaxalone	5–25 mg/kg IM	Anaesthetic induction (adults)
	200 mg/l bath	Anaesthetic induction (adult fire-bellied toads)
	5 mg/l bath	Anaesthetic induction (axolotls)

Table 21.2 (Continued)

Drug	Dose	Main use
Analgesics		
Meloxicam	0.4–1 mg/kg PO, SC or ICe q 24 h	Analgesia
Morphine	38–42 mg/kg SC	Peri-operative analgesia; may provide analgesia for >4 hours
Buprenorphine	38 mg/kg SC	Peri-operative analgesia; may provide analgesia for >4 hours
Lidocaine	Lidocaine 2 mg/kg diluted 3 : 1 with sodium bicarbonate solution and applied topically or as a local infiltration	Local anaesthesia of incision site prior to surgery
Anti-parasitics		
Fenbendazole	30–50 mg/kg PO q24h for 3–5 days 50–100 mg/kg PO	Treatment of nematodes. Repeat treatment after 14–21 days.
Ivermectin	0.2–0.4 mg/kg PO, SC 2 mg/kg topically 10 mg/l × 1 h bath	Treatment of nematodes and mites. Repeat treatment after 14 days. May cause flaccid paralysis with overdose.
Levamisole	10 mg/kg IM, ICe, topically, repeat after 10–14 days 100–300 mg/l × 24 h bath (or 100 mg/l bath × 72 h for resistant nematodes, repeat after 7–14 days 12 mg/l bath × four days	Treatment of nematodes. May cause paralysis in some species at suggested doses.
Praziquantel	8–24 mg/kg PO, SC ICe, topically 10 mg/l × 3 h bath	Treatment of trematodes and cestodes. Repeat treatment after 14 days.
Metronidazole	10–50 mg/kg PO q24h for 3–10 days 100–150 mg/kg PO, repeat in 14–21 days 500 mg/100 g feed for 3–4 treatments 50 mg/l × 24 h bath	Treatment of protozoa. Toxicity may occur at higher doses. Use lower doses for unfamiliar or sensitive species.
Antibiotics		
Ceftazidime	20 mg/kg SC, IM q48–72 h	Broad spectrum.
Enrofloxacin	5–10 mg/kg PO, SC, IM q24h 10 mg/kg topically 500 mg/l × 6–8 h bath q24h	Broad spectrum (except obligate anaerobes).
Oxytetracycline	50 mg/kg PO q12–24 h 1 g/kg feed × 7 days 25 mg/kg SC, IM q24h 50–100 mg/kg IM q48h 100 mg/l × 1 h bath	Broad spectrum, particularly useful for chlamydiosis.
Metronidazole	10–50 mg/kg PO q24–48 h 10 mg/kg IV q24h 12–60 mg/kg topically q24h	Anaerobic infections.
Antifungals		
Itraconazole	0.01% × 5 min bath q 24 h × 11–14 days 0.0025% × 5 min bath q24h × 6 days 0.5–1.5 mg/l × 5 min bath q24h × 7 days 50 mg/l × 5 min bath q24h × 10 days	Treatment of chytridiomycosis (treatment of choice). Care with tadpoles.
Voriconazole	1.25 µg/ml q 24 h via topical spray × 7 days	Treatment of chytridiomycosis.

(Continued)

Table 21.2 (Continued)

Drug	Dose	Main use
Terbinafine	0.005–0.01% in distilled water × 5 min bath q24h for 5 days 0.005–0.01% in distilled water × 5 min bath q48h for 6 treatments	Treatment of chytridiomycosis.
Chloramphenicol	20 mg/kg topically of Chlorsig 1% ointment (Sigma) 10–30 mg/l continuous bath replaced daily for up to 30 days 20 mg/l continuous bath replaced daily for 14 days	Treatment of chytridiomycosis. Risk of aplastic anaemia.
Methylene blue	4 mg/l × 1 h bath q24h	Treatment of saprolegniasis.
Potassium permanganate	1 : 5000 water × 5 min bath q24h	Treatment of saprolegniasis.
Benzalkonium chloride	0.25 mg/l × 72 h bath 2 mg/l × 1 h bath q24h	Treatment of saprolegniasis.

References

Allender, M.C. (2018). Ranaviral disease in reptiles and amphibians. In: *Fowler's Zoo and Wild Animal Medicine*, 9e (eds. R.E. Miller, N. Lamberski and P. Calle), 364–370. St. Louis: Elsevier Saunders.

Amphibian Ark (2017). Husbandry documents. http://www.amphibianark.org/husbandry-documents (accessed 10 October 2017).

Auliya, M., García-Moreno, J., Schmidt, B.R. et al. (2016). The global amphibian trade flows through Europe: the need for enforcing and improving legislation. *Biodiversity and Conservation* 25: 2581–2595.

Baines, F., Chattell, J., Dale, J. et al. (2016). How much UV-B does my reptile need? The UV-Tool, a guide to the selection of UV lighting for reptiles and amphibians in captivity. *Journal of Zoo and Aquarium Research* 4 (1): 42–63.

Baitchman, E. and Herman, T.A. (2015). Caudata (Urodela): tailed amphibians. In: *Fowler's Zoo and Wild Animal Medicine*, 8e (eds. R.E. Miller and M.E. Fowler), 13–20. St Louis: Elsevier Saunders.

Baitchman, E.J. and Pessier, A.P. (2013). Pathogenesis, diagnosis, and treatment of amphibian Chytridiomycosis. *Veterinary Clinics of North America Exotic Animal Practice* 16: 669–685.

Baitchman, E. and Stetter, M. (2014). Amphibians. In: *Zoo Animal and Wildlife Immobilization and Anaesthesia*, 2e (eds. G. West, D. Heard and N. Caulkett), 303–311. Iowa: Wiley-Blackwell.

Barnett, S.L., Cover, J.F., and Wright, K.M. (2001). Amphibian husbandry and housing. In: *Amphibian Medicine and Captive Husbandry* (eds. K.M. Wright and B.R. Whitaker), 35–61. Malabar, FL: Krieger Publishing.

BIAZA RAWG (2018). BIAZA RAWG UV-TOOL. www.uvguide.co.uk/BIAZA-RAWG-UV-Tool.htm (accessed 12 September 2018.)

Blooi, M., Pasmans, F., Longcore, J.E. et al. (2013). Duplex real-time PCR for rapid simultaneous detection of *Batrachochytrium dendrobatidis* and *Batrachochytrium salamandrivorans* in amphibian samples. *Journal of Clinical Microbiology* 51 (12): 4173–4177.

Blooi, M., Martel, A., Haesebrouck, F. et al. (2015a). Treatment of urodelans based on temperature dependent infection dynamics of *Batrachochytrium salamandrivorans*. *Scientific Reports* 5: 8037.

Blooi, M., Pasmans, F., Rouffaer, L. et al. (2015b). Successful treatment of *Batrachochytrium salamandrivorans* infections in salamanders requires synergy between voriconazole, polymyxin E and temperature. *Scientific Reports* 5: 11788.

Chai, N. (2015a). Anurans. In: *Fowler's Zoo and Wild Animal Medicine*, 8e (eds. R.E. Miller and M.E. Fowler), 1–13. St Louis: Elsevier Saunders.

Chai, N. (2015b). Endoscopy in amphibians. *Veterinary Clinics of North America Exotic Animal Practice* 18: 479–491.

Chai, N. (2016). Surgery in amphibians. *Veterinary Clinics of North America Exotic Animal Practice* 19: 77–95.

Clancy, M.M., Clayton, L.A., and Hadfield, C.A. (2015). Hydrocoelom and lymphedema in dendrobatid frogs at National Aquarium, Baltimore: 2003–2011. *Journal of Zoo and Wildlife Medicine* 46 (1): 18–26.

Clayton, L.A. and Gore, S.R. (2007). Amphibian emergency medicine. *Veterinary Clinics of North America Exotic Animal Practice* 10: 587–620.

Courteney-Smith, J. (2016). What is soil? In: *The Arcadia Guide to Bio-activity and the Theory of Wild Re-creation™* (ed. J. Courtney-Smith), 193–199. Horley: Arcadia Products PLC.

Cunningham, A.A., Beckmann, K., Perkins, M. et al. (2015). Emerging disease in UK amphibians. *Veterinary Record* 176: 468.

Densmore, C.L. and Green, D.E. (2007). Diseases of amphibians. *ILAR Journal* 48 (3): 235–254.

Duellman, W.E. and Trueb, L. (1994a). Courtship and mating. In: *Biology of Amphibians* (eds. W.E. Duellman and L. Trueb), 51–86. Baltimore, MD: The Johns Hopkins University Press.

Duellman, W.E. and Trueb, L. (1994b). Food and feeding. In: *Biology of Amphibians*, 229–240. Baltimore, MD: The Johns Hopkins University Press.

Ferrie, G.M., Alford, V.C., Atkinson, J. et al. (2014). Nutrition and health in amphibian husbandry. *Zoo Biology* 33: 485–501.

Gray, M.J., Duffus, A.L.J., Haman, K.H. et al. (2017). Pathogen surveillance in Herpetofaunal populations: guidance on study design, sample collection, biosecurity and intervention strategies. *Herpetological Review* 48 (2): 334–351.

Green, E.D. (2001). Restraint and handling of live amphibians. In: *Standard Operating Procedure. Amphibian Research & Monitoring Initiative*. Madison, WI: National Wildlife Health Center. United States Geological Survey.

Gutleb, A.C., Bronkhorst, M., Vandenberg, J.H.J. et al. (2001). Latex laboratory-gloves: an unexpected pitfall in amphibians toxicity assays with tadpoles. *Environmental Toxicology and Pharmacology* 10: 119–121.

Habidata (2017). http://www.habidata.moonfruit.com/home/4572891200 (accessed 10 October 2017).

Hadfield, C. and Whitaker, B. (2005). Amphibian emergency medicine and care. *Seminars in Avian and Exotic Pet Medicine* 14 (2): 79–89.

Klaphake, E. (2009). Bacterial and parasitic diseases of amphibians. *Veterinary Clinics of North America: Exotic Animal Practice* 12: 597–608.

Klaphake, E. (2010). A fresh look at metabolic bone diseases in reptile and amphibians. *Veterinary Clinics of North America: Exotic Animal Practice* 13: 375–392.

Leary, S., Underwood, W., Anthony, R. et al. (2013). *AVMA Guidelines for the Euthanasia of Animals: 2013 Edition*. Schaumburg, IL: American Veterinary Medical Association.

Lentini, A.M. (2013). Husbandry and care of amphibians. In: *Zookeeping: An Introduction to the Science and Technology* (eds. M.D. Irwin, J.B. Stoner and A.M. Cobaugh), 335–346. Chicago: University of Chicago Press.

Lesbarrères, D., Balseiro, A., Brunner, J. et al. (2012). Ranavirus: past, present and future. *Biology Letters* 8 (4): 481–483.

Leung, W.T., Thomas-Walters, L., Garner, T.W. et al. (2017). A quantitative-PCR based method to estimate ranavirus viral load following normalisation by reference to an ultraconserved vertebrate target. *Journal of Virological Methods* 249: 147–155.

Livingston, S., Lavin, S.R., Sullivan, K. et al. (2014). Challenges with effective nutrient supplementation for amphibians: a review of cricket studies. *Zoo Biology* 33: 565–576.

Martel, A., Adriaensen, C., Bogaerts, S. et al. (2012). Novel Chlamydiaceae disease in captive salamanders. *Emerging Infectious Diseases* 18 (6): 1020–1022.

Martel, A., Spitzen-van der Sluijs, A., Blooi, M. et al. (2013). *Batrachochytrium salamandrivorans* sp. nov. causes lethal chytridiomycosis in amphibians. *Proceedings of the National Academies of Science (PNAS)* 110 (38): 15325–15329.

Martinho, F. and Heatley, J.J. (2012). Amphibian mycobacteriosis. *Veterinary Clinics: Exotic Animal Practice* 15 (1): 113–119.

Michaels, C.J., Gini, B.F., and Preziosi, R.F. (2014a). The importance of natural history and species-specific approaches in amphibian ex-situ conservation. *Herpetological Journal* 24: 135–145.

Michaels, C.J., Antwis, R.E., and Preziosi, R.F. (2014b). Manipulation of the calcium content of insectivore diets through supplementary dusting. *Journal of Zoo and Aquarium Research* 2 (3): 77–81.

Michaels, C.J., Rendle, M., Gibault, C. et al. (2018). *Batrachochytrium dendrobatidis* infection and treatment in the salamanders *Ambystoma andersoni*, *A. dumerilii* and *A. mexicanum*. *Herpetological Journal* 28: 87–91.

Mylniczenko, N. (2008). Amphibians. In: *Manual of Exotic Pet Practice* (eds. M.A. Mitchell and T.N. Tully Jr.), 73–111. St. Louis: Elsevier Saunders.

Odum, R.A. and Zippel, K.C. (2008). Amphibian water quality: approaches to an essential environmental parameter. *International Zoo Yearbook* 42: 40–52.

Pessier, A.P., Mendelson, J.R., Tapley, B. et al. (eds.) (2017). *A Manual for Control of Infectious Diseases in Amphibian Survival Assurance Colonies and Reintroduction Programs*. Apple Valley, MN: IUCN/SSC Conservation Breeding Specialist Group.

PFMA (2019). Pet population 2019. https://www.pfma.org.uk/pet-population-2019 (accessed 21 January 2020).

Poole, V.A. and Grow, S. (eds.) (2012). *Amphibian Husbandry Resource Guide*, 2e. Silver Spring, MD: Association of Zoos and Aquariums.

Reed, K.D., Ruth, G.R., Meyer, J.A. et al. (2000). *Chlamydia pneumoniae* infection in a breeding colony of African clawed frogs (*Xenopus tropicalis*). *Emerging Infectious Diseases* 6 (2): 196–199.

Sabino-Pinto, J., Bletz, M., Hendrix, R. et al. (2015). First detection of the emerging fungal pathogen *Batrachochytrium salamandrivorans* in Germany. *Amphibia-Reptilia* 36 (4): 411–416.

Shaw, S.D., Bishop, P.J., Harvey, C. et al. (2012). Fluorosis as a probable factor in metabolic bone disease in captive New

Zealand native frogs (*Leiopelma* species). *Journal of Zoo and Wildlife Medicine* 43 (3): 549–565.

Spitzen-van der Sluijs, A., Martel, A., Asselberghs, J. et al. (2016). Expanding distribution of lethal Amphibian fungus Batrachochytrium salamandrivorans in Europe. *Emerging infectious diseases* 22 (7): 1286–1288.

Tapley, B., Griffiths, R.A., and Bride, I. (2011). Dynamics of the trade in reptiles and amphibians within the United Kingdom over a ten-year period. *Herpetological Journal* 21: 27–34.

Torreilles, S.L., McClure, D.E., and Green, S.L. (2009). Evaluation and refinement of euthanasia methods for *Xenopus laevis. Journal of the American Association for Laboratory Animal Science* 48 (5): 512–516.

West, J.A. (2017). Therapeutic review Alfaxalone. *Journal of Exotic Pet Medicine* 26: 156–161.

Whitaker, B.R. and McDermott, C.T. (2018). Amphibians. In: *Exotic Animal Formulary*, 5e (ed. J.W. Carpenter), 54–78. St. Louis: Elsevier.

Whitaker, B.R. and Wright, K.M. (2001). Clinical techniques. In: *Amphibian and Captive Husbandry* (eds. K.M. Wright and B.R. Whitaker), 89–110. Malabar, FL: Krieger Publishing.

Williams, D.L. (2012). The amphibian eye. In: *Ophthalmology of Exotic Pets*, 197–210. Chichester, West Sussex, UK: Wiley-Blackwell.

Wright, K.M. (2001a). Restraint techniques and euthanasia. In: *Amphibian and Captive Husbandry* (eds. K.M. Wright and B.R. Whitaker), 111–122. Malabar, FL: Krieger Publishing.

Wright, K.M. (2001b). Diets for captive amphibians. In: *Amphibian and Captive Husbandry* (eds. K.M. Wright and B.R. Whitaker), 63–72. Malabar, FL: Krieger Publishing.

Wright, K.A. (2001c). Idiopathic syndromes. In: *Amphibian and Captive Husbandry* (eds. K.M. Wright and B.R. Whitaker), 239–244. Malabar, FL: Krieger Publishing Company.

Wright, K.M. and Whitaker, B.R. (2001a). Nutritional disorders. In: *Amphibian and Captive Husbandry* (eds. K.M. Wright and B.R. Whitaker), 73–88. Malabar, FL: Krieger Publishing Company.

Wright, K.M. and Whitaker, B.R. (2001b). Pharmacotherapeutics. In: *Amphibian and Captive Husbandry* (eds. K.M. Wright and B.R. Whitaker), 309–330. Malabar, FL: Krieger Publishing Company.

van Zijll Langhout, M., Struijk, R.P.J.H., Könning, T. et al. (2017). Evaluation of bone mineralization by computed tomography in wild and captive European common spadefoots (*Pelobates fuscus*), in relation to exposure to ultraviolet B radiation and dietary supplements. *Journal of Zoo and Wildlife Medicine* 48 (3): 748–756.

22

Koi Carp

Lindsay Thomas

Koi carp are ornamental carp developed from the domestic form of the common carp (*Cyprinus carpio*) in Japan in the early nineteenth century. Known as nishikigoi (brocaded carp) in Japan, these fish have grown in popularity around the world. Two hundred years of selective breeding have produced a wide range of colour and scale pattern variations with new varieties still being developed. The most recent of these are the ghost Koi, developed by crossing Ogon Koi with wild carp to produce a metallic scaled fish, and butterfly Koi, a cross between Koi and Asian carp to produce a fish with long flowing fins. Koi are a different species to goldfish (*Carassius auratus*) and can be distinguished via the paired barbels present on the lips of Koi.

Koi are generally kept in large outdoor ponds to accommodate their adult size; up to 26 in. for normal varieties and up to 36 in. for 'jumbo' varieties. Ponds should be deep enough to allow water temperatures at the bottom of the pond to remain relatively stable throughout the winter. Generally a minimum depth of 1–1.5 m is considered appropriate (Hecker 1993). A filter system including physical and biological filtration as a minimum is essential, as is aeration of the pond using either waterfall or fountain water features or airstone systems. Excessive planting of ponds should be avoided as decaying plant matter can lead to nitrate build ups and algal blooms if regular maintenance is not carried out.

Biological parameters for European and Koi carp are given in Table 22.1.

22.1 The Aquatic Environment

Terrestrial animals live in an environment which can change rapidly and severely, and as a result have evolved multiple defensive mechanisms to maintain internal homeostasis in the face of potentially extreme external conditions. In contrast, aquatic animals such as Koi evolved to live in much more stable environments (with some exceptions), and therefore many of the defensive mechanisms commonly seen in terrestrial animals are lacking in aquatic species. Examples include anatomical features, such as the thin, easily damaged epidermis which overlies fish scales, the delicate gill structure in direct contact with the aquatic environment, and physiological features, such as passive excretion of waste products across the gill epithelium into the surrounding water. This makes species such as Koi very sensitive to changes in their environment.

In open systems such as lakes and rivers, changes in the environment occur very slowly due to the physical properties of water, especially in large volumes, and the constant cycling of water in and out of the system. In a pond situation, where the volume of water available is much smaller and generally static, changes in temperature, pH, salinity, and other parameters can occur much more rapidly and the potential for toxins to build up is much greater. It is therefore important to manage water quality very carefully in pond set ups. This is achieved using a filtration system to remove organic waste products with careful monitoring to detect and allow correction of any extremes of temperature or pH.

Filter systems can vary considerably. There are various modes of filtration that may be employed in various combinations, including physical/mechanical, biological, protein skimmers, chemical, and ultraviolet (UV).

22.1.1 Physical

Physical filtration removes solid waste from the system using mechanical filtration media such as gravel or sponges as a 'sieve' which filter particulate waste from the water. Physical filtration media are usually arranged so water flows through gradually decreasing 'grades', allowing multiple sizes of particulate waste to be removed at different points of the filter system. This helps slow clogging of the

Table 22.1   European and Koi carp biological parameters.

Parameter	European Wild Carp	Koi Carp
Adult Size	Females avg. 20 inches Males avg. 18 inches	Japanese Koi up to 22–26 inches Jumbo Koi up to 30–36 inches
Adult Weight	3–5 kg	3–5 kg in normal varieties, up to 9 kg in jumbo varieties
Lifespan	Females up to 9 years Males up to 15 years	15–25 years on average, up to 50 years
Sex determination	Females slightly more rotund than males. Males display breeding tubercules around spawning	Females slightly more rotund than males. Males display breeding tubercules around spawning.
Reproduction	Spawn when water temperatures reach 18 °C, eggs hatch in 3–4 days at temperatures between 20–23 °C	Spawn when water temperatures reach 18 °C, eggs hatch in 3–4 days at temperatures between 20–23 °C

system over time. Physical filtration media can also provide a surface for adherence of the bacterial colonies necessary for biological filtration. It is therefore important that physical filter media is always cleaned in pond water and never in chlorinated water, as this will destroy the bacteria and disrupt the biological filtration.

22.1.2   Biological

Biological filtration transforms nitrogenous waste products within the pond system. Fish, including Koi, produce ammonia as their primary nitrogenous waste product which is excreted across the gills by a combination of passive and active transport. If ammonia is not removed from the system then passive excretion is compromised and tissue levels of ammonia can rise and lead to ill health (see later). Ammonia is removed from the system by the nitrogen cycle (Figure 22.1), which is the basis of biological filtration. Ammonia is converted to nitrite by *Nitrosomas* spp. bacteria, then from nitrite to nitrate by *Nitrobacter* spp. bacteria. Nitrate, the least toxic of the nitrogenous waste products, is then removed from the system either through water changes, denitrification to nitrogen gas, or uptake by aquatic plants.

The bacteria necessary for biological filtration are very sensitive to chlorine, and therefore all water added to pond systems should be dechlorinated using a commercially available product. The bacteria also need a surface upon which to grow. In small filtration systems this may be the physical filtration media, however as this portion of the filter requires frequent cleaning to prevent clogging there is a risk that the bacteria will be destroyed or removed. Special biological filtration media units with large surface areas for bacterial colony growth are available and can be placed after the physical filtration unit to minimise the risk of clogging. These units should not require routine cleaning

but may need to be replaced over time if they do become clogged. It is important not to replace all the units at the same time as this will cause a dramatic drop in biological filtration capacity, preventing nitrogenous waste products from being removed from the system and can lead to health issues for the fish.

22.1.3   Protein Skimmers

Protein skimmers work by agitating the water to form a proteinaceous foam to which organic waste products and particulate matter are attracted and become trapped. This foam can then be skimmed from the surface of the water, removing the trapped waste material. Protein skimmers can be useful in reducing the workload on the physical and biological filtration units if they are placed first in the filtration system.

22.1.4   Chemical

Chemical filtration removes unwanted chemical compounds from the system. Activated carbon is the most commonly employed chemical filtration media and is frequently used to remove medications from pond systems once the desired course has been given. Ion exchange resins are also available and can be useful to remove organic compounds such as ammonia or nitrates when these compounds have reached dangerous levels and need to be removed quickly. It is important to remove chemical filtration units from the system once the desired effect has been achieved as they can leach compounds back into the water over prolonged time periods.

22.1.5   Ultraviolet

UV filtration is used to decrease water bacterial load and help remove single celled algae from the system, providing

Figure 22.1 The Nitrogen Cycle.

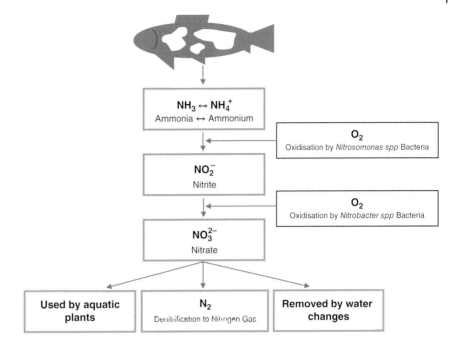

clear water which is aesthetically pleasing. UV is not suitable as a sole filtration unit as it will not remove nitrogenous waste from the water.

22.1.6 Diet

The popularity of Koi means that high quality commercial diets for Koi are widely available, and their use should be encouraged. Specific foods are also available for growth, containing higher protein concentrations, and to improve colour, which may contain algae, bacteria, yeast, fungi, or synthetic carotenoids (Corcoran and Roberts-Sweeney 2014).

Koi are able to metabolise carbohydrates more effectively than other omnivorous fish species, however protein is still more important as an energy source (Corcoran and Roberts-Sweeney 2014). Protein from animal sources, particularly fish meal, is preferred as it has a better essential amino acid profile and is more digestible (Olivia-Teles 2012). General macronutrient requirements for omnivorous fish are protein levels of 35–45%, carbohydrate content of 25–40%, fat levels of 15–25%, and fibre under 5% (Corcoran and Roberts-Sweeney 2014). Energy requirements decrease significantly during the colder months, and therefore feeding amount and frequency should be decreased accordingly (Corcoran and Roberts-Sweeney 2014). Quantities to feed will vary between diets and manufacturer instructions should be followed.

Koi have a requirement for vitamin C (Corcoran and Roberts-Sweeney 2014). This is generally added to commercial feeds in a stabilised form, however careful storage of food for a period of no more than 90 days is still recommended as levels may decrease over time due to oxidation (Olivia-Teles 2012).

22.2 Clinical Examination

As with all species, any Koi presented to the veterinary practice should be given a full clinical examination. In the case of aquatic species this includes full water analysis to determine any underlying water quality issues as well as distant and physical examinations. Table 22.2 provides a useful structure for clinical examination in Koi.

A full management history should be obtained, including filter maintenance routine, pond stocking density, and the presence or absence of vegetation (including algae). Water quality tests can be carried out with a commercial testing kit and a minimum database of ammonia, nitrite, and nitrate levels and pH should be obtained in all cases. Details of pond temperature and dissolved oxygen concentration testing are also useful, especially where the presenting signs may be indicative of a problem in these areas.

Distant examination is most useful in the animals' home environment. The animal's position in the water column, general movement, position within the pond, and opercular movements should all be noted at this point. When performing a physical examination it should be remembered that Koi have a thin, delicate epidermis overlying their scales which can be easily damaged by rough handling. It is advisable therefore to wear gloves whilst handling Koi and to do so in

Table 22.2 Clinical evaluation form.

Date:		Vet:	
Presenting complaint:			
Pond construction:	Length:	Water source:	
	Width:		
	Depth:	Water change regime:	
	Volume:		
Substrate (if any):		Pond last dredged:	
Filtration			
Filter type:		Fitted:	
Filter maintenance regime:			
Contents			
Species present (number):			
Vegetation present (quantity):			
Water Quality			
Ammonia:		Nitrite:	
Nitrate:		pH:	
Temperature:		Dissolved oxygen:	
Clinical Evaluation			
Clinical history:			
Mouth:		Abdomen:	
Eyes:		Skin:	
Gills:		Fins:	
Vent:		Behaviour:	
Samples			
Skin scrapes/impression smears:		Gill clip/impression smears:	
Biopsy:		Blood sample:	
Bacteriology:			

the water as much as possible. Physical examination should include evaluation of the mouth, eyes, gills, skin, abdomen, vent, and fins in detail, making note of any abnormalities.

22.3 Basic Sampling Techniques

Depending on the findings on physical examination it may be desirable to take samples of lesions or general samples to assess fish health. Whilst physical examination in Koi should not require chemical restraint, sedation may be necessary to facilitate handling and sample collection, especially in large Koi. This will be discussed in more detail later in the chapter. Skin scrapes, impression smears of lesions, gill clips, and blood samples can all be collected in the field, however other investigations such as swim bladder aspirates and post mortem examinations should be carried out at the clinic.

22.3.1 Skin Scrapes

Skin scrapes should be considered wherever skin lesions are present or parasites are suspected. Unlike in small animals, the aim of skin scrapes in aquatic species is to remove a small portion of the mucus layer whilst causing minimal damage to the underlying epidermis. The blunt edge of a scalpel blade or the edge of a slide should be used to collect the sample. If taking a scrape from a skin or fin lesion then the edge of the lesion is the ideal sampling site. If generally surveying for parasites the skin directly caudal to the pectoral fin is the preferred site. Once a mucus sample has been obtained it should be transferred to a slide with a drop of the pond water and a cover slip placed over it. Use of tap water or distilled water should be avoided as they may destroy some parasites. Samples should be examined immediately to allow motile organisms to be identified.

441 Sedation and Anaesthesia

22.3.2 Impression Smears

Impression smears carry a much lower risk of iatrogenic trauma than skin scrapes and may be considered in fractious animals where sedation is not possible or undesirable. A dry slide is impressed upon the lesion or area which is being sampled, then prepared as for a scrape with a drop of pond water and a cover slip.

22.3.3 Gill Clip

Gill clips are useful for assessing the presence of gill parasites, fungal infections or localised bacterial infections. Gill clips should only be performed post mortem unless taking only the very tips of a few gill filaments, which can be done in an anaesthetised fish. Gills clips should never be performed in conscious fish, and even gill scrapes and impression smears carry a high risk of iatrogenic damage if the fish moves and should only be considered if sedation is not possible or undesirable, e.g. because the presence of anaesthetic agents is likely to affect the presence of parasites in the sample.

Gill clips are performed by cutting away filaments from the gill arch, making sure not to include any of the cartilage. Gill filaments from the middle of the arch are ideal. These should be placed on a slide with a drop of the pond water and a cover slip placed on top. Samples should be examined immediately to allow motile organisms to be identified.

22.3.4 Blood Sampling

Blood can be most easily obtained from the caudal vein, located just ventral to the vertebral column, using a lateral or ventral approach. For the lateral approach the needle is inserted just ventral to the lateral line on the caudal peduncle. If the needle meets the vertebral column it should be angled slightly ventrally in order to enter the caudal vein. For the ventral approach the needle is inserted on the ventral midline just caudal to the anal fin and advanced until the vertebral column is met, and then withdrawn slightly to enter the caudal vein (Figure 22.2).

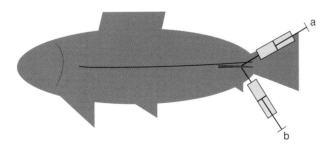

Figure 22.2 (a) Lateral approach and (b) caudal approach to the caudal vein.

22.3.5 Swim Bladder Aspirate

Swim bladder aspirates can be useful where swim bladder infection is suspected, for example when there is over distension of the swim bladder resulting in abdominal distension and/or buoyancy issues. The swim bladder is located in the dorsal coelomic cavity. Sedation of the patient and visualisation of the swim bladder using an ultrasound probe is recommended for this procedure where possible. A needle is inserted between the scales of the flank into the swim bladder and aspirated. If fluid is present a sample can be taken for culture and sensitivity testing, otherwise a small amount of sterile saline can be instilled into the swim bladder then aspirated to provide a sample. Aspiration of gas to allow return the fish to neutral buoyancy may provide temporary relief from the symptoms of swim bladder over-inflation whilst treatment is being initiated, however the vast majority of cases will relapse without appropriate management of the underlying cause (see later).

22.3.6 Bacteriology

Bacterial culture is difficult in fish due to the large numbers of bacteria present in the aquatic environment. In live fish, swabs from skin lesions, blood, and ascitic fluid may all be cultured, however results should be interpreted carefully due to the high risk of environmental contamination. Postmortem, sterile samples obtained from the kidney provide a more reliable indicator of systemic bacterial infection. This can be particularly useful in group situations where multiple animals are affected as it will help in determining the best treatment regime for the remaining animals.

22.4 Sedation and Anaesthesia

Fish often require sedation or anaesthesia for procedures which would be considered minor in canine and feline practice, for example skin scrapes and blood sample collection. However fish anaesthesia also presents a unique set of issues which need to be overcome, foremost being the need for the gills to remain submerged in order for respiration to continue. Fish anaesthesia therefore requires careful planning and preparation.

22.4.1 Pre-Anaesthetic Considerations

Owners should always be asked to bring as much pond water as they can spare when presenting a Koi for anaesthesia or sedation. This is important for recovery, which should be carried out in the animal's own water wherever possible to reduce stress. Any additional water required should be prepared the day before with conditioner added to remove chlorine and chloramines and then be left to stand to come to room temperature.

22.4.2 Induction of Anaesthesia

There are several methods of induction of anaesthesia in fish including immersion (Figure 22.3), intramuscular (Figure 22.4), and intravenous administration. Anaesthetic agents for which there are specific doses available for carp (including Koi) have been exclusively via the immersion method. Doses of anaesthetic agents given via the intramuscular route (for example ketamine, medetomidine, and pentobarbital) and intravenous route (for example propofol) are available for other fish species, but have not been studied in carp. Commonly used anaesthetic agents in carp are shown in the formulary.

22.4.3 Assessing Depth of Anaethesia

Depth of anaesthesia should be carefully monitored, depending on the procedure being performed. For example only light sedation is required for minimally invasive procedures such as skin scrapes whilst a deeper plane of anaesthesia is desirable for more involved surgical procedures

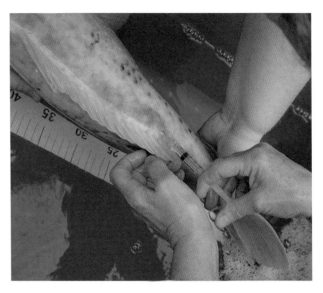

Figure 22.4 Intramuscular injection into the epaxial muscles (*Source:* Photo courtesy of Emily Hall MRCVS).

such as tumour removal or coeliotomy. A scoring system for assessing depth of anaesthesia in fish is shown in Table 22.3.

22.4.4 Maintaining Anaesthesia

For shorter procedures such as skin scrapes or blood sampling, fish can simply be kept moist using a wet towel and eye lubrication. However anaesthesia will need to be actively maintained in any procedure lasting longer than 10 minutes. This involves having a constant flow of water containing an anaesthetic agent over the gills of the fish via the oral cavity. There are three methods by which this can be achieved:

1) *Pump method* – anaesthetic agent is mixed into conditioned water in a container and an electric water pump is used to pump water from the container into the oral cavity of the fish via plastic tubing with resulting movement of water over the gills. This method is not suitable for volatile anaesthetic agents such as isoflurane due to health and safety considerations.
2) *Syringe method* – a syringe is used to draw up water containing an anaesthetic agent and flush it directly into the oral cavity. This method is not suitable for volatile anaesthetic agents such as isoflurane due to health and safety considerations
3) *Drip bag method* – The anaesthetic agent is injected into a bag of sterile saline and mixed well. The drip line is then placed into the animals oral cavity and opened fully. This is a safer method when using volatile agents such as isoflurane, however there is still a risk of anaesthetic agent evolving from the water once it passes over the gills.

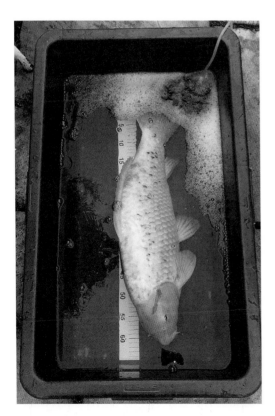

Figure 22.3 Loss of righting reflex during anaesthetic induction (*Source:* Photo courtesy of Emily Hall MRCVS).

Table 22.3   Assessing anaesthetic depth in fish. Modified from Summerfelt and Smith (1990).

Stage	Category	Notes
0	Normal	Reactive to external stimuli; opercular rate and muscle tone normal.
I	Light sedation	Slight loss of reactivity to external visual and tactile stimuli; opercular rate slightly decreased; equilibrium normal.
II	Deep sedation	Total loss of reactivity to external stimuli except strong pressure; slight decrease in opercular rate; equilibrium normal.
III	Partial loss of equilibrium	Partial loss of muscle tone; swimming erratic; increased opercular rate; reactivity only to strong tactile and vibrational stimuli.
IV	Total loss of equilibrium	Total loss of muscle tone and equilibrium; slow but regular opercular rate; loss of spinal reflexes.
V	Loss of reflex reactivity	Total loss of reactivity; opercular movements slow and irregular; heart rate very slow; loss of all reflexes.
VI	Medullary collapse	Opercular movements cease; cardiac arrest usually follows quickly.

22.4.5   Monitoring Anaesthesia

Anaesthetic monitoring can be more difficult in fish compared to other species. Heart rate can be monitored using a Doppler probe, although it should be noted that the heart can continue beating even after cessation of brain function, therefore trends are more important than absolute numbers. Heart rate is also related to buccal flow rate, so increasing the rate of flow through the gills will increase heart rate (Ross 2001).

Respiratory rate can be monitored by watching opercular movements; however these are often much reduced in fish under anaesthesia and will be affected by the method used to maintain anaesthesia, i.e. using a syringe method will disrupt opercular movement.

Temperature can be monitored using a temperature probe inserted into the vent. Fish are poikilotherms and have evolved to live in temperature stable environments, so sudden temperature changes can be very detrimental. It is important therefore to maintain fish as close to the temperature of their home pond as possible during anaesthesia.

Response to manual stimuli can be difficult to assess. Reflexes which are routinely monitored in mammalian species, such as palpebral and corneal reflexes, are not present in fish.

22.4.6   Recovery from Anaesthetic

Where in-water anaesthetic induction has been used, anaesthesia can be reversed simply by placing the fish in fresh, conditioned water, or water from the home pond system, containing no anaesthetic agent. Fish may need to be manually moved around the tank to ensure the fresh water is moved across the gills and recovery time will be dependent on length of anaesthesia and temperature. This is particularly true with drugs such as MS222, as brain and muscle concentrations of this drug will continue to increase even after blood concentration has stabilised.

Intramuscular agents used to induce anaesthesia can have prolonged sedative effects, as seen in domestic mammal species. For this reason, intramuscular anaesthesia induction should be reserved for longer procedures where anaesthesia is likely to be maintained (using the methods described above) for a sufficient period of time following induction to allow the induction agent to be metabolised. Intravenous and immersion methods of induction tend to produce more rapid recovery than intramuscular protocols and are therefore preferred for shorter procedures.

22.5   Analgesia

There is an increasing body of evidence demonstrating the existence of nociceptors and behavioural response to stimulation of these receptors in various fish species (Weber 2011). As such, veterinary surgeons must consider analgesia for fish patients, particularly when carrying out potentially painful procedures such as surgical removal of tumours, gill clips, or other invasive procedures. Unfortunately there is very limited information available on analgesic efficacy in fish species. Butorphanol was found to be effective in one study on Koi at a dose of 0.4 mg/kg whilst ketoprofen had no effect on behaviour post-surgery at a dose of 2 mg/kg (Harms et al. 2005). No other analgesics have been evaluated to date.

22.6   Hospitalisation

Hospitalisation is rarely practical in the veterinary setting as few veterinary practices will see sufficient numbers of fish to justify installing and maintaining a hospital tank of sufficient size to accommodate large Koi carp, even for short periods of time, with a mature biofilter. Difficulties can also arise in a hospital setting as ideally the tank should be emptied, dried and disinfected between patients and the filtration media completely replaced to minimise the risk of spread of pathogens between patients.

Many serious Koi hobbyists will have their own quarantine tank set up for new acquisitions and in most cases this can be converted to a hospital tank if necessary. This solution also has the advantage that the animal's home pond water can be used to fill the tank, and filtration media discarded after the tank has housed an animal with an infectious disease can be replaced from the main pond filtration unit.

22.7 Common Water Quality Issues

There are a huge number of potential water quality issues that can have an impact of the health of fish in a pond system. Derangements of nitrogenous waste levels, rapid temperature fluctuations, heavy metal contaminations, and horticultural run off can all alter water chemistry. A full discussion of water quality issues is beyond the scope of this chapter, however many excellent resources that cover the topic in more detail are listed in the further reading section. The following subsections cover a few of the most commonly encountered water quality issues in Koi pond systems.

22.7.1 Ammonia Toxicity

Ammonia toxicity generally occurs in systems where there are insufficient bacteria present to convert ammonia to nitrite, either because the system is immature (also known as 'new tank syndrome') or because bacteria have been removed through inappropriate cleaning regimes or use of antibacterial medications (Roberts and Palmeiro 2008). High environmental ammonia causes pathology in two ways; first by direct irritation of the gill tissue which causes hyperplastic changes to the branchial arches, decreased diffusion of oxygen across the gill epithelium, with a resulting hypoxia; second by decreasing passive excretion of ammonia across the gills and therefore increasing tissue ammonia concentrations, resulting in increased tissue oxygen consumption, increased blood pH, and disruption of osmoregulation. These biochemical changes manifest as symptoms of respiratory distress (such as gasping at the water surface and gathering near points of increased water aeration), lethargy, anorexia, and mortalities. Skin and fin disease may develop secondary to chronic stress (Svobodová et al. 1993).

High environmental ammonia should be addressed with frequent water changes of 30% to 50% of the total pond volume and by adding zeolite, a chemical which acts as an ammonia sink. Zeolite should only be used as a short-term measure as zeolite left in the pond will eventually start to discharge the ammonia back into the water. Ammonia is released from the zeolite by placing it in saltwater, meaning that sodium chloride should not be added to the pond if using zeolite as an ammonia sink. Other supportive measures for the fish that should be considered include decreased feeding in order to minimise further waste production in the short term, and additional water aeration to help combat hypoxia (Roberts and Palmeiro 2008).

22.7.2 Nitrite Toxicity

Nitrite toxicity is frequently seen in new tank syndrome alongside ammonia toxicity as the biofilter starts to mature. High environmental nitrite levels lead to absorption of nitrite across the gills, where it oxidises haemoglobin to methhaemoglobin (Svobodová et al. 1993). As methhaemoglobin cannot transport oxygen, the primary clinical signs of nitrite toxicity will be due to hypoxia. On clinical examination the brown colour of methhaemoglobin may cause gills to have pale tan or brown appearance. Treatment of nitrite toxicity is similar to ammonia toxicity as it relies primarily on frequent water changes and increasing water aeration whilst the biofilter matures. Addition of sodium chloride increases active transport of nitrite out of the blood across the gills (Roberts and Palmeiro 2008). If both high ammonia and nitrite are present then either zeolite or sodium chloride treatment can be given depending on the clinician's primary concern, but both treatments cannot be given together.

High environmental nitrate is rarely a problem in and of itself as it is the least toxic of the nitrogenous waste products, although eggs and fry may be more sensitive. Instead, nitrate is primarily an issue where it contributes to excessive plant and algal growth and subsequent alterations in oxygen levels.

22.7.3 Low Oxygen Saturation

Although plant life can increase water oxygen saturation through photosynthesis, it should be remembered that plants will respire when there is no sunlight. This can lead to depletion of oxygen overnight to fatally low levels. This phenomenon largely occurs in the summer months when plant life is at its peak and water temperatures are higher, as oxygen saturation of water decreases with increasing temperature (Svobodová et al. 1993). Clinical signs often include overnight mortality of the largest individuals in the pond, animals gathering at points of increased water aeration (e.g. fountains) early in the day, and secondary signs of chronic stress such as skin and fin disease. Water oxygen concentration can be measured using commercially available kits and should ideally be tested at sunrise, then at multiple points over the day to demonstrate rising levels. Treatment involves removing excessive planting and decreasing algae levels, which may be difficult to achieve. Supportive care involves increasing water aeration, particularly overnight, and decreasing stocking densities if possible.

22.7.4 Gas Supersaturation

Heavy algal growth can also less commonly result in gas supersaturation of the water, following excessive oxygen production on hot sunny days. This can also occur where air is forced into water under high pressure and may result from particularly forceful waterfall features or faulty pumps (Boyd 1998). Nitrogen supersaturation is more common than oxygen supersaturation, but is still rare. When fish absorb supersaturated gases from the water, gas bubble disease may occur, where gas emboli form in the fishes' tissue and/or circulation (Boyd 1998). Gas emboli in the eyes are the most commonly recognised symptom. Treatment involves decreasing gas saturation of the water, preventing access of fish to waterfalls or other water features which may cause localised supersaturation of the water, and allowing the fish to reabsorb the gas emboli over time.

22.8 Common Conditions

22.8.1 Skin Trauma

Fish skin is highly susceptible to trauma, both physical and due to poor water quality, and so Koi will commonly be presented to the veterinary clinic showing signs of dermatological disease (Hunt 2006). Physical examination, water quality assessment, impression smears, and skin scrapes are all important in diagnosing the underlying cause of skin disease. Simple trauma cases should be treated before secondary issues can arise. The skin in all fish species has an important role in osmoregulation and breaches can lead to loss of electrolytes and considerable metabolic stress. Aquatic 'bandages' such as commercially available human mouth ulcer gels or Misoprostol/Phenytoin gels (Clarke 2016) can be used to protect trauma sites, both preventing dysregulation of osmosis and protecting against secondary infections. Addition of sodium chloride to the water at a dose of 1–3 mg/l can also help to decrease osmotic stress in these cases (Wangen 2012).

22.8.2 Ectoparasites

The most common ectoparasite of freshwater fish, including Koi, is the protozoan parasite *Ichthyophthirius multifiliis*, commonly known as 'Ich' or white spot disease (Roberts et al. 2009).

I. multifiliis is often carried asymptomatically and only becomes a clinical concern at times of increased stress. Clinical signs include small white spots, evidence of skin irritation such as 'flashing', where fish rub their flanks along the pond bottom and the upper scales catch the sun or 'flash', or leaping from the water, and secondary bacterial and fungal infections. Diagnosis is based on clinical signs of skin irritation and demonstration of the parasites on skin scrapes or impression smears. *I. multifiliis* is only susceptible to treatment in its free-swimming theront life stage and the speed of the lifecycle is temperature dependant, taking between three and six days at 25 °C, 10 days at 15 °C, and up to 28 days at 10 °C (Noga 2010). Therefore treatment should be given multiple times at 5–10 day intervals until no further clinical cases are seen for at least two treatments.

Other common ectoparasites include *Argulus spp.* ('fish lice') (Figure 22.5), *Lernea spp.* ('anchor worm'), *Gyrodactylus spp.* ('skin flukes') and *Dactylogyrus spp.* ('gill flukes'). All cause signs of skin irritation and can result in secondary bacterial and fungal disease. *Dactylogyrus spp.* also cause signs of respiratory distress (see later), and can be diagnosed on gill clips or impression smears. *Argulus spp.* and *Lernea spp.* may be seen with the naked eye and physically removed using fine forceps, whilst *Gyrodactylus spp.* is generally diagnosed via skin scrapes or impression smears (Roberts et al. 2009). The main chemical treatments for *Argulus spp.* and *Lernea spp.*, organophosphates, are now banned in the UK for treatment of fish, making control difficult (Wildgoose 2001). Improving water quality and decreasing stressors to improve overall fish health and decrease the incidence of secondary bacterial and fungal infections are the mainstays

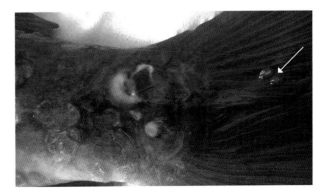

Figure 22.5 Ulcerative lesions (red arrow) associated with *Argulus* spp. infestation (white arrow).

of managing these parasites. Commonly used anti-parasite treatments for *Gyrodactylus spp.*, *Dactylogyrus spp.* and other parasites are summarised in the formulary.

22.8.3 Bacterial Skin Disease

Bacterial infection of skin often occurs secondary to skin trauma or a chronic disease process which causes physiological stress and decreases innate immunity of the skin. Bacterial skin disease most frequently presents as ulcerative skin disease (termed ulcerative dermatitis of Koi) (Figure 22.6) or 'fin-rot' type lesions (Figure 22.7) (Roberts et al. 2009), however the bacteria *Flavobacterium columnare* causes a cotton-wool like growth which is found around the mouth and often mistaken for fungal disease (Wildgoose 2001).

The organisms involved in bacterial skin disease are often opportunistic pathogens found as commensals in the aquatic environment. This makes culture results difficult to interpret as there is also a high risk of environmental contamina-

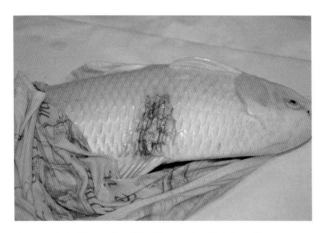

Figure 22.6 Ulcerative Skin Disease in a Koi Carp (*Source:* Photo courtesy of Emily Hall MRCVS).

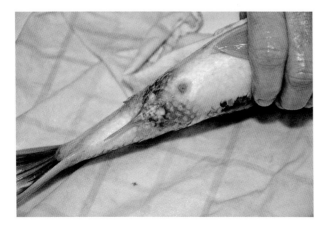

Figure 22.7 Ulceration of the anal fin, colloquially known as 'fin rot' (*Source:* Photo courtesy of Emily Hall MRCVS).

tion during sample collection. Culture is still recommended and treatment should be based on sensitivity testing and concurrently addressing any underlying causes of disease. Skin scrapes or impression smears are also useful to demonstrate the presence of high numbers of bacteria and inflammatory responses at a lesion site, and identify the morphology of those bacteria to help support culture results. Commonly isolated bacterial organisms of pond fish include *Aermonas spp.*, *Pseudomonas spp.*, and *F. columnare* (Wildgoose 2001; Roberts et al. 2009).

22.8.4 Fungal Skin Disease

Similar to bacterial infection, fungal infections of the skin generally occur secondary to skin trauma, where there is a break in the skin barrier which allows colonisation of spores, or poor skin health due to chronic stress from another factor. Samples from fungal lesions should be collected via either skin scrape or impression smears. *Saprolegnia* spp. are the most commonly isolated fungal pathogens of Koi and the main differential is *F. columnare,* as described earlier (Hook et al. 2001). Cytological differentiation of the long bacilli of *F. columnare* from the non-septate hyphae of *Saprolegnia* spp. should always be performed before starting treatment.

Branchiomyces spp. are fungal pathogens that primarily target the gills, causing the presentation known colloquially as 'gill rot'. Cyprinid fish such as Koi appear particularly affected, although infections in many other species have been reported. Ponds are usually endemically infected and disease occurs when water temperature rises above 20 °C. Clinical signs include respiratory distress and pale, necrotic gills on examination (Svobodová et al. 1993). It is extremely difficult to eradicate *Branchiomyces* spp. once a pond has become infected. Strict biosecurity to avoid introduction in the first instance is advisable. If infection is present then careful monitoring of water temperature to allow prediction of high risk periods, control of organic waste (reducing build-up of rotting vegetation, reducing stocking density etc.), and treatment with in-water antifungal agents are indicated. Commonly used antifungal agents are summarised in the formulary. Extended courses of treatment may be necessary.

22.8.5 Exopthalmos

Exophthalmos is a non-specific change commonly referred to as 'pop-eye' by hobbyists. Bilateral exophthalmos usually indicates a systemic condition, e.g. retrobulbar oedema or gas bubble formation, commonly as a result of

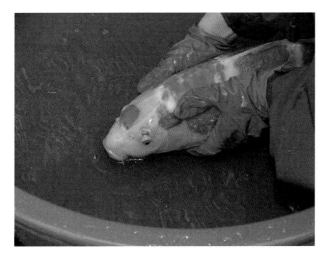

Figure 22.8 Exophthalmos in a Kohaku Koi (*Source:* Photo courtesy of Emily Hall MRCVS).

gas supersaturation (see earlier). Unilateral exophthalmos (Figure 22.8) is more indicative of a localised infection or neoplastic process. Full clinical examination including direct ophthalmoscopy and ocular ultrasonography are indicated in cases of exophthalmos. Treatment will be dependent on the underlying cause, and enucleation may need to be considered in severe cases.

22.8.6 Ocular Trauma

Eye trauma and corneal ulceration often occur in tandem. Similar to approaches in domestic species, fluorescein staining and direct ophthalmoscopy allow the veterinary surgeon to characterise ulcers and target treatment effectively. Treatment can be difficult as topical treatments are quickly removed once the animal is replaced back in the water. Instead in-water treatment can be utilised in these cases. Fish should be hospitalised in a separate tank and water quality monitored extremely closely to prevent further damage to the cornea. Sodium chloride can be added to the water to minimise the development of corneal oedema and antibiotics added directly to the water to prevent infection of the damaged cornea.

22.8.7 Abdominal Distension

Abdominal distension is a non-specific finding which can indicate a wide range of potential pathologies including, amongst others, ascites, reproductive pathology, neoplasia, and swim bladder pathology. Conservative management is almost never effective in these cases, and further investigation is highly recommended. Imaging, including radiography and ultrasonography, fine needle aspirates for cytology

and/or culture of abdominal or swimbladder fluid, and exploratory coeliotomy will help narrow the differential list and guide appropriate treatment. Some of the most common causes of abdominal distension are described in more detail in the following subsecions.

22.8.7.1 Ascites

Ascites can result from a wide range of conditions including cardiac, hepatic, renal, and reproductive pathologies. Radiographs will show poor soft tissue delineation within the coelomic cavity and ultrasonography will reveal the presence of free fluid. Ultrasound guided aspiration of ascitic fluid may be useful for cytological examination and culture and sensitivity testing. Often exploratory coeliotomy will be necessary for diagnosis. Prognosis is dependent on the underlying condition, but is often guarded in cases where major body systems are involved due to a lack of suitable and easily administered treatment options in fish species.

22.8.7.2 Reproductive Pathology

Tumours of both the male and female reproductive tract can be found in Koi species and surgical removal of some ovarian tumours has been described (Raidal et al. 2006; Lewisch et al. 2014; Vergneau-Grosset et al. 2017). Other disorders of the female reproductive tract include 'egg binding', failure to release eggs into the environment resulting in distension of the abdomen (Figure 22.9), and ovarian rupture. Spawning can be induced in carp species using a single injection of GnRH superactive analogue combined with metoclopramide (Drori et al. 1994), or two injections of Carp Pituitary Extract given 12 hours apart (Brzuska and Bialowas 2002). Egg peritonitis of carp is not reported in the literature but has been seen by the author at post-mortem examination.

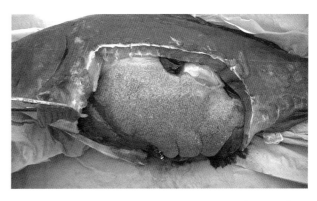

Figure 22.9 Post-mortem examination of a gravid Common Carp.

22.8.7.3 Swimbladder Disorders

Inappropriate buoyancy, both positive (floating) and negative (sinking) are common reasons for Koi hobbyists presenting their animals to the veterinary clinic. Swimbladder conditions are difficult to treat and rarely respond to conservative management, particularly if the underlying cause has not been identified.

Differential diagnoses for increased buoyancy include infection of the swimbladder with gas-producing bacteria or anatomical abnormalities that prevent gas being released from the swimbladder. Radiography of these cases will show a large, gas-filled structure in the dorsal portion of the coelomic cavity. A small amount of sterile saline can be instilled into the swim bladder then aspirated to provide a sample for culture and sensitivity testing. Aspirating some of the gas will provide temporary relief whilst waiting for culture results or initiating treatment. Systemic antibiotic therapy can be coupled with topical application of antibiotics directly into the swimbladder in cases of bacterial infection. Koi carp are physostomous, meaning that the swim bladder is connected to the oesophagus by the pneumatic duct (Stoskopf 1993a). This allows the fish to add and remove air from the swimbladder via the oesophagus. Koi also possess a gas gland, or rete mirabile, which allows gas to be added to the swimbladder from dissolved gases in the blood stream (Stoskopf 1993a). Disorders of either of these anatomical features can lead to altered gas exchange in the swimbladder and resultant overinflation with a poor long-term prognosis.

Decreased buoyancy most often occurs as a result of fluid accumulation within the swimbladder due to an infectious agent. Radiography of these cases will show reduced or even no gas within the dorsal aspect of the coelomic cavity. Ultrasound guided aspiration of fluid for cytological and culture and sensitivity testing will guide treatment. Temporary relief may be given using buoyancy aids, often pieces of cork fitted to a harness, which allow the fish to float in the water column and avoid trauma associated with an extended period resting on the bottom of the tank, however resolution of the underlying cause of fluid accumulation is difficult and long-term prognosis is poor. Other causes of decreased buoyancy, for example abdominal neoplasia impinging on the swimbladder and reducing its volume, also carry a poor prognosis.

22.8.8 Neoplasia

Various neoplasms have been reported in Koi, including papilloma (Wildgoose 1992), squamous cell carcinoma (Wildgoose 1992), chromatophoroma (Murchelano and Edwards 1981), neuroblastoma (Ishikawa et al. 1978), ovarian tumours (Raidal et al. 2006; Lewisch et al. 2014), seminoma (Vergneau-Grosset et al. 2017), and leiomyoma (Vergneau-Grosset et al. 2016).

Many fish will not show any signs of discomfort even with significant tumour development, meaning animals are often not presented to a vet until disease has reached advanced stages. In cases of cutaneous neoplasia, surgical removal is indicated if possible (Figure 22.10). However the inelastic nature of fish skin means large deficits will often remain following removal of large tumours which can cause further issues with osmoregulation and secondary infections. Treatment as for trauma cases can help reduce post-operative complications in these cases. Internal tumours often present as abdominal swelling and require imaging such as radiography, ultrasonography, or computed tomography to diagnose their presence. Exploratory laparotomy and surgical removal have been reported for internal neoplasms, primarily ovarian tumours (Raidal et al. 2006; Lewisch et al. 2014).

Koi are also susceptible to cyprinid herpesvirus which causes carp pox, a benign, virus-induced epidermal neoplasm (Sano et al. 1985). Carp pox appears as smooth, white, raised lesions (Figure 22.11) which are said to resemble drops of candle wax. Lesions typically regress spontaneously once water temperatures rise above 20C and mortality is generally low (Harshbarger 2001), however cyprinid herpesvirus-3 appears to be more pathogenic at higher and variable water temperatures and can cause significant mass mortality events (Takahara et al. 2014).

22.8.9 Notifiable Diseases within the UK

The Fish Health Inspectorate (FHI) lists eight diseases as notifiable in the UK, of which two can affect Koi carp; Spring Viraemia of Carp (SVC) and Koi Herpesvirus (KHV). SVC is caused by the viral agent *Rhabdovirus carpio*. Clinical signs include petechial haemorrhages of the skin, gills and eyes, pale gills, exophthalmos, swelling of the vent, ascites, and lethargy, and mortality can reach 100%. Outbreaks generally occur when water temperatures increase above 5 °C and mortality decreases as temperatures rise above 17–20 °C. Diagnosis is via PCR or virus isolation and there is no known treatment (Ahne et al. 2002).

The causative agent of KHV is Cyprinid Herpesvirus-3, a highly contagious herpes virus which can cause up to 100% mortality. Clinical signs include anorexia, lethargy, necrotic patches on the gills, pale skin patches, and erratic swimming. On histopathology intranuclear inclusion bodies are present in the gill epithelium. Diagnosis

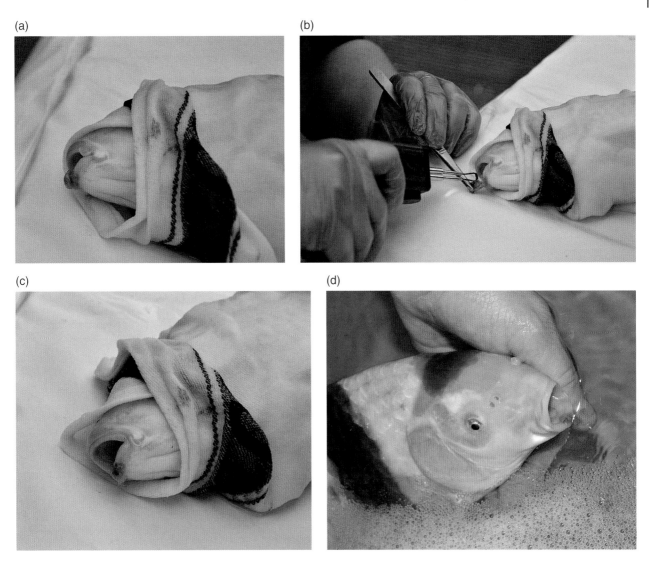

Figure 22.10   (a) Rostral mass in a Koi Carp prior to surgery. (b) The mass is excised. (c) Immediately post-surgery. The surgical wound is left open to heal by secondary intention healing. (d) Three days post-surgery. The wound is healing rapidly (*Source:* Photos courtesy of Emily Hall MRCVS).

is by PCR and there is no known treatment (Pokorova et al. 2005).

22.9 Euthanasia

Humane anaesthesia is a controversial topic in aquatic medicine. For many years standards of euthanasia have been extremely poor, often not involving any veterinary input. There is currently no specific legislation relating to the slaughter of fish for food in the UK as they are not included under The Welfare of Animals at the Time of Killing Regulations for England, Wales, Scotland, or Northern Ireland, which were developed to satisfy EU council regulation (EC) No 1099/2009 on the protection of animals at the time of killing. EC No. 1099/2009 states that '... *as regards fish, only the requirements laid down in Article 3(1) shall apply .... Animals shall be spared any avoidable pain, distress or suffering during their killing and related operations*'.

The only UK legislation regarding the slaughter of fish comes under Schedule 1 of the Animals (Scientific Procedures) Act 1986, which outlines the following methods as suitable for the humane killing of fish:

- Overdose of an anaesthetic agent
- Concussion of the brain by striking the cranium, with destruction of the brain before regaining consciousness

(a)

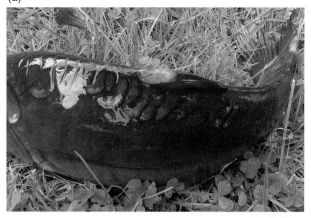

(b)

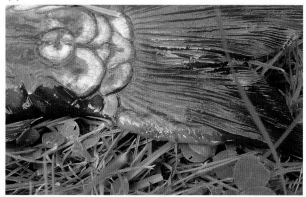

Figure 22.11 (a) Cyprinid herpesvirus lesions in a mirror carp. (b) Cyprinid herpesvirus lesions in a mirror carp.

Humane methods for the euthanasia of fish according to the American Veterinary Medical Association's Guidelines for the Euthanasia of Animals (Leary et al. 2013) include:

- Overdose with an anaesthetic agent
- Blunt force trauma followed by pithing (although this is not considered acceptable in a veterinary setting)
- Decapitation
- Rapid cooling below the lethal threshold in fish <3.8 cm in length.

In the UK euthanasia can be carried out by owners at home using 2-phenoxyethanol (Aquased™). The author recommends using the stated dose on the datasheet (2–2.8 ml/l) and leaving fish in the anaesthetic solution for a minimum of 30 minutes following cessation of opercular movement. After this fish should be immediately placed in a freezer for at least 12 hours to ensure complete destruction of brain tissue prior to disposal. In a veterinary setting, fish should be fully anaesthetised using whichever method is preferred by the veterinary surgeon, then pithed to ensure destruction of brain tissue prior to disposal. It should be noted that a study in goldfish by Balko et al. (2016), there were high recovery rates in fish 'euthanased' with in-water anaesthetic agents following placement in fresh water (85–100% survival using three treatment regimens), and therefore destruction of the brain via pithing should be considered an essential part of euthanasia in all fish following loss on consciousness.

Formulary of selected drugs for Koi carp

Agent	Route	Dose	Notes	References
Anaesthetics				
2-phenoxyethanol	Immersion	0.5–0.7 ml/l (500–700 ppm)	Available under the small animal exemption scheme. For SAES products follow manufacturer guidelines.	Vetark Professional; AquaSed (Vetark 2017a)
Alfaxalone	Immersion	10 mg/l (induction) 2.5 mg/l (maintenance)	2.5 mg/l maintains adequate depth of anaesthesia for surgery but may result in respiratory depression.	Minter et al. (2014)
Eugenol	Immersion	25 mg/l (25 ppm)	Hydrophobic; use a narrow gauge needle to help disperse in water.	Endo et al. (1972)
Isoflurane	Immersion	0.4–0.75 ml/l (induction) 0.25 ml/l (maintenance)	Hydrophobic; use a narrow gauge needle to help disperse in water. Health and safety considerations regarding scavenging of waste gases.	Stetter (2001)
Propofol	Immersion	5 mg/l (induction)	Maintenance of anaesthesia using propofol is associated with prolonged recovery times.	Oda et al. (2014)
Tricaine methanesulphonate (MS-222)	Immersion	20–30 mg/l (sedation) 30–200 mg/l (anaesthesia)	Addition of MS-22 to water can significantly decrease water pH. The pH of the anaesthetic solution should be measured prior to induction and sodium bicarbonate used to buffer the solution if necessary.	Popovic et al. (2011); Pharmaq (2013); R. Killick (personal communication)

(Continued)

Agent	Route	Dose	Notes	References
Antibiotics				
Acriflavine	In-water, topical	4–10 mg/l reported for various species	Available under the small animal exemption scheme. For SAES products follow manufacturer guidelines.	Waddell et al. (1990); Plakas et al. (1998)
Amikacin	Intramuscular, intracoelomic	5 mg/kg IM q72hr × 3		Wildgoose and Lewbart (2001)
Ceftazidine	Intramuscular	20 mg/kg IM q72hr		Roberts et al. (2009)
Chloramine-T	In-water	1 mg/l	Available under the small animal exemption scheme. For SAES products follow manufacturer guidelines.	Vetark Professional: Chloramine-T (Vetark 2017b)
Ciprofloxacin	Intravenous, intramuscular	15 mg/kg		Nouws et al. (1988)
Enrofloxacin	Intracoelomic, per os	5–10 mg/kg ICe q5d 10 mg/kg PO		Lewbart et al. (2005) Fan et al. (2017)
Florfenicol	Intramuscular, per os	25 mg/kg IM q24hr 50 mg/kg PO q24hr	Immersion treatment shown to be ineffective	Yanong et al. (2005)
Methylene blue	Immersion	2 mg/l q48hr for × 3	Immersion treatment for the prevention of infection of fish eggs. Available under the small animal exemption scheme. For SAES products follow manufacturer guidelines.	Noga (2010)
Oxytetracycline	Intramuscular	60 mg/kg IM q7d	Poorly available when given orally in carp species so oral route not recommended.	Grondel et al. (1987)
Potassium permanganate	Immersion	2 mg/l prolonged bath 5 mg/l bath for 30–60 minutes	Available under the small animal exemption scheme. For SAES products follow manufacturer guidelines.	Noga (2010)
Trimathoprim/ sulfamethoxazole	Immersion, per os, intracoelomic	25 mg/l for 6–12 hr bath 50 mg/kg in food q24hr × 10 days 50 mg/kg ICe q24hr × 7 treatments		Noga (2010)
Antifungals				
Bronopol	In water	50 mg/l for 30 minutes (eggs) 20 mg/l q24hr for 14 days (fish)	Licenced for use in Atlantic Salmon and Rainbow trout in the UK, no specific carp doses available.	Elanco Animal Health:Pyceze
Formalin	In water	1500–7500 µl/l 45 minute bath EOD (eggs) 0–400 mg/l flush q48hr (eggs)	Available under the small animal exemption scheme. For SAES products follow manufacturer guidelines. Do not use within 24 hours of hatching. Additional oxygenation of water necessary during treatment of adult fish. Idiopathic deaths may occur after treatment. Do not use if white precipitate (paraformaldehyde) present.	Rach et al. (1997) Khodabandeh and Abtahi (2006)
Hydrogen peroxide	In water	0–6000 µl/l q24hr for 15 days (eggs)	Licenced formulation for the treatment of Sea Lice in Atlantic Salmon available in the UK.	Rach et al. (1998)

(Continued)

(Continued)

Agent	Route	Dose	Notes	References
Itraconazole	Oral/in feed	1–5 mg/kg q24hr in feed q1–7d		Stoskopf (1999)
Ketoconazole	Per os, intramuscular, intracoelomic	2.5–10 mg/kg		Stoskopf (1999)
Malachite green	In water	0.1 mg/l indefinite bath 0.2 mg/l 1 hr bath 67 mg/l 1 minute bath	Available under the small animal exemption scheme. For SAES products follow manufacturer guidelines. CARE: Carcinogenic, mutagenic, respiratory toxin. See Srivastava et al. 2004 for further details.	Noga (2010)
Sodium Chloride	In water	25 000–45 000 mg/l flush BID (eggs)		Khodabandeh and Abtahi (2006)
Antiparasitics				
Chloramine-T	In-water	1 mg/l	Protozoan parasites Available under the small animal exemption scheme. For SAES products follow manufacturer guidelines.	Vetark Professional: Chloramine-T (Vetark 2017b)
Closantel	In water	0.125 mg/l in combination with 0.1875 mg/l mebendazole, once.	Monogenean parasites Available as a combined product licenced for use in sheep in the UK. Equates to 1 ml per 400 L.	Marshall (1999)
Doramectin	Oral, intramuscular	750 µg/kg PO 150 µg/kg IM	Crustacean parasites	Hemaprasanth et al. (2012)
Emamectin benzoate	In water	56ug/1000 L	Crustacean parasites Available under the small animal exemption scheme. For SAES products follow manufacturer guidelines.	Vetark Professional: Lice Solve (Vetark 2017d)
Fenbendazole	In water, oral	2 mg/l q7 days for 3 treatments 50 mg/kg PO q7 days for two treatments 25 mg/l for 12 hr	Nematode parasites (non-encysted) Monogenean parasites	Noga (2010)
Formalin	In water	0.125–0.25 mg/l for 60 min q24hr for 2–3 treatments	Protozoan and metazoan ectoparasites. Available under the small animal exemption scheme. For SAES products follow manufacturer guidelines. Additional oxygenation of water necessary during treatment of adult fish. Idiopathic deaths may occur after treatment. Do not use if white precipitate (paraformaldehyde) present.	Noga (2010)
Formalin/malachite green	In water	25 ppm formalin +0.1 mg/l malachite green	Protozoan ectoparasites Available under the small animal exemption scheme. For SAES products follow manufacturer guidelines.	Noga (2010)

(Continued)

Agent	Route	Dose	Notes	References
Hydrogen peroxide	In water	17.5 mL/l 4 – 10 minute dip once	Ectoparasites Care with smaller fish. Licenced formulation for the treatment of Sea Lice in Atlantic Salmon available in the UK.	Harms (1996)
Ivermectin			**DO NOT USE**	
Levamisole	Oral, intramuscular, in water	10 mg/kg PO q 7 days × 3	Internal nematodes	Harms (1996)
		11 mg/kg IM q 7 days × 2	Internal nematodes	
		1–2 ppm 24 h bath	Internal nematodes	
		50 ppm 2 h bath	External trematodes	
Lufenuron	In water	0.1–0.2 mg/l prolonged immersion	Crustacean parasites	Roberts et al. (2009)
Malachite green	In water	0.1 mg/l indefinite bath 0.2 mg/l 1 hr bath 67 mg/l 1 minute bath	Protozoan ectoparasites Available under the small animal exemption scheme. For SAES products follow manufacturer guidelines. CARE: Carcinogenic, mutagenic, respiratory toxin. See Srivastava et al. 2004 for further details.	Noga (2010)
Mebendazole	In water	0.1875 mg/l in combination with 0.125 mg/l Closantel once.	Monogenean parasites Available as a combined product licenced for use in sheep in the UK. Equates to 1 ml per 400 L.	Marshall (1999)
Methylene blue	In water	1–3 mg/l	Ectoparasites Available under the small animal exemption scheme. For SAES products follow manufacturer guidelines.	Noga (2010)
Metronidazole	Oral, in water	50 mg/kg PO q 24 h × 5 days 7–15 mg/l q24–48 hr for 5–10 days. Change 50% water between treatments	Protozoal flagellates	Harms (1996) Roberts et al. (2009)
Potassium permanganate	In water	5 mg/l 30–60 minutes bath 100 mg/l 5–10 min bath 1 g/l 10–40 second bath	Protozoan and crustacean parasites. **Do not use in ponds containing goldfish – risk of toxicity.** Available under the small animal exemption scheme. For SAES products follow manufacturer guidelines.	Noga (2010)

(Continued)

(Continued)

Agent	Route	Dose	Notes	References
Praziquantel	In water, oral	1 mg/l 90 hour exposure	Flukes and tapeworms	Székely and Molnár (1991)
		2 mg/l minimum 24 hour exposure q3 weeks × 2 treatments	Available under the small animal exemption scheme. For SAES products follow manufacturer guidelines.	Vetark Professional: Fluke Solve (Vetark 2017c)
		10 mg/l 1 hr exposure		Szekely and Molnar (1991)
		50 mg/kg PO once		Noga (2010)
Sodium chloride	In water	1–5 g/l prolonged exposure	Ectoparasites	Noga (2010)
		10 g/l up to 30 minute bath	Available under the small animal exemption scheme. For SAES products follow manufacturer guidelines.	Lewbart (1998)
		30–35 g/l 4–5 minute bath		Noga (2010)
Miscellaneous				
Adrenaline (1 : 1000)	Intravenous, intracoelomic, intramuscular	0.2–0.5 ml/kg	Cardiovascular collapse	Hadfield et al. (2007); Sherrill et al. (2009)
Atropine	Intravenous, intracoelomic, intramuscular	0.03 mg/kg	Bradycardia	Hadfield et al. (2007)
		0.1 mg/kg	Organophosphate toxicity	Stoskopf (1993b)
Carbon (activated)	In filter	—	Available as filter media, use as directed by the manufacturer.	—
Carp Pituitary Extract	Intramuscular	0.3 mg/kg first injection, 2.7 mg/kg second injection given 12 hr apart		Brzuska and Bialowas (2002)
Dexmethasone	Intravenous, intracoelomic	1–2 mg/kg	May improve prognosis in shock, trauma, chronic stress or toxicity issues.	Lewbart (1998) Sherrill et al. (2009)
Doxapram	Intravenous, intracoelomic, intramuscular	5 mg/kg	Respiratory depression. May also be applied topically to the gills.	Hadfield et al. (2007)
Furosemide	Intracoelomic, intramuscular	2–5 mg/kg	Ascites or generalised oedema. Fish do not possess a loop of Henle so questionable efficacy.	Sherrill et al. (2009)
Human chorionic gonadotrophin	Intramucular	400–2000 IU	Poor spawning response in carp even at doses >2000 IU	Yaron et al. (2009)
Hydrogen peroxide	In water	0.25 ml/l 3% solution for 10 min	Acute environmental hypoxia	Sherrill et al. (2009)
Lidocaine	Intravenous	1–2 mg/kg	Cardiac arrhythmias	Sherrill et al. (2009)
Metoclopramide	Intramuscular	20 mg/kg metoclopramide +10 µg/kg sGnRHa	Induction of spawning in common carp	Drori et al. (1994)
Nitrifying bacteria	In water	—	Available as a commercial product to start of filter maturation.	—

(Continued)

Agent	Route	Dose	Notes	References
Oxygen	In water	—	Bubble 100% oxygen through water in cases of hypoxia.	—
salmon gonadotropin-releasing hormone (sGnRHa)	Intracoelomic, intramuscular	10 µg/kg sGnRHa +20 mg/kg metoclopramide	Induction of spawning in common carp. Commercial product available in USA	Drori et al. (1994)
Sodium Chloride	In water	1–3 mg/l continuous bath	To decrease osmotic stress.	Wangen (2012)
Sodium thiosulfate	In water	7–10 mg/l continuous bath	Treatment of chlorine toxicity Available under the small animal exemption scheme as a chlorine/chloramine neutraliser. For SAES products follow manufacturer guidelines.	Hadfield et al. (2007)
Zeolite	In water	—	Commercially available ion exchange resin used to neutralise ammonia. Use as directed by the manufacturer.	—

References

Ahne, W., Bjorklund, H.V., Essbauer, S. et al. (2002). Spring viremia of carp (SVC). *Diseases of Aquatic Organisms* 52: 261–272.

Balko, J.A., Oda, A., and Posner, L.P. (2016). Immersion euthanasia of Goldfish (Carassius auratus). In: *Proceedings of the 47th IAAAM Conference,* Virginia Aquarium. The International Association for Aquatic Animal Medicine.

Boyd, C.E. (1998). Water Quality for Pond Aquaculture, *Research and Development Series No 43 for International Centre for Aquaculture and Aquatic Environments.*

Brzuska, E. and Bialowas, H. (2002). Artifical spawning of carp, *Cyprinus carpio* (L.). *Aquaculture Research* 33: 753–765.

Clarke, E.O. III (2016). Topical Application of Misoprostol and Phenytoin Gel for Treatment of Dermal Ulceration in Teleosts. In: *Proceedings of the 47th IAAAM Conference, Virginia Aquarium.* The International Association for Aquatic Animal Medicine.

Corcoran, M. and Roberts-Sweeney, H. (2014). Aquatic animal nutrition for the exotic animal practitioner. *Veterinary Clinics of North America: Exotic Animal Practice* 17 (3): 333–346.

Drori, S., Ofir, M., Levavi-Sivan, B. et al. (1994). Spawning induction in common carp (*Cyprinus carpio*) using pituitary extract or GnRH superactive analogue combined with metoclopramide: analysis of hormone profile, progress of oocyte maturation and dependence on temperature. *Aquaculture* 119 (4): 393–407.

Elanco Animal Health (2017). Pyceze. www. noahcompendium.

co.uk/?id=-463419&fromsearch=true#iosfirsthighlight (accessed 30 December 2018).

Endo, T., Kenji, O., Hisashi, T. et al. (1972). Studies on the anesthetic effect of eugenol in some fresh water fishes. *Nippon Suisan Gakkaishi* 38 (7): 761–767.

Fan, J., Shan, Q., Wang, J. et al. (2017). Comparative pharmacokinetics of enrofloxacin in healthy and Aeromonashydrophila-infected crucian carp (*Carassius auratus gibelio*). *Journal of Veterinary Pharmacology and Therapeutics* 40: 580–582.

Grondel, J.L., Nous, J.F.M., De Jong, M. et al. (1987). Pharmacokinetics and tissue distribution of oxytetracycline in carp, *Cyprinus carpio* L., following different routes of administration. *Journal of Fish Diseases* 10 (3): 153–163.

Hadfield, C.A., Whitaker, B.R., and Clayton, L.A. (2007). Emergency and critical care of fish. *Veterinary Clinics of North America: Exotic Animal Practice* 10: 647–675.

Harms, C.A. (1996). Treatments for parasitic diseases of aquarium and ornamental fish. *Seminars in Avian and Exotic Pet Medicine* 5 (2): 54–63.

Harms, C.A., Lewbark, G.A., Swanson, C.R. et al. (2005). Behavioral and clinical pathology changes in Koi Carp (*Cyprinus carpio*) subjected to anesthesia and surgery with and without intra-operative analgesics. *Comparative Medicine* 55 (3): 221–226.

Harshbarger, J.C. (2001). Neoplasia and developmental anomalies. In: *BSAVA Manual of Ornamental Fish*, 2e (ed. W.H. Wildgoose), 219–224. Gloucester, UK: British Small Animal Veterinary Association.

Hecker, B.G. (1993). Carp, Koi, and goldfish taxonomy and natural history. In: *Fish Medicine* (ed. M.K. Stoskopf), 442–447. Philadelphia: WB Saunders.

Hemaprasanth, K.P., Kar, B., Garnayak, S.K. et al. (2012). Efficacy of doramectin against natural and experimental infections of Lernaea cyprinacea in carps. *Veterinary Parasitology* 190: 297–304.

Hook, D., Bucke, D., Burgess, P. et al. (2001). Infectious diseases – viruses, bacteria and fungi. In: *Diseases of Carp and Other Cyprinid Fishes* (eds. D. Hoole, D. Bucke, P. Burgess, et al.), 43–62. Oxford: Fishing News Books.

Hunt, C.J.G. (2006). Ulcerative skin disease in a Group of Koi Carp (*Cyprinus carpio*). *Veterinary Clinics of North America Exotic Small Animal Practice* 9: 723–728.

Ishikawa, T., Masahito, P., and Takayama, S. (1978). Olfactory Neuroepithelioma in a domestic carp (*Cyprinus carpio*). *Cancer Research.* 38 (11): 3954–3959.

Khodabandeh, S. and Abtahi, B. (2006). Effects of sodium chloride, formalin, and iodine on the hatching success of common carp (*Cyprinus carpio*) eggs. *Journal of Applied Ichthyology* 22: 54–56.

Leary, S., Underwood, W., Anthony, R. et al. (2013). *AVMA Guidelines for the Euthanasia of Animals: 2013 Edition.* Schaumburg, IL: American Veterinary Medical Association.

Lewbart, G.A. (1998). Emergency and critical care of fish. *Veterinary Clinics of North America Exotic Animal Practice* 11: 233–249.

Lewbart, G.A., Butkus, D.A., Papich, M.G. et al. (2005). Evaluation of a method of intracoelomic catheterization in Koi. *Journal of the American Veterinary Medical Association* 226 (5): 784–788.

Lewisch, E., Reifinger, M., Schmidt, P. et al. (2014). Ovarian tumor in a Koi Carp (*Cyprinus carpio*): diagnosis, surgery, postoperative care and tumour classification. *Tierartzliche Praxis Kleintiere* 42 (4): 257–262.

Marshall, C.J. (1999). Use of Supaverm for the treatment of monogenean infestation in a Koi Carp (*Cyprinus carpio*). *Fish Veterinary Journal* 4: 33–37.

Minter, L.J., Bailey, K.M., Harms, C.A. et al. (2014). The efficacy of alfaxalone for immersion anesthesia in Koi Carp (*Cyprinus carpio*). *Veterinary Anaesthesia and Analgesia* 41: 398–405.

Murchelano, R.A. and Edwards, R.L. (1981). An erythrophoroma in ornamental carp, *Cyprinus carpio*. *Journal of Fish Diseases* 4: 265–268.

Noga, E.J. (2010). *Fish Disease: Diagnosis and Treatment*, 2e. Ames, IA: Wiley-Blackwell.

Nouws, J.F.M., Grondel, J.L., Schutte, A.R. et al. (1988). Pharmacokinetics of ciprofloxacin in carp, African catfish and rainbow trout. *The Veterinary Quarterly.* 10 (3): 211–216.

Oda, A., Bailey, K.M., Lewbart, G.A. et al. (2014). Physiologic and biochemical assessments of koi (*Cyprinus carpio*) following immersion in propofol. *Journal of the American Veterinary Medical Association* 245 (11): 1286–1291.

Olivia-Teles, A. (2012). Nutrition and health of aquaculture fish. *Journal of Fish Diseases* 35: 83–108.

Pharmaq (2013). Summary of product characteristics. http://www.vmd.defra.gov.uk/ProductInformationDatabase/Default.aspx (accessed 6 December 2017).

Plakas, S.M., El Said, K.R., Bencsath, F.A. et al. (1998). Pharmacokinetics, tissue distribution and metabolism of acriflavine and proflavine in the channel catfish (Ictalurus punctatus). *Xenobiotica* 28 (6): 605–616.

Pokorova, D., Vesely, T., Piackova, V. et al. (2005). Current knowledge on Koi herpesvirus (KHV): a review. *Veterinarni Medicina* 50: 139–147.

Popovic, N.T., Strunjak-Perovic, I., Coz-Rakovac, R. et al. (2011). Tricaine methane-sulfonate (MS-222) application in fish anaesthesia. *Journal of Applied Ichythyology* 28: 553–564.

Rach, J.J., Howe, G.E., and Schreier, T.M. (1997). Safety of formalin treatments on warm- and coolwater fish eggs. *Aquaculture.* 149: 183–191.

Rach, J.J., Gaikowski, M.P., Howe, G.E. et al. (1998). Evaluation of the toxicity and effects of hydrogen peroxide treaments on eggs of warm- and coolwater fishes. *Aquaculture* 165: 11–25.

Raidal, S.R., Shearer, P.L., Stephens, F. et al. (2006). Surgical removal of an ovarian tumour in a Koi Carp. *Australian Veterinary Journal* 84 (5): 178–181.

Roberts, H. and Palmeiro, B.S. (2008). Toxicology of aquarium fish. *Veterinary Clinics of North America: Exotic Animal Practice* 11 (2): 359–374.

Roberts, H.E., Palmeiro, B., and Weber, E.S. III (2009). Bacterial and parasitic disease of pet fish. *Veterinary Clinics of North America Exotic Animal Practice* 12: 609–638.

Ross, L.G. (2001). Restraint, anaesthesia and euthanasia. In: *BSAVA Manual of Ornamental Fish*, 2e (ed. W.H. Wildgoose), 75–83. Gloucester, UK: BSAVA.

Sano, T., Fukuda, H., and Furukawa, M. (1985). Herpesvirus cyprinid: biological and oncogenic properties. *Fish Pathology* 20 (2): 381–388.

Sherrill, J., Weber, E.S. III, Marty, G.D. et al. (2009). Fish cardiovascular physiology and disease. *Veterinary Clinics of North America: Exotic Animal Practice* 12: 11–38.

Srivastava, S., Sinha, R., and Roy, D. (2004). Toxicological effects of malachite green. *Aquatic Toxicology* 66: 319–329.

Stetter, M.D. (2001). Fish and amphibian anaesthesia. *Veterinary Clinics of North America: Exotic Animal Practice.* 4 (1): 69–82.

Stoskopf, M.K. (1993a). Anatomy. In: *Fish Medicine*, vol. 1 (ed. M.K. Stoskopf), 2–30. Philadelphia: WB Saunders.

Stoskopf, M.K. (1993b). Appendix II chemotherapeutics. In: *Fish Medicine*, vol. 1 (ed. M.K. Stoskopf), xxviii–xxxv. Philadelphia, PA: WB Saunders.

Stoskopf, M.K. (1999). Fish pharmacotherapeutics. In: *Zoo and Wild Animal Medicine: Current Therapy* (eds. M.E. Fowler and R.E. Miller), 182–189. Philadelphia, PA: WB Saunders.

Summerfelt, R.C. and Smith, L.S. (1990). Anaesthesia, surgery and related techniques. In: *Methods of Fish Biology* (eds. C.B. Schreck and P.B. Moyle), 213–272. Bethesda: American Fisheries Society.

Svobodova, Z., Lloyd, R., and Machova, J. (1993). Water quality and fish health. EIFAC Technical Paper 54. Rome, FAO.

Székely, C. and Molnár, K. (1991). Praziquantel (Droncit) is effective against diplostomosis of grass carp (*Ctenopharyngodon idella*) and silver carp (*Hypophthalmichthys molitrix*). *Diseases of Aquatic Organisms* 11: 147–150.

Takahara, T., Honjo, M.N., Uchii, K. et al. (2014). Effects of daily temperature fluctuation on the survival of carp infected with cyprinid herpesvirus 3. *Aquaculture* 433 (20): 208–213.

Vergneau-Grosset, C., Summa, N., Rodriguez, C.O. et al. (2016). Excision and subsequent treatment of a leiomyoma from the periventiduct of a koi (*Cyprinus carpio Koi*). *Journal of Exotic Pet Medicine.* 25 (3): 194–202.

Vergneau-Grosset, C., Nadeau, M.E., and Groff, J.M. (2017). Fish oncology: diseases, diagnostics, and therapeutics. *Veterinary Clinics of North America: Exotic Animal Practice* 20: 21–56.

Vetark Professional (2017a). Aqua-Sed. www.noahcompendium.co.uk/?id=-459034 (accessed 12 June 2017).

Vetark Professional (2017b). Chloramine-T. www.noahcompendium.co.uk/?id=-459045 (accessed 11 December 2018).

Vetark Professional (2017c). Fluke-Solve. www.noahcompendium.co.uk/?id=-459056 (accessed 31 December 2018).

Vetark Professional (2017d). Lice-Solve. www.noahcompendium.co.uk/?id=-459080 (accessed 31 December 2018).

Waddell, W.J., Lech, J.J., Marlowe, C. et al. (1990). The distribution of [14C] acrylamide in rainbow trout studied by whole-body autoradiography. *Toxicological Sciences.* 14 (1): 84–87.

Wangen, K. (2012). Therapeutic review: sodium chloride. *Journal of Exotic Pet Medicine* 21: 94–98.

Weber, E.S. III (2011). Fish analgesia: pain, stress, fear aversion, or nociception? *Veterinary Clinics of North America: Exotic Animal Practice* 14: 21–32.

Wildgoose, W.H. (1992). Papilloma and squamous cell carcinoma in Koi Carp (*Cyprinus carpio*). *Veterinary Record* 130: 153–157.

Wildgoose, W.H. (2001). Skin disease. In: *BSAVA Manual of Ornamental Fish*, 2e (ed. W.H. Wildgoose), 109–122. British Small Animal Veterinary Association: Gloucester, UK.

Wildgoose, W.H. and Lewbart, G.A. (2001). Therapeutics. In: *Manual of Ornamental Fish*, 2e (ed. W.H. Wildgoose), 237–258. Gloucester, UK: British Small Animal Veterinary Association.

Yanong, P.E., Curtis, E.W., Simmons, R. et al. (2005). Pharmacokinetic studies of Florfenicol in Koi Carp and Threespot gourami Trichogaster trichopterus after Oral and intramuscular treatment. *Journal of Aquatic Animal Health* 17: 129–137.

Yaron, Z., Bogomolnaya, A., Drori, S. et al. (2009). Spawning induction in the carp: past experience and future prospects - a review. *The Israeli Journal of Aquaculture – Bamidgeh* 61 (1): 5–26.

Further Reading

Carpenter, J.W. (2017). *Exotic Animal Formulary*, 5e. St Louis: Elsevier.

Noga, E.J. (2010). *Fish Disease: Diagnosis and Treatment*, 2e. Ames: Wiley-Blackwell.

Stoskopf, M.K. (2010). *Fish Medicine Volume 1*. Philadelphia: WB Saunders.

Stoskopf, M.K. (2010). *Fish Medicine Volume 2*. Philadelphia: WB Saunders.

Wildgoose, W.H. (2001). *BSAVA Manual of Ornamental Fish*, 2e. Gloucester: British Small Animal Veterinary Association.

23

Tarantulas
Sarah Pellett and Steven A. Trim

23.1 Introduction

Theraphosids; commonly referred to as tarantulas, are arthropods belonging to the Order Araneae (spiders), and Family Theraphosidae. There are (as of 2019), 999 recognised species within this family, within 146 genera, and they represent an important group of commonly kept spiders in captivity (Marnell 2016; World Spider Catalogue 2019). Tarantulas appear to be gaining popularity as pets and are often kept in large numbers by enthusiasts. They are also seen frequently at zoological collections and in colleges with animal care courses. Whilst invertebrate medicine is still in its infancy compared with vertebrate medicine, over the last few years there has been more of a demand from both owners and veterinarians seeking advice in treating these animals (Pellett and Kubiak 2017).

23.2 Commonly Kept Species

Arachnid taxonomy is a rapidly changing field as new information is continually emerging, and the recent application of DNA technology in defining taxonomy. This results in controversy between scientists using different techniques and within the hobby. Recent changes include the Mexican red knee tarantula previously known as *Brachypelma smithi* (Integrated Taxonomic Information System Report) which should now be referred to as *Brachypelma hamorii* (Mendoza and Francke 2017). Other changes include complete revision of the *Avicularia* genus in 2017 (Fukushima and Bertani 2017).

Some of the commonly kept species and their basic environmental requirements are listed in Table 23.1.

The Mexican red knee tarantula originates from the central Mexican Pacific coast. This terrestrial species is popular amongst hobbyists due to its attractive colouration and calm nature and is recommended for owners new to keeping tarantulas (Pellett et al. 2014).

The Chilean rose (Figure 23.1) is another terrestrial species, originating from scrubland habitats in Chile and is popular amongst beginners. This spider is popular due to its appearance and is also a slow-growing, hardy species (Pellett et al. 2015).

The Goliath tarantula (Figure 23.2) is a terrestrial species and is fast-growing, with the possibility of reaching a body weight of 115 g and a leg span of up to 300 mm (Herzig and King 2013). This spider is not recommended for inexperienced keepers, due to their larger size, more complex husbandry requirements, and quick defensive dispersal of urticating hairs.

The Pink-toe tarantula, originating from South America, is not an aggressive species but has been reported to be skittish if handled (Pizzi 2012). Along with other arboreal species, the pink-toe tarantula has a slimmer body and longer legs compared with the stocky terrestrial species.

It is not uncommon to see many other species of tarantula for sale at pet shops and invertebrate exhibitions. The knowledge of species presented is important to provide the correct husbandry advice and also to have an understanding of that particular species' venom capabilities before proceeding to clinical examination (Marnell 2016). Many Old world arboreal spiders, such as the baboon (Harpactirinae) and tiger (*Poecilotheria* spp.) spiders, are of concern to handlers as they are often aggressive and bites from these species can cause spastic muscle contractions and intense pain (Ahmed et al. 2009). No fatalities have been associated with tarantula envenomation though allergies to urticating hairs from New World spiders can result in severe symptoms (Castro et al. 1995). Arboreal species also represent a challenge in practice due to their adhesive scopulae giving them the ability to climb smooth vertical surfaces for escape (Pérez-Miles et al. 2017).

Handbook of Exotic Pet Medicine, First Edition. Edited by Marie Kubiak.
© 2021 John Wiley & Sons Ltd. Published 2021 by John Wiley & Sons Ltd.
Companion website: www.wiley.com/go/kubiak/exotic_pet_medicine

Table 23.1 Environmental parameters for common tarantula species (Melidone 2007; Eddy and Clarke 2017).

Common species	Scientific name	Origin	Temperature gradient (°C)	Relative humidity (%)
Chilean Rose	*Grammostola rosea*; *G. porteri*	South America	18–24	60
Mexican Red knee	*Brachypelma hamorii* (formerly *B. smithi*)	Mexico	24–30	60–70
Goliath tarantula	*Theraphosa blondi* and *T. stirmi*	South America	24–29	90
Mexican Painted Red Leg	*Brachypelma emilia*	Mexico	24.4–27.7	60–70
Pink Toe	*Avicularia avicularia*	South America	25.5–30	80–90
Orange Baboon spider	*Pterinochilus murinus*	Central, eastern, and southern Africa	25.5–27.8	65
Cobalt Blue spider	*Cyriopagopus lividus* (previously *Haplopelma lividum*)	Myanmar and Thailand	26–32	85–90

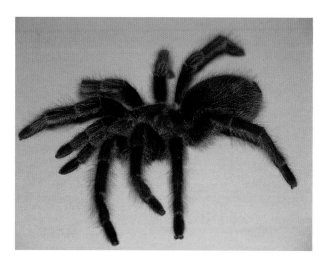

Figure 23.1 The Chilean Rose tarantula (*Source:* copyright Venomtech 2019, reproduced with permission).

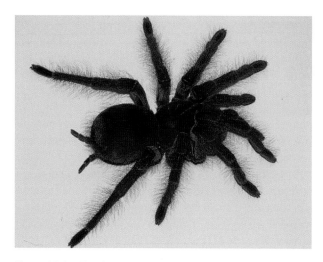

Figure 23.2 The Goliath tarantula (*Source:* copyright Venomtech 2019, reproduced with permission).

23.3 Biological Parameters

In some species, females may live up to 30 years (Bennie et al. 2011) and owners may firmly bond with their pets, especially if they have raised them from spiderling stage (often less than 5 mm in leg span) up to adult size (over 13 cm in leg span for many species) (Marnell 2016). There is a greater demand for female spiders because of their longevity (Pellett et al. 2015). Male spiders generally live for only three to four years and die a few months after their terminal (or ultimate) moult. Some males will live longer and can take 6-7 years to mature with some surviving up to 8 months at the terminal instar stage, and infrequently surviving up to 18 months (Pellett et al. 2015).

23.3.1 Anatomy

The basic external anatomy is shown in Figure 23.3.

Tarantulas have four pairs of legs, one pair of pedipalps, and one pair of chelicerae. The legs are attached to the prosoma, which is equivalent to a fused head and thorax. This prosoma contains the oesophagus and sucking stomach. The sucking stomach leads to the proximal midgut and in the majority of theraphosid species has diverticula that lead to the proximal limbs. The prosoma also contains the central nervous system and attachment muscles for controlling the limbs (Foelix 1996). The chelicerae contain the paired fangs and venom glands (Lewbart and Mosley 2012).

The theraphosid opisthosoma is almost analogous to the abdomen and is separated from the prosoma by the narrow pedicel (Dunlop et al. 1992). Theraphosids have two pairs of book lungs located on the ventral aspect of the opisthosoma, compared to the single pair of book lungs seen in most other spiders (Ruppert et al. 2004). The opisthosoma also contains more of the midgut and diverticula. A large heart is located

Figure 23.3 External anatomy of an adult male Mexican Red Rump tarantula, *Brachypelma vagans* (dorsal view) (*Source:* copyright S.A. Trim 2019, reproduced with permission).

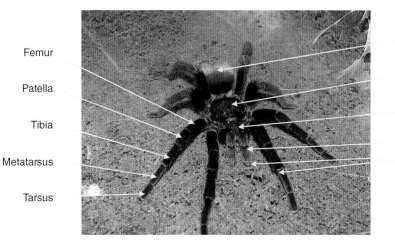

Femur

Patella

Tibia

Metatarsus

Tarsus

Opisthosoma

Prosoma

Chelicera

Pedipalps

Bulbous Pedipalps and tibial spurs present in adult

in the dorsal midline and vessels transport the blood (haemolymph) to tissues and the blood then flows freely in open spaces between organs. The hepatopancreas is located below the heart. Reproductive organs are located on the ventral surface of the opisthosoma and the silk glands are posterior to these. The excretory organs (Malphigian tubules) are located mid-to-posterior and dorsally (Marnell 2016). At the distal end of the opisthosoma either side of the anus there are two pairs of spinnerets responsible for multistrand silk filament formation to create webs.

23.3.2 Ecdysis

Tarantulas have a rigid chitin exoskeleton and undergo moulting (ecdysis) to grow. A new exoskeleton forms beneath the old cuticle from the living epidermal tissue. Behavioural changes may be seen at this time with the spider becoming more defensive, displaying the threat posture, and spending more time in their burrows. The period of ecdysis involves the old exoskeleton splitting to reveal the new cuticle. Normally tarantulas moult on their back and this process may take several hours (Figure 23.4) (Pizzi 2012). Some major structures are shed including the venom ducts, oesophageal lining, book lungs, and the openings to the gonads. It is normal for a tarantula to undergo a period of anorexia before and after moulting (Marnell 2016) and this is partly due to the venom glands not being connected to the old fangs prior to the moulting process. Males emerge from their terminal moult with enlarged palpal organs and, in some species, hooked tibial spurs on the first pair of legs can be seen (Figure 23.3). These are used during mating to secure the female's fangs in many species. Adult theraphosids typically moult annually though the length of time between ecdysis can vary. Owners should be encouraged to record ecdysis so that moulting times can be predicted, and such knowledge may be useful in clinical diagnosis.

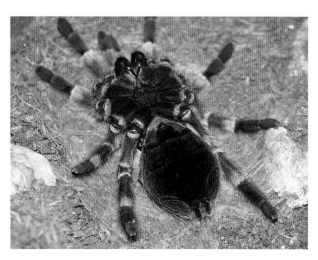

Figure 23.4 Mexican Red Knee tarantula undergoing a normal moult (*Source:* copyright S.A. Trim 2019, reproduced with permission).

23.3.3 Husbandry

In the wild, tarantulas are not generally social and in captivity should be housed singly (Marnell 2016). However, Foelix (1996) reports there are approximately 20 species of spider within the *Poecilotheria* genus that have been observed living together socially in the wild. These species may be maintained together in captivity when raised together as spiderlings, but cannibalism often occurs therefore single-specimen housing is still preferred (Pizzi 2012).

Enclosure size and design varies for theraphosids and individual species requirements must be taken into consideration (Pellett et al. 2015). Enclosures are frequently made out of acrylic, clear plastic, or glass and should be secured against escape. Ventilation holes must be smaller than the prosoma to prevent escape, and ideally smaller than the leg diameter to prevent limbs being trapped. Spiderlings can escape through very small gaps and anorexia can result in a reduction in opisthosoma size so regular assessments of spider and enclosure are necessary.

Terrestrial tarantulas require an enclosure that is approximately three times the spider's legspan in width and depth, and one legspan in height (Wagler 2015). Terrestrial tarantulas have hooks on their feet so mesh top tanks are discouraged as autotomy of the limb may occur if claws become trapped in the mesh (Figure 23.5) (Pizzi 2010). Décor should be secure and terrestrial spiders do not require significant vertical climbing opportunities. A fall from a height of even 30 cm can lead to a fatal opisthosoma trauma. Heavier spiders such as the Goliath tarantula will be more susceptible to traumatic injury from falls.

Arboreal species will require taller enclosures. With these taller enclosures, doors situated both on the front and top of the enclosure are advised (Bennie et al. 2011). At rest, arboreal tarantulas prefer to maintain a vertical position, compared with the terrestrial species who generally rest in a horizontal position, and the enclosure design should accommodate this (Marnell 2016). These arboreal spiders appear to respond positively to environmental

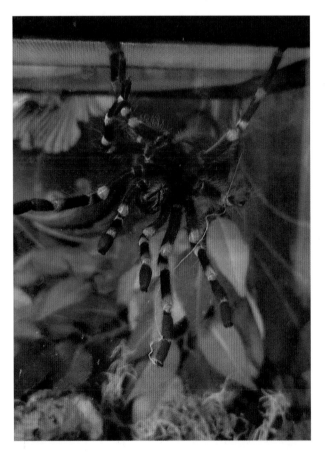

Figure 23.5 Picture of a Giant White Knee spider, *Acanthoscurria geniculata* trapped in mesh insert in an enclosure (*Source:* copyright Christopher Swann 2019, reproduced with permission).

enrichment and thus enclosures should have suitable climbing and hiding structures (Bennie et al. 2011).

Substrate commonly used includes potting soil, peat, coconut coir, and vermiculite, free from pesticides and potential parasites (Bennie et al. 2011). Terrestrial tarantulas require a deep layer of substrate and many old world species such as the Cobalt blue tarantula (*Cyriopagopus lividus*) like to burrow (Marnell 2016). All species require appropriate hiding places and this can be achieved by providing logs, cork bark, roundline guttering or half a flower pot as a hide. Artificial plants can also be provided and frequently spiders will cover this in webbing. Webbing has been considered a sign of naturalistic behaviour and indicative of a well-adapted spider (Bennie et al. 2011).

Recommended temperature ranges for most species of tarantula is within 20–30 °C, but the thermal range for the individual species should be identified and provided, where available (see Table 23.1). A maximum-minimum thermometer is advised for close monitoring of environmental temperatures. Temperature extremes should be avoided and a temperature gradient across the enclosure should be provided to allow thermoregulation. If additional heat is needed, a heat mat (under thermostatic control) can be placed on the exterior of an enclosure side, but never underneath (Pellett et al. 2015). Tarantulas are photophobic and it is believed that they do not require additional lighting. Some collections and owners do use full spectrum lighting (including ultraviolet) and it is not known whether this has an adverse or beneficial effect for the animal. King baboon spiders (*Pelinobius muticus*) exposed to full spectrum lighting showed no difference in burrowing, but significantly more webbing was observed (Somerville et al. 2017). In the same study, cortisol levels were detected for the first time in arachnid haemolymph and were significantly raised after exposure to full spectrum lighting compared with the same period of ambient light.

Tarantulas should not be directly sprayed as this can cause irritation and stress. Instead, the substrate should be moistened for those species requiring a higher humidity and humidity monitored using a hygrometer (Pellett et al. 2015). Water should always be available, provided in a shallow dish. The use of water-soaked sponges should be avoided as these may act as a substrate for bacterial and fungal growth (De Voe 2009; Bechanko et al. 2012). Arboreal species require light spraying of the web or side of the enclosure.

A variety of prey species is important to provide balanced nutrition. Invertebrates such as crickets, locusts, Dubia cockroaches, and mealworms can be offered and should be gut-loaded (i.e. well-fed on varied vegetables or a commercial insect diet) prior to being offered. Wax worms should be fed sparingly due to their high fat content and poor nutritional value. Some larger species, such as *Theraphosa* spp., accept whole killed vertebrates such as small mice, but these often take a long time to consume and this is not advised. The body condition of the tarantula should be monitored carefully and feeding frequency adjusted to this. Overweight tarantulas have a distended opisthosoma which they are unable to lift off the substrate. Tarantulas do not require calcium supplementation as spiders do not incorporate calcium carbonate into their exoskeletons (Pizzi 2010).

23.4 Clinical Evaluation

23.4.1 History-Taking

The clinical approach to a tarantula consultation is no different to that of a more familiar exotic species. A detailed history, emphasising the husbandry aspect is essential as the vast majority of health problems encountered in pet tarantulas are related to suboptimal husbandry and environmental conditions. If the spider is kept in a small enclosure that is easy to transport, then it is helpful to observe the whole set up in the surgery.

History should also include whether the spider was wild caught or bred in captivity as this is important when considering parasitic diseases. Further information such as when the tarantula last ate and last moulted should also be obtained (Pellett et al. 2015).

23.4.2 Handling

It is not recommended to handle any species of tarantula due to the risk of damage to the animal such as haemolymph loss or limb autotomy through rough handling or being dropped, and risk to handlers of envenomation from a bite, or skin and corneal irritation from urticating hairs (Choi and Rauf 2003). Both Old World and New World tarantulas have venom glands and fangs (Figure 23.6), though Old World tarantulas tend to bite more readily than New World tarantulas as they do lack the additional defence of urticating hairs (Blatchford et al. 2011). Approximately 90% of New World tarantula species have the ability to kick off these urticating hairs, which are mostly distributed over the dorsal opisthosoma, in response to a perceived threat (Bertani and Guadanucci 2013). If the hairs penetrate the cornea, they can cause keratitis and uveitis, and hairs penetrating skin and mucus membranes cause localised irritation. Repeated exposure is a risk factor for allergic sensitisation and respiratory protection should be used with active hair kicking spiders (Castro et al. 1995).

Ideally gloves should be worn to handle spiders, but at the very least it is recommended that people wash and dry their hands before handling spiders; this is essential for smokers;

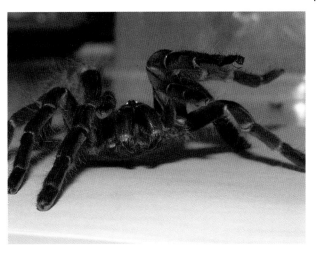

Figure 23.6 Threat pose displaying the fangs in a Cameroon Red Baboon spider, *Hysterocrates gigas* (*Source:* copyright Venomtech 2019, reproduced with permission).

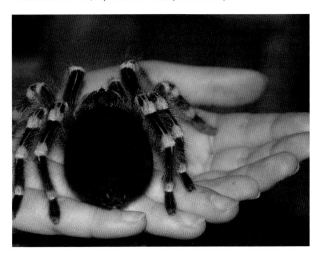

Figure 23.7 Handling session with a Giant White Knee spider (*Acanthoscurria geniculata*) (*Source:* copyright S.A. Trim 2019, reproduced with permission).

nicotine was once used as an insecticide and is harmful to invertebrates (De Sellem 1917; Lovett 1920; Smith 1921). Protective glasses and covering of exposed skin should be considered when handling species with urticating hairs.

Some well-handled tarantulas will walk onto a hand and permit a cursory examination (Figure 23.7), particularly species docile in nature such as *Grammostola rosea* or *Brachypelma* spp. Alternatively, an index finger or a pencil gently placed on the centre of the rigid prosoma will immobilise a spider. The middle finger and thumb are then placed between the second and third pair of legs either side of the prosoma and the spider can be lifted, though a low height and a soft surface should be used to avoid catastrophic falls (Figure 23.8). When held for an examination the spider can be held with its body upside down. This seems to put them in a torpor like state.

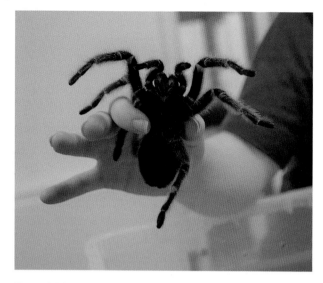

Figure 23.8 Manual restraint of Chilean rose tarantula (*Grammostola rosea*).

Spiders must never be handled during a moult including the pre- to post-moult periods and feeding should resume before they are handled again. Where animals in a vulnerable stage need evaluation, placing a clear container over the spider, or carefully encouraging the animal into the container with a soft paint brush allows close observation. An anaesthetic facemask may be used as the container and the animal can then be anaesthetised for further examination and diagnostic tests if indicated.

23.4.3 Sex Determination

Tibial spurs may be observed in adult males of some species. In males of all species the pedipalps are enlarged at the terminal moult and the presence of palpal balbs is evident, although this may be difficult to observe in some species. In some species the oviductal opening may be seen in the epigastric furrow.

As spiders shed the lining of their reproductive organs during ecdysis, another technique to determine the sex of a theraphosid is to examine the moult (exuvia) to look for the paired spermathecae and uterus externus in the epigynum region in the female (Hancock and Hancock 1999). The exuvia can either be soaked in warm water with a small drop of detergent or left overnight in a wet paper towel. The shed skin is delicate and must be gently parted, starting at the prosoma, using a smooth blunt object such as a seeker or snake sexing probe. The dorsal opisthosoma is then carefully unfurled, to reveal the ventral surface. Often the ventral sides are stuck together so care is required as to not tear the epigynum region. With juvenile and spiderling exuvia, the epigynum can be placed on a microscope slide. Once prepared, the exuvia can be examined to look for the presence of spermatheca

and uterus externus in the female (Figure 23.9). The spermatheca are present in the female to receive the sperm and are situated on the inner surface of the exuvium along the epigastric furrow between the book lungs (Pizzi 2012).

23.4.4 Clinical Examination

The spider can be examined by viewing it from all sides in a clear-walled container. Magnification is recommended to examine the exoskeleton of the tarantula and assess the whole spider for open wounds, masses, ectoparasites, colour changes of the exoskeleton, discharges within the oral cavity, missing appendages, alopecia, and dehydration (Marnell 2016). The gait of the animal should be observed before any anaesthetic agent is given to assess for ataxia or hypermetria. Anaesthesia may be necessary to allow physical examination and further procedures such as diagnostic sampling, supportive care such as fluid therapy, and to allow for treatment such as exoskeleton repair or manual removal of ectoparasites. In an anaesthetised spider, the body can be palpated to assess for masses and firmness. If there is palpal organ enlargement (and tibial spurs for relevant species) the animal may be a mature male and nearing the end of its life.

23.5 Basic Techniques

23.5.1 Sample Collection

23.5.1.1 Blood Sampling
Haemolymph can be sampled with the tarantula under anaesthesia, by using a 30-gauge insulin needle and syringe, collected from the heart with needle placement in the dorsal midline of the opisthosoma. Using larger needles of up to 25G improves cellularity of samples. Volumes of 2 ml/100 g body weight are achievable with suitable fluid replacement (Kennedy et al. 2019), however, the authors advise collecting a smaller volume in unwell theraphosids. Applying pressure with a sterile cotton bud will often seal the wound but a small amount of tissue adhesive can also be applied to the cuticle after sampling to prevent ongoing haemorrhage. An alternative site to collect a small volume of haemolymph is the ventral limb membrane. This is achieved by restraining the spider in dorsal recumbency with a rigid restraint, e.g. using a plastic ruler placed over the spider, to prevent movement (Pizzi 2012). This method may be more challenging but minimises the risk of fatal haemorrhage that may occur from sampling from the heart. If haemorrhage cannot be controlled from the limb site, the leg can be removed by autotomy after recovery from anaesthesia, and tissue adhesive can be applied to the coxal stump to achieve haemostasis (Pizzi 2012).

(a)

(b)

(c)

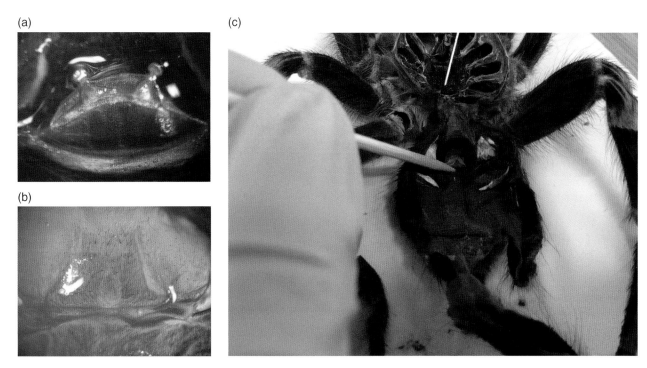

Figure 23.9 (a) Examination of the exuvia to show the paired spermotheca and uterus externus in a female Chilean Rose tarantula, *Grammostola rosea*. (b) Examination of the exuvia to show the epigastric furrow lacking paired spermotheca and uterus externus in a male Chilean Rose tarantula, *Grammostola rosea*. (c) Location of the epigynum on a spider exuvia. *Source:* Photos copyright Venomtech 2019, reproduced with permission.

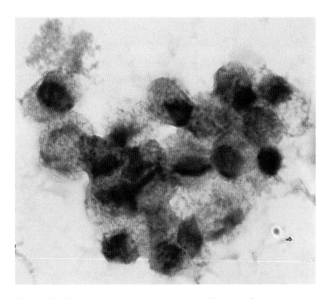

Figure 23.10 Haemolymph smear from Trinidad Chevron spider (*Psalmopoeus cambridgei*) air-dried then stained with Wrights stain (*Source:* Dr. C.M. Trim, reproduced with permission).

Blood smears from haemolymph (Figure 23.10) can be examined but interpretation is still in its infancy with differences in opinion on nomenclature of cell types (Pizzi 2010).

There has been little research in this field and no conclusion has been reached on the most effective anticoagulant to use (Greegoire 1953, Gupta 1985) though both sodium heparin (Kennedy et al. 2019) and sodium citrate have been successfully used by some laboratories.

There is still a lack of validated chemistry reference ranges with variable results being seen in small scale projects, and variation of values between species (Schartau et al. 1983; Zachariah et al. 2007; Soares et al. 2013). Limitations may also occur due to other factors such as the life stage of the tarantula, environmental conditions, and proximity to ecdysis. Two recent studies have assessed plasma biochemistry of haemolymph in Chilean rose tarantulas (Eichelmann and Lewbart 2018; Kennedy et al. 2019). Eichelmann and Lewbart used a commercial dry biochemistry machine, demonstrating that samples can be collected and run within the veterinary practice. Kennedy et al. (2019) raise caution with interpreting albumin and creatine kinase levels through standard techniques as there is no evidence these proteins exist in arachnids. Protein concentration in haemolymph vary between individuals and ecdysis stage, however dramatic changes are seen during dehydration and starvation which are reversible (Paul et al. 1994). Serial sampling may be a useful tool for assessment of hydration status (Zachariah et al. 2007).

23.5.2 Cytology and Histopathology

Cytology can provide useful information in identifying bacterial, fungal, and protozoal infections from the skin surface, discharges, and faeces. Faecal analysis may be useful to identify protozoans and gregarines. Skin scrapings should be performed with care to avoid damage to the exoskeleton, and swab collection of secretions or touch preparations are alternative options.

When collecting tissue samples for histopathology in invertebrates it is advised to discuss fixative choice with the receiving laboratory as formalin, ethanol, or more specialised solutions may be preferred dependent on the area of focus.

23.5.3 Post Mortem Examination

Post-mortem examination and sampling should be carried out immediately as tissues autolyse rapidly, reducing the information available for gross necropsy and histopathology. If immediate necropsy is not possible, the tarantula should be fixed in alcohol (e.g. ethanol) or formalin, with an incision made in the lateral opisthosoma to allow internal fixation (Pizzi 2010). Melanised nodules are a common finding, particularly in the superficial tissues, and are inflammatory responses to trauma and infection. Histopathology of fresh tissue can help differentiate contributing infectious factors in many cases.

23.5.4 Bacterial and Fungal Culture and Sensitivity

Bacterial and fungal culture and sensitivity can be performed on oral or anal discharges or from lesions if cytology is supportive of an infection. Interpretation of results must be taken with caution as some pathogens are often difficult to culture using the standard technique, commensal microbial populations are not described, and culture temperatures may need to be decreased as a result of the poikilothermic nature of tarantulas (Braun et al. 2006).

23.5.5 Fluid Therapy

Dehydration is commonly seen in tarantulas presented to vets (Marnell 2016). Extension of the limbs is dependent on haemolymph pressure so severely dehydrated spiders are unable to extend the limbs and are often observed with their legs pulled inwards towards the prosoma (Ellis 1944). Distortion of the dorsal opisthosoma may also be noted.

If the tarantula remains responsive and has the ability to move, rehydration can be achieved by placing the cranial prosoma in a shallow dish of water taking care not to submerge the ventral surface of the opisthosoma. Alternatively, spiders may take water from a syringe (Braun et al. 2006; Dombrowski and De Voe 2007). Most spiders able to drink will rehydrate within a few hours.

If the spider cannot access or ingest fluids orally then parenteral fluid therapy can be administered directly into the heart located on the dorsal midline of the opisthosoma (Figure 23.11). Alternatively, fluids may also be administered intracoelomically with needle placement from the lateral side of the opisthosoma (Braun et al. 2006). Normal saline or Hartmanns solution has been administered at 2–4% bodyweight, using a 30-gauge insulin needle and syringe (Kennedy et al. 2019). Normal saline is preferred as it appears to have similar osmolarity to arachnid haemolymph (Pizzi 2012). Tissue adhesive should be applied after fluid administration to prevent haemolymph loss from the injection site.

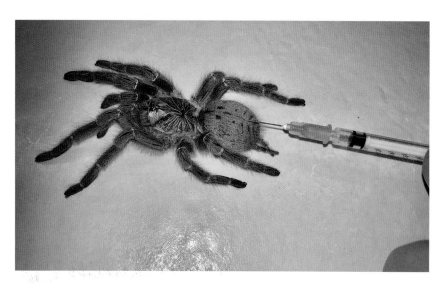

Figure 23.11 Administering fluids to a tarantula; the needle is placed in the dorsal midline of the opisthosoma, such as seen with this anaesthetised orange baboon spider (*Pterinochilus murinus*) using a 27G needle and 1 ml syringe (*Source:* courtesy of Dr. C.M. Trim).

23.5.6 Anaesthesia

Several key obstacles limit successful anaesthetic and analgesic use in invertebrates and these include subjectivity in pain assessment as well as inadequate knowledge of efficacy, safety, and dosing regimens (Sladky 2014).

Volatile or gaseous anaesthetic agents are the method of choice for anaesthetising tarantulas with several studies published. Isoflurane, sevoflurane, and carbon dioxide have been reported to result in anaesthesia in Chilean rose tarantulas (Zachariah et al. 2009; Dombrowski et al. 2013; Zachariah et al. 2014). However, rapid increases in carbon dioxide concentrations have been shown to cause adverse effects such as seizures, stress response and defecation and have also resulted in death in some cases, so its use is not advised (Pizzi 2012; Dombrowski et al. 2013). Isoflurane has been reported to successfully anaesthetise wild-caught *Theraphosa blondi*, and isoflurane and sevoflurane are commonly used for anaesthesia of captive theraphosids (Zachariah et al. 2009; Pellett et al. 2015). Induction can be slow, taking as long as 20 minutes before there is a loss of righting reflex.

The animal is placed under a large anaesthetic facemask or in an induction chamber, and the volatile agent is introduced into the receptacle. The respiratory openings for tarantulas are the book lungs, located on the ventral surface of the opisthosoma and these must be exposed to the anaesthetic agent.

Another method of induction is to place the spider in a closed container with a cotton ball saturated with isoflurane or sevoflurane liquid but control of induction is poor. Care must be taken not to allow the spider to come into direct contact with the saturated cotton wool ball, or for prolonged uptake as excessive depth of anaesthesia or death may result.

Injectable anaesthesia has been studied in Chilean rose tarantulas. Intracardiac alfaxalone at 200 mg/kg resulted in anaesthesia with a median duration of 28 minutes (Gjeltema et al. 2014). The addition of ketamine resulted in greater depth of anaesthesia, and addition of xylazine resulted in increases in both depth and duration of anaesthesia. Morphine addition had no effect on anaesthetic duration (Gjeltema et al. 2014). The authors concluded that all protocols used were safe; all spiders recovered uneventfully but suggested that the ambient temperature and ecdysis were important factors that may alter the response to anaesthesia (Gjeltema et al. 2014).

Monitoring anaesthetic depth can be achieved by assessing the righting reflex, reaction to tactile stimuli and relaxation of the fangs. The chelicerae muscle that hinges the fangs are the last to relax and the first to recover (Figure 23.12). If the oral and prosomal sensilla are visible then these can be observed for movement which indicates a light plane of anaesthesia.

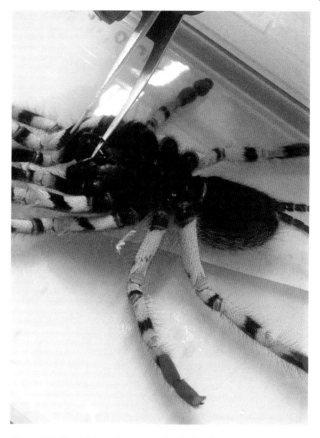

Figure 23.12 Monitoring anaesthetic depth in an Indian Ornamental spider, *Poecilotheria regalis* (*Source:* copyright Venomtech 2019, reproduced with permission).

Cardiac movements can be monitored under anaesthesia, using Doppler probe placement (with a small amount of ultrasound gel) on the dorsal opisthosoma (Braun et al. 2006). Heart rate is 30–70 bpm in larger species and in smaller species can be 200 bpm (Lewbart and Mosley 2012).

Recovery from volatile agents is achieved by withdrawing anaesthetic agents and exposing the animal to oxygen in a mask or chamber.

Little is known about analgesia in invertebrates but many species, especially the cephalopods, have well developed nervous systems that utilise natural opiates and thus are expected to respond to opioids in a similar manner to mammals (Sladky 2014). More research is needed to determine whether invertebrates experience pain, whether the perception of pain is equivalent to that of a vertebrate animal, or whether invertebrates are merely capable of demonstrating a reflexive response to nociceptive stimuli (Elwood 2011; Murray 2012). Evidence in support of invertebrates experiencing pain is inconclusive but it has been shown that tarantulas react to painful thermal stimuli in a similar fashion to vertebrates (Keller et al. 2012; Sladky 2014). Needle insertion into the exoskeleton also incites an apparent pain response with immediate withdrawal reaction followed by limb rubbing at the site of needle insertion. Responses can be affected by administration of morphine or butorphanol indicating potential analgesic effects, but dosages required are relatively high (Sladky 2014). Appropriate anaesthesia should therefore be used to prevent any response to noxious stimuli and analgesia should be considered. Hypothermia is not considered appropriate for analgesia (Pizzi 2012).

23.5.7 Euthanasia

Euthanasia is recommended if the tarantula would be thought to be suffering if kept alive. Common scenarios are severe dysecdysis or a disease process that cannot be resolved. In the UK, invertebrates are not governed by the same legislation as vertebrate species but humane treatment is important on welfare and ethical grounds.

Freezing is not an acceptable method for euthanasia of tarantulas. Anaesthesia using an inhalant agent is recommended prior to injection of pentobarbitone into the haemocoel, the body cavity of arthropods that contains haemolymph (Dombrowski and De Voe 2007; Pellett et al. 2017). Death is confirmed with the absence of cardiac activity using a Doppler ultrasound probe. An overdose of volatile agent, administered into a sealed chamber, has been used in high risk species where handling is to be avoided. Once the theraphosid is non-responsive, the authors advise to then administer pentobarbitone via injection.

Bennie et al. (2012) describe an alternative method for euthanasia in anaesthetised or immobile terrestrial invertebrates. Potassium chloride (KCl) is administered via the anterior sternum into the prosoma ganglia or directly into the heart. Intracardiac delivery is effective for Theraphosidae spiders, but not for Araneomorphae spiders. Death results from terminal depolarisation of the thoracic ganglia and KCl administration under anaesthesia is considered humane and effective (Bennie et al. 2012).

23.6 Common Medical and Surgical Conditions

23.6.1 Lethargy

A common complaint from owners is a change in behaviour with their animal such as reluctance to move, remaining in an abnormally huddled posture and anorexia. Differentials include suboptimal husbandry, infectious

aetiology, trauma, or ageing which are discussed further in this chapter.

23.6.2 Alopecia

Many New World tarantula species are capable of kicking urticating hairs from the opisthosoma as a defensive response to a perceived threat. Alopecia is frequently seen on the dorsal and caudal aspects of the opisthosoma and often indicates environmental stress and repeated defensive displays (Figure 23.13). The hairs will not regrow spontaneously but will be replaced at the next moult. Husbandry issues must be addressed to avoid the stressors responsible. Old-World tarantula species (Asian and African species) do not have urticating hairs and therefore do not develop this alopecia (Pizzi 2012).

23.6.3 Dysecdysis

Normal ecdysis may be misidentified as a problem by inexperienced owners – tarantulas found in dorsal recumbency (Figure 23.4) are likely undergoing a moult. Moribund spiders are normally found in an upright position with the legs contracted beneath them.

True dysecdysis (difficulty moulting) is a common presentation in tarantulas and optimum husbandry with the provision of good nutrition, hydration, and enclosure humidity is important in order to minimise this. Ecdysis may take up to 24 hours and minimal interference is advised as tarantulas in moult are very susceptible to

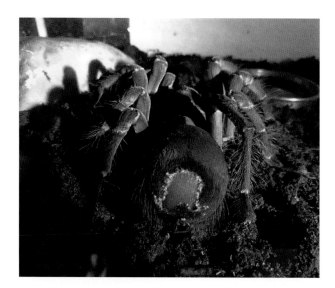

Figure 23.13 Alopecia on the dorsal opisthosoma in the Goliath tarantula (*Theraphosa strimi*) (*Source:* copyright S.A. Trim 2019, reproduced with permission).

trauma. Attempting to assist by pulling the old cuticle is likely to result in damage to the new delicate exoskeleton underneath and haemolymph loss. The new cuticle is initially soft to enable body expansion, having only 50% of its strength 24 hours after ecdysis and taking up to 20 days to reach full strength (Stewart and Martin 1982).

If limbs are trapped in the retained exoskeleton it is recommended to wait until the cuticle has hardened before intervening. Fang colouration helps identify when cuticle hardening is occurring. Immediately post-moult the fangs are white, then become red and finally black when fully hardened. This process takes hours in smaller spiders and days in large theraphosids, progressing from tip to base (Figure 23.14).

Once the cuticle has sclerotised, attempts can be made to remove the old cuticle using mild detergents; the book lungs must be avoided to prevent drowning. A fine tipped artists paint brush has been used to apply small amounts of detergent solutions or glycerine, reducing surface tension and enabling separation of the old and new cuticles (Pizzi 2012). The old cuticle can then be carefully removed with iris scissors but there is a significant risk of haemorrhage if the new cuticle is penetrated (Dombrowski and De Voe 2007). Sutures are inappropriate for spiders as they will further damage the cuticle, and tissue glue is used for repair of minor lacerations (Pizzi 2012). Where limbs cannot be freed, autotomy of the affected limb(s) may be an option.

Intracardiac fluid administration in dysecdysis patients must be done with caution because of an increased risk of trauma to the soft new cuticle. Delayed haemolymph loss from the injection site may occur hours to days after administering fluids as a result of expansion of the new opisthosoma cuticle volume (Pizzi 2012).

23.6.4 Autotomy

Autotomy is a defensive adaptation to physical injury, where an individual sacrifices a limb to escape a dangerous situation, such as capture by a predator. It can be utilised in practice to remove a damaged limb with minimal haemorrhage. This should not be performed under anaesthesia as it is a voluntary action and anaesthesia may prevent the reflex responses that allow the soft tissues to contract and seal the wound. The femur segment of the limb is grasped firmly with forceps and pulled rapidly upwards. Regeneration of the limb will take place, with the limb returning to normal size within the following two to three moults (Pizzi 2002, 2010).

23.6.5 Trauma

Trauma and loss of haemolymph is an emergency situation. Immediate first aid is essential and involves gentle pressure on the wound using cotton-tipped applicators to reduce haemorrhage. If wounds are small in size they can be dried using pure talcum powder (with no added perfume or additive), or wounds can be sealed with tissue glue (Figure 23.15).

Tarantulas have fine hooks and hairs (scopulae) on their feet and if these are caught on clothing fibres or mesh cage panels, limbs can be injured. Complete autotomy may occur or damage may result in loss of haemolymph from the joints. If damaged, the limb should be removed.

After any injury the tarantula should be placed on a paper towel substrate for 24–48 hours to monitor for continued leakage of haemolymph. Haemolymph is clear to

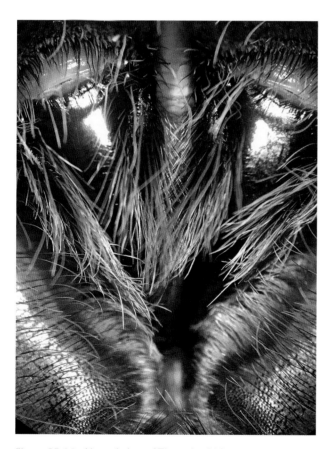

Figure 23.14 Ventral view of Theraphosid fangs several hours post ecdysis. The black tips are where the exoskeleton is fully hardened and the red colouration at the base of the fangs is where the exoskeleton is still maturing. Also visible is the white arthrodial membrane where fangs join the chelicera which remains white even after the fangs have fully hardened to a uniform black. (*Source:* copyright Venomtech 2019, reproduced with permission).

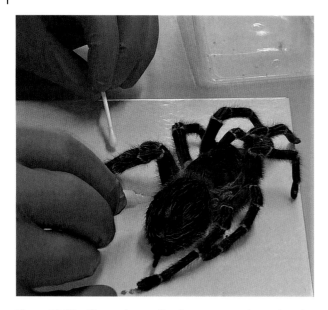

Figure 23.15 Tissue glue application to prevent haemolymph loss in a Brazilian Salmon Pink tarantula, *Lasiodora parahybana* (*Source:* Reprinted with permission from Institute of Animal Technology).

blue in appearance (Pizzi 2012) and should be visible on unpatterned paper towel. Fluid therapy may be necessary after haemolymph loss.

23.6.6 Endoparasites

Wild caught individuals may harbour endo- or ecto-parasites (Pizzi 2012), with those of significance described below.

Acroceridae are a small family of flies, many of which are bee or wasp mimics, and they may parasitise wild-caught spiders. Larvae are deposited onto the spider's body, crawl to the book lungs and penetrate the opisthosoma between the lamellae (Pizzi 2012). Larvae mature inside the spider and the mature fourth instar is the destructive feeding stage, consuming tissues and bursting out of the dorsal opisthosoma to pupate (Pizzi 2012). Diagnosis of acrocercid spider-fly larvae is by identification of larval forms on opisthosomal ultrasonography but prognosis is grave. Ultrasonographic-guided aspiration has been unsuccessful (Pizzi 2012).

Mermithidae nematodes are also seen in wild-caught individuals who may be asymptomatic for months to years. They are uncommon with less than 1% incidence but have been observed in many spider species (Pizzi 2012). Infection is by ingestion of a paratenic host. Clinical signs include an enlarged asymmetrical opisthosoma, malformation of palps and shorter legs. Absence or poor development of male secondary sexual characteristics is also seen. Behavioural changes may be seen, including lethargy and migration towards a water source (Foelix 1996). In more advanced stages the coiled nematode may be visualised through the cuticle. There is no treatment available.

Tarantula hawk wasps, within the family Pompilidae, are parasitoid wasps. The female stings the tarantula to paralyse it, drags it into a brood nest and lays a single egg on the spider's opisthosoma. Developing larva feed on the live tarantula. The spider may remain paralysed or may recover from paralysis depending on the species of wasp. This is rarely seen in captivity, and only where North American tarantula species are kept in regions of North America where the species of spider wasp are also native (Pizzi 2012). Intensive nursing and assist feeding of paralysed wild-caught spiders has proved to be successful in some cases (Breene 1998).

Oral nematodes may be seen in tarantulas, with the most common parasites being *Panagrolaimus* spp. (Pizzi 2009). These nematodes are observed within the mouthparts, with both captive bred and wild-caught specimens affected (Pizzi 2012). This infestation is an important disease of captive spiders in many genera, however the life cycle of these parasites is as yet unknown. Transmission is unknown, but nematodes can sequentially infect animals in a collection and vector transmission from Phoridae flies has been speculated (Pizzi 2012). Other work has speculated that oral Panagrolaimidae nematodes may be related to parasites of beetles such as mealworm beetles (*Tenebrio molitor*) which is a potential food source. Clinical signs include an abnormal posture where spiders are described to stand on the tips of their toes, anorexia, and lethargy. Death often follows several weeks to months after the onset of signs (Pizzi 2012). As the disease process advances, small motile nematodes appearing as a white, thick discharge, may be visualised near the chelicerae. Diagnosis is by full examination under anaesthesia, using an endoscope to visualise the areas between the mouth and chelicerae. Additionally, the mouth can be flushed with physiological saline and cytology of the flush performed. Nematodes are of 0.5–3 mm in length and can be observed under the microscope (Pizzi 2012). Treatment has been trialled with various medications such as ivermectin, fenbendazole, oxfendazole, enrofloxacin, and trimethoprim sulphonamides, but none have been successful (Pizzi 2012). As a result of zoonotic potential and poor prognosis, euthanasia of infected spiders is recommended at this time (Pizzi 2012). Prevention remains the mainstay of managing this condition. All new spiders should be quarantined for a minimum of 30 days, in a separate room from the remaining invertebrate collection (Pizzi 2012). Quarantine duration should be extended if any spiders show signs of anorexia. All spiders should undergo a full examination before ending their quarantine period.

Some related nematodes such as *Halicephalobus* and *Haycocknema* spp. have zoonotic potential, therefore this nematode should also be considered as potentially zoonotic, though the apparently related beetle nematodes are not zoonotic (Pearce et al. 2001; Nadler et al. 2003; Eckert and Ossent 2006; Pizzi 2012).

23.6.7 Dyskinetic Syndrome (DKS)

DKS is a term proposed to cover all tarantulas presenting with ataxia or an unusual gait and is likely due to multiple causes (Draper and Trim 2018). Definitive aetiologies are unknown, but exposure to a neurotoxin such as an insecticide, inherited neurodegenerative disorders, or nutritional deficiencies may be factors (Draper and Trim 2018). Other potential causes include infection, with five cases of suspected DKS testing positive for *Pseudomonas* spp. (Draper and Trim 2018). Further research is necessary to determine normal microbial flora and fauna of the arachnid and to establish whether *Pseudomonas* spp. is a commensal or a true pathogen in spiders. Additional studies are required to investigate viruses amongst spiders.

Clinical signs include anorexia, altered gait, ataxia, incoordination, and twitching. Hydrophobia and lethargy have also been reported (Draper and Trim 2018). Tarantulas displaying these symptoms usually succumb to this condition.

Nursing DKS tarantulas is often challenging; the spider often moves erratically and defensive behaviours can increase. New World species may kick setae from the dorsal surface of the opisthosoma in defence and Old World species may bite. The spider should be isolated from other invertebrates and strict biosecurity and hygiene between enclosures is advised (Draper and Trim 2018). An oral electrolyte solution has been used for spiders with suspected DKS. The solution contains 0.3% sodium chloride (NaCl), 0.3% potassium chloride (KCl), 0.03% calcium chloride (CaCl$_2$) and 0.27% magnesium sulphate (MgSO$_4$) in sterile water and is administered orally. (Draper and Trim 2018). Promising results have been seen with recovery in some cases, but further studies are required to assess efficacy (Draper and Trim 2018).

Suboptimal husbandry must always be addressed and assessment into ecto- and endoparasites such as mites, phorids, and nematodes that may be vectors for transmission (Draper and Trim 2018). Prevention involves avoiding use of potential toxins, such as commercial flea and tick products, cleaning products, nicotine or insecticide treated vegetation for feeding insect prey, (Draper and Trim 2018). Death has occurred in tarantulas due to the residual effects of fipronil remaining on containers several months later after being previously used to house snakes treated for snake mites (Pizzi 2010). Gloves should always be worn when handling these animals and care must be taken in the surgery when using pre-used containers to examine or house individuals.

23.7 Preventative Health Measures

Little preventative medicine is required for single pet tarantulas other than attention to husbandry, environment, and diet. It is vital to consider that prey health is very intimately associated with the health of the tarantula; maintaining a varied and healthy feed source will aid in optimising the health of the tarantula.

When introducing a new individual to a collection, quarantine and screening for Panagrolamidae nematodes is recommended. It is also sensible to perform a clinical examination and assess the whole spider with a hand lens to check for mites before introduction. A quarantine period of at least 30 days with the tarantula kept in a separate room from the existing collection is recommended. The spider should be deemed healthy and have eaten before being moved to the main collection (Pizzi 2012).

23.8 Microchip Identification

Permanent identification is possible in tarantulas and may be useful for valuable animals or for field work (Baker et al. 2018) but requires anaesthesia (Figure 23.16). Reichling and Tabaka (2001) have described the implantation of transponders in the opisthosoma of 12 tarantulas, demonstrating that permanent identification was possible and did not affect ecdysis. Before microchip insertion the setae were removed from the dorsolateral opisthosoma and the area disinfected with 10% povidone-iodine. The microchip was inserted with sterile forceps after a small incision was made with a 20-gauge needle, and the wound was closed using tissue adhesive. Baker et al.

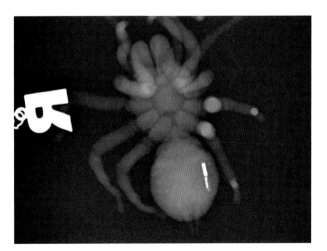

Figure 23.16 Dorsoventral radiograph showing poor soft-tissue differentiation. The transponder can be clearly seen in the opisthosoma of this female salmon pink (*Lasiodora parahybana*) (Baker et al. 2018, *Source:* Reprinted with permission from Institute of Animal Technology).

(2018) used a standard microchip insertion device successfully. Before implanting microchips in theraphosids, a full risk analysis should be discussed with the owner due to potential complications such as haemolymph loss and penetration of organs.

23.9 Imaging

Radiography is of limited value as very little soft tissue differentiation is evident (Figure 23.16). One study has demonstrated that mammography film provides a superior image, but lack of detail remains a concern (Davis et al. 2008). In the same study, use of radiographic contrast media still failed to allow organ differentiation and computed tomography also did not provide diagnostic images. Further studies are needed to assess whether newer digital radiography techniques will improve image quality.

Magnetic resonance imaging shows some promise. This technique has been performed on three tarantulas both with and without contrast and showed good morphology of structures and also provided evidence about regional perfusion (Pohlmann et al. 2007).

Ultrasonography is of value to investigate for the presence of large endoparasitic acrocercid larvae in the opisthosoma (Johnson-Delaney 2006). Use of a 10-MHz curvilinear probe is preferred with the use of ethanol, instead of ultrasound gel to provide a clearer image, however, the use of ethanol may deepen the anaesthesia plane (Pizzi 2012).

Endoscopy is a useful technique when examining oral discharges in tarantulas to assess for panagrolamid nematodes.

23.10 Formulary

Publications of drug dosages for spiders are scarce. The formulary provides a formulary for tarantulas. Consideration into the environmental temperature in which the animal is kept is essential as external temperature will affect metabolism.

Formulary

Medication	Dose	Dosing interval	Comments
Chemical restraint/anaesthetics			
Isoflurane	5% with 1 l/min oxygen for induction, alternatively, place 2 ml on a cotton wool ball.		(Dombrowski et al. 2013; Archibald et al. 2014).
Sevoflurane	5% concentration with an oxygen flow of 1 L/min for induction		(Zachariah et al. 2014)
Alfaxalone	200 mg/kg intracardiac		General anaesthesia for tarantulas (Gjeltema et al. 2014)
Alfaxalone; Ketamine	200 mg/kg; 20 mg/kg via the intracardiac route		Deep anaesthesia plane (Gjeltema et al. 2014)
Alfaxalone; Xylazine	200 mg/kg; 20 mg/kg administered via the intracardiac route		Deep plane of anaesthesia (Gjeltema et al. 2014).
Analgesics			
Butorphanol	20 mg/kg administered intracoelomically		(Sladky 2014)
Meloxicam	0.2 mg/kg administered orally	As a one-off dose (B. Maclean, personal communication) or every 24 hours (B. Kennedy, personal communication)	Efficacy undetermined
Morphine	50-100 mg/kg intracoelomically		(Sladky 2014)
Antimicrobials			
Ceftazidime	20 mg/kg intracardiac	Every 72 hours for up to 3 weeks.	Efficacy not established (Pizzi 2012).
Doxycycline	10 mg/kg PO	Every 24 hours	Efficacy not established (B. Kennedy, personal communication)

(Continued)

Medication	Dose	Dosing interval	Comments
Enrofloxacin	10–20 mg/kg PO	Every 24 hours	Compliance is difficult and most spiders will not take this (B Kennedy, personal communication)
Tetracyclines	No dose provided		Used by hobbyists. Results have been variable and for most cases a diagnosis was not achieved.
Antiparasitics			
Fenbendazole	10–200 mg/kg PO		Not effective at eliminating Panagrolaimidae nematodes (Pizzi 2012)
Ivermectin	Stock solution of 1 : 1 (1% ivermectin and propylene glycol) diluted 1 : 50 with distilled water. Apply topically		This has been used for the treatment of individual parasitic mites. Treatment is applied to mites with artists fine-tipped paint brush (Pizzi 2012). Ivermectin is toxic to spiders so should be used with caution.
Metronidazole	50 mg/kg intracardiac	Given as a single dose	Efficacy undetermined (Pizzi 2012).
Oxfendazole	10–200 mg/kg PO	Dosing intervals from every 24 hours for 10 doses to twice weekly.	This had minimal effect in treating oral nematodes (Pizzi 2012)
Miscellaneous			
Potassium Chloride (300 mg/ml)	0.5 ml /100 g body weight administered centrally via the anterior sternum into the cardiac ganglia or 1 ml/100 g body weight administered via intracardiac delivery		Euthanasia (Bennie et al. 2012)

References

Ahmed, N., Pinkham, M., and Warrell, D.A. (2009). Symptom in search of a toxin: muscle spasms following bites by Old World tarantula spiders (*Lampropelma nigerrimum, Pterinochilus murinus, Poecilotheria regalis*) with review. *QJM* 102 (12): 851–857.

Archibald, K.E., Minter, L.J., Lewbart, G.A. et al. (2014). Semen collection and characterisation in the Chilean rose tarantula (*Grammostola rosea*). *American Journal of Veterinary Research* 75: 929–936.

Baker, S., Knight, E., Pellett, S. et al. (2018). Spider and chips – the use of internal RFID chips as a minimally invasive method to measure internal body temperatures in invertebrates. *Animal Technology and Welfare* 17 (1): 1–7.

Bechanko, R., Hitt, N., O'Malley, K. et al. (2012). Are we aware of microbial hotspots in our household? *Journal of Environmental Health* 75: 12.

Bennie, N.A.C., Loaring, C.D., and Trim, S.A. (2011). Laboratory husbandry of arboreal tarantulas (Theraphosidae) and evaluation of environmental enrichment. *Animal Technology Welfare* 10: 163–169.

Bennie, N.A.C., Loaring, C.D., Bennie, M.M.G. et al. (2012). An effective method for terrestrial arthropod euthanasia. *The Journal of Experimental Biology* 215: 4237–4241.

Bertani, R. and Guadanucci, J.P.L. (2013). Morphology, evolution and usage of urticating setae by tarantulas (Araneae: Theraphosidae). *Zoologia (Curitiba)* 30 (4): 403–418.

Blatchford, R., Walker, S., and Marshall, S. (2011). A phylogeny-based comparison of tarantula spider anti-predator behaviour reveals correlation of morphology and behaviour. *Ethology* 117: 473–479.

Braun, M.E., Heatley, J.J., and Chitty, J. (2006). Clinical techniques of invertebrates. *Veterinary Clinics of North America. Exotic Animal Practice* 9: 205–221.

Breene, R.G. (1998). *The ATS Arthropod Medical Manual: Diagnoses and Treatment*. Carlsbad, NM: American Tarantula Society.

Castro, F.F.M., Antila, M.A., and Croce, J. (1995). Occupational allergy caused by urticating hair of Brazilian spider. *The Journal of Allergy and Clinical Immunology* 95 (6): 1282–1285.

Choi, J.T.L. and Rauf, A. (2003). *Ophthalmia nodosa* secondary to tarantula hairs. *Eye* 17: 433–434.

Davis, M.R., Gamble, K.C., and Matheson, J.S. (2008). Diagnostic imaging in terrestrial invertebrates: Madagascar hissing cockroach (*Gromphadorhina portentosa*), desert millipede (*Orthoporus* sp.), emperior scorpion (*Pandinus imperator*), Chilean rosehair tarantula (*Grammostola spatulata*), Mexican fireleg tarantula (*Brachypelma boehmei*), and Mexican redknee tarantula (*Brachypelma smithi*). *Zoo Biology* 27: 109–125.

De Sellem, F.E. (1917). Nicotine sulfate in codling moth control. *Proceedings of the Washington State Horticultural Association* 13: 111–121.

De Voe, R.S. (2009). Captive invertebrate nutrition. *Veterinary Clinics of North America: Exotic Animal Practice* 12: 349–360.

Dombrowski, D. and De Voe, R. (2007). Emergency care of invertebrates. *Veterinary Clinics of North America: Exotic Animal Practice* 10 (2): 621–645.

Dombrowski, D.S., De Voe, R.S., and Lewbart, G.A. (2013). Comparison of isoflurane and carbon dioxide anaesthesia in Chilean rose tarantulas (*Grammostola rosea*). *Zoo Biology* 32: 101–103.

Draper, E. and Trim, S.A. (2018). Dyskinetic syndrome in tarantula spiders (Theraphosidae). *Veterinary Nursing Journal* 33: 230–232.

Dunlop, J.A., Altringham, J.D., and Mill, P.J. (1992). Coupling between the heart and sucking stomach during ingestion in a tarantula. *Journal of Experimental Biology* 166 (1): 83–93.

Eckert, J. and Ossent, P. (2006). Haycocknema-like nematodes in muscle fibres of a horse. *Veterinary Parasitology* 139: 256–261.

Eddy, S. and Clarke, D. (2017). Theraphosid spiders (bird-eating or tarantula spiders): species care guidelines. TIWG care guidelines for Theraphosid Spiders. https://biaza.org.uk/resources/animal-husbandry/invertebrates (accessed 3 Deember 2018).

Eichelmann, M.A. and Lewbart, G.A. (2018). Hemolymph chemistry reference ranges of the chilean rose tarantula *Grammostola rosea* (Walkenaer, 1837) using the Vetscan biochemistry analyser based on IFCC-CLSI C28-A$_3$. *Journal of Zoo and Wildlife Medicine* 49 (3): 528–534.

Ellis, C.H. (1944). The mechanism of extension in the legs of spiders. *The Biological Bulletin* 86: 41–50.

Elwood, R.W. (2011). Pain and suffering in invertebrates? *ILAR Journal* 52 (2): 175–184.

Foelix, R.F. (1996). Functional anatomy. In: *Biology of Spiders*, 12–37. New York: Oxford University Press.

Fukushima, C.S. and Bertani, R. (2017). Taxonomic revision and cladistic analysis of *Avicularia* Lamarck, 1818 (Araneae, Theraphosidae, Aviculariinae) with description of three new aviculariine genera. *ZooKeys* 659: 1–185.

Gjeltema, J., Posner, L.P., and Stoskopf, M. (2014). The use of injectable alphaxalone as a single agent and in combination with ketamine, xylazine, and morphine in the Chilean rose tarantula, *Grammostola rosea*. *Journal of Zoo and Wildlife Medicine* 45: 792–801.

Greegoire, C.H. (1953). Blood coagulation in arthropods. III. Reactions of insect haemolymph to coagulation inhibitors of vertebrate blood. *The Biological Bulletin* 104: 372–393.

Gupta, A. (1985). Cellular elements in the haemolymph. In: *Comprehensive Insect Physiology, Biochemistry and Pharmacology, Volume 3: Integument, Respiration and Circulation* (eds. J.A. Kerkut and L.I. Gilbert), 401–452. New York: Pergamon Press.

Hancock, J. and Hancock, K. (1999). *Sex Determination of Immature Theraphosid Spiders from their Cast Skins*. Polgate, UK: British Tarantula Society.

Herzig, V. and King, G.F. (2013). The neurotoxic mode of action of venoms from the spider family Theraphosidae. In: *Spider Ecophysiology* (ed. W. Nentwig), 203–215. Berlin, Heidelberg: Springer.

Integrated Taxonomic Information System (2018). Integrated taxonomic information system. www.itis.gov (accessed 25 November 2018).

Johnson-Delaney, C. (2006). Use of ultrasonography in diagnosis of parasitism in goliath bird eater tarantulas (*Theraphosa blondi*). Proceedings British Veterinary Zoological Society, Autumn Meeting 2006, Bristol, UK: 102.

Keller, D.L., Abott, A.D., and Sladky, K.K. (2012). Invertebrate antinociception: are opioids effective in tarantulas? Proceedings of the American Association of Zoo Veterinarians Oakland, CA, 21-26 October: 97.

Kennedy, B., Warner, A., and Trim, S. (2019). Reference intervals for plasma biochemistry of hemolymph in the chilean rose tarantula (*Grammostola rosea*) under chemical restraint. *Journal of Zoo and Wildlife Medicine* 50 (1): 127–136.

Lewbart, G.A. and Mosley, C. (2012). Clinical anaesthesia and analgesia in invertebrates. *Journal of Exotic Pet Medicine* 21: 59–70.

Lovett, A.L. (1920). Insecticide investigations. *Oregon Agricultural Experiment Station Bulletin* 169: 47–52.

Marnell, C. (2016). Tarantula and hermit crab emergency care. *Veterinary Clinics of North America. Exotic Animal Practice* 19: 627–646.

Melidone, R.M. (2007). Tarantula medicine. *UK Vet* 12 (3): 1–8.

Mendoza, J.I. and Francke, O.F. (2017). Systematic revision of Brachypelma red-kneed tarantulas (Araneae: Theraphosidae), and the use of DNA barcodes to assist in the identification and conservation of CITES-listed species. *Invertebrate Systematics* 31 (2): 157–179.

Murray, M.J. (2012). Euthanasia. In: *Invertebrate Medicine* (ed. G.A. Lewbart), 441–443. Oxford: Blackwell Publishing.

Nadler, S.A., Carreno, R.A., Adams, B.J. et al. (2003). Molecular phylogenetics and diagnosis of soil and clinical isolates of *Halicephalobus gingivalis* (Nematoda: Cephalobina: Panagrolaimoidea), an opportunistic pathogen of horses. *International Journal for Parasitology* 33 (10): 1115–1125.

Paul, R.J., Bergner, B., Pfefferseidl, A. et al. (1994). Gas transport in the Haemolymph of arachnids. 1. Oxygen transport and the physiological role of Haemocyanin. *Journal of Experimental Biology* 188: 25–46.

Pearce, S.G., Bouré, L.P., Taylor, J.A. et al. (2001). Treatment of a granuloma caused by *Halicephalobus gingivalis* in a horse. *Journal of the American Veterinary Medical Association* 219 (12): 1735–1728.

Pellett, S., Bushell, M., and Clarke-Williams, J. (2014). Invertebrate care guidelines. *Companion Animal* 20 (1): 50–53.

Pellett, S., Bushell, M., and Trim, S.A. (2015). Tarantula husbandry and critical care. *Companion Animal* 20 (2): 119–125.

Pellett, S. and Kubiak, M. (2017). A review of invertebrate cases seen in practice. Proceedings Veterinary Invertebrate Society Summer Scientific Meeting 2017, Cambridge, UK: 4.

Pellett, S., Kubiak, M., Pizzi, R. et al. (2017). BIAZA recommendations for ethical euthanasia of invertebrates. (Version 3.0, April 2017). http://biaza.org.uk/resources/animal-husbandry/invertebrates (accessed 20 January 2019).

Pérez-Miles, F., Guadanucci, J.P.L., Jurgilas, J.P. et al. (2017). Morphology and evolution of scopula, pseudoscopula and claw tufts in Mygalomorphae (Araneae). *Zoomorphology* 136: 435.

Pizzi, R. (2002). Induction of autotomy in Theraphosidae spiders as a surgical technique. *Veterinary Invertebrate Society Newsletter* 2 (18): 2–6.

Pizzi, R. (2009). Parasites of tarantulas (Theraphosidae). *Journal of Exotic Pet Medicine* 18: 283–288.

Pizzi, R. (2010). Invertebrates. In: *BSAVA Manual of Exotic Pets*, 5e (eds. A. Meredith and C.A. Johnson-Delaney), 373–385. Gloucester, UK: BSAVA Publications.

Pizzi, R. (2012). Spiders. In: *Invertebrate Medicine*, 2e (ed. G.A. Lewbart), 187–221. Oxford: Blackwell Publishing.

Pohlmann, A., Möller, M., Decker, H. et al. (2007). MRI of tarantulas: morphological and perfusion imaging. *Magnetic Resonance Imaging* 25 (1): 129–135.

Reichling, S.B. and Tabaka, C. (2001). A technique for individually identifying tarantulas using passive integrated transponders. *Journal of Arachnology* 29 (1): 117–118.

Ruppert, E.E., Fox, R.S., and Barnes, R.D. (2004). *Invertebrate Zoology: A Functional Evolutionary Approach*, 7e. Belmont, CA: Saunders College Publishing.

Schartau, W., Leidescher, T., Schartau, W. et al. (1983). Composition of the hemolymph of the tarantula *Eurypelma californicum*. *Journal of Comparative Physiology B* 152: 73–77.

Sladky, K.K. (2014). Current Understanding of Fish and Invertebrate Anaesthesia and Analgesia. Proceedings of the Association of Reptilian and Amphibian Veterinarians 18–24 October 2014, Orlando, FL: 122–124.

Smith, R.E. (1921). The preparation of nicotine dust as an insecticide. *California Agricultural Experiment Station Bulletin* 336: 261–274.

Soares, T., dos Santos Cavalcanti, M.G., Ferreira, F.R.D. et al. (2013). Ultrastructural characterisation of the hemocytes of *Lasiodora* sp. (Koch, 1850) (Araneae: Theraphosidae). *Micron* 48: 11–16.

Somerville, S., Baker, S., Baines, F. et al. (2017). Measuring cortisol levels in theraphosids and scorpions. Proceedings Veterinary Invertebrate Society Summer Scientific Meeting 2017, Cambridge, UK: 4.

Stewart, D.M. and Martin, A.W. (1982). Moulting in the tarantula *Dugesiella hentzi*. *Journal of Comparative Physiology* 149: 121–136.

Wagler, R. (2015). A guide for acquiring and caring for tarantulas appropriate for the middle school science classroom. *Science Scope* 38 (8) http://static.nsta.org/connections/middleschool/201504Wagler.pdf (accessed 30 January 2020).

World Spider Catalog (2019). World Spider Catalog. Version 20.0. Natural History Museum Bern. http://wsc.nmbe.ch (accessed 10 February 2019).

Zachariah, T.T., Mitchell, M.A., Guichard, C.M. et al. (2007). Hemolymph biochemistry reference ranges for wild-caught goliath birdeater spiders (*Theraphosa blondi*) and Chilean rose spiders (*Grammostola rosea*). *Journal of Zoo and Wildlife Medicine* 38: 245–251.

Zachariah, T.T., Mitchell, M.A., Guichard, C.M. et al. (2009). Isoflurane anaesthesia of wild-caught goliath birdeater spiders (*Theraphosa blondi*) and Chilean rose spiders (*Grammostola rosea*). *Journal of Zoo and Wildlife Medicine* 40: 347–349.

Zachariah, T.T., Mitchell, M.A., Watson, M.K. et al. (2014). Effects of sevoflurane anaesthesia on righting reflex and haemolymph gas analysis variables for Chilean rose tarantulas (*Grammostola rosea*). *American Journal of Veterinary Research* 75: 521–526.

24

Giant African Land Snails
Sarah Pellett and Michelle O'Brien

24.1 Introduction

Giant African land snails (GALS) are large, terrestrial pulmonate gastropod molluscs, belonging to the Family Achatinidae and Genus Achatina (Integrated Taxonomic Information System 2017). GALS, *Achatina* spp. are frequently kept by hobbyists, zoological collections, teaching colleges, and schools (Cooper and Knowler 1991). Within the pet trade, three species predominate. The most commonly seen species is the East African land snail, *Achatina (Lissachatina) fulica* (Figure 24.1). The West African land snail (Banana Rasp snail or 'Margie'), *Archachatina (Calachatina) marginata* (Figure 24.2), and the Tiger snail, or giant Ghana snail, *Achatina achatina* (Figure 24.3) are also relatively common pets (Pellett et al. 2014).

24.2 Biological Parameters

GALS live for approximately 5–8 years and some may reach 10 years of age (O'Brien 2009). They can be popular pets for children as they are active, simple to keep, and can be carefully handled. They are relatively large, with *A. fulica* averaging 10 cm in length, although some individuals have been reported to be as long as 20 cm (Pizzi 2010). The African land snail is considered to be a significant invasive species around the world (Thiengo et al. 2007), and it is an offence under the Wildlife and Countryside Act (1981) to release captive animals into the wild in the UK.

24.2.1 Anatomy

The most distinctive modification of gastropods is that the body has undergone torsion. When viewed dorsally, the body is twisted 180° counterclockwise, however pulmonate snails (including GALS) have undergone mild detorsion (Ruppert and Barnes 1994). The typical shell is an asymmetrical spiral, containing a visceral mass that spirals around a central axis, the columella. Each spiral is called a whorl, and the head and foot protrude from the aperture of the final whorl (Smolowitz 2012). Dextral (right-handed) shells are more frequently seen (Smolowitz 2012). The palladial cavity lies within the final whorl, which is lined by the mantle, and contains the anus, head and reproductive ostia. The shell is formed by the mantle epithelium (Smolowitz 2012). The head is well-developed with two pairs of bilaterally symmetrical tentacles with the eyes positioned on the upper pair (Figure 24.4) (Smolowitz 2012).

African land snails have a pulmonary sac, formed by the fusion of the mantle edges along the animal's back. Air enters the sac through the pneumostome, a small opening found just beneath the shell rim in the mantle, which can open and close with the ventilatory cycle. The roof of the pulmonary sac has become highly vascularised for gas exchange (Ruppert and Barnes 1994; Smolowitz 2012). The lateral walls of the pharynx are lined by a hardened plate that forms the jaw, the odontophore. The odontophore is covered by the radula, a membrane lined by chitinised teeth produced in the radular sheath (a diverticulum of the pharynx) (Smolowitz 2012). The gastrointestinal tract comprises of an oesophagus, a crop, a scleritised gizzard, a pyloric stomach, a cecum, and intestine leading to the anus (Smolowitz 2012). Gastropods have an open circulatory system with a heart that has a single ventricle (Smolowitz 2012). The heart beats rhythmically, and in an average-sized snail, the heart rate is approximately 25–30 beats per minute (Srivastava 1992). During aestivation, this may reduce to 9–10 beats per minute (Srivastava 1992). The kidney is in the posterolateral part of the mantle cavity, adhering to the mantle and lying parallel to the heart (Srivastava 1992). The excretory lumen of the kidney leads to an opening known as the nephridiopore, exiting into the palladial cavity beside the anus (Smolowitz 2012).

Handbook of Exotic Pet Medicine, First Edition. Edited by Marie Kubiak.
© 2021 John Wiley & Sons Ltd. Published 2021 by John Wiley & Sons Ltd.
Companion website: www.wiley.com/go/kubiak/exotic_pet_medicine

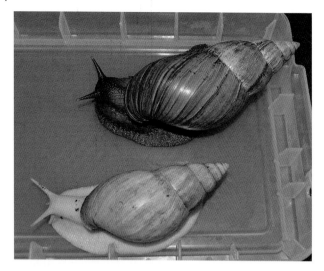

Figure 24.1   East African land snails.

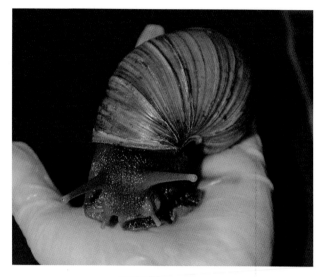

Figure 24.4   Snails have two pairs of retractable tentacles. The eyes are located on the upper tentacles and the lower tentacles detect tactile and chemical stimuli.

24.3 Husbandry

A. fulica and A. marginata require an environment with temperatures of 25–26 °C during the daytime and 21–23 °C at night, to maintain optimum growth (Bazzoni and Pellett 2013). *A. achatina* prefers a higher daytime temperature of 25–30 °C, and a night-time drop of 2–4 °C (Bazzoni and Pellett 2013). A maximum-minimum thermometer is recommended to monitor stability of environmental temperatures. Temperatures can be maintained by placing a heat mat to the side of the enclosure to create a thermal gradient without causing substrate desiccation. Heat mats should not be placed underneath as this will dry the substrate and affect thermoregulatory behaviours. All heat pads should be thermostatically controlled. Snail enclosures should be kept away from direct sunlight and other heat sources to avoid significant temperature fluctuations.

In the wild, the photoperiod is 12:12 hours light to dark and native conditions do not vary much. Additional lighting beyond provisions for a day:night cycle is not recommended for land snail enclosures. Land snails are nocturnal, and generally in the wild, their activities are restricted from dusk till dawn (Srivastava 1992).

Enclosures for GALS can either be glass or plastic tanks. Minimum enclosure guidelines for two land snails are 60 cm long, 45 cm wide and 40 cm high (RSPCA 2017). Snails can be great escape artists so a secure lid must be used at all times. Ventilation is required and holes can be drilled or vents inserted at the top of the tank to allow for this. The walls of the tank should be washed daily to remove mucus and droppings.

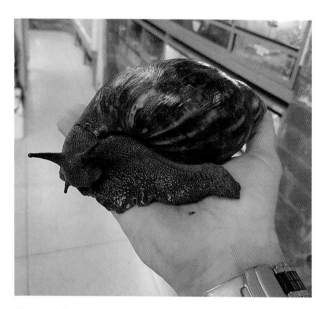

Figure 24.2   West African land snail (*Source:* Courtesy of Lincoln Reptile and Pet Centre).

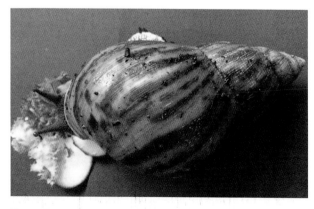

Figure 24.3   Tiger snail (*Source:* Courtesy of Sonja Brown).

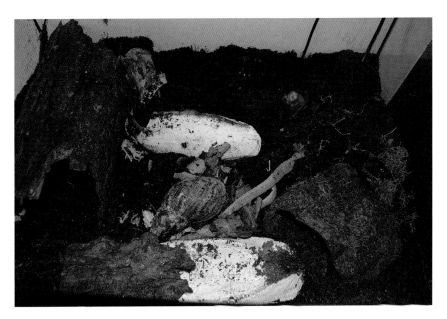

Figure 24.5 Land snails provided with coir substrate and areas to retreat.

The ideal substrate for the enclosure is 3–6 cm of pH neutral peat-free compost or coir. In most cases, coir has been sterilised and minimises the risk of introducing parasites (particularly mites) or pathogens into the enclosure. Ground limestone can be mixed into this substrate to provide calcium. Substrate should allow burrowing and must not be compacted, so clay soils are best avoided. Sandy soils will not retain enough moisture to maintain the required 70–90% relative humidity (80–95% for *A. achatina*). A moist-retaining substrate and lightly misting the enclosure daily with warm water will sustain the humidity required (Bazzoni and Pellett 2013). *A. fulica* are more sensitive to overly wet environments than other species of Achatinidae and any water-logged substrate must be removed immediately. A hygrometer is advised to measure and monitor humidity within the terrarium.

Wide, clean branches should be provided to enable climbing, and terracotta or plastic pots should be provided for hides (Figure 24.5).

24.3.1 Diet

In the wild, GALS are omnivorous, feeding upon a large number of plant species but also carrion, soil, and dung (Olson 1973). In captivity, a variety of dark leafy greens and plants should be offered. Vegetables and fruits, including courgettes, cabbage, cucumber, melon, and apple can also be offered. Spinach and other high oxalate foods should not be given daily as they bind calcium and thereby decrease absorption within the gastrointestinal tract. All foods offered must be washed to ensure the removal of pesticides

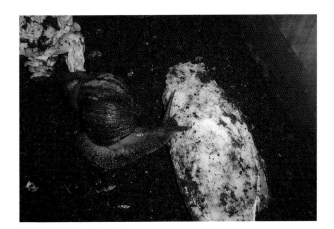

Figure 24.6 Calcium provision must be available.

and toxins. Uneaten food should be removed from the enclosure within 24 hours.

Calcium is essential for normal formation and growth of the shell but powdered supplements are not readily accepted on food. Natural chalk or cuttlefish bone is accepted well and should be provided (Figure 24.6). Calcium deficiency is a commonly seen problem in captivity where a calcium source is not provided. For clinically affected animals, a powdered calcium and vitamin supplement can be added to a small amount of soaked rabbit pelleted food to formulate a calcium-rich paste (Pizzi 2010).

Snails like to climb into water bowls so a shallow bowl of fresh water should be offered daily.

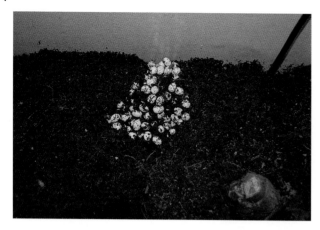

Figure 24.7 Removal of soil to demonstrate buried clutch of *Achatina fulica* eggs.

24.3.2 Reproduction

GALS are obligate outcrossing hermaphrodites. In the wild, the normal breeding time is during the rainy season, from April until July. Sperm can be stored from one mating and successful egg laying can then continue for over a year (Pizzi 2010). Individuals can start laying eggs at around six months of age, and for *A. fulica,* this is when the snail has reached approximately 80 mm in length (O'Brien 2009). Clutch size can be up to 200 eggs and one snail can produce approximately one thousand eggs each year (O'Brien 2009). Eggs are cream in colour, spherical with a mineralised shell, and measure 4.5–5.5 mm in diameter (Figure 24.7). Under optimal conditions, there is a 90% hatch rate hatch after approximately 14 days. Eggs are laid within the substrate, and if breeding is to be encouraged, a deeper substrate is recommended. Once laid, eggs can be carefully buried in a small tank under the same conditions as the adult tank for optimal hatch rate, or left in with the adults. Unwanted eggs can be placed in a deep freezer; they should never be thrown out without destruction as GALS are considered invasive and a threat to native species.

Newly-hatched snails have a globose, very thin and mostly transparent shell. The first whorl is very small, the second one much larger. By the eighth day from hatching, the snail is approximately 6.5 mm and by day 16, at about 8 mm in size, the shell appears thicker and more opaque (Srivastava 1992).

24.4 Clinical Evaluation

24.4.1 History-Taking

A land snail consultation should be approached in a similar way to a consultation of any familiar species. A detailed history, emphasising the husbandry aspect is essential as the vast majority of health problems encountered are related to suboptimal husbandry and environmental conditions. Attention should be paid to ensuring the diet, ambient temperature, and relative humidity provided are appropriate, and whether there has been a recent change in management (Cooper 2004).

If possible, the snail should be brought to the surgery in its home enclosure. If this is not possible, it can be transported in a clear plastic tub with appropriate substrate and a secure lid. If owners cannot bring in the enclosure, digital photographs of the set up should be brought in so the environment can be assessed.

24.4.2 Clinical Examination

Examination can be carried out by gently holding the shell, or allowing the animal to sit on a gloved hand. The use of a hand lens will aid in observing the animal. The snail should be weighed on digital scales and measured as part of routine examination (Cooper 2004). The snail should be examined for any traumatic injuries to the shell, foot or mantle, any signs of prolapse, excess mucus production or any other abnormalities that may indicate the presence of clinical disease.

24.5 Basic Techniques

24.5.1 Anaesthesia and Analgesia

The welfare of invertebrates has to be considered during treatment, particularly for any invasive procedures (Smith 1991). It remains undetermined if invertebrates experience pain or simply demonstrate a reflexive response to a noxious stimuli but many invertebrate species do have well-developed nervous systems and therefore the possibility to perceive pain. Arthropods and molluscs have been shown to have body wall and internal tissues rich with nerve endings or similar sensory structures (Cooper 1998). Given the lack of evidence to the contrary and strong indications that neural pathways exist to allow pain perception, pain management should be considered in Achatinidae where a noxious stimulus is suspected.

Anaesthesia in snails is determined by the absence of body and tentacle withdrawal response to gentle stimulation (Girdlestone et al. 1989; Cooper 2001). In practice, anaesthesia of GALS is challenging and should be regarded as higher risk than that of arthropods. The use of anaesthesia and risks associated with this on land snails should be thoroughly discussed with owners when consent is required (Pizzi 2010). Doppler ultrasonography should be used to monitor anaesthesia and assess for vascular flow. Propylene phenoxytol and MS-222 may cause excitation at induction resulting in excess mucus production and therefore likely stress or discomfort. Gaseous anaesthesia using isoflurane for terrestrial snails is not recommended as this also causes excess mucus production (Pellett et al. 2017). Hypothermia is not considered a humane method of anaesthesia as there is no loss of sensation.

24.5.2 Haemolymph Sampling

GALS blood is referred to as haemolymph and contains haemocyanin, a copper-based respiratory pigment which gives it a pale blue colour (Morton 1958). Haemolymph sampling has been carried out for research purposes (Brockelman 1975; Brockelman 1978; Brockelman and Sithithavorn 1980; Agrawal et al. 1990). However, haemolymph interpretation for veterinary diagnosis is still in its infancy, but samples should be considered as part of a diagnostic approach (Cooper and Knowler 1991).

Several methods have been described where haemolymph can be obtained by drilling into the shell and collecting the sample from the heart (Friedl 1961; Williams 1999), or by incising the mantle and then into the visceral sac (Brockelman 1975). An alternative approach to sampling haemolymph, is described where haemolymph is collected without perforating the shell, or incising soft tissues (Cooper 1994). The snail is washed in cold water to remove soil, faeces and mucus, and gentle pressure is applied to the foot to remove residual mucus. The pneumostome (respiratory opening) is located by observing bubbles over it as it periodically opens when the snail breathes. A 21–25G needle attached to a 1 ml syringe is used, depending upon the size of the snail (Cooper 1994). For Achatina weighing less than 50 g, the insertion site is approximately 5 mm ventral to the pneumostome. For snails weighing 200 g the insertion point is approximately 20 mm ventral to the pneumostome (Cooper 1994). Haemolymph volume is approximately 2 ml per 100 g bodyweight in *Helix* species, though in dormant snails this can reduce significantly (Burton 1964; Barnhart 1986). Approximately 10% of the total volume of haemolymph has been removed in some individuals with no adverse effects (Cooper 1994) so 0.2 ml per 100 g would be considered a safe volume to sample in a metabolically active *Achatina* snail.

24.5.3 Euthanasia

Anaesthesia using phenoxyethanol followed by euthanasia via a sodium pentobarbitone injection for three moribund specimens of *A. marginata* seemed to cause little stress to the animals (pers. comm. R. Saunders, 2013). The method used is a bath of 100% phenoxyethanol (Aqua-Sed,

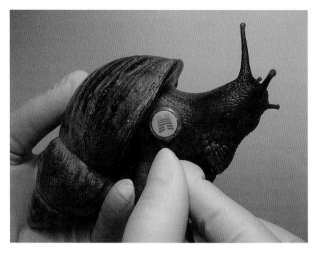

Figure 24.8 Examination with a Doppler probe (*Source:* O'Brien [2008: 293], reprinted with permission from Elsevier).

VETARK Professional) so that the foot is just covered but the pneumostome is not submerged (Pizzi 2010). After 30 minutes the animal was non-responsive and a 400 mg/kg dose of pentobarbital was injected (pers. comm. A. Naylor, 2014). Cessation of vascular flow and a heartbeat can be monitored using an 8 MHz Doppler probe (Rees Davies et al. 2000) (Figure 24.8).

If chemical methods are unavailable or impractical, physical crushing to destroy the nervous centre is regarded as humane due to the speed at which euthanasia is achieved, although the method should be suitable for the size of the animal in question. Animals smaller than 3 cm can be suitably euthanased using this method, although it is recommended to bear in mind the thickness of the shell (Pellett et al. 2017).

24.6 Common Medical and Surgical Conditions

24.6.1 Aestivation

If environmental conditions are suboptimal, such as too hot, cold, or dry, then snails produce a thin, hardened mucus film over the shell aperture to retain moisture and may enter a dormant state (Figure 24.9). The mucous barrier must not be manually broken down as this may cause damage to the snail. Underlying environmental conditions must be addressed and the snail bathed in a shallow dish of warm water or lightly sprayed across the aperture (Pizzi 2010). A Doppler probe applied to the body of the snail can be used to assess heart rate to determine if a retracted snail is in aestivation or is dead.

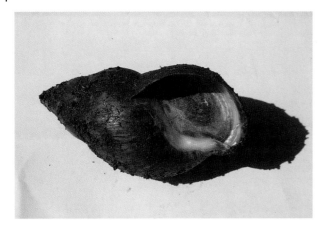

Figure 24.9 When exposed to unfavourable conditions snails may aestivate – sealing the shell aperture and entering a dormant state.

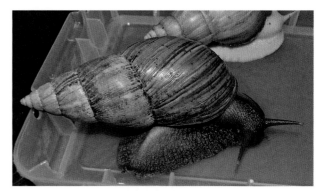

Figure 24.10 Loss of superficial shell as a consequence of rasping by a conspecific. This is often associated with lack of provision of a calcium source.

24.6.2 Trauma

Snails should be handled near to a soft surface as a fall, even from a short distance can result in shell fracture, or damage to the foot with subsequent loss of haemolymph and death (Braun et al. 2006). The protective shell is secreted as a layered structure by the epidermis and is made up of sclerotized protein, with underlying layers being composed of calcium carbonate crystals (Braun et al. 2006). In GALS, trauma usually results in damage to the calcareous shell. Fracture of the shell does not necessarily cause loss of haemolymph but may result in dehydration due to exposure and desiccation to underlying tissues. All wounds should be flushed with sterile saline and then if the damage cannot be repaired immediately, the snail should be placed in a shallow bowl of water or 0.9% saline, pending treatment. Small defects can be covered with a sterile adhesive layer followed by an epoxy resin cover. If the shell fracture is more severe, the two sides of the break can be cleaned, apposed and stabilised using a sterile adhesive layer and then repaired using plaster of Paris or epoxy resin. Roughening of the edges may help with adhesion. Once the plaster of Paris or epoxy resin has dried, clear nail varnish can be applied over the repair to waterproof it. Damage to the tissues of the mantle (near the opening) can lead to shell growth deformities (Zwart and Cooper work in preparation). Dietary calcium supplementation is advised for snails presented with shell injury (Connolly 2004).

Damage to the lip of the shell, unless severe, will often heal with no intervention. If perforation of the soft-body has occurred causing haemolymph leakage then death usually occurs quickly.

In older snails the mantle can separate from the rest of the body. This may repair if the snail is placed in a shallow tank, thus restricting climbing, but usually there are other underlying factors and mortality is high (O'Brien 2009).

24.6.3 Calcium Deficiency

Calcium deficiency can be seen in GALS (O'Brien 2009). The shell of a mollusc is calcium carbonate, not calcium phosphate as found in bones of vertebrates (Williams 2001). Dietary calcium has an important role in shell calcification, with a calcium enriched diet leading to thickening of the shell in a dose-responsive manner (Ireland 1971). Vitamin D, as 25-hydroxycholecalciferol appears to be biologically active in invertebrates (Kriajev et al. 1994). The molluscan metabolite E (a vitamin D metabolite) has been found to accelerate the transfer of calcium from the mantle to the shell (Kriajev and Edelstein 1995). Clinical signs of calcium deficiency include brittle shells leading to a greater chance of fractures, as well as rasping one snail's shell by another (Figure 24.10). Irregular shell growth or slow growth of shells can also be seen. Treatment is by repair of defects and correction of husbandry.

24.6.4 Poisoning

Pesticides and toxins must be removed from all foods before feeding; all foods should be thoroughly washed. Hand-picked lettuce and vegetables should be carefully checked for slug pellets (O'Brien 2009). In the veterinary practice, it is essential that flea sprays or insecticides are not used in any room housing snails, nor containers potentially used for snails. In other invertebrate taxa deaths have occurred following use of containers that had previously housed snakes that had been treated for mites (Pizzi 2010). The containers had been washed before placing the invertebrates in them but the residues remaining were enough to cause fatalities.

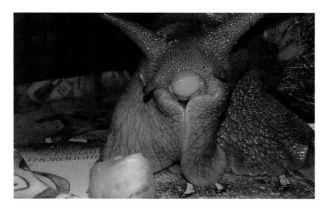

Figure 24.11   Oral prolapse (*Source:* Courtesy of Gemma Bradley).

24.6.5   Ectoparasites

Mites can sometimes be seen on snails, and their pathogenicity varies with the species of mites (O'Brien 2009). In large numbers, they can lead to debilitation and can manually be removed by gently spraying them with water, or removing them with a dampened fine artist's paintbrush. Environmental conditions should then be addressed.

24.6.6   Prolapse

Snails can present with prolapse of organs through their mouthparts, typically comprising the digestive tract. Digestive tract prolapses usually indicate severe systemic disease and are usually seen in chronically unwell or geriatric snails and euthanasia is generally advised. In one case, one author was presented with a snail with an oral prolapse, which was deemed to be part of the radula (Figure 24.11). In this case, the prolapse was replaced with a dampened cotton-tip applicator and the snail went on to make an uneventful recovery without further prolapses. If the bursa copulatrix or dart apparatus has prolapsed, attempts at replacing them using a moistened cotton-tipped applicator can be made (Pizzi 2010).

24.7   Preventative Health Measures

Little preventative medicine is required other than attention to husbandry and environment, adequate calcium supplementation in the diet, and care in preparation of food to ensure all contaminants have been removed.

24.7.1   Zoonotic Considerations

In the wild, GALS may be a potential carrier of *Angiostrongylus cantonensis,* the rat lungworm. In humans, this can cause eosinophilic meningoencephalitis (Latonio

1971; Moreira et al. 2013). African land snails can harbour L_3 larvae, with humans becoming infected through ingestion of larvae deposited on fruit and vegetables in mucus, or through eating raw or undercooked snail meat (Kim et al. 2002; Toma et al. 2002; Neuhauss et al. 2007). The parasite is not seen in pet snails in the UK.

When considering potential zoonosis of GALS, the isolation of potentially pathogenic bacteria must also be factored in. Bacteria isolated in a recent study included the Gram-negative bacteria *Pseudomonas fluorescens, P. putida, Chryseobacterium indologenes, Alcaligenes faecalis, Citrobacter youngae, Klebsiella oxytoca, Enterobacter* spp., *Aeromonas* spp., and *Pantoea* spp. (Williams et al. 2017). Most bacteria isolated are soil-dwelling organisms but *P. putida* and *C. indologenes* have been associated with infections in hospitalised patients (Bayraktar et al. 2007). *P. putida* has also been implicated in causing bacteraemia in patients (Yoshino et al. 2011). Gram-positive bacteria isolated from GALS include *Staphylococcus sciuri* and *Micrococcus* spp. Previous similar studies isolated *Aeromonas liquefaciens* from *A. fulica* (Akinboade et al. 1980; Dean et al. 1970). *A. hydrophila* has also been isolated from *A. fulica* from leucodermal skin lesions (Mead 1979). This bacterium is found within soil, the substrate commonly used for this species, and to cause disease (e.g. cellulitis), mechanical abrasion is usually required (Williams 2001).

Standard hygiene measures are recommended, with diligent hand washing after handling GALS and children supervised at all times, similar to measures for handling any other animal (Williams et al. 2017).

24.8   Imaging

Radiography can provide information on shell fractures and help determine a plan to repair the fracture sites. Snails can also be fed a preferred food item, with barium added to allow visualisation of the gastrointestinal tract (Braun et al. 2006). Gumpenberger and Scmidt-Ukaj (2017) assessed the physical anatomy of four GALS as a reference for radiographic, ultrasonography, and computed tomography (CT) examinations. Contrast media was also administered in food to evaluate the gastrointestinal tract. The shell, heart, and eggs were visualised on radiography and contrast-enhanced radiographs allowed visualisation of the gastrointestinal tract. The respiratory tract, kidney, and contrast-enhanced gastrointestinal tract were visualised on CT examination. The genital tract was not visualised with any imaging methods (Gumpenberger and Scmidt-Ukaj 2017).

Ultrasonography can be useful to assess the oral radula, pharynx, and cranial part of the gastrointestinal tract. Developed eggs can also be visualised (Pizzi 2010).

A 7.5–10MHz curvilinear probe, using a water standoff and not ultrasound gel will provide good definition. Ultrasonography can also aid in determining the origin of a prolapse.

Endoscopy can be performed to examine the snail pneumostome and demonstrate the snail is not infected with parasitic mites or *A. cantonensis* (Braun et al. 2006; Pizzi 2010).

24.9   Formulary

Publications of drug dosages for snails are scarce. A formulary is provided in the formulary. Consideration of the environmental temperature in which the animal is kept is essential as external temperature will affect metabolism.

Formulary; Publications of drug dosages for snails are scarce*

	Dose rate	Notes
Analgesic agents		
Butorphanol	20 mg/kg intracoelomically	Extrapolated from theraphosid doses. Has been shown to attenuate responses to noxious stimuli in theraphosids (Sladky 2014). Butorphanol can also be administered at doses prescribed for fish at 0.05–0.1 mg/kg (Stoskopf 1999) up to 10 mg/kg (Baker et al. 2013)
Morphine	50–100 mg/kg intracoelomically	Extrapolated from theraphosids. (Sladky 2014). Has been shown to attenuate responses to noxious stimuli (Sladky 2014).
Chemical restraint/ anaesthetic agents		
Magnesium sulphate or magnesium chloride	Intracoelomically in sea snails	(Clark et al. 1996). Magnesium ions compete with calcium ions required for synaptic transmission, resulting in immobilisation (O'Brien 2008). Induction is fast (2–5 minutes) and smooth.
Magnesium chloride	10% solution injected around cerebral ganglia	Results in quick relaxation for 5–15 minutes after administering (Runham et al. 1965). However, true anaesthesia may not be provided and the analgesic properties have not been determined (Ross and Ross 1999).
Ethanol	3% solution as a bath	Induced anaesthesia in abalones (Gunkel and Lewbart 2007)
2-phenoxyethanol	1–2 ml/l bath	Induced anaesthesia in abalones (Aquilina and Roberts 2000; Edwards et al. 2000). Fast induction period (1–3 minutes) therefore reducing stress (White et al. 1996; Gunkel and Lewbart 2007).
Benzocaine	100 mg/l bath	Induced anaesthesia in abalones (Aquilina and Roberts 2000; Edwards et al. 2000)
Magnesium sulphate	2–24 mg/100 ml bath	Induced anaesthesia in abalones (Aquilina and Roberts 2000; Edwards et al. 2000). Induction time with magnesium sulphate is fast (5–8 minutes) and smooth.
Sodium pentobarbital	1 ml/l bath	Induced anaesthesia in abalones (Aquilina and Roberts 2000; Edwards et al. 2000)
Methane sulphonate (MS-222)	100 mg/l, as a shallow bath, just covering the foot but avoiding the pneumostome, just beneath the shell rim in the mantle	(Zachariah and Mitchell 2009). Beeman (1969) reported reversible anaesthesia, but Joosse and Lever (1959) reported mortalities after MS-222 use.

*Consideration of the environmental temperature in which the animal is kept is essential as external temperature will affect metabolism.

References

Agrawal, A., Mitra, S., Ghosh, N. et al. (1990). C-reactive protein (CRP) in haemolymph of a mollusc, *Achatina fulica* Bowdich. *Indian Journal of Experimental Biology* 28: 788–789.

Akinboade, O.A., Adegoke, G.O., Ogunji, F.O. et al. (1980). Bacterial isolates from giant snails in Nigeria. *The Veterinary Record* 106: 482.

Aquilina, B. and Roberts, R. (2000). A method for inducing muscle relaxation in the abalone, *Haliotis iris*. *Aquaculture* 190: 403–408.

Baker, T.R., Baker, B.B., Johnson, S.M. et al. (2013). Comparative analgesic efficacy of morphine sulfate and butorphanol tartrate in koi (*Cyprinus carpio*) undergoing unilateral gonadectomy. *Journal of the American Veterinary Medical Association* 243: 882–890.

Barnhart, M.C. (1986). Respiratory gas tensions and gas exchange in active and dormant land snails, Otala lactea. *Physiological Zoology* 59 (6): 733–745.

Bayraktar, M.R., Aktas, E., Ersoy, Y. et al. (2007). Postoperative Chryseobacterium indologenes bloodstream infection. *Infection Control and Hospital Epidemiology* 28: 368–369.

Bazzoni, L. and Pellett, S. (2013). Care guidelines. https://biaza.org.uk/resources/animal-husbandry/invertebrates (accessed 23 July 2017).

Beeman, R.D. (1969). *The Use of Succinylcholine and Other Drugs for Anaesthetising or Narcotising Gastropod Molluscs*. Naples: Publications of the Zoological Station, Naples.

Braun, M.E., Heatley, J., and Chitty, J.C. (2006). Clinical techniques of invertebrates. *Veterinary Clinics of North America: Exotic Animal Practice* 9: 205–221.

Brockelman, C.R. (1975). Inhibition of *Rhabditis maupasi* (Rhabditidae: nematoda), maturation and reproduction by factors from the snail host, *Helix aspersa. Journal of Invertebrate Pathology* 25: 229–237.

Brockelman, C.R. (1978). Effects of parasitism and stress on haemolymph protein of the African giant snail, *Achatina fulica. Zeitschrift für Parasitenkunde* 57: 137–144.

Brockelman, C.R. and Sithithavorn, P. (1980). Carbohydrate reserves and hemolymph sugars of the African giant snail, *Achatina fulica* in relation to parasitic infection and starvation. *Zeitschrift für Parasitenkunde* 62: 285–291.

Burton, R.F. (1964). Variations in the volume and concentration of the blood of the snail, Helix pomatia L., in relation to the water content of the body. *Canadian Journal of Zoology* 42 (6): 1085–1097.

Clark, T.R., Nossov, P.C., and Apland, J.R. (1996). Anaesthetic agents for use in the invertebrate sea snail, *Aplysia californica. Contemporary Topics in Laboratory Animal Science* 35: 75–79.

Connolly, C. (2004). Repair of the shell of a Giant African Landsnail (*Achatina fulica*), using Leucopor tape and Nexabond tissue adhesive. *Veterinary Invertebrate Society Newsletter*: 8–11.

Cooper, J.E. (1994). Bleeding of pulmonate snails. *Laboratory Animals* 28: 277–278.

Cooper, J.E. (1998). Emergency care of invertebrates. *The Veterinary Clinics of North America. Exotic Animal Practice* 1 (1): 251–264.

Cooper, J.E. (2001). Invertebrate anaesthesia. *The Veterinary Clinics of North America. Exotic Animal Practice* 4 (1): 57–67.

Cooper, J.E. (2004). Invertebrate Care. *Veterinary Clinics of North America: Exotic Animal Practice* 7: 473–486.

Cooper, J.E. and Knowler, C. (1991). Snails and snail farming: an introduction for the veterinary profession. *The Veterinary Record* 129: 541–549.

Dean, W.W., Mead, A.R., and Northey, W.T. (1970). *Aeromonas liquefaciens* in the giant African land snail, Achatina fulica. *Journal of Invertebrate Pathology* 16: 346–351.

Edwards, S., Burke, C., and Hindrum, S. (2000). Recovery and growth effects of anaesthetic and mechanical removal on greenlips *(Haliotis laevigata)* and blacklip *(Haliotis rubra)* abalone. *Journal of Shellfish Research* 19: 510.

Friedl, F.E. (1961). Studies on larval *Fascioloides magna*. IV chromatographic analyses of free amino acids in the haemolymph of a host snail. *The Journal of Parasitology* 47: 773–776.

Girdlestone, D., Cruikshank, S.G., and Winlow, W. (1989). The actions of the volatile general anaesthetics on withdrawal responses of the pond snail *Lymnaea stagnalis. Comparative Biochemistry and Physiology C: Comparative Pharmacology* 92: 39–43.

Gumpenberger, M. and Scmidt-Ukaj, S. (2017). Radiography, sonography and computed tomography in giant African landsnails (*Achatina fulica* and *A. albopicta*). How difficult can it be? In: *Proceedings Third International Conference on Avian Herpetological and Exotic Mammal Medicine*. Venice, Italy: International Conference on Avian, Herpetological, and Exotic Mammal Medicine.

Gunkel, C. and Lewbart, G.A. (2007). Invertebrates. In: *Zoo Animal and Wildlife Immobilization and Anesthesia* (eds. G. West, D. Heard and N. Caulkett), 147–157. Iowa: Blackwell Publishing.

Integrated Taxonomic Information System (2017). www.itis.gov (accessed 10 August 2017).

Ireland, M.P. (1971). The effect of dietary calcium on growth, shell thickness and tissue calcium distribution in the snail, *Achatina fulica. Comparative Biochemistry and Physiology* 98A (1): 111–116.

Joosse, J. and Lever, J. (1959). Techniques for narcotisation and operation for experiments with Lymnaea stagnalis (Gastropoda Pulmonata). Proceedings, Koninklijke Nederlandse Akademie van Wetenschappen Amsterdam, Netherlands 2: 145–149.

Kim, D.Y., Stewart, T.B., Bauer, R.W. et al. (2002). *Parastrongylus (=Angiostrongylus) cantonensis* now endemic in Louisiana wildlife. *The Journal of Parasitology* 88 (5): 1024–1026.

Kriajev, L. and Edelstein, S. (1995). Effect of light and nutrient restriction on the metabolism of calcium and vitamin D in land snails. *The Journal of Experimental Zoology* 272: 153–158.

Kriajev, L., Otremski, I., and Edelstein, S. (1994). Calcium cells from snails: response to vitamin D metabolites. *Calcified Tissue International* 55: 204–207.

Latonio, A.A. (1971). The giant African land snail. Achatina fulica. A new threat to public health. *Transactions of the Royal Society of Tropical Medicine and Hygiene* 65: 22.

Mead, A.R. (1979). *Pulmonates: Economic Malacology.* London: Academic Press.

Moreira, V.L.C., Giese, E.G., Melo, F.T.V. et al. (2013). Endemic angiostrongyliasis in the Brazilian Amazon: natural parasitism of Angiostrongylus cantonensis in Rattus rattus and R. norvegicus, and sympatric giant African land snails, Achatina fulica. *Acta Tropica* 125 (1): 90–97.

Morton, J.E. (1958). *Molluscs.* London: Hutchinson.

Neuhauss, E., Fitarelli, M., Romanzini, J. et al. (2007). Low susceptibility of *Achatina fulica* from Brazil to infection with *Angiostrongylus costaricensis* and *A cantonensis*. *Memórias do Instituto Oswaldo Cruz* 102 (1): 49–52.

O'Brien, M. (2008). Invertebrate anaesthesia. In: *Anaesthesia of Exotic Pets* (ed. L. Longley), 279–295. St Louis: Elsevier Saunders.

O'Brien, M. (2009). Dealing with giant African land snails. *Veterinary Times* 39 (18): 36–37.

Olson, F.J. (1973). The screening of candidate Molluscicides against the giant African land snail, Achatina fulica Bowditch (Stylommatophora: Achatinidae). Thesis, University of Hawaii.

Pellett, S., Bushell, M., and Clarke-Williams, J. (2014). Invertebrate care guidelines. *Companion Animal* 20 (1): 50–53.

Pellett, S., Kubiak, M., Pizzi, R. et al. (2017). BIAZA recommendations for ethical euthanasia of invertebrates. Version 3.0, April 2017. http://biaza.org.uk/resources/animal-husbandry/invertebrates (accessed 20 January 2019).

Pizzi, R. (2010). Invertebrates. In: *BSAVA Manual of Exotic Pets*, 5e (eds. A. Meredith and C.A. Johnson-Delaney), 373–385. Gloucester, UK: BSAVA Publications.

Rees Davies, R., Chitty, J.R., and Saunders, R. (2000). Cardiovascular monitoring of an *Achatina* snail using a Doppler ultrasound unit. Proceedings of the British Veterinary Zoological Society Autumn Meeting, November 18–19, RVC London: 101.

Ross, L.G. and Ross, B. (1999). Anaesthesia of aquatic invertebrates. In: *Anaesthetic and Sedative Techniques for Aquatic Animals*, 2e (eds. L.G. Ross and B. Ross), 46–57. Oxford: Blackwell Science.

RSPCA Husbandry Guidelines (2017). Giant African Land Snails. www.rspca.org.uk/adviceandwelfare/pets/other) (accessed 11 August 2017).

Runham, N.W., Isarankura, K., and Smith, B.J. (1965). Methods for narcotizing and anaesthetising gastropods. *Malacologia* 2: 231–238.

Ruppert, E.E. and Barnes, R.D. (1994). The Molluscs. In: *Invertebrate Zoology*, 6e (eds. E.E. Ruppert and R.D.

Barnes), 361–498. Orlando, FL: Saunders College Publishing.

Sladky, K.K. (2014). Current Understanding of Fish and Invertebrate Anaesthesia and Analgesia. Proceedings of the Association of Reptilian and Amphibian Veterinarians. 18–24 October 2014, Orlando, FL: 122–124.

Smith, J. (1991). A question of pain in invertebrates. *ILAR Journal* 33: 25–31.

Smolowitz, R. (2012). Gastropods. In: *Invertebrate Medicine*, 2e (ed. G.A. Lewbart), 95–111. Oxford: Blackwell Publishing.

Srivastava, P.D. (1992). *Problem of Land Snail Pests in Agriculture. A Study of the Giant African Land Snail.* New Delhi: Concept Publishing Company.

Stoskopf, M.K. (1999). Fish pharmacotherapeutics. In: *Zoo and Wild Animal Medicine: Current Therapy*, 4e (eds. M.E. Fowler and R.E. Miller), 182–189. Philadelphia: WB Saunders.

Thiengo, S.C., Faraco, F.A., Salgado, N.C. et al. (2007). Rapid spread of an invasive snail in South America: the giant African snail, *Achatina fulica,* in Brasil. *Biological Invasions* 9 (6): 693–702.

Toma, H., Matsumura, S., Oshiro, C. et al. (2002). Ocular angiostrongyliasis without meningitis symptoms in Okinawa Japan. *The Journal of Parasitology* 88 (1): 211–213.

White, H.I., Hecht, T., and Potgeiter, B. (1996). The effect of four anaesthetics on *Haliotis midae* and their suitability for application in commercial abalone culture. *Aquaculture* 140: 145–151.

Williams, D. (1999). Sample taking in invertebrate veterinary medicine. *The Veterinary Clinics of North America. Exotic Animal Practice* 2 (3): 777–801.

Williams, D. (2001). Integumental disease in invertebrates. *The Veterinary Clinics of North America. Exotic Animal Practice* 4 (2): 309–320.

Williams, D., Haverson, V., and Chandler, M. (2017). Proceedings Veterinary Invertebrate Society Summer Scientific Meeting 2017, Cambridge, UK: 5.

Yoshino, Y., Kitazawa, T., Kamimura, M. et al. (2011). Pseudomonas putida bacteraemia in adult patients: five case reports and a review of the literature. *Journal of Infection and Chemotherapy* 17: 278–282.

Zachariah, T. and Mitchell, M.A. (2009). Invertebrates. In: *Manual of Exotic Pet Practice* (eds. M.A. Mitchell and T. Tully), 11–38. St. Louis, MO: Saunders-Elsevier.

Zwart, P. and Cooper, J.E. (in preparation). Shell deformities in the European edible snail (*Cornu aspersum*) andthe giant African snail (*Achatina achatina*) In preparation for the Veterinary Invertebrate Society Journal.

Index

Note: Page numbers in *italic* refer to figures.
Page numbers in **bold** refer to tables.

a

abdominal distension, Koi carp 447–448
abscesses
    aural, terrapins 397–398
    geckos 251–252
    retrobulbar
        chameleons 271
        sugar gliders 134
    subcutaneous, African
        tortoises 373
    subspectacular 293, 319
Acanathocephalus ranae 427
acariasis *see* mites
accelerated growth, Mediterranean
        tortoises 341
acetylcysteine
    Mediterranean tortoises **356**
    rats 110, **118**
Achatina (spp.) *see* giant African land
        snails
Acroceridae 470
activated carbon filters 418, 438
    Koi carp **454**
acupuncture 7
acyclovir
    Columbid herpesvirus-1 198
    Mediterranean tortoises 345, **355**
    terrapins **406**
adenoviruses, *see also* agamid
        adenovirus-1
    birds of prey 198–199
    renal disease from, cockatiels 149
adrenocortical neoplasms,
        hamsters 88, 91
Aeromonas hydrophila 483

aestivation
    Mediterranean tortoises 330
    snails 481, *482*
African clawed frog, biological
        parameters **416**
African horned frog, biological
        parameters **416**
African land snails *see* giant African
        land snails
African pygmy hedgehogs 13–26
    anaesthesia 19, **24**
    breeding 16
    common conditions 20–24
    euthanasia 20
    examination 17
    fluid therapy 19
    formulary **24**
    handling 16–17
    history-taking 16
    hospitalisation requirements 20
    husbandry 14–16
    imaging 23–24
    neoplasms 22
    neutering 24
    nutritional support 18–19
    sampling from 17–18
    sex determination 17
African spurred tortoise *see* Sulcata
        tortoise
African tortoises 361–386
    anaesthesia 369–372
    analgesia 370
    common conditions 371–377
    euthanasia 370
    examination 367
    fluid therapy 369

    formulary **378–380**
    handling 366
    history-taking 366
    hospitalisation requirements 370
    imaging 378
    neoplasms 376–377
    nutritional support 368–369
    sampling from 367–368
    sex determination 366–367
    species 361–366
agamid adenovirus-1 229, 232
aglepristone
    hamsters 91
    rats **118**
Aldabran tortoise **362**, 365
    thyroxine values 376
aldose reductase, degus 64
Aleutian disease, skunks 49
alfaxalone
    African tortoises 369, **378**
    amphibians 425, **432**
    bearded dragons 224, **298**
    boas 312, **321**
    chameleons **277**
    corn snakes 288, **298**
    geckos 248, **256**
    hedgehogs 19, **24**
    Koi carp **450**
    marmosets 37
    Mediterranean tortoises 337, **354**
    pythons 312, **321**
    rats **116**
    tarantulas 467, **472**
    terrapins **395**
alkaline phosphatase, adrenal disease,
        hamsters 91

Handbook of Exotic Pet Medicine, First Edition. Edited by Marie Kubiak.
© 2021 John Wiley & Sons Ltd. Published 2021 by John Wiley & Sons Ltd.
Companion website: www.wiley.com/go/kubiak/exotic_pet_medicine

allergies, to rodents   113
allopreening   **175**, *see also* barbering
alopecia
    degus   64
    gerbils   78
    hamsters   89
    tarantulas   468
alpha-linolenic acid levels, birds   173
Alzheimers-like disease, degus   65
amantadine
    budgerigars and cockatiels   158, **159**
    grey parrots   **177**, 179
    rats   **116**
amdoparvovirus, skunks   49
ammonia   110, 418, 438, 444
amphibians   415–436
    anaesthesia   423–425
    common conditions   425–430
    euthanasia   425
    examination   421–422
    fluid therapy   423
    formulary   432
    handling   419, *420*
    history-taking   419
    husbandry   415–422
    imaging   430–431
    nutritional support   423
    sampling from   422–423
    sex determination   419–421
    surgery   429–430
Amphibiocystidium spp.   428
amputation
    limb
        amphibians   429–430
        terrapins   400
    phallus
        Mediterranean tortoises   345
        terrapins   399
amyloidosis
    degus   65
    hamsters   90
    marmosets   36
anaesthesia *see under specific animals*
anal glands, skunks   45
    excision   48
    pathology   48–49
analgesia
    African tortoises   370
    bearded dragons   223
    birds of prey   197, **208, 209**
    boas and pythons   312
    chameleons   268

Koi carp   443
    rats   105, 107
    tarantulas   467–468
    terrapins   396
aneurysms, bearded dragons   231
Angiostrongylus cantonensis   483
Angusticaecum holopterum   372
anorexia
    bearded dragons   223–225
    boas and pythons   314
    chameleons   267–268
    corn snakes   287, 289, **290**
    geckos   247, 249
    Mediterranean tortoises   340
    royal python   312
    tarantulas   461
    terrapins   392, 394
anti-inflammatory drugs, respiratory
        tract infections, rats   110
antibiotics
    hamsters   92, **94**
    psittacosis   152
    rats, respiratory tract infections
        109–110
anticoagulants for blood samples
    birds of prey   195
    corn snakes   287
    rats   105
anting *see* self-anointing
anurans *see* amphibians
apex beat, ground squirrels   5
APMV-1 (Newcastle disease)   197
apnoea, corn snakes, blood
        circulation   292–293
aquaporin APQ-2, degus   58
arboreal spiders   459
    enclosures for   462
Argulus spp.   445
arrhythmias, grey parrots   173
arthritides, *see also* osteoarthritis
    sciuromorphs   7
    septic arthritis, bearded
        dragons   230
ascarids, African tortoises   372–373
ascites, Koi carp   447
aspartate transaminase
    chameleons   270
    in kidneys, budgerigars   150
aspergillosis
    air sacs   178, *201*
    birds of prey   200
    grey parrots   177

Astroturf   197
ataxia, hedgehogs   22
atherosclerosis
    birds of prey   205
    grey parrots   173–174
atrial thrombosis, hamsters   90
atropine, Mediterranean tortoises
        338, **356**
aural abscesses, terrapins   397–398
auscultation, grey parrots   170–171
autotomy
    geckos   253
    tarantulas   469
avian bornavirus   157, 178
avian gastric yeast   153
avian influenza, birds of prey   197
aviaries
    batons   189, *192*
    birds of prey   189
axillary dermatitis, grey parrots
        176–179
axolotls   415
    anaesthesia   424
    biological parameters   **416**
aylmeri   189
baboon spider   459

b

bacteria, *see also* biological water filters
    amphibians   425
    giant African land snails, zoonotic
        diseases   483
    Koi carp   441, 446, 448
    spiral   150–151
    tarantulas, culture   466
bandages, pododermatitis   202
barbering, *see also* allopreening
    degus   63
    gerbils   77
    rats   111
barium studies
    boas   320
    corn snakes   297
        dosage   **299**
    grey parrots   179, 181
        proventricular dilation disease
            178–179
    hamsters   94
    Mediterranean tortoises   350
        dosage   **356**
    pythons   320
barn owls   *191*

basal metabolic rate, *see also* standard
 metabolic rate
 birds of prey 196
basilar vein *see* superficial ulnar vein
basking
 bearded dragons 219–220
 chameleons 264, 269
basking lamps, Mediterranean
 tortoises 329
bathing
 amphibians 423
  for chytridiomycosis 426
  medication 432
 boas and pythons 311
 Mediterranean tortoises **337**
batons, aviaries 189, *192*
Bauchstreich response 314
Baylisascaris spp., skunks 50
beak trimming
 African tortoises 375
 birds of prey 194
 budgerigars and cockatiels 147
 Mediterranean tortoises 350
bearded dragons 219–240
 anaesthesia 223–224, **234**
 analgesia 223
 breeding 221
 common conditions 224–232
 euthanasia 224
 examination 222
 fluid therapy 223
 formulary **234–236**
 handling 221
 history-taking 221
 hospitalisation requirements 224
 husbandry 219–222
 imaging 233–236
 neoplasms 227–228
 nutritional support 223
 sampling from 222
 sex determination 221–222
benzocaine
 abalones **484**
 amphibians 425, **432**
benzodiazepines, *see also specific*
 drugs
 for feather damaging
  behaviour 176
beta blockers, birds 174
betamethasone, rats **116**
biliverdinuria, Mediterranean
 tortoises 336

biochemistry
 hedgehogs, reference intervals **18**
 tarantulas 465
biological water filters 418, 438
biopsy
 kidney, birds 150
 liver, geckos 249
 proventricular dilation disease 158,
  178–179
 skin, bearded dragons 228
birds of prey 189–218
 anaesthesia 196–197
 common conditions 197–207
 euthanasia 197
 examination 193–195
 fluid therapy 195–196
 formulary **208–211**
 handling 192–193
 history-taking 192
 hospitalisation requirements 197
 husbandry 189–192
 imaging 207
 nutritional support 196
 sampling from 195
 sex determination 193
birth weight, marmosets 28
bites
 from cats 148
 from geckos 254
 on marmosets 36
 from sugar gliders 127
black rat 99
bladder prolapse, Mediterranean
 tortoises 344
blindness, Mediterranean
 tortoises 348
blood loss, rats 107
blood pressure monitoring
 boas and pythons 312
 grey parrots 171
boa constrictors 305, **306**
boas 305–307
 taxonomy **307**
boas and pythons 305–325
 anaesthesia 312–314, **321**
 common conditions 314–319
 examination 310–311
 fluid therapy 311
 formulary **321–322**
 handling 310
 history-taking 310
 hospitalisation requirements 314

 husbandry 309–310
 imaging 319–320
 nutritional support 311–312
 sampling from 311
 sex determination 310
body condition score, rats 102, 104
body wraps, rats 107
book lungs, tarantulas 467
bornavirus, avian 157, 178–179
borreliosis, Siberian chipmunks 8–9
bow perches *193*
 tibiotarsal fractures and 206
brachial vein, African tortoise 368
brainstem destruction
 African tortoises 370
 amphibians 425
 boas and pythons 314
 chameleons 268
 corn snakes 289
 euthanasia 396
 Koi carp 449
 Mediterranean tortoises 338–339
 reptiles 224, 249
Branchiomyces spp. 446
brassicas, Mediterranean tortoises
 and 329
breeder frustration 174
breeding *see under specific animals*
bronchoalveolar lavage, African
 tortoises 372
brown rat 99
brumation
 bearded dragons 225
 corn snakes, induction 285
bubonic plague, sciuromorphs 8
budgerigars and cockatiels 141–164
 anaesthesia 147, **159**
  salpingotomy 156
 breeding 142–143
 common conditions 147–158
 euthanasia 147
 examination 144–145
 fluid therapy 147
 formulary **159–160**
 handling 143–144
 history-taking 143
 hospitalisation requirements 147
 husbandry 141–142
 imaging 158
 medication administration
  145–146
 neoplasms 154–155

budgerigars and cockatiels (*cont'd*)
    nutritional support   146
    sampling from   146
    sex determination   144
bumblefoot *see* pododermatitis
buoyancy
    Koi carp   448
    terrapins   391
burns
    boas and pythons   318
    corn snakes   289
bursa copulatrix prolapse   483
butorphanol
    bearded dragons   223, **235**
    corn snakes   288, **298**
    ground squirrels   10
    Koi carp   443
    sugar gliders   129, **130**
    terrapins   396
buttercups, Mediterranean tortoises
        and   329

C

cabergoline, rats   109, **118**
cable ties, shell fractures, terrapins   **401**
caesarean section
    boas and pythons   317
    degus   65
    marmosets   37
cages
    birds of prey, hospitalisation   *197*
    budgerigars and cockatiels   141, *142*
        for hospitalisation   147
    grey parrots   165
        hospitalisation   171–172
    hamsters   83
    Mediterranean tortoises,
        hospitalisation   *339*
    rats   99–101
    sugar gliders   125
        for hospitalisation   130
calcitonin
    bearded dragons   230, **236**
    skunks   47
calcium
    deficiency
        African tortoises   373–374
        bearded dragons   228–229
        budgerigars and cockatiels   148
        chameleons   269
        geckos   243
        snails   482

    excess, budgerigars and
        cockatiels   149
calcium (blood levels)
    African tortoises   373
    chameleons   270
    grey parrots   172
    nutritional secondary
        hyperparathyroidism   32
calcium borogluconate
    grey parrots   **182**
    Mediterranean tortoises   **356**
calcium (diet)
    bearded dragons   221
    degus
        dental disease   61
        excretion   64
    giant African land snails   479
    hedgehogs   16
    sugar gliders   130
    supplements
        amphibians   419, 431
        geckos   243, 258
        Mediterranean tortoises   330
        terrapins   399
calcium gluconate, amphibians   429
calcium : phosphorus ratio (diet)
    African tortoises   373
    Mediterranean tortoises   329
calculi *see* cholelithiasis; stones;
        uroliths
callitrichid hepatitis   35
Campbell's hamster   **84**
Campylobacter spp., rats   113
candidiasis
    birds of prey   201
    cockatiels   153
cannibalism
    hamsters   85
    hedgehogs   16
Capillaria hepatica   35
Capillaria spp., birds of prey   199
capnography
    African tortoises   370
    birds   170
    terrapins   395
carbon dioxide, tarantulas, anaesthesia
        with   467
carbon dioxide monitoring, birds   170
cardiac arrest, Mediterranean
        tortoises   338
cardiocentesis
    amphibians   422

boas and pythons   310, *311*
    corn snakes   287
cardiomegaly, birds of prey   205
cardiomyopathy, *see also* dilated
        cardiomyopathy
    corn snakes   292
    hamsters   90
    hedgehogs   22
caries, *see also* periodontal disease
    degus   62
    hamsters   90
    sugar gliders   131
Carolina anole   263
carotene, for geckos   250
carp *see* Koi carp
carp pituitary extract   447, **454**
carp pox   448
carpet python   **306**
carprofen
    degus   **66**
    geckos   **256**
    gerbils   **79**
    grey parrots   **181**
    marmosets   **39**
    Mediterranean tortoises   **355**
    rats   **116**
    sugar gliders   **137**
Caryospora infections   199–200
cast pellets   190, *192*
castration *see* orchidectomy
cat bites   148
cataracts
    birds of prey   205
    degus   64
    hedgehogs   20
    Mediterranean tortoises   347–348
    sugar gliders   131
cauda equina compression,
        skunks   48
caudal coiling syndrome, boas and
        pythons   316
caudal vein, Koi carp   441
ceftiofur, red-tail hawks   **209**
celecoxib
    budgerigars and cockatiels   158, **159**
    grey parrots   179, **182**
cephalic vein, degus   60
ceramic lamps   220, 329
cerebral xanthomatosis, geckos   251
cestodes
    amphibians   427
    rats   113

chameleons 263–281
  anaesthesia 268, **277**
  breeding 265–266
  common conditions 269–276
  endoparasites 275–276
  euthanasia 269
  examination 266–267
  fluid therapy 268
  formulary **277–278**
  handling 266
  history-taking 266
  hospitalisation requirements 269
  husbandry 263–265
  imaging 276–278, *276*
  neoplasms 271
  neutering 277
  non-specific debilitation 269
  nutritional support 267–268
  sampling from 267
  sex determination 266
cheek pouch conditions, hamsters 90
cheek teeth
  degus 61, 62
  rat 113
chelation therapy 156
chelicerae, spiders 460
chemical water filters 418, 438
Chilean rose tarantula 459, 460
Chinese finger trap suture *394*
Chinese hamster **84**, 89
Chinese softshell turtles, ranavirus
    infection 396
chipmunks 1, *see also* Siberian
    chipmunks
  hospitalisation 5
Chlamydia psittaci 151–152,
    173, 177
Chlamydia spp., amphibians 425
chloramines, in water 417
chlorhexidine, surgery for
    amphibians 430
chlorine, in water 417
cholelithiasis, bearded dragons 233
cholesteatomas, gerbils 77
cholesterol, *see also* xanthomas, grey
    parrots 173
chromatophoromas, chameleons 271
chromodacryorrhoea, rats 104, 110
Chryseobacterium indologenes 483
Chrysosporium anamorph,
    Nannizziopsis vriesii 228,
    254, 272

chytridiomycosis
  amphibians 426
  swabbing for 422
cider vinegar, megabacteria and 153
circovirus, painted turtles 397
Citrobacter freundii 398
claws
  Mediterranean tortoises,
    clipping 352
  rats, trimming 113
cleaning, enclosures for marmosets 27
cloaca
  birds of prey 194
  prolapse
    Mediterranean tortoises 343–345
    sugar gliders 134
cloacal wash, amphibians 422
cloacoscopy, terrapins 391
clomipramine, cockatoos 176
clonidine, African tortoises 370
cloth, rat bedding 100
coccidia
  amphibians 428
  bearded dragons 231–232
  birds of prey 199–200
  chameleons 275
  skunks 49
cockatiels *see* budgerigars and
    cockatiels
coconut fibre, for amphibians
    415–416
coelioscopy
  boas and pythons 320
  terrapins 391
coeliotomy
  amphibians 429
  boas and pythons 319
  corn snakes 295, *296*
  hamsters 91
  Mediterranean tortoises 343,
    348–349
    cloacal prolapse 345
  terrapins, ventilation for 396
coelomic cavity, parrots 156
coiling syndrome (caudal), boas and
    pythons 316
colchicine, budgerigars and cockatiels
    150, **160**
colitis
  protozoal, geckos 254
  sugar gliders 134
collapsed bird 147–148, 170

colonic prolapse
  hamsters 91
  Mediterranean tortoises 344
colour changes, chameleons 265
Columbid herpesvirus-1, birds of
    prey 198
common iliac vein, budgerigars and
    cockatiels 149
common marmosets 27–42
  anaesthesia 31, **39**
  breeding 28
  common conditions 32–35
  euthanasia 31
  examination 30
  fluid therapy 30–31
  formulary **39**
  handling 29
  history-taking 28–29
  hospitalisation requirements 31–32
  husbandry 27–28
  imaging 38–39
  neutering 37
  nutritional support 30
  sampling from 30
  sex determination 29
computed tomography
  African tortoises 377
  amphibians 431
  boas and pythons 315, 320
  Mediterranean tortoises 352
  rats 115
  terrapins 404
congestive heart failure
  grey parrots 172–174
  hamsters 90
  rats 110
Congo grey parrots *166*
conjunctivitis, chameleons 271
constipation, bearded dragons 230
contraceptive implants, marmosets
    37–38
copepods, amphibians 428
coprophagy, degus 57
cor pulmonale, grey parrots 172
coracoid fractures, birds of prey 206
corn snakes 283–304
  anaesthesia 287–288, **298**
  breeding 285
  common conditions 289–297
  euthanasia 288–289
  examination 286
  fluid therapy 287

corn snakes (*cont'd*)
  formulary **298–299**
  handling 286
  history-taking 286
  hospitalisation requirements 289
  husbandry 283–285
  imaging 297
  neoplasms 295, **296**
  nutritional support 287
  preventive health measures 297
  sampling from 287
  sex determination 286
cornea
  amphibians, lipid keratopathy 429
  ulceration
    Koi carp 447
    owls 205
corneal reflex, birds 170
corneospectacular space, boas and
        pythons 319
corticosteroids, birds and 179
cortisol
  excess, hamsters 91
  spiders 462
Corynebacterium kutscheri, rats 112
cowpox 9
crabbing, sugar gliders 127
cranial vena cava access
  degus 60
  gerbils 74
  ground squirrels 4
  hamsters 74
  hedgehogs 17, *18*
  rats 104
  sugar gliders 128
creatinine phosphokinase, hamsters
        90–91
creatinine (serum), hamsters **91**
crested geckos
  ambient temperature 242
  biological parameters **244**
  conditions for **243**
critical care formulae, amphibians 423
crop, birds of prey 203
crop tube placement
  feeding 196
  medication 145, 169
crown vetch 157
cryptococcal enteritis, marmosets 34
Cryptosporidium infections
  African tortoises 373
  bearded dragons 231
  birds of prey 200

chameleons 275
corn snakes 294
Cryptosporidium saurophilum 254
Cuora flavimarginata 390
curved multiplanar reformatting
        software 320
cyprinid herpesvirus 448
cystitis, hedgehogs 22
cystocentesis, rats 105

d

Dactylogyrus spp. 445
daffodils, Mediterranean tortoises
        and 329
dart apparatus prolapse 483
death confirmation, Mediterranean
        tortoises 339
degloving injury to tail
  degus 63
  gerbils 78
degus 57–69
  anaesthesia 60, **61**
  breeding 58
  common conditions 61–65
  euthanasia 60
  examination 59–60
  fluid therapy 60
  formulary **61**
  handling 59
  history-taking 58
  hospitalisation requirements 61
  husbandry 57–58
  imaging 66
  neoplasms 64
  neutering 65
  nutritional support 60
  sampling from 60
  sex determination 59
dehydration
  African tortoises 369
  amphibians 421–422
  bearded dragons 223
  budgerigars and cockatiels 149
  chameleons 265
  gerbils 74, 77
  hamsters 87
  marmosets 30–31
  Mediterranean tortoises 336
Demodex spp., Syrian hamster 89
densitometry (shell), tortoises 378
dental disease
  chameleons 271
  degus 61–63

hamsters 89
hedgehogs 20–21
marmosets 35, *36*
rats 112–113
sciuromorphs 6
  imaging 9–10
skunks 48
sugar gliders 131
dental formulae
  African pygmy hedgehogs 13
  common marmosets 35
  degus 61
  hamsters 89
  rats **100**
  sciuromorphs 6
  striped skunks 43
  sugar gliders 131
Dentostomella translucida
  gerbils 78
  hamsters 92
dermatitis
  bearded dragons 228–229
  chameleons 272–273
  corn snakes 289–291
  geckos 254
  grey parrots 176–177
  hamsters 89
  hedgehogs 20
  rats 111
  ulcerative
    grey parrots 176–177
    Koi carp 446
    rats 111
dermatology
  bearded dragons 228–229
  degus 63
  gerbils, neoplasms 76
  hedgehogs 20
  rats 111–113
    examination 104
  sugar gliders 133
dermatophytosis
  degus 63
  sugar gliders 133–134
dermatosepticaemia, amphibians 425
desflurane, birds of prey 196–197
deslorelin
  budgerigars, Sertoli cell
        neoplasms 155
  budgerigars and cockatiels **148**
  geckos and 253
  marmosets 38
  Mediterranean tortoises 352–353

rats **118**

skunks 52, **54**

detergents, for dysecdysis,
tarantulas 469

Devriesea agamarum 228

deworming, skunks 51

diabetes mellitus, *see also*
hyperglycaemia

budgerigars and cockatiels 154

hamsters 92

diarrhoea

hamsters 92

hedgehogs 21

marmosets 34

rats 112

skunks 49

diet

amphibians 418–419

supplementation 418–419

bearded dragons 220–221, 223

boas 310

budgerigars and cockatiels 142, 146

chameleons 268

corn snakes 285

degus 57, 63–64

gastrointestinal disease 65

geckos 243–244, 247

gerbils 71–72

giant African land snails 479

grey parrots 165–166

hamsters 84, 87

hedgehogs 15–16

Koi carp 439

Mediterranean tortoises
329–330, 336

plants 365

prairie dogs 2

pythons 310

rats 102, 103

Siberian chipmunks 1

sugar gliders 125–126, 129

terrapins 389

Testudo graeca 363

dihydrostreptomycin, gerbils and **79**

1 alpha, 25-dihydroxyvitamin D3,
marmosets 32

dilated cardiomyopathy

marmosets 36

prairie dogs 7

dirofilaria, in skunks 48

disinfection

megabacteria 153

ranaviruses 426

distemper, vaccination, skunks 50

Djungorian hamsters 84

anaesthesia **94**

DMSA (meso-2,3-dimercaptosuccinic
acid), budgerigars and
cockatiels 156, **159**

dominance hierarchy, marmosets 27

dorsal coccygeal vein

Mediterranean tortoises 335

terrapins 392

dorsal tail vein, African tortoises 368

doxapram

Koi carp **454**

Mediterranean tortoises 338, **356**

doxycycline

budgerigars and cockatiels 153, **159**

psittacosis 152–153

dressings

pododermatitis 111, 201–202

rats 107, 111

terrapins 400, **401**

tibiotarsal fractures in birds 148

drink patches, anurans 419

drip bag method, fish anaesthesia 442

drowning, Mediterranean
tortoises 347

Dumbo rats **101**

duprasi (fat-tail girds) 71

dwarf hamsters 83

dysecdysis

bearded dragons 229

boas and pythons 317

corn snakes 289

geckos 250, *251*

tarantulas 468–469

dyskinetic syndrome, tarantulas 471

dyspnoea

birds, respiratory obstruction 151

birds of prey 194

Mediterranean tortoises 346

sciuromorphs, hepatic carcinoma 7

dystocia

African tortoises 376

boas 316–317

budgerigars and cockatiels
156–157

chameleons 274–275

corn snakes 294–295

degus 65

marmosets 36–37

Mediterranean tortoises 342–343

pythons 316–317

terrapins 399

e

ear mites, rats 111

Eastern box turtles

biological parameters **388**

ranavirus infection 396

Eastern river cooters, herpesvirus
infection 397

ecdysis

corn snakes, anorexia 289

tarantulas 461, *see also* exuvia

echocardiography

bearded dragons 233

birds of prey 205

boas 315, 320

corn snakes 293, 297

geckos 255

grey parrots 173

pythons 315, 320

terrapins 404

euthanasia 396

eclampsia, hedgehogs, postpartum 22

ecological niches 242

ectopic pregnancy, hamsters 91

EDTA (sodium calcium edetate)

budgerigars and cockatiels
155–156, **159**

calcium disodium ethylene
diaminetetracetate, falcons **211**

egg(s), giant African land snails 480

egg binding

bearded dragons 226–227

budgerigars and cockatiels 156

chameleons 274–275

corn snakes 294

Koi carp 448

Mediterranean tortoises 342–343

terrapins 399

egg laying

chameleons 265–266

chronic 157

egg laying disorders, geckos 252

egg peritonitis, carp 447

egg yolk coelomitis 157

electrocardiography

corn snakes 292

grey parrots 173

Mediterranean tortoises 338

elementary bodies, psittacosis 151

Elizabethan collars, rats 107

elodontomas

degus 62–63

imaging 10

sciuromorphs 6

emboli, gas bubble disease   445
emerald tree boa   305, **306**
emodepsid
    African tortoises   **380**
    Mediterranean tortoises   **356**
Emydid herpesvirus 1   397
Encephalitozoon hellem,
    budgerigars   149
enclosures *see* husbandry *under specific*
    animals
end tidal CO$_2$, birds   170
endoscopy
    amphibians   431
    boas and pythons   320
    giant African land snails   484
    Mediterranean tortoises   350
      respiratory tract   346
    terrapins   391
endotracheal intubation
    bearded dragons   224
    birds of prey   196
    boas   313
    budgerigars and cockatiels   147
    chameleons   268
    corn snakes   288
    degus   60
    geckos   248
    gerbils   75
    hamsters   87–88
    marmosets   31
    Mediterranean tortoises   336
    pythons   313
    rats   106
    skunks   46–47
    sugar gliders   129
    terrapins   395
      for aural abscess removal   398
endurance test, birds of prey   194
energy intake
    amphibians   423
    birds of prey   197
    corn snakes   287
    degus   60
    gerbils   74
    grey parrots   169
enrichment (environmental)
    budgerigars and cockatiels
      141–142
    grey parrots   166, *167*, 174–176
    rats   100
    skunks   44
Entamoeba invadens   254

Entamoeba ranarum   427
Entamoeba spp., bearded
    dragons   232
enteral fluid therapy, Mediterranean
    tortoises   **337**
enteritis
    hamsters   92
    marmosets   33–34
    protozoal
      corn snakes   294
      geckos   254
    sugar gliders   134
enterotomy, bearded dragons   227
epi-coelomic space
    Mediterranean tortoises, medication
      via   **354**
    terrapins, fluid therapy via   394
erythrocytes, boas and pythons   311
erythromycin
    marmosets   **39**
    rats   **117**
ethanol
    anaesthesia for abalones   **484**
    for ultrasound, tarantulas   472
etonogestrel, marmosets   38
Eublepharid geckos, eyelids   251
eugenol, Koi carp   **450**
European Union, Invasive Alien
    Species Regulation   1
euthanasia *see under specific*
    animals
exophthalmos (proptosis)
    chameleons   272
    hamsters   89
    hedgehogs   20
    Koi carp   446–447
external jugular vein, terrapins   392
external skeletal fixators, tibiotarsal
    fractures   206
extraction, degus teeth   62
exuvia, spiders, sex
    determination   464
eyelids
    amphibians   421
    geckos   251
    terrapins, vitamin A deficiency
      399–400
eyes, *see also* Harderian glands; ocular
    conditions
    amphibians, enucleation   430
    birds of prey   194
    protection, rats   107

f
F10 disinfectant
    grey parrots   **182**
    tortoises   372
facemasks, anaesthesia, rats   106
faecal smears, tortoises   377
falconid adenovirus-1   198–199
falcons   189–217
false map turtles, biological
    parameters   **388**
fang colouration, tarantulas   469
fasting, preoperative, anurans   430
fat tail geckos
    biological parameters   **244**
    conditions for   **243**
fat-tail girds (duprasi)   71
feather damaging behaviour   174–176
feather dystrophy   153–154
feathers
    birds of prey
      examination   195
      protection for hospitalisation   197
    psittacine beak and feather
      disease   177
    trauma to   148
feeding, *see also* gavage feeding;
    nutritional support *under*
    specific animals
    amphibians   423
    bearded dragons   221, 223
    birds of prey   196, 203
    boas and pythons   310, 311–312
    budgerigars   146
    chameleons   268
    corn snakes   287
    degus   60
    geckos   243, 247
    grey parrots   169
    ground squirrels   4
    hedgehogs   18–19
    Mediterranean tortoises   336
    sugar gliders   129, 135
femoral artery haematoma,
    marmosets   36
femoral vein
    degus   60
    marmosets   30
    rats   104
    skunks   45–46
femur, fractures, birds of prey   206
Ferguson zones   417
fibroadenomas, rats   108

fibrosarcomas, grey parrots   177
filaria
    amphibians   427
    chameleons   275–276
filters, *see also* activated carbon filters
    for water   418, 437–439
fin rot   446, *446*
fipronil
    bearded dragons   232, **235**
    tarantulas and   471
fireflies, poisoning of bearded
        dragon   231
fish slaughter   449
fixation, tibiotarsal fractures   206
flaked foods, amphibians   418
flashing, fish   445
flavobacteriosis, amphibians   425
Flavobacterium columnare   446
fleas
    marmosets   35
    skunks   50
floating, terrapins   391
flock mortality   148
flotation technique, tortoise
        faeces   377
fluconazole, megabacteria   153
fluffed-up appearance, budgerigars   *143*
fluid requirements
    African tortoises   369
    amphibians   423
    bearded dragons   223
    birds of prey   196
    boas   311
    budgerigars and cockatiels   142, 147
    chameleons   268
        renal disease   **277–278**
    corn snakes   287
    degus   57–58, 60
    geckos   247–248
    gerbils   72, 74
    grey parrots   170
    hamsters   85, 87
    hedgehogs   19
    Mediterranean tortoises   336
    primates   30–31
    pythons   311
    rats   102, 105
    sciuromorphs   4
    skunks   46
    sugar gliders   129
    terrapins   394
fluid therapy *see under specific animals*

fluoxetine, for feather damaging
        behaviour   176
Foleyella spp.   275
follicular stasis *see* pre-ovulatory stasis
footing (handling birds of prey)   192
foraging enrichment, grey parrots   166
forelimb pumping, Mediterranean
        tortoises   346
forked penis, sugar gliders   134
Fowl adenovirus-4   199
fractures
    birds of prey   206–207
    budgerigars and cockatiels   148
    hamsters   92
        incisors   89
    Mediterranean tortoises   347
    nutritional secondary
        hyperparathyroidism
        marmosets   32
        skunks   47
    terrapins   400, **401**
freezing (euthanasia)
    amphibians   425
    Koi carp   450
    terrapins   396
fret marks, birds of prey   195
fridges, Mediterranean tortoises   331
frogs *see* amphibians
fructosamine, psittacine   154
frusemide *see* furosemide
fungal infections
    amphibians   426–427
    bearded dragons   228
    birds   151
    chameleons   272–273
        periodontal osteomyelitis   272
    corn snakes   291
    geckos   254
    Koi carp   *447*
    rats   111
    tarantulas, culture   466
fur mites, rats   111
furosemide
    boas and pythons   315–316
    grey parrots   173, **182**

g
galactomannan, aspergillosis   178
galvanised bars, rat cages   99
gapeworm, birds of prey   199
gas bubble disease   445
gas gland, Koi carp   448

gas supersaturation, water quality   445
gastric dilatation, sugar gliders   134
gastric neuroendocrine carcinoma,
        bearded dragons   227
gastric volume, terrapins   394
gastric yeast, avian   153
gastritis, corn snakes, *Cryptosporidium*
        infections   294
Gastrografin, Mediterranean tortoises
        350, **356**
gastrointestinal disease, *see also* colitis;
        diarrhoea; enteritis
    corn snakes   294
    degus, diet   65
    impaction, bearded dragons   227
    rats   112
    sugar gliders   134
    terrapins   404
gastrointestinal tract, African land
        snails   477
gastropods
    anatomy   477
    pain   480
gavage feeding, *see also* crop tube
        placement
    African tortoises   368–369
    amphibians   423
    bearded dragons   223
    chameleons   268
    corn snakes   287
    Mediterranean tortoises
        fluid therapy   **337**
        medication administration   **353**
    rats   105
    terrapins   392–394
geckos   241–262
    anaesthesia   248–249
    breeding   244–245
    common conditions   249–253
    euthanasia   249
    examination   246–247
    fluid therapy   247–248
    formulary   **256–258**
    handling   245
    history-taking   245
    hospitalisation requirements   249
    husbandry   241–245
    imaging   255
    neoplasms   253
    nutritional support   247
    sampling from   247
    sex determination   245–246

gerbils *see* Mongolian gerbils
geriatric
    rats, skin   111, *111*
gestation
    degus   58
    gerbils   73
    sugar gliders   126
giant African land snails   477–486
    anaesthesia   480–481
    anatomy   477
    breeding   480
    common conditions   481–483
    euthanasia   481
    examination   480
    formulary   **484**
    history-taking   480
    husbandry   478–480
    poisoning   482
    sampling from   481
giant cell nephritis, corn snakes   297
giant day geckos
    biological parameters   **244**
    conditions for   **243**
gill clips   441
gill rot   446
gingiva, boas and pythons   314
glass tanks
    bearded dragons and   219
    gerbils   71
glaucoma, owls   205
gliding membranes
    sugar gliders   125
    trauma   131
glomerular filtration rate,
        chameleons   270
gloves
    handling amphibians   419
    handling marmosets   29
glycopyrolide, rats   **116**
goitre, budgerigars   149
Goliath tarantula   459, 460
gonadotropin-releasing hormone, Koi
        carp   448, **454**
gonadotropin-releasing hormone
        analogues, budgerigars and
        cockatiels   157
gout
    bearded dragons   230
    birds   150
    Mediterranean tortoises   341
grading, water filters   437–438
granulomatous disease, chameleons
        272–273

green anaconda   305, **306**
green tree python   **306**, 308–309
green urates, Mediterranean
        tortoises   336
grey parrots   165–189
    anaesthesia   170–171, **181–182**
    breeding   167
    common conditions   172–180
    euthanasia   171
    examination   168–169
    fluid therapy   169–170
    formulary   **181–182**
    handling   168
    history-taking   168
    hospitalisation
        requirements   171–172
    husbandry   165–167
    imaging   178–180
    medication administration   169
    neoplasms   176
    nutritional support   169
    sampling from   169
    sex determination   168
grit, for lead poisoning   156
ground squirrels   1–12
    anaesthesia   4, **10**
    common conditions   5–9
    euthanasia   5
    examination   3–4
    fluid therapy   4
    formulary   **10–11**
    handling   3
    history-taking   3
    hospitalisation requirements   5
    husbandry   1–2
    imaging   9–10, *11*
    neoplasms   5
    neutering   9
    nutritional support   4
    sampling from   4
    sex determination   3
gular movement, amphibians   424
gum, for marmosets   27–28
gut-loading, prey   243, 250, 462
gyr falcon   190
    tetanus   201
Gyrodactylus (spp.)   445

h

H5N1 (avian influenza), birds of
    prey   197
haematology, hedgehogs, reference
    intervals   **18**

haemochromatosis
    hepatic, marmosets   32–33
    sugar gliders   130
haemolymph
    snails, sampling   481
    tarantulas   469–470
        sampling   464–465
haemoparasites
    African tortoises   373
    birds of prey   200
hairless rats   **101**
Halicephalobus spp.   471
haloperidol, for feather damaging
        behaviour   176
halothane, degus and   60
hammocks, rats   100
hamster papova virus   89
hamsters   83–98
    anaesthesia   87–88, **94**
    breeding   85
    common conditions   88–94
    euthanasia   88
    examination   86
    fluid therapy   87
    formulary   **94–95**
    handling   85
    history-taking   85
    hospitalisation requirements   88
    husbandry   83–85
    imaging   94–95
    neoplasms   88–89
    neutering   94
    nutritional support   87
    sampling from   86–87
    sex determination   85, 86
hand-rearing
    budgerigars and cockatiels   143
    grey parrots   167, 174
    sugar gliders   135
handling
    African pygmy hedgehogs   16–17
    African tortoises   366
    amphibians   419, *420*
    bearded dragons   221
    birds of prey   192
    boas   310
    budgerigars and cockatiels
        143–144
    chameleons   266
    common marmosets   29
    corn snakes   286
    degus   59
    geckos   245

grey parrots   168
ground squirrels   3
hamsters   85
Mediterranean tortoises   332
Mongolian gerbils   73
pythons   310
rats   103
striped skunks   45
sugar gliders   127
tarantulas   463–464
terrapins   389–390
hantaviruses   113
Harderian glands
   gerbils   77
   rats   110
Harris' hawks   *193*
   tibiotarsal fractures   206
hawks   189–218
Haycocknema spp.   471
hearing, rats   102
heart, *see also* cardiomyopathy;
      congestive heart failure
   boas and pythons
      disease   315–316
      monitoring   313
   corn snake   292–293
   gastropods   477
   grey parrots, radiography   181
   sampling from *see* cardiocentesis
   tarantulas, fluid therapy via   466, 469
heart rate
   amphibians   425
   Koi carp   444
   tarantulas   467
heat mats, Mediterranean tortoises
      and   329
heating
   amphibians   416–417
   bearded dragons   219–220
   boas and pythons   309
      recovery from anaesthesia   313
   chameleons   264
   corn snakes   283–284
      burns   289
   geckos   242
      anaesthesia   248
   giant African land snails   478
   marmosets   27
   Mediterranean tortoises
      328–329, *339*
   Sulcata tortoise   365
   terrapins   387–389
   tortoises, shell necrosis   376

hedgehogs   13–26
Helicobacter pylori, gerbils   77
Helicobacter septicaemia, African
      tortoises   372
heliotherms   328
hemipenes
   disorders, geckos   253–254
   prolapse, chameleons   275
hepadnavirus hepatitis   6
hepatic carcinoma, sciuromorphs   6, 8
hepatic disease, African tortoises, on
      calcium homeostasis   **374**
hepatic failure, hedgehogs   22
hepatic haemochromatosis, marmosets
      32–33
hepatic lipidosis
   bearded dragons   225, 233
   geckos   249
   tortoises, computed tomography   377
hepatitis
   callitrichid   35
   hepadnavirus   6
   renal disease from, cockatiels   149
   terrapins   397
hepatomegaly, budgerigars and
      cockatiels   158
herpes simplex virus   29, 35
herpes tamarinus virus   35
herpesviruses
   African tortoises   374
   birds of prey   199
   chelonian   345
   Koi carp   448
   psittacine   158
   terrapins   397, 398
hibernation
   African tortoises   366
   Mediterranean tortoises   330–331
hides
   bearded dragons   224
   degus   62
   geckos   241, 242
   hamsters   88
   marmosets   *28*
   rats   *101*
   snails   479
   snakes   309, 311, 314
   sugar gliders   125
   tarantulas   462
hindleg degeneration, rats   112
hindlimb paralysis, sugar gliders   130
hingeback tortoises   **362**, 365
   handling   366

histoplasmosis, skunks   51
hoarding food, hamsters   84
hockey stick probe, amphibians   431
hospitalisation requirements *see under*
      specific animals
humane slaughter   449
humeral fractures, birds of prey   207
humidity
   amphibians   417–418
   boas and pythons   309
   chameleons   265
   geckos   241
   marmosets   27
   tarantulas   462
   terrapins   389
hyalinosis, pulmonary, sugar
      gliders   133
hydronephrosis, rats   111
Hymenolepis diminuta, rats   112
Hymenolepis nana   9
hypercalcaemia, African tortoises   375
hypercapnia, birds   170
hyperglycaemia, degus   65–66
hyperimmune bovine colostrum
   corn snakes   294, **298**
   geckos   254, **257**
hyperparathyroidism *see* nutritional
      secondary hyperparathyroidism;
      renal secondary
      hyperparathyroidism
hyperthyroidism, corn snakes   289
hypocalcaemia
   grey parrots   172
   Mediterranean tortoises   343
hypoglycaemia, marmosets   37
hypothermia
   marmosets   37
   rats, prevention   106–110
hypothyroidism
   hamsters   93
   tortoises   376
hypromellose drops, corn snakes   289

i

Ichthyophonus spp.   428
Ichtyopthirius multifiliis   445
imaging *see under specific animals*
impaction, intestinal, bearded
      dragons   230
impression smears, Koi carp   441
incisors
   degus   62
   hamsters   89

incisors (*cont'd*)
  rats   112
  sciuromorphs   6
  sugar gliders   131
inclusion body disease, boas and
     pythons   316
inclusion disease of boids   297
incubation, chameleon eggs   266
indomethacin, geckos   253
infections, *see also Cryptosporidium*
     infections; fungal infections;
     upper respiratory infections;
     specific organisms
  African tortoises   371–373
  amphibians   425–427
    prevention   431
  bearded dragons, skin   228–229
  boas   314
  grey parrots, dermatitis
    176–179
  Mediterranean tortoises,
    kidneys   341
  pythons   314
  renal disease, budgerigars and
    cockatiels   149
  respiratory, *see also* nebulisation
    treatment
     boas and pythons   315
     budgerigars and cockatiels   150
     hamsters   89–90
     rats   109–110, 114–115
     sugar gliders   131–133
  skin, rats   111
  sugar gliders   134
  terrapins   396–398
influenza
  avian   197
  skunks   50
injection sites, budgerigars and
    cockatiels   146
insects
  for bearded dragons   221
  for chameleons   265, 268
  for geckos   243
  parasitising tarantulas   470
  retinol rich diet for   270
insulin
  degus   65, **66**
  hamsters   **94**
  rats   **119**
interferon gamma, grey parrots
    177, **182**

intermittent positive pressure
    ventilation
  African tortoises   370
  birds   147
  boas and pythons   312
  chameleons   268
  Mediterranean tortoises   337–338
  terrapins   396
intervertebral disc disease
  hedgehogs   22
  skunks   48
intervertebral disc rupture, prairie
    dogs   *8*
intestinal impaction, bearded
    dragons   227
intoxications, budgerigars and
    cockatiels   156
intracardiac injection
  ground squirrels   10
  Mediterranean tortoises   338
intracoelomic fluid therapy
  amphibians   423
  corn snakes   287
  geckos   248
  tarantulas   466
intracoelomic medication
  amphibians   432
  Mediterranean tortoises   **354**
intradermal tuberculin test,
    marmosets   34
intramedullary pins, fracture fixation
    206–207
intramuscular medication
  amphibians   432
  Koi carp   442, 444
  Mediterranean tortoises   **353**
intranasal anaesthesia, terrapins   406
intraocular teratoid medulloepithelioma
    (malignant)   155
intraosseous catheter placement,
    marmosets   31
intraosseous fluid therapy
  amphibians   423
  bearded dragons   223
  birds of prey   195
  budgerigars and cockatiels   147
  chameleons   268
  degus   60
  geckos   248
  gerbils   74
  grey parrots   170
  hamsters   87

  hedgehogs   19
  Mediterranean tortoises   **337**
  rats   **106**
  skunks   46
  sugar gliders   129
  terrapins   394
intraosseous medication,
    Mediterranean tortoises   **354**
intraperitoneal fluid therapy
  hedgehogs   19
  rats   **106**
intravenous fluid therapy
  amphibians   423
  bearded dragons   223
  birds of prey   195
  boas   311
  chameleons   268
  corn snakes   287
  grey parrots   169–170
  Mediterranean tortoises   **337**
  pythons   311
  rats   **106**
  skunks   46
  terrapins   394
intravenous medication
  amphibians   432
  Mediterranean tortoises   **353**
intussusception, marmosets   34
Invasive Alien Species Regulation,
    European Union   1
iodine deficiency, budgerigars   149
iohexol, Mediterranean tortoises
    350, **356**
iohexol clearance test,
    chameleons   270
ion exchange resins, water filters   438
iridoviruses
  Mediterranean tortoises   345–346
  tortoises   371
iron, hepatic haemochromatosis,
    marmosets   33
isoflurane
  amphibians   424, **432**
  bearded dragons   224, **234**
  birds of prey   196, **208**
  boas   313
  degus   60, **66**
  marmosets   31
  pythons   313
  rats   105–106, **116**
  tarantulas   467, **472**
Isospora amphiboluri   231

isoxsuprine
  grey parrots   174, **182**
  for wing tip oedema   204
itraconazole
  amphibians   427, **433**
  grey parrots   178, **181**
ivermectin, Mediterranean tortoises
        and   352
Ixodes frontalis, birds of prey   199

j

Jackson ratio curve, weight/length,
        Mediterranean tortoises   333
jesses   189
jugular veins
  African tortoises   368
  birds of prey   195
  budgerigars and cockatiels   146
  degus   60
  gerbils   74
  grey parrots   169
  hamsters   86
  Mediterranean tortoises   335
  rats   104
  sugar gliders   128
  terrapins   392
juvenile diarrhoea, hamsters   93–94

k

ketamine
  corn snakes   288, **298**
  geckos   248, **256**
ketoprofen
  on kidneys, budgerigars   150
  Koi carp and   443
kidney, gastropods   477
kidney diseases, *see also* renal
        secondary hyperparathyroidism
  African tortoises, on calcium
        homeostasis   **374**
  budgerigars, neoplasms   148, 155
  budgerigars and cockatiels
        149–150
  chameleons   270
  corn snakes   297
  degus   64
    ultrasound   66
  gerbils   77
  hamsters   91
  hedgehogs   22
  marmosets   36
  Mediterranean tortoises   341

rats   110
  sevoflurane poisoning   106
skunks   49
sugar gliders   133
Knemidokoptes pilae   151
Koi carp   437–457
  anaesthesia   441–445
    stages   **443**
  analgesia   443
  aquatic environment   437–439,
        443–444
  common conditions   445–449
  euthanasia   449–450
  examination   439–440
  formulary   **450–455**
  neoplasms   448
  notifiable diseases   448–449
  sampling from   440–441
  sedation   441–448
Koi herpesvirus   448–449

l

laboratory rats   99
lameness
  birds   148, 150
  hedgehogs   22
land snails *see* giant African land snails
lateral sinuses, boas and pythons   311
lateral veins, tail, rat   104–105, **106**
Lawsonia intracellularis   92
lead poisoning, birds   156, 202–203
Leadbeater's mix   **126**
leeches, amphibians   427
leopard geckos   241
  biological parameters   **244**
  breeding   244
  environmental conditions for   **243**
  midazolam   248
  neurological diseases   251
  vitamin A deficiency diseases   250
leopard tortoises   **362**, 365, *367*
  Plasmodium spp.   373
  upper respiratory infections
        371, 372
leptospirosis
  marmosets   34
  rats   113
Lernea spp.   445
leukaemia, bearded dragons   227
leuprolide, budgerigars and
        cockatiels   155, 157, **160**
lice, rats   111

lidocaine
  African tortoises   **379**
  amphibians   **433**
  boas and pythons   **321**
  geckos   **249**
  Koi carp   **447**
  Mediterranean tortoises   **355**
  terrapins   **395**
lighting, *see also* ultraviolet-A light;
        ultraviolet-B light
  bearded dragons   225
  tarantulas   462
  tortoises   361
limb swelling, bearded dragons   230
lingual myolysis, hamsters   91
lipid keratopathy, amphibians   429
lipomas, budgerigars and cockatiels
        154, *154*
liposarcomas, budgerigars and
        cockatiels   154
liquid diets
  African tortoises   368
  amphibians   423
  bearded dragons   223
  budgerigars and cockatiels   146
  chameleons   268
  corn snakes   287
  geckos   247
  grey parrots   169
  ground squirrels   4
  hamsters   87
  rats   105
  skunks   46
  sugar gliders   129
  terrapins   394
listeriosis
  bearded dragons   231
  sugar gliders   134
litter training, *see also* potty training
  rats   99
liver, *see also entries beginning* hepat.
  tumours, bearded dragons   227, *228*
lungworms
  amphibians   427
  giant African land snails   483
lures   189–190
lymph sacs, amphibians, medication
        via   432
lymphocytic choriomeningitis virus   35
lymphodilution of blood samples
  African tortoises   368
  Mediterranean tortoises   334, 335

lymphoma
grey parrots   176
hamsters   89
lymphosarcoma, Sulcata tortoise   376

m

Macrorhabdus ornithogaster   153
maggots, tortoise trauma   347
magnetic resonance imaging
boas and pythons   320
Mediterranean tortoises   352
rats   115
tarantulas   472
terrapins   404
malignant intraocular teratoid
medulloepithelioma   155
malnutrition
budgerigars and cockatiels   149
grey parrots, feather damage   **175**
sugar gliders   130
malocclusion
degus   62
incisors
hamsters   89
sciuromorphs   6
mammary gland tumours, rats
108–109
mandibular symphysis, rat   112
map turtles, herpesvirus infection   397
marmoset jellies   30
marmosets *see* common marmosets
maropitant   111
masks, anaesthesia, rats   106
mass mortality (flock mortality)   148
Mediterranean tortoises   327–359
anaesthesia   336–338, **354**
common conditions   340–350
euthanasia   338–339
examination   333–334
fluid therapy   336
formulary   353–356
handling   332
history-taking   331–332
hospitalisation requirements
339–340
husbandry   327–330
imaging   350–352
medication administration   **353–354**
nutritional support   336
sampling from   334–336
sex determination   333
species identification   **328**

megabacteria   155
megestrol acetate
marmosets   37–39
skunks   **54**
melanomas, hamsters   89
melarsomine, falcons   **210**
meloxicam
bearded dragons   223, **235**
budgerigars and cockatiels   150, **159**
grey parrots   **179, 181**
terrapins   **396, 405**
Mermithidae (nematodes)   470
mesenchymal neoplasms, budgerigars
and cockatiels   154
meso-2,3-dimercaptosuccinic acid
(DMSA)   **156**, 159
metabolic bone disease, *see also*
nutritional secondary
hyperparathyroidism; renal
secondary hyperparathyroidism
African tortoises   373–375
amphibians   429
computed tomography   431
bearded dragons   229–230
chameleons   269
hedgehogs   16
Mediterranean tortoises   340–341
terrapins   398
Metarhizium granulomatis   272–273
Metarhizium viride   272
metatarsal vein access, birds of
prey   195
methaemoglobin   444
metoclopramide
grey parrots   **179, 182**
Koi carp   **447, 454**
metronidazole
amphibians   428, **433**
geckos   **254, 258**
rats   **117**
Mexican red knee tarantula   459, **460**
Mexican red leg tarantula   **460**
mice, for corn snakes   285
microchipping
African tortoises   377
boas and pythons   321
Mediterranean tortoises   349–350
tarantulas   471–472
Microsporidium (spp,)   232, 427
milbemycin, skunks, praziquantel
with   **47**, 52
milk replacers, skunks   44

minimum alveolar concentrations,
anaesthetics
marmosets   31
rats   105–106
misoprostol/phenytoin gels, Koi
carp   445
mites
amphibians   428
bearded dragons   232
boas   317–318
budgerigars and cockatiels   151
corn snakes   297
hedgehogs   20
marmosets   35
pythons   317–318
rats   111
snails   483
tarantulas   471
mobility, rats, examination   104
molars *see* cheek teeth
molluscan metabolite E   482
Mongolian gerbils   71–82
anaesthesia   74–75, **79**
breeding   72–73
common conditions   75–78
euthanasia   75
examination   73
fluid therapy   74
formulary   **79**
handling   73
history-taking   73
hospitalisation requirements   75
husbandry   71–72
imaging   93
neoplasms   75–77
nutritional support   74
sampling from   73–74
sex determination   73
monkeypox   9
morphine
bearded dragons   223, **235**
corn snakes   288, **298**
terrapins   396
tortoises   370
morphs, snakes   308
moss, for amphibians   415
mourning geckos
ambient temperature   242
biological parameters   **244**
breeding   244–245
conditions for   **243**
mouth rot, corn snakes   293

mouth ulcer gels (human), Koi
    carp   445
MS-222 *see* tricaine methanesulfonate
Mucor ramosissimus   254
musk, skunks   43
Mycobacterium avium avium,
    Richardson's ground squirrel   9
Mycobacterium spp.
  amphibians   425
  budgerigars and cockatiels   151
  marmosets   34
  osteomyelitis, bearded dragons   230
Mycoplasma pulmonis, rats   109, 110
Mycoplasma spp.
  Eastern box turtles   396
  tortoises   371
myocarditis, hamsters   91
myopathy, hamsters   90
myxozoa   428

n

nails
  blood samples from, birds   146, 169
  prairie dogs   9
naltrexone
  dosage for grey parrots   **182**
  for feather damaging behaviour   176
nandrolone, bearded dragons   **236**
Nannizziopsis dermatitidis   272
Nannizziopsis vriesii, Chrysosporium
  anamorph   228, 254, 272
nasal dermatitis, gerbils   77
nasal discharge
  chameleons   272
  leopard tortoises   *371*
  Mediterranean tortoises   346
nasolacrimal duct obstruction, corn
  snakes   293
nebulisation treatment
  grey parrots   178
  Mediterranean tortoises   **354, 356**
  rats   109
  with terbinafine   291
nematodes
  amphibians   427
  birds of prey   199
  chameleons   275
  marmosets   35
  Mediterranean tortoises   352
  tarantulas   470
  zoonotic diseases   471
neonatal rejection, sugar gliders   135

neonates, *see also* hand-rearing
  chameleons   266
  corn snakes   285
  sugar gliders   126–127
neoplasms *see under specific animals*
nephridiopore, gastropods   477
nephrocalcinosis, rats   111
nephrotoxicity, sevoflurane, rats   106
nesting areas, Mediterranean
  tortoises   343
neuroendocrine carcinoma, bearded
  dragons   227
neutering *see under specific animals*
new tank syndrome   444
Newcastle disease   197–198
nifedipine, birds   174
nitrate pollution   444
nitrifying bacteria   418
nitrite toxicity, fish   444
non-steroidal anti-inflammatory drugs
  boas   312
  budgerigars and cockatiels   150, 158
  Mediterranean tortoises   338
  for proventricular dilation
    disease   179
  pythons   312
normal saline, tarantulas   466
normal values *see* reference intervals
North African hedgehog   *14*
notifiable diseases
  Koi carp   448–449
  West Nile disease   198
nuclear scintigraphy, corn snakes   297
nutritional secondary
  hyperparathyroidism
  African tortoises   373–374
  amphibians   429
  bearded dragons   229–230, *234*
  chameleons   269
  geckos   249–250, *255*
  grey parrots   172
  marmosets   32, 35
  Mediterranean tortoises   340–341
  skunks   47–48
  sugar gliders   130
  terrapins   398
nystatin, megabacteria   153

o

obesity
  amphibians   429
  bearded dragons   225

ground squirrels   4
hedgehogs   15, *23*
skunks   46, 47
sugar gliders   130
tarantulas   463
occipital plexus, African tortoises   368
ocular conditions
  birds of prey   205
  boas   318–319
  chameleons   272
  corn snakes   293
    ultrasound   297
  geckos   251
  hamsters   89
  hedgehogs   20
  Koi carp   446
  Mediterranean tortoises
    347–348
  pythons   318–319
  sugar gliders   134
odontogenic fibroma, hedgehogs   21
odontophores, African land
  snails   477
oedema syndrome, amphibians
  428–429
oesophagostomy tubes
  Mediterranean tortoises   **337**, 349
  terrapins   393–394
oestrous cycle
  degus   58
  hamsters   85
  marmosets   28
oophoritis, geckos   252
open water systems   417
opercula, birds of prey   194
Ophidascaris robertsi, sugar
  gliders   133
ophidian paramyxovirus
  boas and pythons   316
  corn snakes   291
Ophidiomyces ophiodiicola   291
Ophionyssus natricis   232, 297,
  317–318
ophthalmology *see* ocular conditions
opioid antagonists, for feather
  damaging behaviour   176
opioids, *see also specific drugs*
  amphibians   425
  boas and pythons   312
opisthosoma, spiders   460
Orabase Protective Paste   428
Orajel, amphibians   424

oral examination
African tortoises   367
amphibians   421
boas and pythons   310
geckos   247
Mediterranean tortoises   332
rats   104
oral gland obstruction, geckos   250
oral medication, amphibians   432
oral prolapse, snails   483
orange baboon spider   **460**
orchidectomy
birds   155
degus   65
gerbils   78
hamsters   92
hedgehogs   *23*
marmosets   37
rats   113
Siberian chipmunks   9
skunks   50
sugar gliders   135
oscillometric blood pressure monitoring,
boas and pythons   313
osteoarthritis
rats   112
sciuromorphs   7
osteomyelitis
chameleons   271
Mycobacterium spp., bearded
dragons   230
otitis externa, hedgehogs   *21*
otitis media/interna, rats   113
outdoor enclosures, marmosets   27
ovariectomy
bearded dragons   226
budgerigars and cockatiels   155
chameleons   273, 275
geckos   252
Mediterranean tortoises   343, 352
rats   114
terrapins   399
ovaries
corn snakes, ultrasound   297
cysts and tumours
budgerigars and cockatiels   155
gerbils   78
ovariohysterectomy
degus   65
gerbils   78
hamsters   91
rats   114

skunks   51
sugar gliders   135
overgrooming   48, 63, *see also*
barbering
overwintering, Mediterranean
tortoises   330, 331
oviducts
bearded dragons, surgery   227
budgerigars and cockatiels
156–157
corn snakes, surgery   295
geckos, inertia   252
Mediterranean tortoises, prolapse
344, 345
ovocentesis, geckos   252–253
ovulation, hedgehogs   16
owls   189–217
corneal ulceration   205
ocular common conditions   205
oxfendazole
African tortoises   **380**
Mediterranean tortoises   352, **356**
tarantulas   **473**
oxygen, low and high levels, water
quality   444
oxygen consumption,
amphibians   423
oxygen therapy
bearded dragons   224
budgerigars and cockatiels   148
oxytocin
bearded dragons   227, **236**
Mediterranean tortoises   343, **356**
terrapins   399, **406**
oxyurids *see* pinworms

p

Pacheco's disease   158
Pacific pond turtles, herpesvirus
infection   397
Paecilomyces infection   254
pain
African tortoises   370
birds of prey   197
boas and pythons   312
fish   443
gastropods   480
invertebrates   467–468
Mediterranean tortoises   338
painted turtles, herpesvirus
infection   397
palatopharyngeal arch, degus   60

palpation, amphibians   421
palpebral intradermal tuberculin test,
marmosets   34
Panagrolaimus spp.   470
pancake tortoise   **362**, 366
plastronotomy   376
upper respiratory infections   371
pancreas, diseases in degus   64
paper, rat bedding   100
paracloacal gland cyst, sugar
gliders   131
paracostal incisions, chameleons   274
paramyxovirus
boas and pythons   316
corn snakes   292, 293
parathyroid hormone, African
tortoises   373
parenteral rehydration, *see also*
intravenous fluid therapy
bearded dragons   223
chameleons   268
paromomycin
bearded dragons   232, **236**
geckos   254, **257**
paroxetine
for feather damaging
behaviour   176
grey parrots   **182**
parrot cages   141
parrots *see* budgerigars and cockatiels;
grey parrots
parvovirus, skunks   49
Pasteurella multocida, cat bites   148
Pasteurella spp.
hamsters   *90*
sciuromorphs   7
Pasteurella testudinis   371
patagial dermatitis, grey parrots
176–177
pecten oculi   194, 204
penis, *see also* phallus
prolapse
degus   59
Mediterranean tortoises   344
sugar gliders   134
terrapins   400
pentastomes   254
peracute dyspnoea, birds   151
perches
birds of prey   *193*, 197
tibiotarsal fractures and   206
budgerigars and cockatiels   141

peregrine falcon 190, *191*
pericarditis, marmosets 36
periocular Harderian gland,
    gerbils 77
periodontal disease, *see also* caries
    bearded dragons 231
    chameleons 271
periorbital neoplasms, grey
    parrots 176
peritoneal fluid, skunks 51
permethrin, corn snakes and 297
pethidine, African tortoises
    370, **379**
pH, tortoise urine 336
phacoemulsification, birds of
    prey 205
phallus, *see also* penis
    amputation
        Mediterranean tortoises 345
        terrapins 400
    prolapse, Mediterranean
        tortoises 345
pharyngitis, Mediterranean tortoises
    345–346
pharyngostomy tubes, rats 105
phenoxyethanol
    African land snails 481
    Koi carp 450, **450**
phosphates (blood levels)
    chameleons, kidney diseases 270
    marmosets, nutritional secondary
        hyperparathyroidism 32
phosphates (diet)
    African tortoises, on calcium
        homeostasis **374**
    degus, dental disease 61
    hedgehogs 16
physostomous fish 448
picornaviruses, tortoises 371
    renal secondary
        hyperparathyroidism 375
pink-toe tarantula 459
pinna, hedgehogs, dermatitis 21
pinworms, *see also Dentostomella*
    translucida
    African tortoises 372
    bearded dragons 231–232
    chameleons 275
    geckos 254
    Mediterranean tortoises 352
    rats 111
    zoonotic 78

pithing *see* brainstem destruction
pituitary extract, carp 447, **454**
pituitary neoplasms
    budgerigars and cockatiels 155
    rats 108, 113
plants
    for amphibian enclosures 418
    tortoise diets 329, 363, 365
    toxic to budgerigars 156
Plasmodium spp.
    birds of prey 200
    leopard tortoises 373
plastronotomy
    Mediterranean tortoises *343,*
        348–349
    pancake tortoise 376
pneumatic duct, Koi carp 448
pneumonia
    hamsters 90
    marmosets 34
pneumostomes, African land snails
    477, 481
pododermatitis
    birds of prey 201–202
    rats 111, 113
poisoning, budgerigars and
    cockatiels 156
polycystic disease, hamsters 91
polycystic renal disease, degus 64
polymerase chain reaction (PCR)
    agamid adenovirus-1 229
    Mediterranean tortoises, upper
        respiratory infections 346
    psittacine beak and feather
        disease 177
    psittacosis 152
polymyxin E, amphibians 427
polyoma virus, budgerigars and
    cockatiels 154
polyostotic hyperostosis, birds 158
ponds, for Koi carp 437
pop-eye, Koi carp 446
popping, corn snakes 286
post-hibernation anorexia,
    Mediterranean tortoises 340
post-mortem examination,
    tarantulas 466
post-ovulatory stasis *see* egg
    binding
posthitis, hedgehogs 22
potassium chloride, spiders,
    euthanasia 468, **473**

potty training, *see also* litter training
    rats 102
povidone–iodine solution, surgery for
    amphibians 430
poxvirus, birds of prey 198
prairie dogs 1–2
    dilated cardiomyopathy 7
    elodontomas 6
    infections 8, 9
    nails 9
    neoplasms 5–6
pre-femoral surgical approach
    African tortoises 376
    Mediterranean tortoises **354**
pre-ovulatory stasis/follicular stasis
    African tortoises 376
    bearded dragons 225–227
    chameleons 273–274
    Mediterranean tortoises 343
    terrapins 399
preen gland carcinoma 155
preening, grey parrots 176
preferred optimum temperature zone
    (POTZ)
    Mediterranean tortoises 328
    terrapins 387–389
pregnancy
    ectopic, hamsters 91
    marmosets 28, 36–37
    Mediterranean tortoises,
        handling 332
premedication
    birds of prey 196
    gerbils 75
    grey parrots 170
    sugar gliders 129
prey
    boas and pythons 309
    corn snakes **290**
    gut-loading of 243, 252, 462
    tarantulas 462–463
progestagen implants, marmosets 38
prolapse, *see also under* penis
    cloaca
        Mediterranean tortoises
            343–345
        sugar gliders 134
    colonic
        hamsters 92
        Mediterranean tortoises 344
    rectal *see* rectal prolapse
    snails 483

proliferative spinal osteopathy, boas and pythons   318
propofol
  bearded dragons   224, **234**
  boas   312
  corn snakes   288, **298**
proptosis *see* exophthalmos
propylene phenoxytol   480–481
prosoma, spider   460
protein, for Koi carp   439
protein skimmers   438
protozoa
  amphibians   427
  marmosets   34, 35
protozoal enteritis
  corn snakes   294
  geckos   254
proventricular dilation disease   157–158, 178–179
pseudogout
  bearded dragons   230–231
  terrapins   399
Pseudomonas putida   483
Pseudomonas spp., tarantulas   471
PsHV-1 (psittacine herpes virus) infection   158
psittacine beak and feather disease   153, **175**, 177
psittacine herpes virus infection   158
psittacosis   151–152, 177–178
pterygosomid mites   232
PTFE (Teflon)   155
pulmonary hyalinosis, sugar gliders   133
pulmonary sac, African land snails   477
pulse oximetry, grey parrots   171
pump method, fish anaesthesia   442
pupils, amphibians   421
pyometra, hamsters   91
pythons   305, 307–308, *see also* boas and pythons
  biological parameters   **306**
  breeding parameters   **314**

q
quarantine
  amphibians   431
  boas and pythons   320–321
  Koi carp   444
  tarantulas   470, 471
quills, hedgehogs   13

r
rabies, skunks   50
radula, African land snail   477
rainwater   417
ranavirus infection
  amphibians   426
  geckos   254
  Mediterranean tortoises   345–346
  terrapins   397
ranching, snakes   308
raptors *see* birds of prey
rasburicase *see* urate oxidase
rat bite fever   113
rats   99–123
  anaesthesia   105–107
  breeding   102
  common conditions   108–113
  for corn snakes   285
  euthanasia   107
  examination   104
  fluid therapy   105
  formulary   **116–119**
  handling   103
  history-taking   102–103
  hospitalisation requirements   107–108
  husbandry   99–102
  imaging   114–115
    respiratory tract infections   109
  neoplasms   108–109
  neutering   114
  nutritional support   105
  sampling from   104–105
  sex determination   103
recombinant urate oxidase *see* urate oxidase
rectal prolapse
  marmosets   34
  skunks   49
  sugar gliders   134
red-eared sliders
  biological parameters   **388**
  pre-ovulatory stasis   399
  ranavirus infection   396
red leg syndrome   425
reference intervals
  African tortoises
    metabolic bone disease   373, 375
    thyroxine   376
  birds
    diabetes mellitus   154
    hypocalcaemia   172

boas   311
hamsters, endocrine   91
hedgehogs   **18**
pythons   312
tarantulas   465
reflex monitoring, birds   170
reflexes, amphibians   421
refugia   416
rehydration
  parenteral, *see also* intravenous fluid therapy
    bearded dragons   223
    chameleons   269
    tarantulas   466
renal biopsy, birds   150
renal cysts, chameleon case   271
renal portal valve, budgerigars and cockatiels   149
renal secondary hyperparathyroidism
  African tortoises   375
  bearded dragons   228
  Mediterranean tortoises   341
reovirus
  geckos   255
  grey parrots   179
reproduction *see* breeding *under specific animals*
respiratory arrest, Mediterranean tortoises   338
respiratory distress
  budgerigars and cockatiels   148
  fish   444
respiratory tract disease
  African tortoises   372
  aspergillosis   178
  birds of prey, examination for   194
  boas   315
  budgerigars and cockatiels   151
  chameleons   272
  corn snakes   292
  hamsters   91–92
  Mediterranean tortoises   346–347
    nebulisation for   **354, 356**
  pythons   315
  rats   109–110
    radiography   114–115
  sciuromorphs   6
  sugar gliders   131–133
  terrapins   397
respiratory tract obstruction, birds   151
resuscitation, Mediterranean tortoises   338

rete mirabile, Koi carp   448
reticulated python   **306**, 308
retrobulbar abscesses
   chameleons   271
   sugar gliders   134
reverse osmosis water   417
rhinitis, degus   65
rhododendron, Mediterranean tortoises
      and   329
rhubarb, Mediterranean tortoises
      and   329
Richardson's ground squirrel   2
   elodontomas   7
   Mycobacterium avium avium   9
   neoplasms   5
Ringer's solution
   amphibians   423, 429
   reptiles   423
Roborovski hamster   **84**
rodent control, enclosures for
      marmosets   27, 35
Rodentolepsis nana
   gerbils   78
   rats   112
rostral abrasions, amphibians   428
rosuvastatin, birds   174
rosy boa   **306**, 307
royal python   **306**, 307–308, *see also*
      spider morphs
   feeding   311
runny nose syndrome, Mediterranean
      tortoises   346
Russian winter white hamster   **84**

s

salamanders, *see also* amphibians
   blood sampling   422
   chytridiomycosis   426
   clinical examination   421
   handling   419
   protozoa   427
   sex determination   420–421
salbutamol, rats   **119**
Salmonella spp.
   bearded dragons   232
   boas and pythons   311
   geckos   256
   sugar gliders   134
   terrapins   390
   zoonosis   134, 232, 256, 310
salpingectomy
   corn snakes   295
   parrots   156

salpingotomy
   budgerigars and cockatiels,
      anaesthesia   156
   corn snakes, sutures   *295*
   geckos   252
sand, geckos   241–242
sand baths
   gerbils   71
   hamsters   83
saprolegniasis   427, 446
sarcoptic mange, skunks   50
scent glands
   gerbils, neoplasms   76
   sugar gliders   135
sciuromorphs   1–12
scrapes, amphibian skin   422–423
scruff restraint
   hamsters   85
   sugar gliders   127
sebaceous Zymbals gland, rats,
      carcinoma   109
sedation
   African tortoises   369
   hedgehogs   19
   Koi carp   441–443
   rats, postoperative   107
seizures
   gerbils   75
   grey parrots, hypocalcaemia   172
selective serotonin reuptake inhibitors,
      for feather damaging
      behaviour   176
selenium deficiency, geckos   251
self-anointing, hedgehogs
      13–14, *15*
self-mutilation, sugar gliders   133
self-trauma, parrots   174–176
semi-closed water systems   417–418
Sendai virus
   hamsters   90
   marmosets   35
septic arthritis, bearded dragons   230
septicaemia
   Helicobacter, African tortoises   372
   marmosets   34
   Mediterranean tortoises   348
septicaemic cutaneous ulcerative
      disease, terrapins   398
serology, psittacosis   152
Serratospiculum spp., birds of
      prey   199
Sertoli cell neoplasms, deslorelin,
      budgerigars   155

sevoflurane
   amphibians   424, **432**
   bearded dragons   224
   birds of prey   197, **208**
   boas   313
   marmosets   31
   pythons   313
   rats   105, 105–106, **107**
   tarantulas   467, **472**
sex of neonates, chameleons   266
shell necrosis, tortoises   376
shell pyramiding
   African tortoises   375
   Mediterranean tortoises   341
shell wounds
   African tortoises   375
   Mediterranean tortoises   347
   terrapins   400
shock, birds   147
short tongue syndrome,
      amphibians   429
shunting blood from lungs
   bearded dragons   224
   corn snakes   292
Siberian chipmunks   1
   borreliosis   8
   neutering   9
sildenafil, rats   110, **118**
sinoatrial arrest, grey
      parrots   173
sinus venosus, corn snake   292
sinusitis, cockatiels   150
skin, *see also* dermatology
   amphibians, sampling from
      422–423
   Koi carp
      bacterial diseases   446
      fungal infections   446
      neoplasms   448
      sampling from   440
      trauma   445–446
skin glue, rats   107
skunks *see* striped skunks
sleeping areas, hamsters   83
snails *see* giant African land
      snails
snakes *see* boas and pythons; corn
      snakes
sodium benzoate, budgerigars and
      cockatiels   153, **159**
sodium calcium edetate (EDTA),
      budgerigars and cockatiels
      156, **159**

sodium chloride
  as antifungal **451**
  Koi carp   445, **455**
  for parasites   **453**
  zeolite and   444
somatostatin, neuroendocrine
      carcinoma, bearded
      dragons   227
sour crop   203
spatulas, dental examination,
      degus   62
spectacles
  boas and pythons   318–319
  corn snakes   289
  geckos, disorders   251
Sphinx rats   **101**
spider morphs, wobble
      syndrome   308, 316
spiders *see* tarantulas
spinach
  giant African land snails and   479
  Mediterranean tortoises and   329
spines, hedgehogs   13
spiral bacteria, budgerigars and
      cockatiels   150
splenomegaly, budgerigars and
      cockatiels   158
splinting, tibiotarsal fractures in
      birds   148
spontaneous cutaneous lymphoma,
      hamsters   88
spontaneous degenerative
      radiculoneuropathy, rats   113
spring viraemia of carp   448
spur-thigh complex, Mediterranean
      tortoises   **328**
spur-thighed tortoises   361–363
  hibernation   366
spurs, degus teeth   61, 62
squamous cell carcinoma
  bearded dragons   227
  chameleons   271, 272
  grey parrots   177
  hedgehogs, oral   21, *23*
squirrels *see* ground squirrels
stages of anaesthesia, fish   **443**
standard metabolic rate, *see also* basal
      metabolic rate
  African tortoises   368
  bearded dragons   223
  geckos   247
Staphylococcus aureus, birds of
      prey   202

statins, birds   174
stethoscopes, grey parrots   170–171
stomach tubes, *see also* gavage feeding
  boas and pythons   311
stomatitis
  boas   314–315
  chameleons   271
  corn snakes   293
    subspectacular abscess   293
  geckos   250–251
  Mediterranean tortoises   345–346
  pythons   314–315
  terrapins   396–397
stones, *see also* uroliths
  biliary, bearded dragons   233
  terrapins   404
Streptococcus equisimilis, skunks   50
Streptococcus pneumoniae,
      hamsters   90
streptomycin, gerbils and   **79**
stress
  feather damaging behaviour   174
  sugar gliders   133
striped skunks   43–56
  anaesthesia   46–47
  breeding   43–44
  common conditions   47–50
  euthanasia   47
  fluid therapy   46
  formulary   52, **53–54**
  handling   45
  history-taking   45
  hospitalisation requirements   47
  husbandry   44–45
  imaging   52
  neoplasms   49
  neutering   51–52
  nutritional support   46
  sampling from   45–46
  sex determination   45
subcarapacial sinus
  African tortoise   370
  Mediterranean tortoise   335
  terrapin   392
subcutaneous abscess, African
      tortoises   377
subcutaneous anaesthesia,
      terrapins   395
subcutaneous fluid therapy
  bearded dragons   223
  birds of prey   195–196
  boas   311
  corn snakes   287

  degus   60
  geckos   248
  gerbils   74
  hamsters   87
  hedgehogs   19
  pythons   312
  rats   **106**
  sugar gliders   129
subcutaneous medication
  amphibians   432
  Mediterranean tortoises   **353**
subspectacular abscess   293, 319
substrates
  African tortoises   364
  amphibians   415–416
  bearded dragons   219, 226, 227
  boas   309–310
  chameleons   263–264, 266, 269
  corn snakes   285, 289
  degus   57, 61
  geckos   241–242
  gerbils   71, 75
  ground squirrels   1, 2
  hamsters   83
  land snails   479, 480
  Mediterranean tortoises
      329, *339*, 343
  pythons   309–310
  rat cages   100
  sugar gliders   125
  tarantulas   462
sucking stomach, spiders   460
sugar gliders   125–139
  anaesthesia   129, **137**
  breeding   126–127
  common conditions   130–135
  euthanasia   130
  examination   127–128
  fluid therapy   129
  formulary   **137**
  handling   127
  history-taking   127
  hospitalisation requirements   130
  husbandry   125–126
  imaging   135, *136*
  neoplasms   131, **132**
  neutering   135
  nutritional support   129
  sampling from   128–129
  sex determination   127
Sulcata tortoise   **362**, 363–365, *367*
  thyroxine values   376
  uroliths   375

sunlight, for marmosets 27
superficial ulnar vein
   birds 146
   birds of prey 195
   grey parrots 169
sutures
   amphibians 430
   bearded dragons 227
   boas 319
   Chinese finger trap suture *394*
   corn snakes, salpingotomy *295*
   Mediterranean tortoises 348
     cloacal prolapse 345
   pythons 319
   rats 107, 114
swabs, amphibians 422
swim bladder aspirates, Koi carp 441
swim bladder disorders, Koi
    carp 448
Syngamus trachea, birds of prey 199
Syrian hamster **84**
   ectoparasites 89
   teddy bear variety *92*
syringe method, fish anaesthesia 442

t
tadpoles
   diet for 418
   swabbing 422
tailless rats **101**, 113
tails
   bearded dragons 222
   birds of prey, protection for
     hospitalisation 197
   corn snakes, dysecdysis 289
   degloving injury
     degus 63
     gerbils 78
   geckos 245, 253
   rats
     constricting rings 111
     lateral veins 104–105, **106**
   sugar gliders, trauma 131
tamoxifen
   geckos 253
   rats 108–109
tanks
   bearded dragons 219
   geckos 241
   gerbils 71
   giant African land snails 478
   Koi carp 443–444
   tarantulas 462

tapeworms, gerbils 78
tarantula hawk wasps 470
tarantulas 459–475
   anaesthesia 467–468, **472**
   anatomy 460–461
   common conditions 468–471
   euthanasia 468
   examination 464
   fluid therapy 466
   formulary **472–473**
   handling 463–464
   history-taking 463
   husbandry 461–463
   imaging 472
   lethargy 468
   sampling from 464–466
   sex determination 464
   species 459
taxonomy
   arachnids 459
   boas **307**
teddy bear variety, Syrian
    hamster *92*
Teflon 155–156
temperature (ambient)
   amphibians 416
   bearded dragons 219–220
   budgerigars and cockatiels 141
   chameleons 264
   geckos 244
     sex determination 242, 244
   giant African land snails 478
   hedgehogs 14, 20
   hingeback tortoises 365
   marmoset anaesthesia 31
   Mediterranean tortoises
     328–329, *339*
     hibernation 331
   skunks 44
   spur-thighed tortoises 361
   sugar gliders 125
   tarantulas 462
   terrapins 387–389
temperature (body)
   birds 147
   boas and pythons, anaesthetic
     monitoring 313
   grey parrots 171
   hamsters 84
   rats, measurement 104
tentacles, snails *478*
teratoid medulloepithelioma
    (malignant intraocular) 155

terbinafine
   amphibians **434**
   corn snakes **277**, 291
terrapene herpesvirus 1 396–397
terrapins 387–413
   anaesthesia 395
   analgesia 396
   common conditions 396–401
   euthanasia 396
   examination 391
   fluid therapy 394
   formulary **405–406**
   handling 389–390
   hospitalisation requirements 396
   husbandry 387–391
   imaging 401–404
   neoplasms **402–403**
   nutritional support 392–394
   sampling from 391–392
   sex determination 390–391
terraria, amphibians 415
testes
   removal *see* orchidectomy
   tumours, budgerigars and
     cockatiels 155
testudinid herpesviruses 345
Testudo graeca **362**
   diet 363
   subspecies **363**
tetanus, gyrfalcon 201
tetany, amphibians 429
tethering
   birds of prey 189
     tibiotarsal fractures 206
theraphosids *see* tarantulas
thigmotherms 242
thyroid neoplasms, hamsters 89
thyroxine, corn snakes **299**
thyroxine (levels)
   corn snakes 289
   tortoises 376
tibiotarsal fractures
   birds of prey 206
   budgerigars and cockatiels 207
ticks
   birds of prey 199, *199*
   skunks 49
tie-in hybrid fixator, tibiotarsal
    fractures 206
tiger spider 459
Timneh grey parrots 165, *166*
   neoplasms 176
tissue glue, boas and pythons 319

toads *see* amphibians
Tokay geckos
  biological parameters **244**
  conditions for **243**
  eye infections 251
  handling 245
toltrazuril 200
torpor
  ground squirrels 2
  hamsters 84
  hedgehogs 14, 22
  prairie dogs 2
  Siberian chipmunks 1
torsion, oviduct, parrots 156
tortoise tables 327, 328
tortoises *see* African tortoises;
    Mediterranean tortoises
Toxocara canis, skunks 50
Toxoplasma gondii
  birds of prey 200
  marmosets 35
  skunks 50
  sugar gliders 134
trachea
  African tortoises, sampling
      from 368
  boas and pythons,
      obstruction 315
  intubation *see* endotracheal
      intubation
Trachemys spp. 387–413
tramadol
  African tortoises 370, **379**
  bearded dragons 223, **234**
  terrapins 396, **405**
transdermal fentanyl patches, boas and
      pythons 312
transdermal fluid therapy,
      amphibians 423
transillumination, geckos 247
transponder identification *see*
    microchipping
trauma, *see also* bites; fractures
  Koi carp 445
    ocular 447
  Mediterranean tortoises 347
  snails 482
  sugar gliders 131
  tarantulas 469–470
  terrapins 400–401
trematodes, amphibians 427

tricaine methanesulfonate
  amphibians 423–425
  Koi carp 443, **450**
  snails 480–481
Trichomonas gallinae 199
trichomoniasis
  budgerigars and cockatiels 150
  geckos 254
Trichophyton mentagrophytes 63
trombiculid mites 428
Trypanosoma cruzi
  degus 65
  in skunks 48
trypanosomiasis
  amphibians 428
  sugar gliders 134
tubal ligation, marmosets 37
tuberculin test, marmosets 34
tuberculosis, marmosets 34
tularaemia, sciuromorphs 9
tunnelling
  degus 57
  gerbils 71
  hamsters 83
Turkmenian eagle owl *191*
Turtles *see* terrapins
tympanic membranes, terrapins 391
Tyzzers disease, rats 112

u

ulcerative dermatitis
  grey parrots 176–177
  Koi carp 446
  rats 111
ulcers, amphibians 428
ulnar vein *see* superficial ulnar vein
ultrasound
  amphibians 430–431
  bearded dragons 233
    pre-ovulatory stasis 226
  boas 320
  chameleons, follicles **274**
  corn snakes 297
  degus, kidney diseases 66
  geckos 255
  giant African land snails 483–484
  hamsters 94
  Mediterranean tortoises 350
  pythons 320
  rats 115
  tarantulas 472

terrapins 404
tortoises 378
ultrasound frequencies, rat
      hearing 102
ultraviolet-A light
  chameleons 264–265
  corn snakes 285
  spur-thighed tortoises 361
ultraviolet-B light
  African tortoises 373
  amphibians 416, 417, 431
  bearded dragons 220
  boas 309
  chameleons 264–265, 269
  corn snakes 284–285
  degus 58
  geckos 242–243
  grey parrots 165
  marmosets 27
  Mediterranean tortoises 328,
      329, *339*
  pythons 309
  spur-thighed tortoises 361
  terrapins 389
ultraviolet water filters 438–439
uncurling, hedgehogs 16–17
upper respiratory infections
  cockatiels 151
  Mediterranean tortoises 346
  tortoises 371, 372
urate oxidase
  budgerigars and cockatiels 149, **160**
  Mediterranean tortoises 341, **356**
  red-tail hawks **211**
urea (serum)
  birds 150
  hamsters **91**
ureters, vitamin A deficiency,
      budgerigars 149
urethrostomy, sugar gliders 134
uric acid (serum)
  birds 149
  Mediterranean tortoises 341
urine
  collection
    gerbils 74
    hamsters 86
    hedgehogs 17–18
  hamsters 91
  Mediterranean tortoises 336
  rats 105

specific gravity
  gerbils   77
  hamsters   86, **91**
  Mediterranean tortoises   336
  sugar gliders   133
  sugar gliders   133
uroliths
  bearded dragons   230
  Mediterranean tortoises   342
  Sulcata tortoise   375
uropygial gland, birds of prey   195
urticating hairs, spiders   463
  loss   468
uterus, gerbils, neoplasms   76
UV-Tool (online document)   417

V

vaccinations
  raptors   197, 198
  skunks   50–51
vacuum-assisted closure, shell wounds,
    tortoises   376
vagal response, bearded dragons   221
vasectomy, marmosets   37
ventilation (pulmonary), *see also*
    intermittent positive pressure
    ventilation
  bearded dragons   224
  boas and pythons   313
  chameleons   268
  corn snakes   288
  Mediterranean tortoises   337–338
  terrapins   395
ventral abdominal vein,
    amphibians   422
ventral coccygeal sinus, bearded
    dragons   222
ventral coccygeal vein,
    chameleons   267
ventral limb membrane, tarantulas,
    blood sampling   464
ventral scent gland, gerbils,
    neoplasms   76–77
ventral tail vein
  amphibians   422
  boas and pythons   311
ventricular dilatation, cardiomyopathy
  hamsters   90–91
  marmosets   36
verapamil, birds   174
Vibravenos (doxycycline)   153

viral diseases, *see also specific viruses*
  African tortoises   371
  amphibians   426
  birds of prey   197–199
  boas   316
  budgerigars and cockatiels
    157–158
  corn snakes, respiratory   292
  geckos   254
  inclusion disease of boids   297
  marmosets   35
    neoplasms from   36
  Mediterranean tortoises   345–346
  pythons   316
vitamin(s), Mediterranean
    tortoises   352
vitamin A, parenteral   269–270
vitamin A deficiency
  amphibians   430
  budgerigars   149
  chameleons   269–270
  cockatiels   149
  geckos   250
  grey parrots   172
  terrapins   400
vitamin A excess, cockatiels   149
vitamin C
  for Koi carp   439
  for marmosets   28
vitamin C deficiency, marmosets   33
vitamin D
  excess, African tortoises   375
  reference values, tortoises   374
  snails   482
vitamin D deficiency
  geckos   249
  grey parrots   165
vitamin D levels, grey parrots   172
vitamin D3
  African tortoises   373
  amphibians   417, 429, 431
  excess, budgerigars and
    cockatiels   149
  levels, marmosets   32
  for marmosets   27, 28
vitamin E deficiency, geckos   251
vivaria
  chameleons   263
  corn snakes   283
  geckos   241
    hospitalisation   249

hospitalisation
  bearded dragons   224
  boas and pythons   314
  corn snakes   289
  snake mites and   318
volvulus, sugar gliders   134
voriconazole
  amphibians   427, **433**
  corn snakes   292
  grey parrots   178, **181**

W

wasps, parasitising tarantulas   470
wasting marmoset syndrome   33
water, for tortoises   329
water heaters   389
water quality, *see also* filters
  amphibians   417–418
  for Koi carp   437, 444–445
    testing   439
  terrapins   389
weaning, hedgehogs   16
weight (body)
  grey parrots, proventricular dilation
    disease   181
  ground squirrels   4
  marmosets, at birth   28
  Mediterranean tortoises   333
    hibernation   331
  rats   102, 104
weight loss, wasting marmoset
    syndrome   33
well water   417
West Nile disease   198
wet tail, hamsters   92
Whitaker-Wright solution   429
White's tree frog, biological
    parameters   **416**
whorls, gastropods   477
wing tip oedema, birds of prey
    203–204
wiring, shell fractures   **401**
wobble syndrome, spider morphs
    308, 316
wobbly hedgehog syndrome   22
wound closure, rats   107

X

xanthomas
  budgerigars and cockatiels   154
  geckos   251

y

yeast, avian gastric   153
yellow-bellied sliders, biological
      parameters   **388**
yellow fungus disease *see Nanniziopsis*
      vriesii
Yersinia pseudotuberculosis
  marmosets   33
    vaccine   37
  rats   113
yersiniosis, sciuromorphs   9

z

zeolite   444, **455**
zoonotic diseases   9
  Angiostrongylus cantonensis   483
  Baylisascaris spp.   50
  Encephalitozoon hellem   149
  ground squirrels   8
  Mycobacterium spp.   34
  nematodes   471
  pentastomes   254
  pinworms   78
  prairie dogs   9
  primates   29
  psittacosis   177–178
  rats   113
  Rodentolepsis nana   112
  salmonellosis   134, 233,
    256, 310
  Staphylococcus aureus   202
  Trichophyton mentagrophytes   63
Zymbals gland, rats, carcinoma   109